Contagious and Infectious Diseases of Livestock

Contagious and Infectious Diseases of Livestock

Editor: Salvador Barker

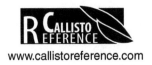

www.callistoreference.com

Callisto Reference,
118-35 Queens Blvd., Suite 400,
Forest Hills, NY 11375, USA

Visit us on the World Wide Web at:
www.callistoreference.com

ISBN: 978-1-64116-842-7 (Hardback)

Cataloging-in-Publication Data

Contagious and infectious diseases of livestock / edited by Salvador Barker.
    p. cm.
Includes bibliographical references and index.
ISBN 978-1-64116-842-7
1. Communicable diseases in animals. 2. Livestock--Infections. 3. Livestock--Diseases.
4. Veterinary medicine. I. Barker, Salvador.
SF781 .C66 2023
636.089 69--dc23

Table of Contents

Preface

Every book is a source of knowledge and this one is no exception. The idea that led to the conceptualization of this book was the fact that the world is advancing rapidly; which makes it crucial to document the progress in every field. I am aware that a lot of data is already available, yet, there is a lot more to learn. Hence, I accepted the responsibility of editing this book and contributing my knowledge to the community.

Contagious and infectious diseases are those diseases of livestock that are caused by pathogens, such as fungi, bacteria and viruses. They can be transmitted from one animal to another, and can also spread from insects and vectors such as mosquitoes, ticks, midges, and flies. Some infectious diseases may also occur due to the consumption of contaminated water or feed, or exposure to micro-organisms in the environment. Some of the common infectious diseases in livestock include foot and mouth disease, blue tongue, black quarter, pox, Johne's disease, bovine rhinotracheitis, and theileriosis. The measures to prevent infectious diseases in animals are divided into three categories, which include animal husbandry, biosecurity, and vaccinations. The adoption of good practices of animal husbandry involve providing clean water, clean housing, good quality feed, and isolating the sick animal. This book aims to shed light on some of the unexplored aspects of contagious and infectious diseases of livestock and the recent researches on them. Those with an interest in these diseases would find it helpful.

While editing this book, I had multiple visions for it. Then I finally narrowed down to make every chapter a sole standing text explaining a particular topic, so that they can be used independently. However, the umbrella subject sinews them into a common theme. This makes the book a unique platform of knowledge.

I would like to give the major credit of this book to the experts from every corner of the world, who took the time to share their expertise with us. Also, I owe the completion of this book to the never-ending support of my family, who supported me throughout the project.

Editor

1

Association between Infectious Agents and Lesions in Post-Weaned Piglets and Fattening Heavy Pigs with Porcine Respiratory Disease Complex (PRDC)

Jessica Ruggeri[1], Cristian Salogni[1], Stefano Giovannini[1], Nicoletta Vitale[1],
Maria Beatrice Boniotti[1], Attilio Corradi[2], Paolo Pozzi[3], Paolo Pasquali[4] and
Giovanni Loris Alborali[1]*

[1] Istituto Zooprofilattico Sperimentale della Lombardia e dell'Emilia Romagna [Experimental Zooprophylactic Institute of Lombardia and Emilia Romagna], Brescia, Italy, [2] Department of Veterinary Sciences, University of Parma, Parma, Italy, [3] Department of Veterinary Sciences, University of Torino, Turin, Italy, [4] Department of Food Safety, Nutrition and Veterinary Public Health, Istituto Superiore di Sanità, Rome, Italy

*Correspondence:
Giovanni Loris Alborali
giovanni.alborali@izsler.it

Porcine Respiratory Disease Complex (PRDC) is a multifactorial syndrome that causes health problems in growing pigs and economic losses to farmers. The etiological factors involved can be bacteria, viruses, or mycoplasmas. However, environmental stressors associated with farm management can influence the status of the animal's health. The role and impact of different microorganisms in the development of the disease can be complex, and these are not fully understood. The severity of lesions are a consequence of synergism and combination of different factors. The aim of this study was to systematically analyse samples, conferred to the Veterinary Diagnostic Laboratory (IZSLER, Brescia), with a standardized diagnostic protocol in case of suspected PRDC. During necropsy, the lungs and carcasses were analyzed to determine the severity and extension of lesions. Gross lung lesions were classified according to a pre-established scheme adapted from literature. Furthermore, pulmonary, pleural, and nasal lesions were scored to determine their severity and extension. Finally, the presence of infectious agents was investigated to identify the microorganisms involved in the cases studied. During the years 2014–2016, 1,658 samples of lungs and carcasses with PRDC from 863 farms were analyzed; among them 931 and 727 samples were from weaned piglets and fattening pigs, respectively. The most frequently observed lesions were characteristic of catarrhal bronchopneumonia, broncho-interstitial pneumonia, pleuropneumonia, and pleuritis. Some pathogens identified were correlated to specific lesions, whereas other pathogens to various lesions. These underline the need for the establishment of control and treatment programmes for individual farms.

Keywords: porcine respiratory disease complex (PRDC), pig, lung lesion, multifactorial disease, diagnostic protocol

INTRODUCTION

Porcine Respiratory Disease Complex (PRDC) is a multifactorial disease that affects growing pigs in different stages of production, causing economic losses. This complex syndrome is influenced by the presence of several types of pathogens (porcine reproductive and respiratory syndrome virus (PRRSV), porcine circovirus (PCV)-type 2, *Mycoplasma hyopneumoniae*, *Mycoplasma hyorhinis*, *Pasteurella multocida*, *Haemophilus parasuis*, etc.), along with environmental conditions, as temperature, dust, ammonia, carbon dioxide and airborne bacteria and farm management (1–4).

PRDC is a major burden in piggeries worldwide because of the consequent economic losses. In affected farms, considerable costs are associated with high percentages of mortality (2–20%) and morbidity (10–40%), therapy, and limited growth performances (5, 6). Reportedly, infection with *M. hyopneumoniae* causes major economic losses to the pig industry, mainly because of reduced performance, uneven growth, increase in the number of days to reach slaughter weight, treatment and control, and increase in mortality rate when complicated infections occur (7). However, the economic impact of *M. hyopneumoniae* subclinical infection was inferred only once based on the difference in average daily weight gain (ADWG) (38 g/day) between seropositive and seronegative pigs from 18 different cohorts (8). Various studies have demonstrated the economic impact of lung lesions on growth performances. The results were mostly based on the relationship between lung lesions observed at the slaughterhouse and ADWG (9). Some authors have reported a reduction of 6–16% in the growth rate of finishing pigs (10, 11). The main study on respiratory diseases in Italian piggeries started with the observation of lung and pleural lesions (and correspondent scores) while slaughtering. The results demonstrated that diseases affecting the respiratory tract greatly prevail, and they are very likely underestimated in live animals (12, 13). Inspection while slaughtering is a valid tool to estimate the incidence of PRDC in pigs. The most commonly recorded lesion corresponds to catarrhal bronchopneumonia mainly affecting cranial lobes. This is frequently associated with interstitial pneumonia and pleuritis (14). In Italy, the percentage of catarrhal bronchopneumonia associated with enzootic pneumonia is 46.4% and that of pleuritis is 47.5% (13). These lesions indicate the evolution or exacerbation of respiratory diseases affecting pigs during the farrow-finishing period.

On the contrary, the evaluation of lesions in piglets or pigs during PRDC outbreaks is a valid tool to estimate the type of acute lesions, their extension, and the possible involvement of serosa and nasal mucosa. Furthermore, the isolation of etiological pathogens is easier in acute lesions than in chronic ones. As a

TABLE 1 | Data on samples analyzed during 2014–2016, presented as number of animals, number of investigated cases, and production stage.

Year	N° of animals	N° of investigated cases	Weaned piglets	Growing/fattening pigs
2014	510	257	295 (57.8%)	215 (42.2%)
2015	622	320	334 (53.7%)	288 (46.3%)
2016	524	286	301 (57.5%)	223 (42.5%)
Total	1,656	863	930 (56.2%)	726 (43.8%)

consequence, treatment or the control of each outbreak should be addressed according to the specific farm situation to limit the generic use of antimicrobials.

The aim of this study was to investigate the association between lesions and infectious agents and to assess the association between nasal, pleural, and lung scores, in order to gain insights about the etiological agents associated with PRDC. The novelty of this study is to assess the etiology and lesions in samples from dead pigs with clinical suspect of respiratory disease.

MATERIALS AND METHODS

Samples

A standardized diagnostic protocol was applied to growing pigs that died because of respiratory diseases, conferred to the Veterinary Diagnostic Laboratory (IZSLER, Brescia), during 2014–2016. **Table 1** shows the total number and the production stage of the sampled pigs. A further distinction per year was made to carry out a temporal assessment.

The protocol used for the qualitative and quantitative evaluation of the lung, pleura, and nasal lesions is associated with a systematic monitoring of pathogens. It was applied to carcasses or organs (lungs) submitted to the Diagnostic Laboratory of Istituto Zooprofilattico Sperimentale della Lombardia e dell'Emilia-Romagna with the suspicion of respiratory disease, which was then confirmed during necropsy.

Lung, pleural, and nasal lesion scores were registered during necropsy with other information such as that on the productive stage and laboratory investigations performed.

Classification of Lung Lesions

The scheme for the classification of lesions was adapted from published methods (15).

The lesions of the organs were identified to be associated with the following diseases/conditions: catarrhal bronchopneumonia (CBP), purulent bronchopneumonia (PBP), interstitial pneumonia (IP), interstitial bronchopneumonia (BIP), pleuropneumonia (PP), pleuritis (PL), pericarditis (PE), and pleuro-pericarditis (PL-PE).

CBP is characterized by lesions of parenchyma and bronchi affecting principally the cranial, cardiac, and anterior portions of diaphragmatic lobes. It is characterized by mucus and catarrhal exudate in the lumen of the bronchus tree, by parenchymal consolidation and by interstitial space thickening.

Abbreviations: PRDC, Porcine Respiratory Disease Complex; PRRSV, Porcine Reproductive and Respiratory Syndrome Virus; PCV, type 2: Porcine Circovirus Type 2; ADWG, Average Daily Weight Gain; CBP, Catarrhal Bronchopneumonia; PBP, Purulent Bronchopneumonia; IP, Interstitial Pneumonia; BIP, Interstitial Bronchopneumonia; PP, Pleuropneumonia; PL, Pleuritis; PE, Pericarditis; PL-PE, Pleuro-pericarditis; SD, standard deviation; SPES, Slaughterhouse Pleuritis Evaluation System; SIV, Swine Influenza Virus; PCR, Polymerase Chain Reaction; CI, Confidence Interval; OR, Odds Ratio.

The appearance of the lungs varies from red to light brown and changes to a grayish color during chronic infection.

PBP is characterized by lesions of lung parenchyma and bronchi, which are characterized by mucus and catarrhal-purulent exudate in the lumen of the bronchus tree. Generally, it is a totally disseminated complication of CPB or BIP. Hence, cellular detritus and stagnated exudates favor the replication of pyogenic bacteria. These lesions develop abscess formations detectable with palpation.

IP is characterized by serosal exudation into alveolar walls and by interstitial oedema. Parenchyma suffers from incremented consistency, and the color changes from light red to purple red during the acute phase and to light pink during the chronic phase. These lesions are commonly associated with viral infections and involve the entire affected lung. Unfortunately, this lesion can be masked (by other lesions) or be complicated, and it can evolve into broncho-interstitial pneumonia. BIP is a complication of IP because it also involves the bronchus tree. In particular, serosal exudation is found in the lumen of bronchi and bronchioles.

PP is a fibrinous/necrotising pneumonia associated with pleuritis and affects the dorso-caudal portions of the diaphragmatic lobes. A hyperacute lesion is characterized by an increased consistency and by a color variation of the parenchyma that ranges from brown to red. An acute lesion is characterized by an increased consistency of the affected portions of parenchyma and by an alternation of the red area with a lighter pink area, which is a result of fibrin deposition. The chronic evolution is characterized by abscess formations and sequestrum, complicated by fibrous adherences between lung lesions and chest wall.

PL, PE, and PL-PE are characterized by inflammation of the pleura and pericardium (or both) and by fibrinous exudation that can evolve in adherences.

Lung, Pleural, and Nasal Scores

Here, irrespectively. to the character of the lung lesion (as above assessed), we scored (0–4 points) the extension of the lesion in each lobe, according to Madec and Derrien (16) and Madec and Kobish (17). SPES (Slaughterhouse Pleuritis Evaluation System) was applied to score (0–4 points) pleural lesions (18). Nasal lesions were scored on a 6-point scale (0–5 points) according to the system described by de Jong (19).

Laboratory Investigations

The lung, heart, pericardium, lymph nodes, pericardial and pleural fluids, and tracheobronchial swabs were processed to conduct, histology, microbiological examinations, and molecular identification.

For bacteriological examination, we inoculated the processed samples into blood agar and Gassner agar (Reparto Produzione Terreni – IZSLER, Brescia) and incubated the culture plates for 24–48 h at 37°C and 5% CO_2 to identify *Actinobacillus pleuropneumoniae*, *P. multocida*, *Streptococcus* spp., and *Actinomyces pyogenes*, the bacterial cultures were subjected to Gram's staining and confirmation with biochemical identification and serotyping. Furthermore, to isolate NAD-dependent pathogens (*A. pleuropneumoniae* and *H. parasuis*), blood agar cultures were cross-streaked with a *Staphylococcus intermedius* to evaluate colony-satellitism. Furthermore, DNA extraction was applied to pure cultures of *A. pleuropneumoniae* in order to serotype each isolated strain by an end-point PCR, as described below.

Viral isolation of SIV (Swine Influenza Virus) was performed. A lung fragment was homogenized with Minimum Essential Medium Eagle (Sigma-Aldrich) containing Streptomycin, Penicillin G, and Sulfate Streptomycin. The solution was centrifuged at 1,500 rpm for 5 min. An aliquot of supernatant was used to infect cells (MDBK or Caco-2).

Molecular identification of PRRSV, PCV-type 2, *M. hyopneumoniae*, *M. hyorhinis*, *H. parasuis*, and *A. pleuropneumoniae* was performed.

Several commercial kits were used for Nucleic Acid Extraction: NucleoMag Vet 200 (Macherey-Nagel) for PRRSV and PCV-type 2; Rneasy mini kit (Qiagen) for SIV; Dneasy Blood & Tissue kit (Qiagen) for *M. hyopneumoniae*, *M. hyorhinis,* and *H. parasuis*. Finally, DNA boiling extraction was applied to a pure cultures of *A. pleuropneumoniae* (98°C for 10 min with 1,050 rpm oscillation).

An end-point PCR was performed to confirm the presence of *H. parasuis* according to the protocol described by Oliveira et al. (20), and *A. pleuropneumoniae* serotyping was performed according to the protocol described by Xie et al. (21).

A Real Time RT-PCR for PRRSV detection from blood and lung tissue homogenate was performed using the[1] following the manufacturer's instructions.

A Real Time PCR for PCV-type2 detection from lung tissue homogenate and inguinal lymph node homogenate was performed in accordance with the protocol described by Olvera et al. (22).

A Real Time RT-PCR for SIV detection was performed from lung tissue homogenate in accordance with the protocol described by Spackman et al. (23).

A Real Time PCR for *M. hyopneumoniae* detection was performed from lung tissue homogenate in accordance with the protocol described by Marois et al. (24).

A Real Time PCR for *M. hyorhinis* detection was performed from lung tissue homogenate in accordance with the protocol described by Tocqueville et al. (25).

Finally, a Real Time PCR for *A. pleuropneumoniae* detection from trachea-bronchial swabs and lung tissue homogenate was performed in accordance with the protocol described by Tobias et al. (26).

Statistical Analysis

The proportion of each type of lesion was calculated, and the binomial exact method was used to compute 95% confidence intervals (95% CI). The association of the production stage and pathological lesions with pathogens was assessed by Fisher's exact test (FET). For *A. pyogenes, A. pleuropneumoniae, Streptococcus spp.,* and PCV-type 2, multivariate logistic regression models were employed, with pathogens as dependent variables and production stage and pathological lesions as covariate. To

---

[1]LSI VetMAX (TM) PRRSV EU/NA Real-Time PCR kit (Thermo Fisher).

identify a possible association among different scores and to a verify score distribution, Spearman's correlation coefficient (r) was calculated between different scores (lung vs. pleural scores, lung vs. nasal scores, and pleural vs. nasal scores). Furthermore, a Chi-square test (3 × 2) was performed to compare the scores according to the different classes. The classes identified were: slight (0–9), moderate (10–19), and severe (20–28) for the lung score; slight (0–2) and severe (3, 4) for the pleural score; and slight (0–2) and severe (3–5) for the nasal score. The Chi-square test (2 × 2) was also performed to compare pleural and nasal scores. For each test a $p <0.05$ was considered statistically significant. All analyses were performed using R software (R version 3.3.1, R Core Team, R Foundation for Statistical Computing. R: A language and environment for statistical computing, http://www.R-project.org/; 2016 [accessed 31/05/2017]).

RESULTS

The proportions of weaned piglets and growing/fattening pigs with PRDC were 57.8 and 42.2%, respectively, in 2014; 53.7 and 46.3%, respectively, in 2015; and 57.5 and 42.5%, respectively, in 2016 (**Table 1**). Four hundred sixty-one farms conferred pigs 863 times for diagnostic investigations, with a cumulative number of 1,656 pigs. The mean number of pigs conferred for each farm was 3.6 (SD 4.4) and the mean of times each farm conferred pigs was 1.9 (SD 1.9).

Pleuritis Is the Most Frequently Observed Lesion in Both Groups of Animals Affected by PRDC

The frequencies of lesion distribution in the lungs, pleura, and pericardium are depicted in **Figure 1** (number of pigs with lesions). PL was recorded in the highest number of samples (469; 28.3%), followed by pleuropneumonia (PP) (286; 17.2%), catarrhal bronchopneumonia (CBP) (273; 16.5%), and BIP (265; 16.0%).

The frequencies of lesion distributions in the organs of weaned piglets and growing/fattening pigs are depicted in **Table 2**. PL was the most frequent lesion observed in both the groups (253 and 216 cases, respectively). Other frequent lesions corresponded to CBP (184), BIP (122), PP (125), PE (119), and PL-PE (77) in weaned piglets. On the contrary, PP and BIP were frequently observed in fattening pigs (161 and 143, respectively). The association between the production stage and pathological lesions was statistically significant for IP, PP, PBP, PL, and PE. The post-weaning group showed a lower probability of developing pathological lesions associated with PP, PBP, and PE and a higher probability to developing pathological lesions associated with IP and PL than did the growing group.

Detection of Respiratory Pathogens

The proportions of respiratory pathogens in the samples collected from weaned piglets or fattening pigs are depicted in **Table 3**. The association between the production stage and the isolated pathogen was statistically significant for *Streptococcus*

suis, P. multocida, A. pleuropneumoniae, PRRSV, PCV-type 2, *M. hyopneumoniae, M. hyorhinis*, and *H. parasuis*. The post-weaning group was more likely to show *S. suis*, PRRSV, *M. hyorhinis*, and *H. parasuis* than was the growing group. *M. hyorhinis* was the most commonly detected pathogen in the lungs of weaned piglets with lesions (98.7%). In the lungs of weaned piglets with and without lesions, PRRSV (75 and 59.6%), *H. parasuis* (61.3 and 38.2%), and *Streptococcus* spp. (45.3 and 34.8%) were the most commonly detected pathogens.

Differently, the growing group was more likely to show *P. multocida, A. pleuropneumoniae*, PCV-type 2, and *M. hyopneumoniae*.

M. hyopneumoniae (68.5%) and PCV-type 2 (43.7%) were the most commonly detected pathogens in the organs of fattening pigs with lesions, whereas, in the organs of fattening pigs with and without lesions, PRRSV (55.1 and 41.3%), *Streptococcus* spp. (41 and 18.7%), and *P. multocida* (26.3 and 14.7%) were the most frequently detected pathogens.

Distribution Between a Single Lesion and Respiratory Pathogen Detection in Weaned Piglets and Fattening Pigs

The distribution between pathogen detection and each single lesion in samples collected from weaned piglets and fattening pigs are depicted in **Figure 2**.

P. multocida was detected in the organs of weaned piglets affected by the lesions associated with the following diseases/conditions: PBP (28.6%); PL (26%); CBP (25.9%); and PE (25%). This pathogen was detected in different proportions in the organs of fattening pigs with the lesions associated with the following diseases/conditions: CBP (37.8%); PL (29.9%); BIP (28%); PBP (28%); and IP (23.3%). *A. pleuropneumoniae* was detected in the organs of weaned piglets affected by the lesions associated with the following diseases/conditions: PP (64.4%); PL (16.7%); and PBP (14.3%). This pathogen was detected in different proportions in the organs of fattening pigs with the lesions associated with the following diseases/conditions: PP (81%); PL (38.10%); PBP (28%); BIP (24%); and PE (20.8%).

H. parasuis was detected in the organs of weaned piglets affected by the lesions associated with the following diseases/conditions: BIP (76.9%); PP (73.3%); PE (70.4%); and PL (60.7%). This pathogen was detected in different proportions in the organs of fattening pigs with the lesions associated with the following diseases/conditions: PBP (66.3%); CBP (58.3%); BIP (52.8%); IP (50%); PL (50%); and PE (50%).

Streptococcus spp. was detected in the organs of weaned piglets affected by the lesions associated with the following diseases/conditions: IP (83%); BIP (59%); PL (61%); and PE (50%). The pathogen was also detected in high proportions in the organs of fattening pigs with the lesions associated with the following diseases/conditions: IP (63%); CBP (60%); PBP (52%); BIP (51%); PE (63%); and PL (57%).

A. pyogenes was detected in the organs of both groups affected by purulent bronchopneumonia (21% in weaned piglets and 20% in fattening pigs). The pathogen was also detected in the organs with the lesions associated with the following

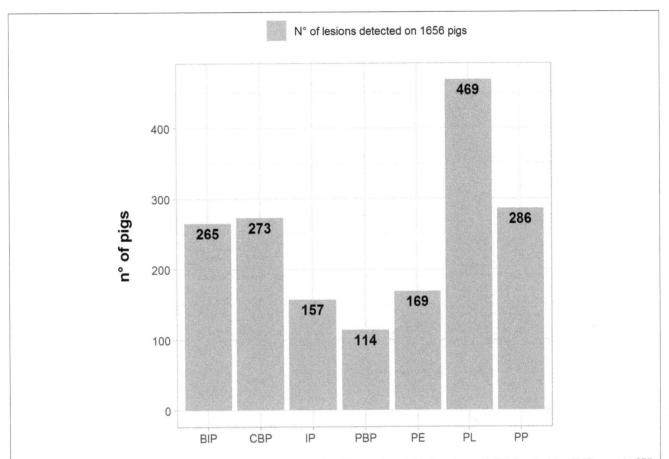

FIGURE 1 | Number (left axes/gray bars) and percentage (right axes/black lines) of different pathological lesions observed in BIP, Broncho-Interstitial Pneumonia; CBP, Catarrhal Bronchopneumonia; IP, Interstitial Pneumonia; PBP, Purulent Bronchopneumonia; PE, Pericarditis; PL, Pleuritis; and PP, Pleuropneumonia.

TABLE 2 | Number, percentage (%), and 95% CI of pathological lesions detected in pigs according to production stage.

Pathological Lesions	N°	Growing/fattening			Post-weaning			p-value	OR	OR CI 95%
		N°	%	CI95%	N°	%	CI 95%			
CBP	273	89	32.6	27–38.1	184	67	61.8–72.9	0.0000	1.76	1.33–2.35
IP	157	83	52.8	45–60.6	74	47	39.3–54.9	0.0179	0.67	0.47–0.94
BIP	265	143	53.9	47.9–59.9	122	46	40–52	0.0003	0.62	0.47–0.81
PP	286	161	56.2	50.5–62	125	44	37.9–49.4	0.0000	0.55	0.42–0.71
PBP	114	59	51.7	42.5–60.9	55	48	39–57.4	0.0792		
PL	469	216	46	41.5–50.5	253	54	49.4–58.4	0.2717		
PE	169	50	29.5	22.7–36.4	119	70	63.5–77.2	0.0001	1.98	1.39–2.86

The association between the pathological lesions and the production stage was calculated by Fisher's exact test; when the association was statistically significant (p < 0.05), the odds ratio (OR) was calculated using the growing group as the source of baseline data.

diseases/conditions: CBP (14% in weaned piglets and 18% in fattening pigs); BIP (12% in weaned piglets and 11% in fattening pigs); and PL (12% in weaned piglets and 10% in fattening pigs).

M hyorhinis was detected in high proportions in the organs of weaned piglets (percentage range 70–90%) and in low proportions in the lungs affected by BIP (53.8%). The pathogen was detected in low proportions in the organs of fattening pigs showing lesions associated with the following

diseases/conditions: CBP (66.7%); PBP (60%); PL-PE (85.7%); and PE (38.9%).

M. hyopneumoniae was scarcely detected in the lung and serosal lesions of weaned piglets (38.9% in PBP and 30.9% in CBP). On the contrary, it was detected in high proportions in the lung and serosal lesions of fattening pigs (percentage range 65–90%) with the exception of those associated with IP (44.4%) and pleuropneumonia.

TABLE 3 | Pathogens detected, proportion and 95% CI according to production stage.

Respiratory pathogen	N° isolated	Growing/fattening			Post-weaning			p-value	OR	OR CI 95%
		N°	%	CI 95%	N°	%	CI 95%			
Streptococcus spp	372	160	43	38.0–48.0	212	57	52.0–62.0	0.722		
Streptococcus suis	17	3	18	0.5–35.8	14	82	64.2–100	0.046	3.68	1.02–20.05
A. pyogenes	72	31	43	31.6–54.5	41	57	45.5–68.4	0.904		
P. multocida	213	109	51	44.5–57.9	104	49	42.1–55.5	0.021	0.71	0.53–0.96
A. pleuropneumoniae	264	167	63	57.4–69.1	97	37	30.9–42.6	0.001	0.39	0.29–0.52
PRRS	946	344	36	33.3–39.4	602	64	60.6–66.7	0.001	2.24	1.79–2.80
PCV-type2	455	251	55	50.6–59.7	204	45	40.3–49.4	0.001	0.47	0.37–0.60
SIV	192	94	49	41.9-56.0	98	51	44.0-58.1	0.16		
M. hyopneumoniae	141	99	70	62.7–77.8	42	30	22.2–37.3	0.001	0.15	0.09–0.25
M. hyorhinis	217	43	20	14.5–25.1	174	80	74.9-85.5	0.001	23.85	6.54–131.94
H. parasuis	185	58	31	24.7–38.0	127	69	62.0–75.3	0.016	1.75	1.09–2.82

The association between the pathogens isolated and the production stage was calculated using Fisher's exact test; when the association was statistically significant (p < 0.05), OR was calculated using the growing group as the source of baseline data.

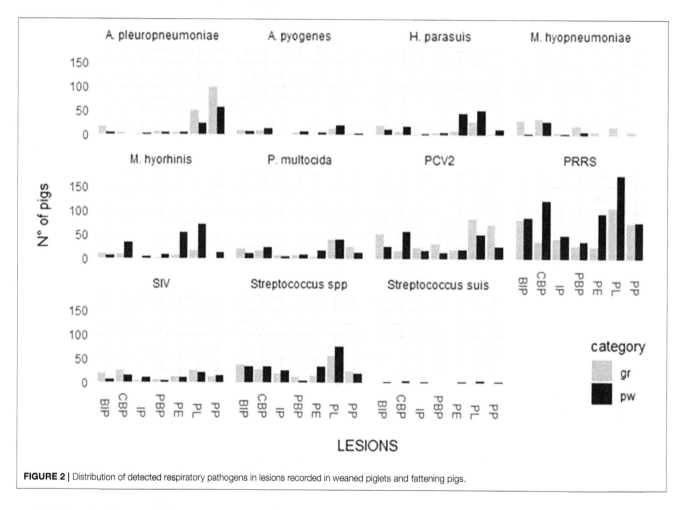

FIGURE 2 | Distribution of detected respiratory pathogens in lesions recorded in weaned piglets and fattening pigs.

PRRSV was highly associated with lung and serosal lesions of both the groups. The detection percentages of different lesions were higher in weaned piglets than in fattening pigs. The rate of detection in weaned piglets varied from 65.8% (PP) to 84.7% (PE) and that in fattening pigs varied from 45.6% (CBP) to 66.7%

(PL). The highest percentages of detection were associated with PL (66.7%) and BIP (62.5%).

SIV was associated with PL in weaned piglets (30.8%) and CBP (30.4%), PE (26.1%), and PL (33.3%) in fattening pigs.

TABLE 4 | Number of pathogens isolated from pathological lesions detected in weaned piglets and fattening pigs.

Pathogens	Isolated	CBP	IP	BIP	PP	PBP	PL	PE
Streptococcus spp.	372	58	44	72	41*I	18	129*I	49*I
Streptococcus suis	17	4	1	1	1	0	4	3
A. pyogenes	72	20*I	1*D	15	5*D	11*I	32*I	4
P. multocida	213	39	11*D	31	39	15	79*I	21
A. pleuropneumoniae	264	5*D	4*D	23*D	153*I	11	74	10*D
PRRSV	946	157	89	165	147	62	279	118*I
PCV-type2	455	73	38	78	94*I	45*I	132	38*D
SIV	192	39	14	24	26	12	46	23
M. hyopneumoniae	141	62	6	32	7	26*I	18	6
M. hyorhinis	217	41	4	17*D	13	11	86	60
H. parasuis	185	23	4	29	13	8	79	52

The association between the detected pathogen (yes/no) and pathological lesions (yes/no) was calculated by Fisher exact test.
* Statistically significant association. I = presence of pathogens increased the probability of detecting a lesion. D = the presence of pathogens decreased the probability of detecting a lesion.

PCV-type 2 was more associated with lung and serosal lesions in fattening pigs than with those in weaned piglets. The rate of detection in weaned piglets varied from 17.6% (PE) to 37.3% (CBP) and that in fattening pigs varied from 25.4% (CBP) to 65.3% (PBP).

As reported in **Table 4**, *A. pyogenes* was associated with the following: CBP (FET: $p < 0.05$; OR, 2.02; 95% CI, 1.12–3.52), IP (FET: $p < 0.05$; OR, 0.13; 95% CI, 0.003–0.754), PP (FET: $p < 0.05$; OR, 0.35; 95% CI, 0.11–0.86), PBP (FET: $p < 0.05$; OR, 2.6; 95% CI, 1.20–5.17), and PL (FET: $p < 0.001$; OR, 2.1; 95% CI, 1.3–3.5). The detection of *A. pyogenes* made the detection of PP and IP lesions twice less probable and CBP, PBL, and PL lesions it twice more probable.

A. pleuropneumoniae was associated with the following: CBP (FET: $p < 0.0001$; OR, 0.08; 95% CI, 0.03–0.2), IP (FET: $p < 0.0001$; OR, 0.13; 95% CI, 0.03–0.33), BIP (FET: $p < 0.0001$; OR, 0.45; 95% CI, 0.28–0.72), PP (FET: $p < 0.0001$; OR, 13.0; 95% CI, 9.53–17.85), and PE (FET: $p < 0.0001$; OR, 0.31; 95% CI, 1.20–5.17). The detection of *A. pleuropneumoniae* made the detection of CBP, IP, BIP, and PE lesions 13 times less probable and that of PP lesions 13 times more probable.

M. hyopneumoniae was associated with PBP (FET: $p < 0.001$; OR, 2.91; 95% CI, 1.38–6.45). The detection of *M. hyopneumoniae* doubled the probability of detection of PBP lesions.

M. hyorhinis was associated with BIP (FET: $p < 0.0001$; OR, 0.14; 95% CI, 0.05–0.45). The detection of *M. hyorhinis* decreased the probability of detection of BIP lesions.

P. multocida was associated with IP (FET: $p < 0.05$; OR, 0.49; 95% CI, 0.23–0.91) and PL (FET: $p < 0.01$; OR, 1.59; 95% CI, 1.16–2.17). The detection of *P. multocida* decreased the probability of detection of IP lesions and nearly doubled the probability of detection of PL lesions.

PCV-type 2 was associated with pathological lesions of PP (FET: $p < 0.01$; OR, 1.47; 95% CI, 1.08–1.99), PBP (FET: $p < 0.001$; OR, 1.92; 95% CI, 1.23–3.01), and PE (FET: $p < 0.05$; OR, 0.65; 95% CI, 0.43–0.96). The detection of PCV-type 2 decreased the probability of detection of PE pathological

lesions and increased the probability of detection of PP and PBP pathological lesions.

PRRSV was associated with PE pathological lesions (FET: $p < 0.001$; OR, 1.84; 95% CI, 1.24–2.76). The detection of PRRSV nearly doubled the probability of detection of BIP lesions.

Streptococcus spp. was associated with pathological lesions of PP (FET: $p < 0.0001$; OR, 0.52; 95% CI, 0.36–0.75), PL (FET: $p < 0.001$; OR, 1.47; 95% CI, 1.14–1.90), and PE (FET: $p < 0.05$; OR, 1.47; 95% CI, 1.01–2.12). The detection of *Streptococcus* spp. decreased the probability of detection of PP lesions and increased the probability of detection of PL and PE lesions by one and an half times (**Table 4**).

Multivariate Analysis

Multivariate regression logistic models were applied, with pathogens (*A. pyogenes, A. pleuropneumoniae, Streptococcus spp.,* and PCV-type 2) as dependent variables and production stage and pathological lesions as covariates. The results of the multivariate regression analysis are shown in **Table 5**. For *A. pyogenes*, the best model (LRT, 33.99; df = 3; $p < 0.0001$) included CBP, PBP, and PL lesions. The detection of *A. pyogenes* was four times more probable with CBP, PBL, and PL lesions.

For *A. pleuropneumoniae*, the best model ($p < 0.0001$) included all factors that were found to be statistically significant by FET, as well as production stage. The presence of *A. pleuropneumoniae* was more likely to occur in the growing group than in the post-weaning group with PP lesions and without CBP, IP, BIP, and PE lesions.

For PCV-type 2, the best model (LRT, 48.3; df = 2; $p < 0.0001$) included PCP lesion and production stage. The presence of PCV-type2 was more likely to occur in the growing group than in the post-weaning group with PCP lesions.

Finally, for *Streptococcus* spp. the best model (LRT, 14.3; df = 1; $p < 0.0001$) included PP lesion. The presence of *Streptococcus* spp. was more likely to occur in the absence of PP lesions.

TABLE 5 | Factors that were found to be statistically significant by multivariate regression analysis for *A. pyogenes*, *A. pleuropneumoniae*, *Streptococcus* spp., and PCV-type 2 pathogens.

Pathogens	Factor	Baseline	OR	OR 95% CI		p-value
A. pyogenes	CBP	Lesion detected	4.40	2.27	8.61	<0.0001
	PBP	Lesion detected	3.77	1.77	7.46	<0.0001
	PL	Lesion detected	3.55	2.01	6.44	<0.0001
A. pleuropneumoniae	CBP	Lesion not detected	7.61	3.36	21.89	<0.0001
	IP	Lesion not detected	6.62	2.67	21.95	<0.0001
	BIP	Lesion not detected	1.70	1.05	2.85	0.03
	PP	Lesion detected	7.21	5.16	10.14	<0.0001
	PE	Lesion not detected	2.51	1.33	5.28	<0.0001
	Production stage	Growing	2.27	1.66	3.10	<0.0001
PCV-type2	PBP	Lesion detected	1.82	1.18	2.80	0.001
	Production stage	Growing	2.08	1.65	2.62	<0.0001
Streptococcus spp.	PP	Lesion not detected	1.90	1.35	2.74	0.001

OR and 95% CI were calculated by multivariate logistic regression.

TABLE 6 | Frequency (n) and percentage (%) of detection of respiratory pathogens in samples without lesions are shown at global level (overall) and by production stage (growing/post-weaning).

Pathogen	Overall			Growing		Post-weaning		p-value
	Without lesions	Positive	%	n	%	n	%	
Streptococcus spp.	234	46	19.7%	11	23.9%	35	76.1%	0.288
Streptococcus suis	234	6	2.6%	3	50.0%	3	50.0%	0.379
A. pyogenes	234	4	1.7%	2	50.0%	2	50.0%	0.591
P. multocida	234	20	8.5%	6	30.0%	14	70.0%	1.000
A. pleuropneumoniae	**234**	**19**	**8.1%**	**11**	**57.9%**	**8**	**42.1%**	**0.017**
PRRSV	204	133	65.2%	35	26.3%	98	73.7%	0.058
PCV-type2	185	45	24.3%	15	33.3%	30	66.7%	0.572
SIV	202	40	19.8%	12	30.0%	28	70.0%	1.000
M. hyopneumoniae	**18**	**7**	**38.9%**	**6**	**85.7%**	**1**	**14.3%**	**0.049**
M. hyorhinis	**56**	**51**	**91.1%**	**7**	**13.7%**	**44**	**86.3%**	**0.000**
H. parasuis	66	41	62.1%	7	17.1%	34	82.9%	0.535

p-value was calculated using Fisher's exact test to assess the association between the occurrence of pathogens and the production stage.

Isolation of Single Pathogens in Organs Without Lesions

Among 1,656 lung samples, 234 non-lesioned samples were observed (14.1%, 95% CI, 12.5–15.9%); in particular, among these 234 samples, 161 (68.8%, 95% CI, 62.4–74.7%) and 73 (31.2%, 95% CI, 25.3–37.6%) were identified in the post-weaning and growing groups. The association between the production stage and the lesions was statistically significant (FET: $p < 0.0001$), with the post-weaning group showing a lower probability of presenting lesions (OR, 0.53; 95% CI, 0.39–0.73). **Table 6** shows the frequencies and percentages of the pathogens detected in the lungs without lesions according to the production stage. The p-value obtained by FET indicates the association between the pathogen and the production stage. Statistically significant associations of the production stage were found with *A. pleuropneumoniae* (FET: $p = 0.017$), *M. hyopneumoniae* (FET: $p = 0.049$), and *M. hyorhinis* (FET: $p < 0.001$). The post-weaning group showed lower probabilities of detection of *A. pleuropneumoniae* (OR, 0.3; 95% CI, 0.1–0.8) and *M. hyopneumoniae* (OR, 0.1; 95% CI, 0.1–0.9) than did the growing group. A different pattern was observed for *M. hyorhinis*; it was mostly detected in the post-weaning group (OR, 3.14; 95% CI, 4.4–∞).

Relation Between Nasal, Pleural, and Lung Scores

The mean lung score was 13.53 in weaned piglets and 12.14 in fattening pigs With 14.7% of the samples being non-lesioned (equaly distributed between weaned and fattening pigs). The mean pleural score was 1.46 and 1.48, in the weaned and fattening pigs, respectively, with 42.71 and 39.10% of the samples, respectively, being non-lesioned. The mean nasal score was 0.50 and 0.78 in the weaned and fattening pigs, respectively, with 61.82 and 42.71% of the samples, respectively, being non-lesioned.

Data distributions and correlations between the different scores are shown in **Figure 3**. The results indicate that the difference was statistically significant among scores ($p < 0.0001$, lung score vs. pleural score; $p = 0.0039$, lung score vs. nasal score; $p = 0.0023$, pleural score vs. nasal score). However, the Spearman r value was low, indicating a discrete/limited correlation ($r = 0.39$; $r = 0.14$; $r = 0.15$, respectively). On the contrary, Chi-square test showed that there was a statistically significant relationship between lung and pleural scores (3×2; $p < 0.0001$) and that there was no statistically significant relationship between the lung and nasal scores (3×2) and between the pleural and nasal scores (2×2); however, p was 0.0572 in the case relationship between the lung and nasal scores (**Supplementary Material**).

DISCUSSION

The systematic application of the standardized protocol during 2014–2016 allowed the identification of the principal lesions and pathogens associated with PRDC outbreaks in growing pigs and the comparison of different situations. Our results indicate that the PRDC percentages recorded during the 3 years of study were almost constant between the weaned and the fattening pigs and that PRDC principally affects the weaned pigs (53–58 vs. 42–47%) causing high mortality. The proportion of lung lesions was high with values comparable to those reported by previous investigations at slaughterhouses (12, 13, 27–29). Nevertheless, it is important to highlight that the frequency of pleuritis, BIP, and pleuropneumonia along with that of IP and purulent bronchopneumonia was similar between piglets and pigs. Conversely, catarrhal bronchopneumonia, pericarditis, and pleuro-pericarditis affected principally weaned piglets. Generally, pleuritis lesions were more frequently detected in weaned piglets. The comparison between these results and the data obtained from slaughtered pigs with catarrhal bronchopneumonia and pleuropneumonia (12, 13), highlighted an evolution of the lesions from the growing stage to the slaughtering stage.

The analysis of the association between lesions and the pathogens involved showed that the presence of *A. pleuropneumoniae* is largely associated with pleuropneumonia in fattening pigs. *A. pleuropneumoniae* is the agent associated with porcine pleuropneumonia, a contagious respiratory disease capable of causing significant economic losses to the swine industry worldwide (30).

Frequently, pigs that overcome acute diseases remain chronically infected, showing no clinical signs, but likely harboring chronic lung alterations, such as fibroblastic pleurisy and lung tissue sequesters surrounded by fibrotic tissue (13, 31). In this study, in fact, *A. pleuropneumoniae* was strongly associated with lesions characteristic of pleuropneumonia with a minor involvement of pleura. In addition, we isolated *A. pleuropneumoniae* from non-lesioned lungs in 8.1% of the cases; this finding suggests that *A. pleuropneumoniae* is unlikely to be associated with a subclinical lung condition.

Streptococcus spp. and *S. suis* were associated with pleural and pericardial lesions, mainly in post-weaning pigs. Fibrinous

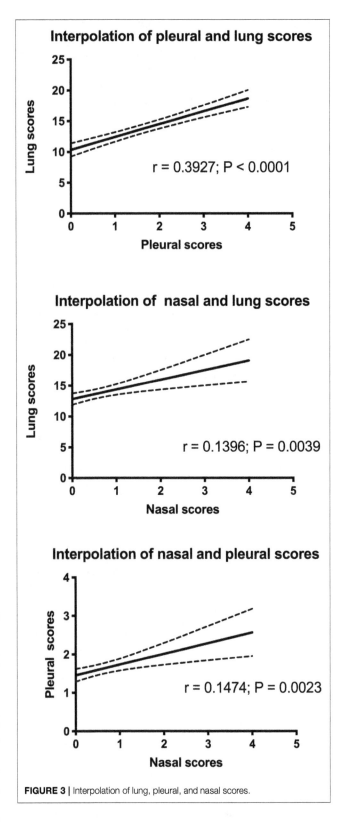

FIGURE 3 | Interpolation of lung, pleural, and nasal scores.

or fibrinopurulent pleuritis, peritonitis, or polyserositis were identified in pigs infected with both *S. suis* and *H. parasuis*. Pigs in which only *S. suis* was isolated had a more extensive suppurative exudation than that was associated with *H. parasuis*.

S. suis in pigs with pleuritis, peritonitis, and polyserositis should be considered first during differential diagnosis, especially when the exudate was more suppurative than fibrinous (32). In this study, the frequency of *Streptococcus* spp. and *S. suis* detection in non-lesioned lungs was 19.7 and 2.6%, respectively. This finding is partly in contrast with other published data, which showed that asymptomatic colonization of *S. suis* in the upper respiratory tract as well as in the intestinal and genital tract was common (33).

M. hyopneumoniae was significantly more prevalent in cases of purulent bronchopneumoniae and even more apparently prevalent in catarrhal bronchopneumoniae. The lesions were more frequent in fattening pigs than in weaned piglets. *M. hyopneumoniae* is an important respiratory pathogen capable of causing the disease by itself or in combination with other pathogens (34, 35). A combination was observed between *M. hyopneumoniae* and PRRSV or *S.* suis (36, 37). Different studies have demonstrated that disease severity in growing pigs is correlated with several factors (38, 39). The fact that *M. hyopneumoniae* was frequently found in organs without lesions corroborates the finding that it is a common pathogen with effects that are likely dependent on other triggering factors, however we cannot exclude that *M. hyopneumoniae* has been detected in the first stage of the infection.

The correlation between lung and pleural scores was found to be linear with $p < 0.0001$. However, it was a moderate correlation because Spearman's r-coefficient was low ($r < 0.4$). Probably, this aspect is associated with a wide distribution of lung scores in each class of pleural scores. For this reason, a further comparison between scores was performed using the Chi-squared test. Lung scores were divided into three categories, while pleural scores were divided into two categories. The results indicated that the frequency of severe lesions in lungs corresponded to a high frequency of severe pleural lesions. Therefore, the results suggest that the proposed scoring approach could be a reliable system to evaluate lesions in the respiratory tracts during pathological investigations.

In conclusion, these data shed light on the impact of different pathogens on the respiratory disease of pigs and highlight the need for a systematic diagnostic approach to manage the respiratory disease in pig farms.

AUTHOR CONTRIBUTIONS

JR, PPa, and GA contributed to the conception and design of the study, acquisition of data, analysis and interpretation of data, and drafting of the article. CS, SG, and NV contributed to the acquisition of data, analysis and interpretation of data, and drafting of the article. BB contributed to the acquisition of data, analysis and interpretation of data, and revise revisions of the article. AC and PPo contributed to the analysis and interpretation of data and revision of the article. All authors contributed to the revision of the manuscript and furthermore they read and approved the submitted version.

ACKNOWLEDGMENTS

Special thanks to E. language editing service for the English writing assistance.

REFERENCES

1. Chae C. Porcine respiratory disease complex: interaction of vaccination and porcine circovirus type 2, porcine reproductive and respiratory syndrome virus, and *Mycoplasma hyopneumoniae. Vet J.* (2016) 212:1–6. doi: 10.1016/j.tvjl.2015.10.030
2. Fablet C, Marois-Créhan C, Simon G, Grasland B, Jestin A, Kobisch M, et al. Infectious agents associated with respiratory diseases in 125 farrow-to-finish pig herds: a cross-sectional study. *Vet Microbiol.* (2012) 157:152–63. doi: 10.1016/j.vetmic.2011.12.015
3. Opriessnig T, Giménez-Lirola LG, Halbur PG. Polymicrobial respiratory disease in pigs. *Anim Health Res Rev.* (2011) 12:133–48. doi: 10.1017/S1466252311000120
4. Stärk KDC. Epidemiological investigation of the influence of environmental risk factors on respiratory diseases in swine – a literature review. *Vet J.* (2000) 159:37–56. doi: 10.1053/tvjl.1999.0421
5. Harding JC, Halbur PG. PMWS or a group of PCV2-associated syndromes: ever-growing concerns. In: *Proceedings of the 17th International Pig Veterinary Society Congress. PMWS and PCV2 Diseases, Beyond the Debate, Keynotes on the Merial Symposium and Brief Epidemiological Updates.* Ames. (2002).
6. Harms PA, Halbur PG, Sorden SD. Three cases of porcine respiratory disease complex associated with porcine circovirus type 2 infection. *J Swine Health Prod.* (2002) 10:27–30. Available online at: https://www.aasv.org/shap/issues/v10n1/v10n1p27.pdf.
7. Holst S, Yeske P, Pieters M. Elimination of *Mycoplasma hyopneumoniae* from breed-to-wean farms: A review of current protocols with emphasis on herd closure and medication. *J Swine Health Prod.* (2015) 23:321–30.

8. Regula G, Lichtensteiger C, Mateus-Pinilla N, Scherba G, Miller G, Weigel R. Comparison of serologic testing and slaughter evaluation for assessing the effects of subclinical infection on growth in pigs. *J Am Vet Med Assoc.* (2000) 217:888–95. doi: 10.2460/javma.2000.217.888
9. Maes D, Sibila M, Kuhnert P, Segalés J, Haesebrouck F, Pieters M. Update on *Mycopasma hyopneumoniae* infections in pigs: knowledge gaps for improved disease control. *Transbound Emerg Dis.* (2018) 65(Suppl. 1):110–24. doi: 10.1111/tbed.12677
10. Pointon A, Byrt D, Heap P. Effect of enzootic pneumonia of pigs on growth performance. *Aust Vet J.* (1985) 62:13–8. doi: 10.1111/j.1751-0813.1985.tb06032.x
11. Rautiainen W, Virtala A, Wallgren P, Saloniemi H. Varying effect of infections with *Mycoplasma hyopneumoniae* on the weight gain recorded in three different multisource fattening pig herds. *J Vet Med B Infect Dis Vet Public Health.* (2000) 47:461–9. doi: 10.1046/j.1439-0450.2000.00370.x
12. Ostanello F, Dottori M, Gusmara C, Leotti G, Sala V. Pneumonia disease assessment using a slaughterhouse lung-scoring method. *J Vet Med A Physiol Pathol Clin Med.* (2007) 54:70–5. doi: 10.1111/j.1439-0442.2007.00920.x
13. Merialdi G, Dottori M, Bonilauri P, Luppi A, Gozio S, Pozzi P, et al. Survey of pleuritis and pulmonary lesions in pigs at abattoir with a focus on the extent of the condition and herd risk factors. *Vet J.* (2012) 193:234–9. doi: 10.1016/j.tvjl.2011.11.009
14. Hansen MS, Pors SE, Jensen HE, Bille-Hansen V, Bisgaard M, Flachs EM, et al. An investigation of the pathology and pathogens associated with porcine respiratory disease complex in Denmark. *J Comp Path.* (2010) 143:120–31. doi: 10.1016/j.jcpa.2010.01.012

15. Segalés J, Sibila M. Viral pulmonary lesions at slaughter. In: Leneveu P, Pommier P, Pagot E, Morvan H, Lewandowski E, editors. *Slaughterhouse Evaluation of Respiratory Tract Lesions in Pigs*. Plérin: RoudennGrafik-Guingamp (2016). p. 102–3.

16. Madec F, Derrien H. Fréquence, intensité et localisation deslésions pulmonaires chez le porc charcutier. *Journées Rech Porcine en France*. (1981) 13:231–6.

17. Madec F, Kobisch M. Bilan lesionnel des poumons de porcs charcutiers a l'abattoir. *J Rech Porc Fr*. (1982) 14:405–12.

18. Dottori M, Nigrelli A, Bonilauri P, Merialdi G, Gozio S, Cominotti F. Proposta di un nuovo sistema di punteggiatura delle pleuriti suine in sede di macellazione La griglia S.P.E.S. (Slaughterhouse Pleuritis Evaluation System). *Large Anim Rev*. (2007) 13:161–5. Available online at: https://www.vetjournal.it/riviste/item/21673-dottori-m-,-nigrelli-a-d-,-bonilauri-p-,-merialdi-g-,-gozio-s-,-cominotti-f.html

19. De Jong MF. Progressive and nonprogressive atrophic rhinitis. In: Straw BE, Zimmerman JJ, D'Allaire SD, Taylor DJ, editors. *Diseases of Swine. 9th Edn*. Blackwell Publishing (2006). P. 577–602.

20. Oliveira S, Galina L, Pijoan C. Development of a PCR test to diagnose *Haemophilus parasuis* infections. *J Vet Diagn Invest*. (2001) 13:495–501. doi: 10.1177/104063870101300607

21. Xie F, Lei L, Du C, Li S, Han W, Ren Z. Genomic differences between *Actinobacillus pleuropneumoniae* serotypes 1 and 3 and the diversity distribution among 15 serotypes. *FEMS Microbiol Lett*. (2010) 303:147–55. doi: 10.1111/j.1574-6968.2009.01870.x

22. Olvera A, Sibila M, Calsamiglia M, Segalés J, Domingo M. Comparison of porcine circovirus type 2 load in serum quantified by a real time PCR in post weaning multisystemic wasting syndrome and porcine dermatitis and nephropathy syndrome naturally affected pigs. *J Virol Methods*. (2004) 117:75–80. doi: 10.1016/j.jviromet.2003.12.007

23. Spackman E, Senne DA, Myers TJ, Bulaga LL, Garber LP, Perdue ML, et al. Development of a real-time reverse transcriptase PCR assay for type A influenza virus and the avian H5 and H7 hemagglutinin subtypes. *J Clin Microbiol*. (2002) 40:3256–60. doi: 10.1128/JCM.40.9.3256-3260.2002

24. Marois C, Dory D, Fablet C, Madec F, Kobisch M. Development of a quantitative real-time TaqMan PCR assay for determination of the minimal dose of *Mycoplasma hyopneumoniae* strain 116 required to induce pneumonia in SPF pigs. *J Appl Microbiol*. (2010) 108:1523–33. doi: 10.1111/j.1365-2672.2009.04556.x

25. Tocqueville V, Ferré S, Nguyen NH, Kempf I, Marois-Créhan C. Multilocus sequence typing of *Mycoplasma hyorhinis* strains identified by a real-time TaqMan PCR assay. *J Clin Microbiol*. (2014) 52:1664–71. doi: 10.1128/JCM.03437-13

26. Tobias TJ, Bouma A, Klinkenberg D, Daemen AJ, Stegeman JA, Wagenaar JA, et al. Detection of *Actinobacillus pleuropneumoniae* in pigs by real-time quantitative PCR for the apxIVA gene. *Vet J*. (2012) 193:557–60. doi: 10.1016/j.tvjl.2012.02.004

27. Maes D, Deluyker H, Verdonck M, Castryck F, Miry C, Vrijens B, et al. Non-infectious factors associated with macroscopic and microscopic lung lesions in slaughter pigs from farrow-to-finish herds. *Vet Rec*. (2001) 148:41–6. doi: 10.1136/vr.148.2.41

28. Meyns T, Van Steelant J, Rolly E, Dewulf J, Haesebrouck F, Maes D. A cross-sectional study of risk factors associated with pulmonary lesions in pigs at slaughter. *Vet J*. (2011) 187:388–92. doi: 10.1016/j.tvjl.2009.12.027

29. Christensen G, Enoe C. The prevalence of pneumonia, pleuritis, pericarditis and liver spots in Danish slaughter pigs in 1998, including comparison with 1994. *Dansk Veterinaertidsskrift*. (1999) 82:1006–15.

30. Sassu EL, Bossé JT, Tobias TJ, Gottschalk M, Langford PR, Hennig-Pauka I. Update on *Actinobacillus pleuropneumoniae*-knowledge, gaps and challenges. *Transbound Emerg Dis*. (2018) 65(Suppl. 1):72–90. doi: 10.1111/tbed.12739

31. Liggett AD, Harrison LR, Farrell RL. Sequential study of lesion development in experimental Haemophilus pleuropneumonia. *Res Vet Sci*. (1987) 42:204–12. doi: 10.1016/S0034-5288(18)30687-8

32. Reams RY, Glickman LT, Harrington DD, Thacker HL, Bowersock TL. *Streptococcus suis* infection in swine: a retrospective study of 256 cases. Part II Clinical signs, gross and microscopic lesions, and coexisting microorganisms. *J Vet Diagn Invest*. (1994) 6:326–34. doi: 10.1177/104063879400600308

33. Goyette-Desjardins G, Auger JP, Xu J, Segura M, Gottschalk M. *Streptococcus suis*, an important pig pathogen and emerging zoonotic agent-an update on the worldwide distribution based on serotyping and sequence typing. *Emerg Microbes Infect*. (2014) 3:e45. doi: 10.1038/emi.2014.45

34. Sørensen V, Jorsal SE, Mousing J. Diseases of the respiratory system. In: Straw BE, Zimmerman JJ, D'Allaire SD, Taylor DJ, editors. *Diseases of Swine, 9th Edn*. Oxford: Blackwell Publishing (2006). p. 149–77.

35. Opriessnig T, Thacker EL, Yu S, Fenaux M, Meng XJ, Halbur PG. Experimental reproduction of postweaning multisystemic wasting syndrome in pigs by dual infection with *Mycoplasma hyopneumoniae* and porcine circovirus type 2. *Vet Pathol*. (2004) 41:624–40. doi: 10.1354/vp.41-6-624

36. Thanawongnuwech R, Thacker B, Halbur P, Thacker EL. Increased production of proinflammatory cytokines following infection with porcine reproductive and respiratory syndrome virus and *Mycoplasma hyopneumoniae*. *Clin Diagn Lab Immunol*. (2004) 11:901–8. doi: 10.1128/CDLI.11.5.901-908.2004

37. Halbur P, Thanawongnuwech R, Brown G, Kinyon J, Roth J, Thacker E, et al. Efficacy of antimicrobial treatments and vaccination regimens for control of porcine reproductive and respiratory syndrome virus and *Streptococcus suis* coinfection of nursery pigs. *J Clin Microbiol*. (2000) 38:1156–60. doi: 10.1128/JCM.38.3.1156-1160.2000

38. Garza-Moreno L, Segalés J, Pieters M, Romagosa A, Sibila M. Acclimation strategies in gilts to control *Mycoplasma hyopneumoniae* infection. *Vet Microbiol*. (2018) 219:23–9. doi: 10.1016/j.vetmic.2018.04.005

39. Maes D, Segales J, Meyns T, Sibila M, Pieters M, Haesebrouck F. Control of *Mycoplasma hyopneumoniae* infections in pigs. *Vet Microbiol*. (2008) 126:297–309. doi: 10.1016/j.vetmic.2007.09.008

2

First Report of *Chlamydia* Seroprevalence and Risk Factors in Domestic Black-Boned Sheep and Goats in China

Li-Xiu Sun[1], Qin-Li Liang[1], Xiao-Hui Hu[1], Zhao Li[2], Jian-Fa Yang[2], Feng-Cai Zou[2]* and Xing-Quan Zhu[1]*

[1] State Key Laboratory of Veterinary Etiological Biology, Lanzhou Veterinary Research Institute, Chinese Academy of Agricultural Sciences, Lanzhou, China, [2] Key Laboratory of Veterinary Public Health of Yunnan Province, College of Veterinary Medicine, Yunnan Agricultural University, Kunming, China

Correspondence:
Feng-Cai Zou
zfc1207@vip.163.com
Xing-Quan Zhu
xingquanzhu1@hotmail.com

The Gram-negative bacteria of the genus *Chlamydia* cause a wide range of diseases in humans and animals. The seroprevalence of *Chlamydia* in domestic black-boned sheep and goats in China is unknown. In this survey, a total of 481 serum samples were collected randomly from domestic black-boned sheep and goats from three counties in Yunnan province, southwest China, from July to August 2017. The sera were examined by an indirect hemagglutination assay (IHA). Antibodies to *Chlamydia* were detected in 100/481 [20.79%, 95% confidence interval (CI), 17.16–24.42] serum samples (IHA titer ≥1:64). The *Chlamydia* seroprevalence ranged from 12.21% (95% CI, 7.81–16.61) to 30.89% (95% CI, 22.72–39.06) across different regions in Yunnan province, and the differences were statistically significant ($P < 0.01$). The seroprevalence in male domestic black-boned sheep and goats (28.64%; 95% CI, 22.36–34.92) was significantly higher than that in the females (15.25%; 95% CI, 11.05–19.45) ($P < 0.01$). However, there was no statistically significant difference in *Chlamydia* seroprevalence in domestic black-boned sheep and goats between ages and species ($P > 0.05$). To our knowledge, this is the first report of *Chlamydia* seroprevalence in domestic black-boned sheep and goats in Yunnan Province, southwest China. These data provide baseline information for future implementation of measures to control *Chlamydia* infection in these animals.

Keywords: *Chlamydia*, domestic black-boned sheep and goats, indirect hemagglutination assay, seroprevalence, China

INTRODUCTION

Chlamydia, an obligate intracellular Gram-negative pathogen, is responsible for a broad spectrum of diseases in animals and humans (1, 2). *Chlamydia* grows and reproduces in the respiratory, urogenital, and gastrointestinal tracts (2). Two species of the genus *Chlamydia*, namely *Chlamydia abortus* and *Chlamydia pecorum*, can cause serious infections in sheep and goats (1). *Chlamydia* is a leading cause of abortion in sheep and goats, which caused significant economic losses to livestock industry (3–6). Additionally, as a zoonotic pathogen, humans can be infected via exposure to *Chlamydia* infected animals (7).

Chlamydia infection is prevalent in sheep and goats all over the world, especially in sheep-rearing areas, such as in Northern Europe and North America (8, 9). In China, *Chlamydia* infection in sheep has been reported in many provinces, such as Qinghai, Shandong, and Hubei (10). However, data about *Chlamydia* infection in domestic black-boned sheep and goats have been limited. Domestic black-boned sheep and goats have dark tissue compared to ordinary sheep and goats, which has been attributed to the presence of excessive melanin in domestic black-boned sheep and goats (11).

Domestic black-boned sheep and goats are indigenous animals to the Lanping County of Yunnan Province, China (11–13). Because of their unique characteristics of these breeds, black-boned sheep and goats have a strong adaptability, and they have been introduced into other provinces of China, such as Shandong, Henan, and Hebei (14). Therefore, in this study, we examined the seroprevalence and risk factors of *Chlamydia* infection in domestic black-boned sheep and goats in Yunnan Province, southwest China. Our results provide baseline data for future control strategies of *Chlamydia* infection in domestic black-boned sheep and goats in China.

MATERIALS AND METHODS

Ethical Statement

This study was approved by the Animal Administration and Ethics Committee of Lanzhou Veterinary Research Institute, Chinese Academy of Agricultural Sciences (approval no.: LVRIAEC-2017-06). Domestic black-boned sheep and goats, from which the blood samples were collected, were handled humanely in accordance with the requirements of the Animal Ethics Procedures and Guidelines of the People's Republic of China.

The Study Sites

The survey was conducted in Shilin County, Lanping County, and Yongsheng County in Yunnan Province, southwest China (**Figure 1**). Yunnan Province is the major producing region of domestic black-boned sheep and goats in China. In the present study, the sampling sites are all large-scale farms, which implement a free-range breeding mode for 5–8 h in daytime. The annual temperature difference in Yunnan Province is small, but the daily temperature difference is large.

Serum Samples

Between July and August 2017, a total of 481 blood samples were collected randomly from domestic black-boned sheep and goats from four intensive farms ($n = 6,100$), two of which were from Lanping county ($n = 213$), followed by Yongsheng county ($n = 145$) and Shilin county ($n = 123$), Yunnan province, southwest China. A standardized questionnaire was used to collect information about the region, gender, age, and species of each animal. Blood samples were transported to the laboratory, kept at room temperature for 2 h, and centrifuged at 3,000 g for 10 min, and the supernatants, which represent the serum samples, were collected and stored at −20°C until further analysis.

Serological Examination

A commercially available indirect hemagglutination assay (IHA) kit (Lanzhou Veterinary Research Institute, Chinese Academy of Agricultural Sciences) was used to determine the level of *Chlamydia* antibodies in the serum of domestic black-boned sheep and goats. As a mature technology for detecting *Chlamydia* antibodies, the sensitivity and specificity of the IHA kit used in this study have been verified by the Ministry of Agriculture of China (NY/T 562-2002), which were 100% and 95%, respectively (15). The serological analysis was carried out according to the manufacturer's recommendations as previously described (16–19). Briefly, serum samples were added to 96-well V-bottomed polystyrene plates, which were diluted fourfold serially from 1:4 to 1:1,024. The detection antigen was added to each well, and the plate was then shaken slightly for 2 min followed by incubation at 37°C for 2 h. The samples were considered positive for *Chlamydia* antibodies when the agglutinated erythrocytes were formed in wells at dilutions of 1:64 or higher. Samples that had agglutination results between 1:4 and 1:64 were considered "suspect" and were retested.

Statistical Analysis

Differences in the seroprevalence of *Chlamydia* among domestic black-boned sheep and goats of different regions, genders, ages, and species were analyzed by a χ^2 test using the SPSS software (release 23.0 standard version; SPSS Inc., Chicago, IL, USA). $P < 0.05$ was considered statistically significant. Odds ratios (ORs) with 95% confidence intervals (CIs) were also determined.

RESULTS

In the present study, 100 of the examined 481 serum samples of domestic black-boned sheep and goats (20.79%; 95% CI, 17.16–24.42) were seropositive for *Chlamydia* by IHA test at the cutoff titer of 1:64. The 100 positive samples included 26 samples (of 213) from Lanping Country (12.21%; 95% CI, 7.81–16.61), 36 (of 145) from Yongsheng Country (24.83%; 95% CI, 17.80–31.86), and 38 (of 123) samples from Shilin Country (30.89%; 95% CI, 22.72–39.06). The differences in *Chlamydia* seroprevalence between these regions were statistically significant ($\chi^2 = 18.59$, $df = 2$, $P < 0.01$; **Table 1**). As shown in **Table 1**, the investigation revealed that the seroprevalence in female and male animals was 15.25% (43/282; 95% CI, 11.05–19.45) and 28.64% (57/199; 95% CI, 22.36–34.92), respectively. The difference in *Chlamydia* seroprevalence was statistically significant between genders ($\chi^2 = 12.71$, $df = 1$, $P < 0.01$) of domestic black-boned sheep and goats. Seropositive black-boned sheep and goats were found in all four age groups and varied from 16.41% (21/128; 95% CI, 10.00–22.83) to 25.40% (48/189; 95% CI, 19.19–31.61). In terms of species, the seroprevalence was 22.76% (71/312; 95% CI, 18.11–27.41) in black-boned sheep and 17.16% (29/169; 95% CI, 11.48–22.84) in black-boned goats. There was no statistically significant difference in *Chlamydia* seroprevalence observed between age groups ($\chi^2 = 4.63$, $df = 3$, $P > 0.05$) and species ($\chi^2 = 2.09$, $df = 1$, $P > 0.05$) in domestic black-boned sheep and goats (**Table 1**).

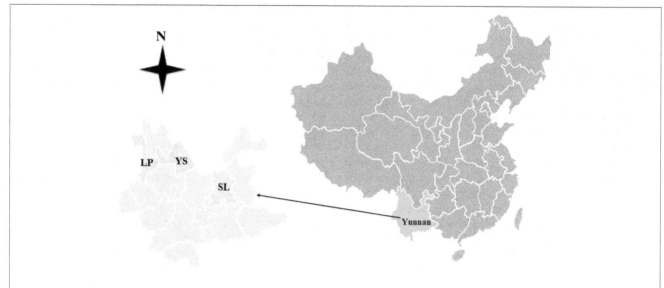

FIGURE 1 | The map of China showing the geographical regions in Yunnan province, where domestic black-boned sheep and goats were sampled. LP, Lanping County; SL, Shilin County; YS, Yongsheng County.

The antibody titers were diverse in domestic black-boned sheep and goats of different regions, genders, ages, and species, with the most frequent titers being 1:64 (87.00%), followed by 1:256 (10.00%) and 1:1,024 (3.00%; **Table 1**).

DISCUSSION

In this study, the seroprevalence of *Chlamydia* in domestic black-boned sheep and goats in Yunnan province was 20.79%, which was higher than the 8.45% reported in goats in Hunan Province, China (20), but was lower than that reported in sheep in Xinjiang Province (40.13%) in China (10). *Chlamydia* seroprevalence has been reported in sheep and goats worldwide. For example, 10.60% seroprevalence has been reported in sheep in India (21), and 33% seroprevalence has been reported in Spain (22). The different seroprevalences in different counties in our study is probably attributed to the differences in sanitation, husbandry practices, and animal welfare. In addition, other reasons for the variations of prevalence may include different ecological and geographical factors including temperature, rainfall, altitude, or level of vegetation. Furthermore, differences in the serological methods and cutoff titers used may be other factors that influence the seroprevalence of *Chlamydia* in different regions.

The overall *Chlamydia* seroprevalence in domestic black-boned sheep and goats in Shilin County was 30.89%, which was higher than the seroprevalence in Yongsheng County (24.83%) and in Lanping County (12.21%). There was significant difference in *Chlamydia* seroprevalence in domestic black-boned sheep and goats of different regions (P < 0.01). This result is consistent with a previous study that reported an 18.65% *Chlamydia* seroprevalence in Tibetan sheep in Gansu province (15). *Chlamydia* is significantly resistant under dry, cold (5–10°C), and dark conditions (23). Yunnan Province has a generally mild climate as diverse as its terrain. Shilin

Country has an average annual temperature of 15°C and a mean annual rainfall of 1,010 mm. The warm temperature and appropriate precipitation in Shilin Country are favorable for the survival of *Chlamydia*. Therefore, the differences in *Chlamydia* seroprevalence in domestic black-boned sheep and goats across different regions are probably attributed to the variable climatic conditions in Yunnan Province.

Statistically, the *Chlamydia* seroprevalence in male (28.64%) domestic black-boned sheep and goats was significantly higher than in the females (15.25%). Statistical analysis showed a significant difference between genders (P < 0.01). Gender-related differences in *Chlamydia* seroprevalence were related to variations in immune response or antibody persistence between males and females (24). The result was different from a previous study, which reported no effect of the gender on the prevalence of *Chlamydia* infection in sheep (17).

The seroprevalence of *Chlamydia* varied across the different age groups of domestic black-boned sheep and goats. The highest seroprevalence was 25.40% in black-boned sheep and goats of the 0 < years ≤ 1 age group, and the lowest prevalence was 16.41% in the 2 < years ≤ 3 age group. But the differences were not statistically significant among different age groups (P > 0.05), which disagree with the study of Qin et al. (15), which reported positive association of *Chlamydia* seroprevalence with the ages of Tibetan sheep in Gansu Province. The higher seroprevalence in domestic black-boned sheep and goats of the 0 < years ≤ 1 age group may be due to the low levels of antibodies, which makes them more susceptible to infection. The different prevalence in different age groups indicates the possibility of horizontal transmission in investigated black-boned sheep and goat herds (25).

The seroprevalence of *Chlamydia* in domestic black-boned sheep (22.76%) was slightly higher than that in domestic black-boned goats (17.16%), which may be

TABLE 1 | Seroprevalence and risk factors for *Chlamydia* in domestic black-boned sheep and goats in Yunnan Province, southwest China, determined by indirect hemagglutination (IHA) test.

Variables	Categories	Antibody titers			No. tested	No. positive	Prevalence (%) (95% CI)	OR (95% CI)	P-value
		1:64	1:256	1:1.024					
Region	Lanping	22	1	3	213	26	12.21 (7.81–16.61)	Reference	<0.01
	Yongsheng	33	3	0	145	36	24.83 (17.80–31.86)	2.38 (1.36–4.15)	
	Shilin	32	6	0	123	38	30.89 (22.72–39.06)	3.22 (1.84–5.63)	
Gender	Female	40	1	2	282	43	15.25 (11.05–19.45)	Reference	<0.01
	Male	47	9	1	199	57	28.64 (22.36–34.92)	2.23 (1.43–3.49)	
Age (years)[a]	<0 to ≤1	42	6	0	189	48	25.40 (19.19–31.61)	1.73 (0.98–3.07)	0.2013
	1< to ≤2	17	1	0	103	18	17.48 (10.15–24.81)	1.08 (0.54–2.15)	
	2< to ≤3	18	1	2	128	21	16.41 (10.00–22.83)	Reference	
	>3	10	2	1	61	13	21.31 (11.03–31.59)	1.38 (0.64–2.98)	
Species	BBG[b]	28	0	1	169	29	17.16 (11.48–22.84)	Reference	0.1487
	BBS[c]	59	10	2	312	71	22.76 (18.11–27.41)	1.42 (0.88–2.30)	
	Total	87	10	3	481	100	20.79 (17.16–24.42)		

[a] *Year.*
[b] *Domestic black-boned goat.*
[c] *Domestic black-boned sheep.*
OR, odds ratio; CI, confidence interval.

related to the different susceptibility of goats and sheep to *Chlamydia*. Statistical analysis suggested that species may not be a crucial factor for *Chlamydia* infection in black-boned sheep and goats. The difference in *Chlamydia* seroprevalence in domestic black-boned sheep and goats may be caused by the sample bias, where more domestic black-boned sheep samples were examined than black-boned goats.

There are some limitations to the present investigation. The serum samples of black-boned sheep and goats examined in this study were collected from July to August 2017, a relatively short sampling time; thus, the reported *Chlamydia* seroprevalence may not fully reflect the true situation of long-term infection of *Chlamydia* in domestic black-boned sheep and goats. Given that domestic black-boned sheep and goats have been introduced into other provinces of China (14), further research should investigate *Chlamydia* seroprevalence in domestic black-boned sheep and goats in these provinces, which will provide global baseline data for the prevention of *Chlamydia* infection in black-boned sheep and goats in China.

CONCLUSION

The present study revealed that *Chlamydia* seroprevalence (20.79%) is relatively high in domestic black-boned sheep and goats in Yunnan Province, southwest China. This study also demonstrated that region and gender are the main risk factors for *Chlamydia* seroprevalence between domestic black-boned sheep and goats. To our knowledge, the present survey is the first to document the seroprevalence of *Chlamydia* infection in domestic black-boned sheep and goats in China, which provided baseline data for future prevention and control of *Chlamydia* in domestic black-boned sheep and goats.

AUTHOR CONTRIBUTIONS

X-QZ and F-CZ conceived and designed the experiments. L-XS performed the experiments, analyzed the data, and wrote the paper. ZL, J-FY, and F-CZ participated in the collection of serum samples. Q-LL and X-HH participated in the implementation of the study. X-QZ and F-CZ critically revised the manuscript. All authors have read and approved the final version of the manuscript. All authors contributed to the preparation of the manuscript.

ACKNOWLEDGMENTS

The authors would like to thank Associate Professor Hany M. Elsheikha from the Faculty of Medicine and Health Sciences, University of Nottingham, UK, for improving the English of the manuscript.

REFERENCES

1. Longbottom D, Coulter LJ. Animal chlamydioses and zoonotic implications. *J Comp Pathol.* (2003) 128:217–44. doi: 10.1053/jcpa.2002.0629

2. Rohde G, Straube E, Essig A, Reinhold P, Sachse K. Chlamydial zoonoses. *Dtsch Arztebl Int.* (2010) 107:174–80. doi: 10.3238/arztebl.2010.0174

3. Wang FI, Shieh H, Liao YK. Prevalence of *Chlamydophila abortus* infection in domesticated ruminants in Taiwan. *J Vet Med Sci.* (2001) 63:1215–20. doi: 10.1292/jvms.63.1215

4. Szeredi L, Bacsadi A. Detection of *Chlamydophila* (*Chlamydia*) *abortus* and *Toxoplasma gondii* in smears from cases of ovine and caprine abortion by the streptavidin-biotin method. *J Comp Pathol.* (2002) 127:257–63. doi: 10.1053/jcpa.2002.0591

5. Sharma SP, Baipoledi EK, Nyange JFC, Tlagae L. Isolation of *Toxoplasma gondii* from goats with history of reproductive disorders and the prevalence of Toxoplasma and Chlamydial antibodies. *Onderstepoort J Vet Res.* (2003) 70:65–8. doi: 10.1046/j.1365-2915.2003.00404.x

6. Masala G, Porcu R, Sanna G, Tanda A, Tola S. Role of *Chlamydophila abortus* in ovine and caprine abortion in Sardinia, Italy. *Vet Res Commun.* (2005) 29:117–23. doi: 10.1007/s11259-005-0842-2

7. Schautteet K, Vanrompay D. *Chlamydiaceae* infections in pig. *Vet Res.* (2011) 42:29. doi: 10.1186/1297-9716-42-29

8. Seth-Smith HMB, Busó LS, Livingstone M, Sait M, Harris SR, Aitchison KD, et al. European *Chlamydia abortus* livestock isolate genomes reveal unusual stability and limited diversity, reflected in geographical signatures. *BMC Genomics.* (2017) 18:344. doi: 10.1186/s12864-017-3657-y

9. Campos-Hernández E, Vázquez-Chagoyán JC, Salem AZM, Saltijeral-Oaxaca JA, Escalante-Ochoa C, López-Heydeck SM, et al. Prevalence and molecular identification of *Chlamydia abortus* in commercial dairy goat farms in a hot region in Mexico. *Trop Anim Health Prod.* (2014) 46:919–24. doi: 10.1007/s11250-014-0585-6

10. Zhou JZ, Li ZC, Lou ZZ, Fei YY. Prevalence, diagnosis, and vaccination situation of animal chlamydiosis in China. *Front Vet Sci.* (2018) 5:88. doi: 10.3389/fvets.2018.00088

11. Deng WD, Yang SL, Huo YQ, Gou X, Shi XW, Mao HM. Physiological and genetic characteristics of black-boned sheep (*Ovis aries*). *Anim Genet.* (2006) 37:586–8. doi: 10.1111/j.1365-2052.2006.01530.x

12. Deng WD, Shu W, Yang SL, Shi XW, Mao HM. Pigmentation in Black-boned sheep (*Ovis aries*): association with polymorphism of the MC1R gene. *Mol Biol Rep.* (2009) 36:431–6. doi: 10.1007/s11033-007-9197-9

13. Deng, WD, Xi DM, Gou X, Yang SL, Shi XW, et al. Pigmentation in Black-boned sheep (*Ovis aries*): association with polymorphism of the *Tryosinase* gene. *Mol Biol Rep.* (2008) 35:379–85. doi: 10.1007/s11033-007-9097-z

14. Chen D, Wang SS, Zou Y, Li Z, Xie SC, Shi LQ et al. Prevalence and multi-locus genotypes of *Enterocytozoon bieneusi* in black-boned sheep and goats in Yunnan Province, southwestern China. *Infect Genet Evol.* (2018) 65:385–91. doi: 10.1016/j.meegid.2018.08.022

15. Qin SY, Yin MY, Cong W, Zhou DH, Zhang XX, Zhao Q, et al. Seroprevalence and risk factors of *Chlamydia abortus* infection in Tibetan sheep in Gansu Province, northwest China. *Sci World J.* (2014) 2:1–6. doi: 10.1155/2014/193464

16. Cong W, Huang SY, Zhang XY, Zhou DH, Xu MJ, Zhao Q, et al. Seroprevalence of *Chlamydia psittaci* infection in market-sold adult chickens, ducks and pigeons in north-western China. *J Med Microbiol.* (2013) 62:1211–4. doi: 10.1099/jmm.0.059287-0

17. Huang SY, Wu SM, Xu MJ, Zhou DH, Danba C, Gong G, et al. First record of *Chlamydia abortus* seroprevalence in Tibetan sheep in Tibet, China. *Small Rumin Res.* (2013) 112:243–5. doi: 10.1016/j.smallrumres.2012.12.012

18. Wu SM, Huang SY, Xu MJ, Zhou DH, Song HQ, Zhu XQ. *Chlamydia felis* exposure in companion dogs and cats in Lanzhou, China: a public health concern. *BMC Vet Res.* (2013) 9:104. doi: 10.1186/1746-6148-9-104

19. Zhang NZ, Zhou DH, Shi XC, Nisbet AJ, Huang SY, Ciren D, et al. First report of *Chlamydiaceae* seroprevalence in Tibetan pigs in Tibet, China. *Vector Borne Zoonotic Dis.* (2013) 13:196–9. doi: 10.1089/vbz.2012.1208

20. Hu SF, Li F, Zheng WB, Liu GH. Seroprevalence and risk factors of *Chlamydia abortus* infection in goats in Hunan province, subtropical China. *Vector Borne Zoonotic Dis.* (2018) 18:500–3. doi: 10.1089/vbz.2017.2183

21. Chahota R, Gupta S, Bhardwaj B, Malik P, Verma S, Sharma AM. Seroprevalence studies on animal chlamydiosis amongst ruminants in five states of India. *Vet World.* (2015) 8:72–5. doi: 10.14202/vetworld.2015.72-75

22. Tejedor-Junco MT, González-Martín M, Corbera JA, Santana Á, Hernández CN, Gutiérrez C. Preliminary evidence of the seroprevalence and risk factors associated with *Chlamydia abortus* infection in goats on the Canary Islands, Spain. *Trop Anim Health Prod.* (2019) 51:257–60. doi: 10.1007/s11250-018-1654-z

23. Reinhold P, Sachse K, Kaltenboeck B. *Chlamydiaceae* in cattle: commensals, trigger organisms, or pathogens? *Vet J.* (2011) 189:257–67. doi: 10.1016/j.tvjl.2010.09.003

24. Zhang NZ, Zhang XX, Zhou DH, Huang SY, Tian WP, Yang YC, et al. Seroprevalence and genotype of *Chlamydia* in pet parrots in China. *Epidemiol Infect.* (2015) 143:55–61. doi: 10.1017/S0950268814000363

25. Zhou DH, Zhao FR, Xia HY, Xu MJ, Huang SY, Song HQ, et al. Seroprevalence of chlamydial infection in dairy cattle in Guangzhou, southern China. *Ir Vet J.* (2013) 66:2. doi: 10.1186/2046-0481-66-2

3

Estimation of the Basic Reproduction Numbers of the Subtypes H5N1, H5N8 and H5N6 during the Highly Pathogenic Avian Influenza Epidemic Spread between Farms

Woo-Hyun Kim and Seongbeom Cho*

College of Veterinary Medicine and Research Institute for Veterinary Science, Seoul National University, Seoul, South Korea

*Correspondence:
Seongbeom Cho
chose@snu.ac.kr

It is important to understand pathogen transmissibility in a population to establish an effective disease prevention policy. The basic reproduction number (R_0) is an epidemiologic parameter for understanding the characterization of disease and its dynamics in a population. We aimed to estimate the R_0 of the highly pathogenic avian influenza (HPAI) subtypes H5N1, H5N8, and H5N6, which were associated with nine outbreaks in Korea between 2003 and 2018, to understand the epidemic transmission of each subtype. According to HPAI outbreak reports of the Animal and Plant Quarantine Agency, we estimated the generation time by calculating the time of infection between confirmed HPAI-positive farms. We constructed exponential growth and maximum likelihood (ML) models to estimate the basic reproduction number, which assumes the number of secondary cases infected by the index case. The Kruskal-Wallis test was used to analyze the epidemic statistics between subtypes. The estimated generation time of H5N1, H5N8, and H5N6 were 4.80 days [95% confidence interval (CI) 4.23–5.38] days, 7.58 (95% CI 6.63–8.46), and 5.09 days (95% CI 4.44–5.74), respectively. A pairwise comparison showed that the generation time of H5N8 was significantly longer than that of the subtype H5N1 ($P = 0.04$). Based on the ML model, R_0 was estimated as 1.69 (95% CI 1.48–2.39) for subtype H5N1, 1.60 (95%CI 0.97–2.23) for subtype H5N8, and 1.49 (95%CI 0.94–2.04) for subtype H5N6. We concluded that R_0 estimates may be associated with the poultry product system, climate, species specificity based on the HPAI virus subtype, and prevention policy. This study provides an insight on the transmission and dynamics patterns of various subtypes of HPAI occurring worldwide. Furthermore, the results are useful as scientific evidence for establishing a disease control policy.

Keywords: avian influenza, basic reproduction number, Korea, H5N1, H5N6, H5N8

INTRODUCTION

Highly pathogenic avian influenza (HPAI) is a highly contagious viral disease that infects domestic poultry and wild birds (1). The HPAI virus can cause an epidemic that may spread rapidly, has a high mortality rate among domestic birds, and devastates the poultry industry (2). Outbreaks of distinct subtypes of HPAI, including H5N1, H5N8, and H5N6, are continually reported worldwide (3–5), and this global HPAI virus dissemination is caused by migratory wild birds (6). The HPAI crisis appears to be a great threat to not only animal health but also public health worldwide. Furthermore, the World Health Organization reported 860 human infection cases of avian influenza A subtype H5N1 (7) after the first human case of HPAI subtype H5N1, which was reported in Hong Kong in 1997 (8).

In South Korea, outbreaks of three different subtypes of HPAI occurred between 2003 and 2018. The first outbreak of H5N1 occurred from December 2003 to February 2004 and had a high mortality rate at poultry farms, especially among chickens (9). Since then, outbreaks of H5N1 have occurred in 2006, 2008, and 2010 (10–12). The novel HPAI subtype, H5N8, was first reported in January 2014 at South Korean poultry farms (13). Genetic analyses of viruses isolated from wild birds and poultry farms showed that migratory birds could be responsible for the first wave of H5N8 outbreaks between January and May 2014 (14). After the first wave, two waves of subtype H5N8 occurred during September 2014 to June 2015 and during September 2015 to November 2015 (15). It was reported that these sporadic outbreaks were caused by viruses reintroduced into Korea by migratory waterfowl (16). In November 2016, a novel genotype of H5N6 that was first detected in wild birds in Korea and HPAI infectious cases was reported at poultry farms (17). Another novel H5N8 virus co-circulated with H5N6 virus during the outbreaks in 2016, from February to June 2017 (18). In November 2017, the novel H5N6 virus was detected at a broiler duck farm and in wild mallards, with infection spreading to poultry farms (19).

The main strategies used to prevent and control HPAI outbreaks are based on the prohibition of movement, preemptive culling, and vaccinations in infected areas (20). Therefore, it is important to understand pathogen transmissibility in a population to establish an effective disease prevention policy. The basic reproduction number (R_0) is one of the important epidemiologic parameters necessary to understand the characterization of disease and the dynamics in a population (21). R_0 is generally defined as the average number of secondary cases caused by one infectious individual during the entire infectious period in an uninfected population (22). If each infected individual infects more than one other individual, on an average, at any time point, then the epidemic will be sustainable (23). Various methods are used to estimate the reproduction number (24–26), and these have been implemented in the R program (27) and Excel (28) as ready-made procedures.

Reproduction number estimation has been used to understand HPAI epidemic characteristics and to provide insight regarding control measures for epidemics. These farm-to-farm reproduction number estimations were targeted to

the HPAI subtype H5N1 and were conducted in Nigeria (29), Romania (30), Thailand (31), Bangladesh (32), India (33), Italy, Canada, and the Netherlands (34). In Korea, there was a mathematical modeling study of the reproduction number for HPAI from 2016 to 2017, but this was limited to the local reproduction number and did not include all epidemics from South Korea (35). We aimed to estimate the serial interval and R_0 of HPAI subtypes H5N1, H5N8, and H5N6, which were associated with nine outbreaks from 2003 to 2018 in Korea, and demonstrate the characterization of each subtype by analyzing HPAI characteristics, including the epidemic days, number of farms, species distribution, serial interval, and R_0. It is expected that the results of the present study will become a foundation for demonstrating the disease dynamics of each HPAI subtype and its characteristics, as well as for establishing effective HPAI control, not only for traditional HPAI subtype H5N1 but also the emerging subtypes H5N8 and H5N6.

MATERIALS AND METHODS
Data Collection

The epidemic data of HPAI outbreaks in Korea were collected by the Animal and Plant Quarantine Agency (APQA) in Gimcheon, Korea (**Table 1**). In Korea, three HPAI subtypes occurred from 2003 to 2017, HPAI subtype H5N1 occurred in a total of 214 poultry farms, H5N8 occurred in 469 farms, and H5N6 occurred in total 362 farms. The livestock owner (including the manager) or veterinarian who found an animal with clinical signs and suspected HPAI was required to report the case to the APQA according to the Prevention of Contagious Animal Disease Act. Cloacal, fecal, and blood samples were collected from sick or dead poultry in reported poultry farms, and HPAI virus was confirmed using reverse-transcriptase polymerase chain reaction at the Avian Influenza Research and Diagnosis Department of the APQA. If the suspected farm was confirmed as HPAI-positive and deemed an infected premise (IP), then depopulation of farms with infected poultry and depopulation of all poultry farms in the protection zone were conducted. If a depopulated farm was found to be positive, then it was defined as a positive premise (PP) (36). Both IP and PP were considered cases in this study. The epidemic curve of these HPAI cases was depicted using the "incidence" package in R (37) to illustrate the weekly reported number of poultry farms in the International Organization for Standardization (ISO) week date system (37) (**Figure 1**). In Korea, there were no poultry farms infected with two HPAI subtypes simultaneously, and each farm only had one subtype in each outbreak.

Based on the APQA epidemiology reports, the HPAI outbreaks were classified as waves when the period between cases was longer than 1 month (38). As a result of this classification, outbreaks of the subtype H5N8, which occurred in 2014 and 2016, were classified as four and two waves, respectively. Four outbreaks, including the H5N1 outbreak in 2003, outbreak in 2006, the fourth wave of the H5N8 outbreak in 2014, and the second wave of the H5N8 outbreak in 2016, were excluded from the analysis because the samples were too small to calculate R_0.

TABLE 1 | HPAI epidemic in Korea from 2003 to 2018.

Subtype	Year of epidemic	Clade	Date	Days of epidemic	Total number of Farms	Cases per day	No. of chicken farms (%)	No. of duck farms (%)	No. of other poultry farms (%)
H5N1	2003	2.5	10/12/2003–05/02/2004	58	18	0.310	7 (38.9)	11 (61.1)	0 (0.0)
	2006	2.2	25/11/2006–06/03/2007	103	7	0.068	4 (57.1)	2 (28.6)	1 (14.3)
	2008	2.3.2	01/04/2008–24/05/2008	54	98	1.815	80 (81.6)	17 (17.3)	1 (1.0)
	2010	2.3.2	29/12/2010–23/05/2011	146	91	0.623	38 (41.8)	50 (54.9)	3 (3.3)
H5N8	2014 1st	2.3.4.4	16/01/2014–29/07/2014	194	212	1.093	39 (18.4)	166 (78.3)	7 (3.3)
	2014 2nd	2.3.4.4	24/09/2014–10/06/2015	260	162	0.623	39 (24.1)	117 (72.2)	6 (3.7)
	2014 3rd	2.3.4.4	14/09/2015–15/11/2015	63	17	0.270	0 (0.0)	14 (82.4)	3 (17.6)
	2014 4th	2.3.4.4	23/03/2016–05/04/2016	14	2	0.143	0 (0.0)	2 (100.0)	0 (0.0)
	2016 1st	2.3.4.4	06/02/2017–14/04/2017	58	40	0.690	16 (40.0)	23 (57.5)	1 (2.5)
	2016 2nd	2.3.4.4	02/06/2017–19/06/2017	18	36	2.000	30 (83.3)	0 (0.0)	6 (16.7)
H5N6	2016	2.3.4.4	16/11/2016–18/02/2017	95	340	3.579	192 (56.5)	140 (41.2)	8 (2.4)
	2017	2.3.4.4	19/11/2017–18/03/2018	121	22	0.182	8 (36.4)	14 (63.6)	0 (0.0)

Serial Interval and Generation Time

A serial interval is the time between successive cases in a chain of transmission, estimated from the interval between clinical onsets in patients (25). We estimated the serial interval of HPAI as the time between the reported date of the first farm with infected cases and secondary farm with infected cases. This estimation was based on the investigation of the epidemic pathway of HPAI transmission, which shows the epidemiologic relationship between the infector and infectee. According to the APQA investigations, HPAI transmission could be possible through wild migratory birds, wild animals, farm owners, managers, staff, vehicles related to the poultry industry, and airborne transmission from nearby infected farms. The epidemic transmission pathway investigation was conducted by an APQA epidemiologic investigator visiting and interviewing the places suspected to be associated with the infected farms, including animal facilities such as hatcheries, feed factories, and live bird markets. The APQA investigated vehicles, people, livestock, and their products that entered an infected farm from 21 days prior to infection and estimated the disease transmissions.

In addition to investigating via interview, the APQA used geographic information to identify HPAI viral transmission by vehicles. In Korea, vehicles related to the poultry industry transporting poultry, poultry products, medicines, feed, and feces must be registered with the Korea Animal Health Integrated System (KAHIS; http://www.kahis.go.kr). The movements of livestock-related vehicles are reported to the KAHIS, making it possible to track the movement of vehicles, people, livestock, and animal products.

Through these interviews and vehicle information, the disease transmission pathway via transportation and human movement was identified. If a clear epidemiologic link to the infected farm could not be found through interviews and movement tracking, then we hypothesized that the farm might have been infected with HPAI by wild migratory birds or wild animals. We then excluded infection thought to be caused by wild birds or wild animals during the estimation of the serial interval because it is not possible to observe the serial interval of virus transmission from wild birds and animals.

The generation time is the modeling term describing the time duration from the onset of transmittable infection in a primary case to the onset of infection in a secondary case infected from the primary case. We defined the generation time as the difference between suspected infection days of the primary farm and secondary farm, which was measured through epidemiologic investigation (**Figure 2**). The suspected infection day was estimated according to the day reported by the farm owner after clinical symptoms were found in the poultry and the period between the infection and latent period of each HPAI subtype in the poultry species. We estimated the suspected infection date from the day the clinical symptoms were reported by subtracting the periods between infection and clinical symptoms. For H5N1, the periods between infection and clinical symptoms were assumed to be 2 days for chickens (9), 4 days for ducks (39), and 3.8 days for other poultry species (9). For H5N8, the periods were 3.2 days for chickens (40), 8.0 days for ducks (15), and 2.0 days for other species (41). For H5N6, the periods were 2.6 days for chickens (42), 4.6 days for ducks (43), and 3.0 days for other species (43).

Based on the generation time between case farms, we calculated the discretized generation time distribution using a function (est.GT) in the R0 package (27). Discretization is performed on the grid [0, 0.5), [0.5, 1.5), [1.5, 2.5), etc... where the unit is time interval of days (27). Time-to-event data were assumed to follow a parametric distribution with a probability density function (PDF). The distribution of generation time is expressed in the form of parametric distribution such as "gamma," "lognormal," or "Weibull," using maximum likelihood. The mean and standard deviation of generation time is provided in the desired time units. The calculated distribution of the generation time in each subtype and outbreaks is depicted in **Figure 3**.

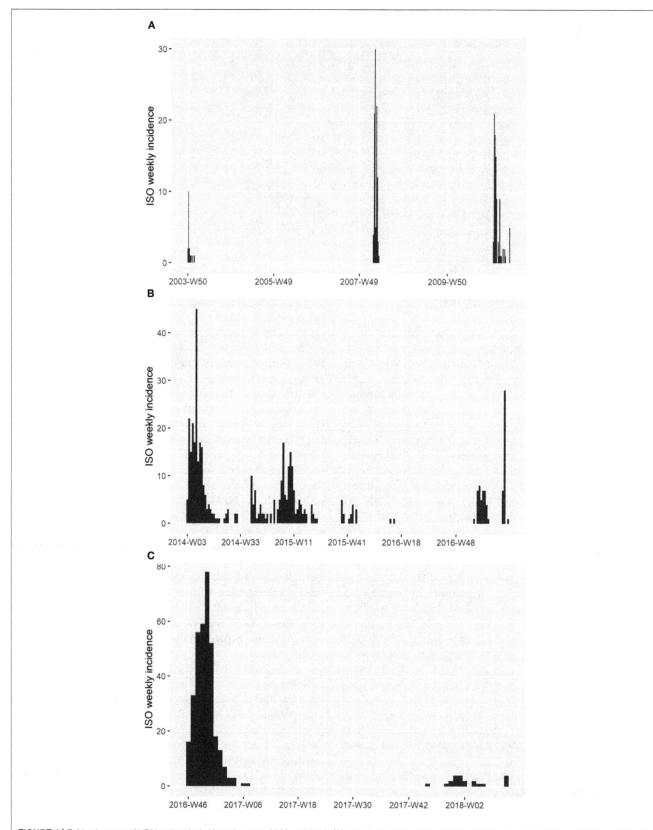

FIGURE 1 | Epidemic curve of HPAI outbreaks in Korea between 2003 and 2018. **(A)** Weekly epidemic case number of HPAI subtype H5N1 from 2003 to 2011. **(B)** Weekly epidemic case number of HPAI subtype H5N8 from 2014 to 2017. **(C)** Weekly epidemic case number of HPAI subtype H5N6 from 2016 to 2018. The x-axis represents the week numbers, which were based on the ISO 8601 week date system.

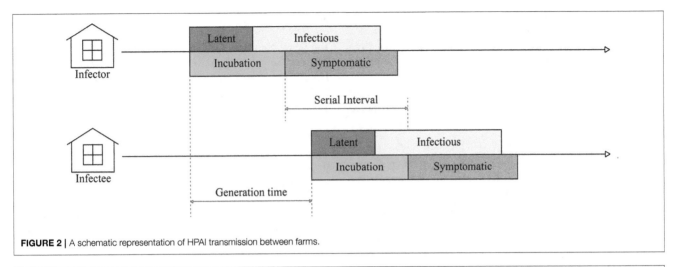

FIGURE 2 | A schematic representation of HPAI transmission between farms.

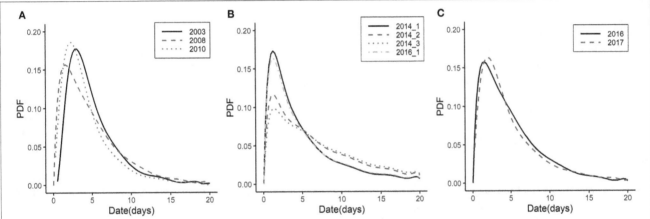

FIGURE 3 | Generation time distribution of HPAI outbreaks from 2003 to 2018 in Korea by HPAI subtype. **(A)** Generation time distribution of HPAI subtype H5N1 in 2003, 2008, and 2010. **(B)** Generation time distribution of HPAI subtype H5N8 during the 2014 first wave, second wave, and third wave and during the 2016 first wave. **(C)** Generation time distribution of HPAI subtype H5N6 in 2016 and 2017. The x-axis represents the days for generation time. The y-axis represents the probability density function (PDF).

Model Assumption and Data Analysis

The study model is based on the susceptible-infected-removed (SIR) compartmental model (44), which divides poultry farms into compartment. A susceptible farm (S) becomes infectious (I) through contact with the possible disease and is then removed (R) by depopulation. The dynamics of an epidemic can be described as the equation given below when N is the sum of S, I, and R.

$$\frac{dS}{dt} = -\frac{\beta IS}{N}$$
$$\frac{dI}{dt} = \frac{\beta IS}{N} - \gamma I$$
$$\frac{dR}{dt} = \gamma I$$

In this model, β is a parameter, which controls how much the disease can be transmitted through the exposure of HPAI virus, and γ is a parameter, which expresses how many poultry farms can be removed in a specific period. In this model, the average number of secondary infections caused by an infected host, R_0, equals β / γ (45).

We constructed exponential growth (EG) and maximum likelihood (ML) models to estimate early reproduction numbers using the R0 package (27) in R (version 3.3.0). The EG model assumes that the initial reproduction ratio can be associated with the EG rate during the early epidemic phase (24). The formula is $R_0 = 1/M (-r)$, where r denotes the initial EG rate and M stands for the moment generating function of generation time distribution. In the initial EG model, a period from day 1 to day 14 of the epidemics was chosen when the outbreak's growth was exponential. The 14-day interval was selected based on Korea's standstill policy (38). When HPAI outbreaks are reported in South Korea, a standstill policy is implemented for the vehicles, to reduce the spread of HPAI. This policy is intended to minimize the contact between vehicles and suppress the HPAI dissemination. We determined that this intervention affects the basic reproduction number of HPAI. Therefore, we specified the exponential growth for the first 14 days of the epidemic wave in each case.

A function (est.R0.EG) in the R0 package was used (27). We used a sensitivity test in EG to select the period during which growth is exponential as optimized time windows. We used the "sensitivity analysis" function to compute the deviance R-squared statistic over a range of periods.

The ML estimation model assumes that the number of secondary cases caused by an index case is Poisson-distributed with the expected value R_0 (25). The log-likelihood (LL) of R_0 was defined as $LL(R_0) = \sum_{t=1}^{T} \log(\frac{e^{-\mu_t}\mu_t^{N_t}}{N_t!})$, where $\mu_t = R_0 \sum_{i=1}^{t} N_{t-i} w_i$. This model assume that the number of new cases at indexing time t as $N = \{N_t\}$, $t = 0,...T$, a generation time distribution w, and μ_t which represent the total number of cases produced by the earlier case N_t. The likelihood must be calculated on a period of exponential, and the deviance R-squared measure may be used to select the best period that maximized the likelihood. In this study, the range was set as 0.01–50, in which the maximum must be searched. A function (est.R0.ML) in the R0 package was used (27). The goodness of fit of each model was calculated using the chi-square goodness of fit test in R.

The Kruskal-Wallis test was used to determine the statistical differences in epidemics between subtypes (46). The epidemic days, number of farms, cases per day, poultry species distribution of farms, generation time, and R_0 estimated by EG and ML of the three subtypes H5N1, H5N8, and H5N6 were analyzed. The significance level was $\alpha = 0.05$. These statistical analyses were performed using SPSS 22.0 (IBM, Armonk, NY, USA).

RESULTS

HPAI Epidemic in Korea

We investigated 12 HPAI outbreaks of three subtypes, H5N1, H5N8, and H5N6, that occurred from 2003 to 2018 in Korea. Table 1 presents a summary of the epidemic data, including the period of outbreaks and the number of infected farms that were investigated. The weekly epidemic curves of HPAI outbreaks are shown in Figure 1 based on the ISO 8601 week date system. The H5N1 HPAI outbreaks (except for the 2008 outbreaks) began between November and February, when the lowest temperature drops below 0°C (Figure 1A). Regarding H5N8 in 2014, the second and third waves recurred in September 2015 and 2016, respectively (Figure 1B). However, the second wave of H5N6 in 2016 occurred in June (Figure 1C). The longest outbreak was the second wave of H5N8 in 2014, which occurred over 260 days. The shortest outbreak was the fourth wave of H5N8 in 2014, which occurred over 14 days. The outbreaks with the most cases (340 poultry farms) and cases per day (3.579 cases per day) were the H5N6 outbreaks in 2016. Regarding H5N8 in 2014, more than 72% of the occurrences were in ducks; however, there was no apparent species specificity for subtypes H5N1 and H5N6.

Serial Interval and Basic Reproduction Number of HPAI in Korea

We selected nine outbreaks with sufficient number of premises to calculate R_0 and analyzed the generation time and initial R_0 using the EG and ML methods (Table 2). Generation time distributions are illustrated by each HPAI subtype as the PDF in Figure 3. Generation time of H5N1 were estimated between

4.58 and 5.24 days (Figure 3A), generation time of H5N8 were estimated to have 6 days or more (6.01–8.23 days) (Figure 3B), and generation time of H5N6 were estimated between 5.02 and 5.91 days (Figure 3C). R_0 was estimated as 1.65–2.20 for subtype H5N1, 0.03–1.56 for subtype H5N8, and 1.03–1.24 for subtype H5N6 using EG methods. Using ML methods, R_0 was estimated as 1.68–1.95 for subtype H5N1, 1.03–1.83 for subtype H5N8, and 1.37–1.60 for subtype H5N6.

Most of the R_0 in the EG and ML methods were similar, except for the second and third waves of H5N8 in 2014. The R value obtained by the EG method was <1 for the second and third waves of H5N8 in 2014. To select the optimal time windows, sensitivity results of the time windows and R_0 were used (Table 2). Optimized time windows selected by sensitivity tests accounted for 69.14% of the outbreak periods, on an average, and the optimal R_0 values in optimized time windows were <1 for the subtypes H5N1 and H5N6 outbreaks.

Epidemic Statistics Between Subtypes

The average values of the number of epidemic days, infected poultry farms, species distribution, and infected farms per day for the three subtypes of nine selected outbreaks were determined (Table 3). The average numbers of epidemic days were 86.0 for H5N1, 108.0 for H5N6, and 143.8 for H5N8. The average numbers of farms were 69.0 for H5N1, 107.8 for H5N8, and 181.0 for H5N6. Regarding the species distribution, subtype H5N8 was more highly distributed among duck farms (74.2%) than other subtypes (37.7% for H5N1 and 42.5% for H5N6).

The Kruskal-Wallis H test showed a statistically significant difference in mean generation time among the different subtypes [$\chi^2(2) = 6.444$; $p = 0.040$], with mean rank scores of 2.33 for subtype H5N1, 7.50 for H5N8, and 4.00 for H5N6. The pairwise comparison showed that the mean H5N8 generation time (7.58 days) was significantly longer than the H5N1 generation time (4.80 days) ($P = 0.03$) (Table 3). There were no significant differences among subtypes in epidemic days, number of farms, cases per day, species distributions, or reproduction number.

DISCUSSION

HPAI outbreaks occur continually worldwide and have become a major threat to animal and human public health. In South Korea, eight outbreaks with multiple waves of infections occurred between 2003 and 2018; these involved three different HPAI subtypes, H5N1, H5N8, and H5N6, and massively damaged the poultry industry. Therefore, it is important to understand the HPAI transmissibility at poultry farms to control outbreaks by establishing an effective prevention policy. An effective tool for understanding disease characteristics is the R_0, which is generally defined as the average number of secondary cases caused by one infected individual (21). Therefore, we investigated the transmission dynamics of the HPAI subtypes H5N1, H5N8, and H5N6 by estimating the generation time and R_0. To the best of our knowledge, no previous study has attempted to estimate R_0 of various HPAI subtypes and perform comparative analyses among them. This could be the first study to investigate the disease transmission dynamics of HPAI subtypes H5N1, H5N8, and H5N6, which are emerging worldwide.

TABLE 2 | Generation time and reproduction number of HPAI by EG and ML method.

Subtype	Year of epidemic	Distribution	Mean generation time (95% CI) (Days)	Initial R_0 by EG Method (95% CI)	χ^2 of EG Method	Initial R_0 by ML Method (95% CI)	χ^2 of ML Method	Optimal time windows (percent in total period)	R_0 by EG Method (optimal) (95% CI)
H5N1	2003	Lognormal	5.24 (3.51–6.97)	2.02 (1.02–3.76)	0.33	1.95 (0.81–3.86)	0.33	9–46 (65.52%)	0.18 (0.01–0.51)
	2008	Gamma	4.98 (4.15–5.81)	1.65 (1.02–2.49)	0.33	1.68 (0.92–2.76)	0.34	9–54 (85.19%)	0.74 (0.65–0.82)
	2010	Gamma	4.58 (3.76–5.40)	2.20 (1.51–3.16)	0.30	1.93 (1.10–3.10)	0.30	9–138 (89.04%)	0.77 (0.72–0.83)
H5N8	2014 1st	Lognormal	7.45 (5.83–9.07)	1.56 (0.95–2.23)	0.31	1.83 (1.11–2.81)	0.31	14–125 (57.73%)	0.72 (0.65–0.79)
	2014 2nd	Weibull	8.23 (6.94–9.52)	0.35 (0.00–1.38)	0.36	1.56 (0.70–2.97)	0.35	10–248 (91.92%)	1.01 (0.99–1.03)
	2014 3rd	Weibull	7.39 (4.39–10.39)	0.03 (0.00–0.98)	0.36	1.03 (0.22–2.88)	0.38	10–50 (65.08%)	2.17 (1.26–3.67)
	2016 1st	Weibull	6.01 (4.57–7.45)	1.23 (0.50–2.31)	0.34	1.70 (0.75–3.22)	0.37	2–45 (75.86%)	1.37 (1.13–1.16)
H5N6	2016	Gamma	5.02 (4.56–5.48)	1.24 (0.87–1.73)	0.36	1.60 (1.09–2.25)	0.36	14–94 (85.26%)	0.71 (0.67–0.74)
	2017	Lognormal	5.91 (3.14–8.68)	1.03 (0.01–2.45)	0.38	1.37 (0.34–3.56)	0.38	14–107 (77.69%)	0.90 (0.78–1.01)

SD, standard deviation; EG, exponential growth; ML, maximum likelihood estimation; CI, confidence interval.

TABLE 3 | Epidemic characteristics, mean generation time, and R_0 in two models by HPAI subtype H5N1, H5N8, and H5N6.

Subtype	Average epidemic days	Average number of farms	Cases per day	Chicken (%)	Duck (%)	Etc. (%)	Mean generation time (days)	R_0 by EG Method (95% CI)	R_0 by ML Method (95% CI)
H5N1	86.0	69.0	0.802	41.7 (60.4)	26.0 (37.7)	2.0 (2.9)	4.80 (4.23–5.38)	1.96 (1.48–2.39	1.69 (1.10–2.28)
H5N8	143.8	107.8	0.750	23.5 (21.8)	80.0 (74.2)	4.3 (3.9)	7.58*(6.63–8.46)	1.49 (1.19–1.79)	1.60 (0.97–2.23)
H5N6	108.0	181.0	1.676	100.0 (55.2)	77.0 (42.5)	4.0 (2.2)	5.09 (4.44–5.74)	1.14 (0.76–1.51)	1.49 (0.94–2.04)

EG, exponential growth; ML, maximum likelihood estimation; CI, confidence interval.
*Mean generation time of subtype H5N8 is significantly longer than subtype H5N1 (P = 0.03).

The R_0 of HPAI H5N1 in Korea estimated in this study was between 1.68 and 1.95, according to the ML method (**Table 1**). The R_0 of subtype H5N1 has previously been estimated in countries such as Italy (1.2–2.7), Canada (1.4–2.7), the Netherlands (1.0–3.0) (34), Romania (1.95–2.68) (30), Bangladesh (0.85–0.96) (32), and Thailand (1.27–1.60) (47). Despite being the same subtype of HPAI, the estimated R_0 subtype H5N1 varied across countries. We assumed that several factors, such as geographic distribution of poultry farms, mixed farming systems, poultry product supply system, and climate, were associated with this difference.

We believe that unique characteristics of the poultry industry in Korea and climatic differences are the major causes for these observed differences. We speculate that the estimated R0 may be related to characteristics of the Korean poultry industry, such as the coexistence of large-scale commercial farms and small family farms. Among the Organization for Economic Cooperation and Development (OECD) countries, Korea has the lowest availability of arable land per capita (0.03 hectare in 2016) (48). This land scarcity is an important factor leading to high stocking densities (49). A previous study suggested that farms with large flocks and the presence of a neighboring farm within

500 m were risk factors of HPAI at Korean broiler duck farms (50). This high stocking and local density of large-scale poultry farms could increase the likelihood of massive infections when HPAI outbreaks occur in Korea.

Small family poultry farms also represent a biosecurity risk during HPAI outbreaks. Most of these small farms sell live poultry to local markets without going through slaughterhouses; this could be a pathway for the spread of HPAI viruses. Additionally, there was an obvious lack of information regarding the official statistics of poultry farms too small to be defined as agricultural holders in Korea (51). This includes establishments with <0.1 hectares of land or with sales of agricultural products per year or value of agricultural animals less than KRW 1.2 million (USD 1,090).

Secondly, we hypothesize that climate factors during the epidemic period may affect R_0 in these countries. Climate factors could affect HPAI transmission and persistence by altering bird migration, virus shedding between hosts, and virus survival outside the host (52). Climate change is considered to influence the wild bird species composition and their migration cycle, and these changes will affect the transmission intensity of disease (53). Furthermore, temperature and humidity could be related to viral persistence in the host and environment. An influenza virus transmission experiment using a guinea pig model suggested that relative low humidity and cold temperature were favorable for spreading influenza (54). Liu et al. (55) showed that the environmental temperature decreased shortly before HPAI H5N1 outbreaks in domestic poultry in Eurasia between 2005 and 2006. Additionally, AI viral infectivity remained at lower temperatures ($<17°C$) during an *in vivo* test (56). Therefore, it is assumed that our estimated R_0 in Korea is higher than the R_0 in Thailand and Bangladesh, where the average annual temperatures and humidity are higher. Based on these results, we assumed that the climate factors were closely related to the R_0 estimated in several countries in terms of virus transmission and survivability.

In 2016, two novel HPAI subtypes, H5N6 and H5N8, occurred simultaneously. HPAI H5N6 occurred from November 2016 to February 2017, whereas subtype H5N8 occurred from February to April 2016; the first wave and second wave occurred in June. Although these two subtypes occurred simultaneously, both were novel viruses. The genetic clade analysis suggested that Korean H5N6 viruses are novel reassortments of multiple virus subtypes, and it is difficult for H5N6 virus reassortment to occur during outbreaks that could increase the possibility of viral subtype mutation (5). Additionally, an infection experiment involving wild mandarin ducks demonstrated a difference in viral shedding and viral tropism in H5N8 and H5N6 viruses within the same clade of 2.3.4.4 H5 HPAI viruses (57). Based on these findings, both subtypes were independent of each other, and the virus infectivity could also be different; therefore, different R_0 was expected.

However, our estimated initial R_0 value in 2016 suggested a similarity between the reproduction number represented in subtypes H5N8 (1.70) and H5N6 (1.60) (**Table 2**). Apart from the difference in transmissibility of each virus subtype, the level of transmission between farms in the field may be similar between the two subtypes. However, this presumes that the values of R_0 of the two subtypes were similarly calculated because the biosecurity policy implemented during the outbreaks was identical. The basic reproductive number is affected by the rate of contacts in the host population, the probability of infection being transmitted during contact, and the duration of infectiousness (58). Therefore, it can be estimated that the R_0 of two different subtypes were similar due to the reduction of the poultry population through preemptive culling and the reduction of contact between farms because of the standstill (59).

The quarantine against HPAI in Korea has changed over 14 years after the first HPAI epidemic in 2003. The HPAI prevention policy changed dramatically, especially before and after H5N8 epidemics in 2014. Before the outbreaks, Korea Animal Health Integrated System (KAHIS) was established in 2013 to monitor livestock vehicle movement. In this system, all poultry-related vehicles must be registered with KAHIS and equipped with a global positioning system mandatorily (60). Also during the epidemics, the preemptive depopulation of the protective zone was changed from a radius of 500 m−3 km, and inspections were conducted more than once before releasing poultry and poultry products (36), The influence of these quarantine policy can also be seen in the changes in the R_0 values of each wave of subtype H5N8 that occurred between 2014 and 2016. For H5N8 in 2014, the initial R_0 of each wave showed a tendency to decrease as the outbreak progressed gradually (**Table 2**). This would indicate that the effectiveness of control measures for HPAI were increasing while the waves were passing.

In the Kruskal-Wallis model, H5N1 and H5N8 subtypes showed statistically significant differences in generation time ($P = 0.03$) (**Table 3**). However, there were no significant differences in the epidemic characteristics of the subtypes. There was also no statistical significance in the R_0 obtained through the EG and ML models. This generation time difference in the two subtypes might be associated with subtype pathogenicity in the poultry species. The spread of H5N1 viruses in the field was quickly controlled as a result of the rapid diagnosis of the infections due to the high pathogenicity of these viruses in poultry. In contrast, subtypes H5N6 and H5N8 clustered as clade 2.3.4. H5NX viruses are usually mild in ducks, leading to delayed diagnosis of infections and persistent spread in the wild (61). Therefore, the H5N8 subtype could possibly spread the HPAI virus over a relatively longer period than the H5N1 subtype which could be driven by sub-clinical spread in ducks.

In conclusion, this study showed the characterization of each subtype by analyzing the HPAI characteristics, including the epidemics, number of farms, species distribution, generation time, and R_0 of HPAI subtypes H5N1, H5N8, and H5N6, which were associated with nine outbreaks in Korea between 2003 and 2018. R_0, which is estimated by the generation time, index case, and secondary cases, is essential for identifying the characteristics of HPAI. In particular, our findings suggest that the estimated R_0 might be influenced by the HPAI subtype and might be associated with the seasonal aspects during the early stage, species specificity by virus subtype, and prevention policy. We believe that the results of the present study are helpful for demonstrating the disease dynamics of each HPAI subtype and its characteristics and, thus greatly assist in better disease control strategies. It could be possible to establish systematic quarantine policies to reduce the socio-economic losses caused by HPAI, Especially differences observed between countries with different poultry raising systems and climatic conditions. This study provided insight regarding HPAI transmission of the traditional subtype H5N1 and newly emerging subtypes H5N8 and H5N6. Further research on the basic reproduction numbers of the HPAI subtypes occurring worldwide is required to understand the global dynamics of HPAI transmission.

AUTHOR CONTRIBUTIONS

W-HK designed the study, investigated data collection, reviewed the data, performed data analysis, and participated in manuscript preparation. SC supervised the project, administrated the project, acquired funds, and participated in the manuscript review.

ACKNOWLEDGMENTS

The authors would like to express deep gratitude to Dr. Jeff Bender, professor of the School of Public Health, University of Minnesota, for his comments on the manuscript.

REFERENCES

1. Alexander DJ. An overview of the epidemiology of avian influenza. *Vaccine.* (2007) 25:5637–44. doi: 10.1016/j.vaccine.2006.10.051

2. Short KR, Richard M, Verhagen JH, van Riel D, Schrauwen EJ, van den Brand JM, et al. One health, multiple challenges: the inter-species transmission of influenza A virus. *One Health.* (2015) 1:1–13. doi: 10.1016/j.onehlt.2015.03.001

3. Gu M, Zhao G, Zhao K, Zhong L, Huang J, Wan H, et al. Novel variants of clade 2.3. 4 highly pathogenic avian influenza A (H5N1) viruses, China. *Emerg Infect Dis.* (2013) 19:2021. doi: 10.3201/eid1912.130340

4. DeJesus E, Costa-Hurtado M, Smith D, Lee D-H, Spackman E, Kapczynski DR, et al. Changes in adaptation of H5N2 highly pathogenic avian influenza H5 clade 2.3. 4.4 viruses in chickens and mallards. *Virology.* (2016) 499:52–64. doi: 10.1016/j.virol.2016.08.036

5. Si Y-J, Lee IW, Kim E-H, Kim Y-I, Kwon H-I, Park S-J, et al. Genetic characterisation of novel, highly pathogenic avian influenza (HPAI) H5N6 viruses isolated in birds, South Korea, November 2016. *Euro Surveill.* (2017) 22:30434. doi: 10.2807/1560-7917.ES.2017.22.1.30434

6. Verhagen JH, Herfst S, Fouchier RA. How a virus travels the world. *Science.* (2015) 347:616–7. doi: 10.1126/science.aaa6724

7. World Health Organization. *Cumulative Number of Confirmed Human Cases for Avian Influenza A(H5N1) Reported to WHO, 2003-2019.* (2019). Available online at: https://www.who.int/ (accessed 24 May, 2019).

8. De Jong J, Claas E, Osterhaus A, Webster R, Lim W. A pandemic warning? *Nature.* (1997) 389:554. doi: 10.1038/39218

9. Lee C-W, Suarez DL, Tumpey TM, Sung H-W, Kwon Y-K, Lee Y-J, et al. Characterization of highly pathogenic H5N1 avian influenza A viruses isolated from South Korea. *J Virol.* (2005) 79:3692–702. doi: 10.1128/JVI.79.6.3692-3702.2005

10. Kim H-R, Park C-K, Lee Y-J, Woo G-H, Lee K-K, Oem J-K, et al. An outbreak of highly pathogenic H5N1 avian influenza in Korea, 2008. *Vet Microbiol.* (2010) 141:362–6. doi: 10.1016/j.vetmic.2009.09.011

11. Lee Y-J, Choi Y-K, Kim Y-J, Song M-S, Jeong O-M, Lee E-K, et al. Highly pathogenic avian influenza virus (H5N1) in domestic poultry and relationship with migratory birds, South Korea. *Emerg Infect Dis.* (2008) 14:487. doi: 10.3201/eid1403.070767

12. Kim H-R, Lee Y-J, Park C-K, Oem J-K, Lee O-S, Kang H-M, et al. Highly pathogenic avian influenza (H5N1) outbreaks in wild birds and poultry, South Korea. *Emerg Infect Dis.* (2012) 18:480. doi: 10.3201/1803.111490

13. Lee Y. Novel Reassortant Influenza A (H5N8) Viruses, South Korea, 2014. *Emerg Infect Dis. J.* (2014) 20:1087–9. doi: 10.3201/eid2006.1 40233

14. Jeong J, Kang H-M, Lee E-K, Song B-M, Kwon Y-K, Kim H-R, et al. Highly pathogenic avian influenza virus (H5N8) in domestic poultry and its relationship with migratory birds in South Korea during 2014. *Vet Microbiol.* (2014) 173:249–57. doi: 10.1016/j.vetmic.2014.08.002

15. Animal and Plant Quarantine Agency. *2014-2016 Epidemiologic Reports of Highly Pathogenic Avian Influenza.* Animal and Plant Quarantine Agency (2016) .

16. Kwon J-H, Lee D-H, Swayne DE, Noh J-Y, Yuk S-S, Erdene-Ochir T-O, et al. Highly pathogenic avian influenza A (H5N8) viruses reintroduced into South Korea by migratory waterfowl, 2014–2015. *Emerg Infect Dis.* (2016) 22:507. doi: 10.3201/eid2203.151006

17. Lee E-K, Song B-M, Lee Y-N, Heo G-B, Bae Y-C, Joh S-J, et al. Multiple novel H5N6 highly pathogenic avian influenza viruses, South Korea, 2016. *Infect Genet Evol.* (2017) 51:21–3. doi: 10.1016/j.meegid.2017.03.005

18. Kim Y-I, Park S-J, Kwon H-I, Kim E-H, Si Y-J, Jeong J-H, et al. Genetic and phylogenetic characterizations of a novel genotype of highly pathogenic avian influenza (HPAI) H5N8 viruses in 2016/2017 in South Korea. *Infect Genet Evol.* (2017) 53:56–67. doi: 10.1016/j.meegid.2017.05.001

19. Lee E-K, Lee Y-N, Kye S-J, Lewis NS, Brown IH, Sagong M, et al. Characterization of a novel reassortant H5N6 highly pathogenic avian influenza virus clade 2.3. 4.4 in Korea, 2017. *Emerg Microbes Infect.* (2018) 7:103. doi: 10.1038/s41426-018-0104-3

20. Yee KS, Carpenter TE, Cardona CJ. Epidemiology of H5N1 avian influenza. *Comp Immunol Microbiol Infect Dis.* (2009) 32:325–40. doi: 10.1016/j.cimid.2008.01.005

21. de Jong MC. Mathematical modelling in veterinary epidemiology: why model building is important. *Prev Vet Med.* (1995) 25:183–93. doi: 10.1016/0167-5877(95)00538-2

22. Thomas JC, Thomas JC, Weber DJ. *Epidemiologic Methods for the Study of Infectious Diseases.* Oxford: Oxford University Press (2001) p. 64–5.

23. Dietz K. The estimation of the basic reproduction number for infectious diseases. *Stat Methods Med Res.* (1993) 2:23–41. doi: 10.1177/096228029300200103

24. Wallinga J, Lipsitch M. How generation intervals shape the relationship between growth rates and reproductive numbers. *Proc R Soc B.* (2006) 274:599–604. doi: 10.1098/rspb.2006.3754

25. Forsberg White L, Pagano M. A likelihood-based method for real-time estimation of the serial interval and reproductive number of an epidemic. *Stat Med.* (2008) 27:2999–3016. doi: 10.1002/sim.3136

26. Wallinga J, Teunis P. Different epidemic curves for severe acute respiratory syndrome reveal similar impacts of control measures. *Am J Epidemiol.* (2004) 160:509–16. doi: 10.1093/aje/kwh255

27. Obadia T, Haneef R, Boëlle P-Y. The R0 package: a toolbox to estimate reproduction numbers for epidemic outbreaks. *BMC Med Inform Decis Mak.* (2012) 12:147. doi: 10.1186/1472-6947-12-147

28. Cori A, Ferguson NM, Fraser C, Cauchemez S. A new framework and software to estimate time-varying reproduction numbers during epidemics. *Am J Epidemiol.* (2013) 178:1505–12. doi: 10.1093/aje/kwt133

29. Bett B, Henning J, Abdu P, Okike I, Poole J, Young J, et al. Transmission rate and reproductive number of the H 5 N 1 highly pathogenic avian influenza virus during the December 2005–July 2008 Epidemic in Nigeria. *Transbound Emerg Dis.* (2014) 61:60–8. doi: 10.1111/tbed.12003

30. Ward M, Maftei D, Apostu C, Suru A. Estimation of the basic reproductive number (R 0) for epidemic, highly pathogenic avian influenza subtype H5N1 spread. *Epidemiol Infect.* (2009) 137:219–26. doi: 10.1017/S0950268808000885

31. Marquetoux N, Paul M, Wongnarkpet S, Poolkhet C, Thanapongtharm W, Roger F, et al. Estimating spatial and temporal variations of the reproduction number for highly pathogenic avian influenza H5N1 epidemic in Thailand. *Prev Vet Med.* (2012) 106:143–51. doi: 10.1016/j.prevetmed.2012.01.021

32. Ssematimba A, Okike I, Ahmed G, Yamage M, Boender G, Hagenaars T, et al. Estimating the between-farm transmission rates for highly pathogenic avian influenza subtype H5N1 epidemics in Bangladesh between 2007 and 2013. *Transbound Emerg Dis.* (2018) 65:e127–34. doi: 10.1111/tbed.12692

33. Pandit PS, Bunn DA, Pande SA, Aly SS. Modeling highly pathogenic avian influenza transmission in wild birds and poultry in West Bengal, India. *Sci Rep.* (2013) 3:1–8. doi: 10.1038/srep02175

34. Garske T, Clarke P, Ghani AC. The transmissibility of highly pathogenic avian influenza in commercial poultry in industrialised countries. *PLoS ONE.* (2007) 2:e349. doi: 10.1371/journal.pone.0000349

35. Lee J, Ko Y, Jung E. Effective control measures considering spatial heterogeneity to mitigate the 2016–2017 avian influenza epidemic in the Republic of Korea. *PLoS ONE.* (2019) 14:e0218202. doi: 10.1371/journal.pone.0218202

36. Oh S-m. *Self-Declaration of the Recovery of Freedom From Highly Pathogenic Avian Influenza in Poultry by Republic of Korea: OIE Delegate for Republic of Korea, Ministry of Agriculture, Food and Rural Affairs.* (2018). Available online at: http://www.oie.int (accessed 27 May, 2019).

37. Kamvar ZN, Cai J, Pulliam JR, Schumacher J, Jombart T. Epidemic

curves made easy using the R package incidence. *F1000Res.* (2019) 8:139. doi: 10.12688/f1000research.18002.1

38. Animal and Plant Quarantine Agency. *High Pathogenic Avian Influenza; The Blue Book.* Yong-Sang K, editor. Noida, IN: Imun Company (2015).

39. Jeong O-M, Kim M-C, Kim M-J, Kang H-M, Kim H-R, Kim Y-J, et al. Experimental infection of chickens, ducks and quails with the highly pathogenic H5N1 avian influenza virus. *J Vet Sci.* (2009) 10:53–60. doi: 10.4142/jvs.2009.10.1.53

40. Lee E-K, Song B-M, Kang H-M, Woo S-H, Heo G-B, Jung SC, et al. Experimental infection of SPF and Korean native chickens with highly pathogenic avian influenza virus (H5N8). *Poult Sci.* (2016) 95:1015–9. doi: 10.3382/ps/pew028

41. Lee D-H, Kwon J-H, Noh J-Y, Park J-K, Yuk S-S, Erdene-Ochir T-O, et al. Pathogenicity of the Korean H5N8 highly pathogenic avian influenza virus in commercial domestic poultry species. *Avian Pathol.* (2016) 45:208–11. doi: 10.1080/03079457.2016.1142502

42. Park S-C, Song B-M, Lee Y-N, Lee E-K, Heo G-B, Kye S-J, et al. Pathogenicity of clade 2.3. 4.4 H5N6 highly pathogenic avian influenza virus in three chicken breeds from South Korea in 2016/2017. *J Vet Sci.* (2019) 20:e27. doi: 10.4142/jvs.2019.20.e27

43. Animal and Plant Quarantine Agency. *2016-2017 Epidemiologic Reports of Highly Pathogenic Avian Influenza.* Animal and Plant Quarantine Agency (2017).

44. Iwami S, Takeuchi Y, Liu X. Avian–human influenza epidemic model. *Math Biosci.* (2007) 207:1–25. doi: 10.1016/j.mbs.2006.08.001

45. Ridenhour B, Kowalik JM, Shay DK. Unraveling r 0: Considerations for public health applications. *Am J Public Health.* (2018) 108:S445–54. doi: 10.2105/AJPH.2013.301704r

46. Breslow N. A generalized Kruskal-Wallis test for comparing K samples subject to unequal patterns of censorship. *Biometrika.* (1970) 57:579–94. doi: 10.1093/biomet/57.3.579

47. Retkute R, Jewell CP, Van Boeckel TP, Zhang G, Xiao X, Thanapongtharm W, et al. Dynamics of the 2004 avian influenza H5N1 outbreak in Thailand: the role of duck farming, sequential model fitting and control. *Prev Vet Med.* (2018) 159:171–81. doi: 10.1016/j.prevetmed.2018.09.014

48. Bank W. *World Bank Open Data Online.* (2020). Available online at: https://data.worldbank.org/indicator/AG.LND.ARBL.HA.PC (accessed 12 May, 2020).

49. Statistics Korea. *Livestock Statistics Survey Korea.* (2015). Available online at: http://kosis.kr/statisticsList/statisticsListIndex.do?menuId=M_01_01&vwcd=MT_ZTITLE&parmTabId=M_01_01?menuId=M_01_01&vwcd=MT_ZTITLE&parmTabId=M_01_01&parentId=F#SubCont (accessed 12 May, 2020).

50. Kim WH, An JU, Kim J, Moon OK, Bae SH, Bender JB, et al. Risk factors associated with highly pathogenic avian influenza subtype H5N8 outbreaks on broiler duck farms in South Korea. *Transbound Emerg Dis.* (2018) 65:1329–38. doi: 10.1111/tbed.12882

51. OECD. *Producer Incentives in Livestock Disease Management.* Paris: OECD (2017).

52. Gilbert M, Slingenbergh J, Xiao X. Climate change and avian influenza. *Rev Sci Tech.* (2008) 27:459. doi: 10.20506/rst.27.2.1821

53. Tian H, Zhou S, Dong L, Van Boeckel TP, Pei Y, Wu Q, et al. Climate change suggests a shift of H5N1 risk in migratory birds. *Ecol Model.* (2015) 306:6–15. doi: 10.1016/j.ecolmodel.2014.08.005

54. Lowen AC, Mubareka S, Steel J, Palese P. Influenza virus transmission is dependent on relative humidity and temperature. *PLoS Pathog.* (2007) 3:e151. doi: 10.1371/journal.ppat.0030151

55. Liu C-M, Lin S-H, Chen Y-C, Lin KC-M, Wu T-SJ, King C-C. Temperature drops and the onset of severe avian influenza A H5N1 virus outbreaks. *PLoS ONE.* (2007) 2:e191. doi: 10.1371/journal.pone.0000191

56. Brown JD, Goekjian G, Poulson R, Valeika S, Stallknecht DE. Avian influenza virus in water: infectivity is dependent on pH, salinity and temperature. *Vet Microbiol.* (2009) 136:20–6. doi: 10.1016/j.vetmic.2008.10.027

57. Son K, Kim YK, Oem JK, Jheong WH, Sleeman J, Jeong J. Experimental infection of highly pathogenic avian influenza viruses, clade 2.3. 4.4 H5N6 and H5N8, in mandarin ducks from South Korea. *Transbound Emerg Dis.* (2018) 65:899–903. doi: 10.1111/tbed.12790

58. Delamater PL, Street EJ, Leslie TF, Yang YT, Jacobsen KH. Complexity of the basic reproduction number (R0). *Emerg Infect Dis.* (2019) 25:1. doi: 10.3201/eid2501.171901

59. USDA Foreign agricultural service. *Status of Highly Pathogenic Avian Influenza in South Korea Seoul.* (2016). Available online at: https://kr.usembassy.gov/wp-content/uploads/sites/75/2017/01/KS-1648-Status-of-Highly-Pathogenic-Avian-Influenza-in-South-Korea_12-19-2016.pdf (accessed 6 May, 2020).

60. Kim E-T, Pak S-I. The contribution of farm vehicle movements for a highly pathogenic avian influenza epidemic in 2014 in the Republic of Korea. *J Prev Vet Med.* (2019) 43:182–8. doi: 10.13041/jpvm.2019.43.4.182

61. Kwon H-i, Kim E-H, Kim Y-i, Park S-J, Si Y-J, Lee I-W, et al. Comparison of the pathogenic potential of highly pathogenic avian influenza (HPAI) H5N6, and H5N8 viruses isolated in South Korea during the 2016–2017 winter season. *Emerg Microbes Infect.* (2018) 7:–29. doi: 10.1038/s41426-018-0029-x

Epidemiology of Bovine Tuberculosis and its Zoonotic Implication in Addis Ababa Milkshed, Central Ethiopia

Begna Tulu[1,2*], Aboma Zewede[3], Mulugeta Belay[4], Miserach Zeleke[1], Mussie Girma[1], Metasebia Tegegn[5], Fozia Ibrahim[5], David A. Jolliffe[4], Markos Abebe[5], Taye Tolera Balcha[5], Balako Gumi[1], Henny M. Martineau[6], Adrian R. Martineau[4] and Gobena Ameni[1,7]

[1] Aklilu Lemma Institute of Pathobiology, Sefere Selam Campus, Addis Ababa University, Addis Ababa, Ethiopia, [2] Department of Medical Laboratory Sciences, Bahir Dar University, Bahir Dar, Ethiopia, [3] Ethiopian Public Health Institute, Addis Ababa, Ethiopia, [4] Barts and the London School of Medicine and Dentistry, Queen Mary University of London, London, United Kingdom, [5] Armeur Hansen Research Institute, Addis Ababa, Ethiopia, [6] Department of Pathology, The Royal Veterinary College, Hatfield, United Kingdom, [7] Department of Veterinary Medicine, College of Food and Agriculture, United Arab Emirates University, Al Ain, United Arab Emirates

*Correspondence:
Begna Tulu
tulubegna@gmail.com

Bovine tuberculosis (bTB) continues to be one of the most widely distributed chronic infectious diseases of zoonotic importance, which causes a significant economic loss in animal production. A cross-sectional study was conducted to estimate the prevalence of bTB and its associated risk factors and type the *Mycobacterium bovis* isolated in central Ethiopia. A total of 65 dairy farms and 654 cattle were tested for bTB using a single intradermal comparative cervical tuberculin (SICCT) test. Data on farm management, animal-related characteristics, and the owner's knowledge of the zoonotic importance of bTB were collected using a structured questionnaire. In addition, a total of 16 animals from different farms were identified for postmortem examination. Lowenstein Jensen (LJ) culture was also conducted, and spoligotyping was used to type the *M. bovis* strains isolated. Chi-square test and logistic regression models were used to analyze the herd- and animal-level risk factors. Herd- and animal-level prevalence rates of bTB were 58.5% (95% CI: 46.2%–69.2%) and 39.3% (95% CI: 35.5%–43.5%), respectively. At the herd level, poor farm management was the predictor for bTB positivity ($p < 0.05$). Animal breed, poor BCS, farm type, and poor farm management conditions were significant predictors of bTB positivity ($p < 0.05$) at an individual animal level. All animals identified for postmortem examination were found to have gross TB-like lesions. A total of 14 *M. bovis* strains were identified from 12 animals that were positive for LJ culture. The strain with the largest number of clusters (five isolates) was SB1176, followed by SB0134 (three isolates), SB0192 (two isolates), and SB2233 (two isolates), and two new strains, each consisting of only one isolate. The majority (58.5%) of the respondents did not know the zoonotic importance of bTB. The result of this study showed a high prevalence of bTB in the Addis Ababa milkshed and a low level of consciousness of the owners on its transmission to humans. Therefore, the launching of acceptable control measures of bTB and the creation of public awareness about its zoonotic transmission and prevention measures are required.

Keywords: bovine tuberculosis, Addis Ababa milkshed, zoonotic implication, spoligotyping, farm management

BACKGROUND

Bovine tuberculosis (bTB) is caused by *Mycobacterium bovis*, a member of *Mycobacterium tuberculosis* complex (MTBc). It is a chronic infectious disease of animals characterized by the formation of granulomas primarily in the lungs, lymph nodes, intestine, and kidney. *M. bovis* has the widest host ranges of all MTBc organisms and can readily be transmitted to humans or a variety of domestic and wild animals (1). The most common route of transmission to people is through the consumption of unpasteurized dairy products and inhalation of infectious droplet nuclei (2). In 2019 alone, the World Health Organization (WHO) reported that *M. bovis* was responsible for 143,000 new human TB cases and 12,300 deaths (3). More than 91.0% of the deaths were from the African and Asian countries, where the highest prevalence of bTB has been reported (4).

Many developed nations have reduced or eliminated bTB from their cattle population by implementing effective control strategies that include testing and culling of infected animals, active surveillance, and restrictions of movement in affected areas (5–7). However, in poor and marginalized communities, bTB still continues to cause a significant impact on livestock productivity and on livelihoods of communities (1, 6).

Ethiopia has the largest cattle population in Africa (8) and is also the second most populous country in Africa, with more than 108 million inhabitants (9). The majority of the Ethiopian economy relies on agriculture that depends on traditional farming using cattle force and cattle husbandry (10). Earlier reports showed that in Ethiopia, the prevalence of bTB can reach up to 50% in intensive dairy production systems that are known to serve a large number of people in the urban setup with milk and other dairy products (11, 12).

Therefore, understanding the magnitude of bTB infection and the molecular epidemiology in animal and human populations in the peri-urban area that supplies the major city of Addis Ababa is a key priority. Additionally, information about the knowledge of dairy farm owners or farm workers about the bTB and its zoonotic importance is essential in designing the control strategy and for policy recommendation. To this effect, the objectives of this study were to determine the prevalence of bTB both at the herd and animal level, type the *M. bovis* strains isolated, and assess the knowledge of farm owners or workers about bTB and its zoonotic importance in Addis Ababa milkshed, the capital of Ethiopia.

MATERIALS AND METHODS

Study Setting and Area

The study was conducted between December 2017 and March 2019 in the milkshed of the capital Addis Ababa, central Ethiopia, situated in a range of 80 km toward the North West and North East, namely, Chanco Woreda, Laga-Tafo Laga-Dadi Town, Muka Turi Town, Sandafa-Bake Woreda, and Suluta Town (**Figure 1**). The area has the largest concentration of intensive dairy farms supplying milk to the capital Addis Ababa. In addition to their proximity to the capital Addis Ababa City, where

there is a huge demand for dairy products, these localities are known for their conducive climatic conditions for dairy products.

Study Subjects

The study subjects were dairy cattle managed in the selected dairy farms in the study area. The farms were characterized by a mix of small holders at household level and intensive and semi-intensive farms owned by members of private investors (11). Dairy cattle in the selected herds were the study units, and their breed compositions were one of the following: crosses of Holstein Friesian (HF) and Zebu, crosses of Jersey and Zebu, or pure Zebu. The husbandry and farm setting differed somewhat from one study site to the other depending on the level of awareness, educational status of farmers, and access of extension services. The following inclusion and exclusion criteria were used for farms and individual animals.

Farms were included if they had been established for over a year, owned at least five cattle, gave written informed consent for cattle to have SICCT test, and agreed that at least one strong reactor could be slaughtered in return for financial compensation. Individual animals were excluded if they were calves younger than 4 weeks, clinically sick cattle with diseases not suggestive of bTB, or cows in the last 2 months of pregnancy.

Study Design and Sample Strategy

A cross-sectional study was conducted in the farms located in the milkshed of Addis Ababa City, central Ethiopia. Lists of intensive dairy farms with more than five cattle with HF and/or crossbreed were obtained from the local Livestock and Fishery Department offices in the study area. The farms were grouped into three categories; small (<10 animals per farm), medium (10–50 animals per farm), and large (>50 animals per farm). From each study area, the farms and the animals were randomly selected. The farms were approached for their willingness to participate in bTB testing and those farms that agreed were tested. New farms with less than 1 year since establishment were excluded.

A total of 65 farms and 654 individual animals were screened for bTB infection using a single intradermal comparative cervical tuberculin (SICCT) test. After the farms were identified and written informed consent was obtained from the owners for their cattle to undergo SICCT test, study staff administered intradermal injections of purified protein derivatives (PPDs) from *M. bovis* and *Mycobacterium avium* tuberculin to cattle on the day of consent and returned 72 h later to read the tests. A total of 16 highly reactive cows using SICCT test were purchased (one animal per farm), and further laboratory examinations were performed.

Risk factors associated with bTB positivity both at animal and herd levels were recorded before PPD injection. Body condition score (BCS) of the animals was determined as good, medium, or poor according to Nicholson and Butterworth (13). Good BCS was considered for the animals when the fat cover is easily observed in critical areas and the transverse process was not visible or felt. Animals with visible ribs having a little fat cover and barely visible dorsal spines were classified as medium BCS. Poor BCS was considered when there is an extremely lean animal

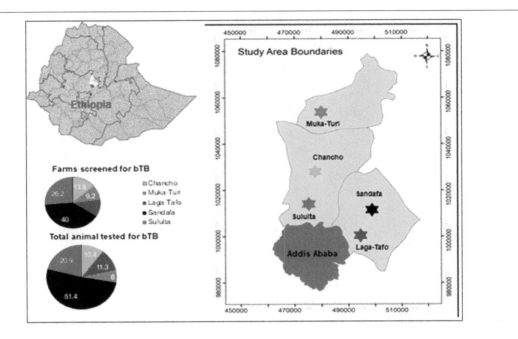

FIGURE 1 | Study area. Source: https://en.wikipedia.org/wiki/Districts_of_Ethiopia.

with projecting dorsal spines pointed to the touch and individual noticeable transverse processes.

The management condition of the farms was categorized based on Ameni et al. (14) as poor, medium (satisfactory), or good. The classification of management condition depends on the housing condition (such as neatness, waste drainage, nature and cleanness of the floor and animals, light source, ventilation, presence of confinement), feeding practice (concentrate and hay), possession of an exercise yard, and contact with other nearby herds and provision with clean water.

Questionnaire Data

Data were collected by study staff using a paper Case Report Format (CRF). Each page of the CRF bears a study ID number unique for each participant farm. Either the owner or the farm manager was interviewed using a predesigned questionnaire about the awareness of bTB transmission, habits of raw milk and meat consumption, and recent TB cases identified from family or workers.

Single Intradermal Comparative Cervical Tuberculin Test

For each cattle selected in this study, SICCT tests were performed using PPDs from *M. bovis* (PPDb) and *M. avium* (PPDa) according to a published protocol (15).

Sample Collection, Processing, and Culturing of Mycobacteria

For all cattle tested by the SICCT test, information about age, sex, type of breeds, and BCS was recorded. Selected positive cattle were purchased and subjected to postmortem examination performed. The criteria used to select the purchased animals

were based on the strong PPD response, one animal per farm, and based on the willingness of the farmer to sell the animal. The postmortem examination was done using standard protocols (16).

Seven lymph nodes with suspicious gross lesions were collected per animal, placed in individual 50-ml sterile universal tubes, and transported at 4°C to Aklilu Lemma Institute of Pathobiology (ALIPB) for further processing. At ALIPB laboratory, samples were stored at −22°C, and all samples were processed and cultured for mycobacteria as previously described by the World Organization for Animal Health protocols (17). The tissues were sectioned using sterile blades and were then homogenized with a mortar and pestle. The homogenate was decontaminated by adding an equal volume of 4% NaOH and by centrifugation at 1,865 g for 15 min. The supernatant was discarded, and the sediment was neutralized by 1% (0.1N) HCl using phenol red as an indicator. Neutralization was considered to have been achieved when the color of the solution changed from purple to yellow. Thereafter, 0.1 ml of suspension from each sample was spread onto a slant of Löwenstein–Jensen (LJ) medium. Duplicate slants were used, one enriched with sodium pyruvate and the other enriched with glycerol. Cultures were incubated aerobically at 37°C for at least 8 weeks and with a weekly observation of the growth of colonies.

Identification and Molecular Typing of Mycobacteria

Slants with no growth at week 8 were considered culture negative. Bacterial colonies from culture-positive samples were stained by the Ziehl–Neelsen staining technique to identify acid-fast bacilli (AFB). Spoligotyping was performed following the standard operating procedure that was used by Berg et al. (12) and primarily developed by Kemerbeek et al. (18). The

DNA released by heat killing of the colonies was used as a template to amplify the direct repeat (DR) region of *M. tuberculosis* complex by polymerase chain reaction (PCR) using oligonucleotide biotin-labeled primers derived from the DR sequence, RDa (5′GGTTTTGGGTTTGAACGAC3′) and RDb (5′CCGAGAGGGGACG GAAAC3′) (18).

A total volume of 25 μl and reaction mixtures of 12.5 μl of HotStarTaq Master Mix (Qiagen), a final concentration of 1.5 mM MgCl$_2$, 200 μM of each deoxynucleotide triphosphate, 2 μl of each primer (20 pmol each), 5 μl suspension of heat-killed cells (approximately 10–50 ng), and 3.5 μl distilled water were used. The mixture was heated for 15 min at 96°C and then subjected to 30 cycles of 1 min denaturation at 96°C, annealing at 55°C for 1 min and extension at 72°C for 30 s. And the final stabilization stage at 72°C for 10 min. Immediately before running spoligotyping, the PCR product was denatured using thermocyler at 96°C for 10 min and then removed from the thermocycler and kept on ice so as to prevent renaturing of the PCR products. Thereafter, the denatured PCR product was loaded onto a membrane covalently bonded with a set of 43 oligonucleotides, each corresponding to one of the unique spacer DNA sequences within the DR locus of *M. tuberculosis* complex and then hybridized at 60°C for 1 h. After hybridization, the membrane was washed twice for 10 min in 2× SSPE [1× SSPE is 0.18 M NaCl, 10 mM NaH$_2$PO$_4$, and 1 mM EDTA (pH 7.7)]-0.5% sodium dodecyl sulfate (SDS) at 60°C and then incubated in 1:4,000 diluted streptavidin peroxidase (Boehringer) for 1 h at 42°C. The membrane was washed twice for 10 min in 2× SSPE-0.5% SDS at 42°C and rinsed with 2× SSPE for 5 min at room temperature. Hybridizing DNA was detected by the enhanced chemiluminescence (ECL) method (Amersham, Biosciences, Amersham, UK) and by exposure to X-ray film (Hyperfilm ECL, Amersham). A mixture of 10 ml of ECL reagent 1 and 10 ml of ECL reagent 2 was prepared and then added onto the membrane, and the membrane was rinsed in the solution for 5 min at room temperature. Then, the membrane was attached onto a film in the dark room and placed in the cassette and incubated for 15 min at room temperature. The film was removed and placed in a developer solution for 2 min, removed from the developer, and rinsed with tap water for 15 s and then placed in a fixer solution for 1 min. Finally, the film was dried and used for interpretation of the result. The presence of the spacer was identified as a black square, while absence of the spacer was identified as a white square on the film. The black squares were converted to 1 while the white squares were converted to 0 and then transferred to the spoligotype international type (SIT)-VNTR international type (VIT) database for the identification of the SITs and the lineages of the isolates.

Statistical Analysis

SICCT test and other questionnaire data were entered and analyzed by SPSS version 21.0. Descriptive statistics like mean, median, and standard deviation were used to summarize data. For both herd and animal levels, prevalence was calculated by dividing the number of reactors to the total number tested. One-sample nonparametric test was used to compute the 95% confidence interval of the prevalence. A chi-square test was used to compare the proportions. Univariable and multivariable logistic regressions were used to rule out the risk factors associated with bTB at the herd and animal levels. Statistical significance was indicated using 95% confidence intervals and *p*-values <0.05.

Ethical Considerations

The study obtained ethical approval from the Armauer Hansen Research Institute (AHRI) Ethics Review Committee (Ref P018/17); the Ethiopian National Research Ethics Review Committee (Ref 310/253/2017); the Queen Mary University of London Research Ethics Committee, London UK (Ref 16/YH/0410); and the ALIPB, Addis Ababa University (Ref ALIPB/IRB/011/2017/18). Written informed consent was obtained from all the owners of the farms.

RESULTS

Herd- and Animal-Level Prevalence

A total of 65 dairy farms in the milkshed of Addis Ababa City, central Ethiopia, were screened for bTB using SICCT test. The overall prevalence of bTB at herd level was 58.5% (95% CI: 45.6–70.6) at a cutoff value >4.0 mm. When the study sites were considered, 50.0% (19/38) of the positive herds were recorded at Sandafa followed by Sululta (23.7%), Chancho (13.2%), Laga-Tafo (10.5%), and Muka-Turi (2.6%). The overall animal-level prevalence was 39.3% (95% CI: 35.5–43.2) at a cutoff value >4.0 mm. The highest proportion (63.8%) of bTB-positive animals was reported from Sandafa area, followed by Sululta area 19.8% (51/257), Laga-Tafo area 10.5% (27/257), Chancho area 3.1% (8/257), and Muka-Turi area 2.7% (7/257) (**Table 1**).

Herd-Level Risk Factors

Results on the farms' characteristics including the type of farms whether they are traditional or commercial, herd size of the farms, and the farms' management conditions are summarized in **Table 2** below.

In order to identify factors associated with bTB at herd level, binary logistic regression analysis was conducted. The univariable logistic regression analysis showed that the type of farm, management condition, and herd size were factors associated with the presence of bTB in the farms (p < 0.05). The multivariable logistic regression analysis showed that farm management conditions remain the predictors for bTB positivity at the herd level (*p* < 0.05) (**Table 2**).

Animal-Level Risk Factors

The mean age of the animals included in this study was 5.1 years (SD = 2.21), the majority of them were in the age group 4.0–9.0 years of age. Eighty-eight percent of the animals were cows, and 93.0% of the animals belong to crossbreed between either HF or Jersey and the local Zebu (**Table 3**).

At the individual animal level, univariable logistic regression showed that factors like the location of animals, being a cow, crossbreed, medium and poor farm management conditions, poor BCS, animals from commercial farms, and animals from medium and large herd size were significantly associated with

TABLE 1 | Herd and animal prevalences of bTB using SICCT test at >4.0mm cut-off.

bTB status	Level	Chancho		Laga-Tafo		Muka-Turi		Sandafa		Sululta		Total	
		No.	%	No.	%	No.	%	No.	%	No.	%	No.	Prevalence (95 % CI)
Negative	Herd	4	44.4	3	42.9	5	83.3	7	26.9	8	47.1	27	41.5 [30.8–53.8]
	Animal	60	88.2	47	63.5	32	82.1	172	51.2	86	62.8	397	60.7 [56.9–64.7]
Positive	Herd	5	55.6	4	57.1	1	16.7	19	73.1	9	52.9	38	58.5 [46.2–96.2]
	Animal	8	11.8	27	36.5	7	17.9	164	48.8	51	37.2	257	39.3 [35.3–43.1]

TABLE 2 | Risk factors associated with bTB in selected dairy farms in the Addis Ababa milkshed, central Ethiopia.

Risk factors		Total (%)	bTB status					
			N (%) positive	Crude OR (95% CI)	P-value	Adjusted OR [95% CI]	P-value
Locations	Chancho	9 (13.8)	5 (13.2)	1		-	
	Laga-Tafo	7 (10.8)	4 (10.5)	1.1(0.1–7.8)	0.949	-	-
	Muka-Turi	6 (9.2)	1 (2.6)	0.2(0.01–1.9)	0.154	-	-
	Sandafa	26 (40.0)	19 (50.0)	2.2(0.4–10.5)	0.334	-	-
	Sululta	17 (26.2)	9 (23.7)	0.9(0.2–4.5)	0.899	-	-
Farm type	Traditional	44 (67.7)	20 (52.6)	1		-	-
	Commercial	21 (32.3)	18 (47.4)	7.2(1.8–28.0)	0.004	-	-
Management condition	Good	15 (23.1)	6 (15.8)	1		1	
	Medium	17 (26.2)	13 (34.2)	4.8(1.1–22.4)	0.042	9.0(1.1–73.2)	0.040
	Poor	33 (50.8)	19 (50.0)	2.0(0.6–7.1)	0.262	6.7(1.0–43.1)	0.045
Herd size	Small (< 10 animals)	21 (32.3)	8 (21.1)	1		-	-
	Medium (11-50 animals)	29 (44.6)	16 (42.1)	2.0(0.6–6.2)	0.235	-	-
	Large (> 50 animals)	15 (23.1)	14 (36.8)	22.7(2.5–207.7)	0.006	-	-

bTB infection ($p < 0.05$). According to the multivariable logistic regression location of the animals, breed, poor body condition, animals in a commercial farm, and farm management conditions were significant predictors of bTB positivity ($p < 0.05$) (**Table 3**).

Spoligotype Patterns of Cattle Isolates

A total of 16 cows, one cow from each farm were purchased based on their higher SICCT test result. The mean SICCT score was 22.5 mm (SD = 15.59), 8.7 and 71.0 mm being the lowest and the highest score, respectively. Out of the 16 animals that showed gross TB lesions, 12 of them were positive for *M. bovis* culture on LJ medium with a culture positivity rate of 75.0%. All the samples have shown growth on the LJ media supplemented with sodium pyruvate, and only three samples have shown growth on the LJ media supplemented with glycerol. The spoligotype pattern of 14 isolates was shown in **Figure 2**. The isolates from two animals have shown two different spoligotype patterns, which indicate the possibility of double infection. The isolates were grouped into four clusters of *M. bovis* strains of which two were new strains. The genotype with the largest of isolates (five isolates) was SB1176, followed by SB0134 (three isolates), SB0192 (two isolates), and SB2233 (two isolates) and two new strains each with one isolate.

Cattle Owners' Awareness About Bovine Tuberculosis and Its Zoonotic Importance

Farm owners or managers were interviewed to assess their awareness about bTB and its zoonotic transmission. Out of 65 respondents, 31.0% did not know what bTB was, and 58.5% did not know the zoonotic importance of bTB. The participants responded that they had a habit of eating raw meat 83.0% and drinking raw milk 86.2%. Similarly, 87.7% of owners' families or their workers share the same room with their cattle. Finally, 13.8% reported a history of TB in either the owners' family or their workers (**Table 4**).

DISCUSSION

This study reports the epidemiology of bTB and its zoonotic implication in Addis Abba milkshed, central Ethiopia. The country is known to have a high burden of TB in its human (3) and cattle populations (19). In Ethiopia, there are no control and prevention policies of bTB. In addition, human behaviors like drinking raw milk (unpasteurized) and eating raw meat are highly practiced.

In the present study, the herd and animal prevalence rates of bTB using SICCT test were 58.5 and 39.3%, respectively. This is one of the highest reports regarding bTB in the country.

TABLE 3 | Risk factors associated with bTB positive animals from selected dairy farms in the Addis Ababa milkshed, central Ethiopia.

Characteristics		Total (%)	bTB status				
			N (%) positive	Crude OR (95% CI)	P-value	Adjusted OR (95% CI)	P-value
Locations	Chancho	68 (10.4)	9 (3.1)	1		1	
	Laga-Tafo	74 (11.3)	27 (10.5)	4.31(1.79–10.35)	0.002	8.54(2.91–25.04)	<0.001
	Muka-Turi	39 (6.0)	7 (2.7)	1.64(0.54–4.94)	0.378	-	-
	Sandafa	336 (51.4)	164 (63.8)	4.46(1.97–10.05)	<0.001	5.58(2.01–15.45)	<0.001
	Sululta	137 (20.9)	51 (19.8)	7.15(3.32–15.42)	<0.001	12.96(4.94–34.00)	<0.001
Sex	Male	80 (12.2)	16 (6.2)	1		-	-
	Female	574 (87.8)	241 (93.8)	2.89(1.63–5.13)	<0.001	-	-
Breed	Zebu	27 (4.1)	2 (0.8)	1		1	
	Cross breed	613 (93.7)	253 (98.4)	8.78(2.06–37.42)	0.003	6.15(1.26–26.98)	0.025
	HF	14 (2.1)	2 (0.8)	2.08(0.26–16.63)	0.489	-	-
Body condition	Good	93 (14.2)	21 (8.2)	1		1	
	Medium	411 (62.8)	118 (45.9)	1.38(0.81–2.35)	0.234	-	-
	Poor	150 (22.9)	118 (45.9)	12.64(6.77–23.58)	<0.001	12.38(5.96–25.73)	<0.001
Farm type	Traditional	333 (50.9)	64 (24.9)	1		1	
	Commercial	321 (49.1)	193 (75.1)	6.34(4.46–9.02)	<0.001	9.33(4.65–18.68)	<0.001
Management condition	Good	108 (16.5)	64 (24.9)	1		1	
	Medium	268 (41.0)	133 (51.8)	3.29(2.29–4.76)	<0.001	1.86(1.13–3.08)	0.016
	Poor	278 (42.5)	64 (24.9)	4.18(2.61–6.69)	<0.001	-	-
Herd size	<10 animals	95 (14.5)	13 (5.1)	1		-	-
	11–50 animals	273 (41.7)	76 (29.6)	2.43(1.28–4.63)	0.007	-	-
	>50 animals	286 (43.7)	168 (65.4)	8.98(4.78–16.87)	<0.001	-	-

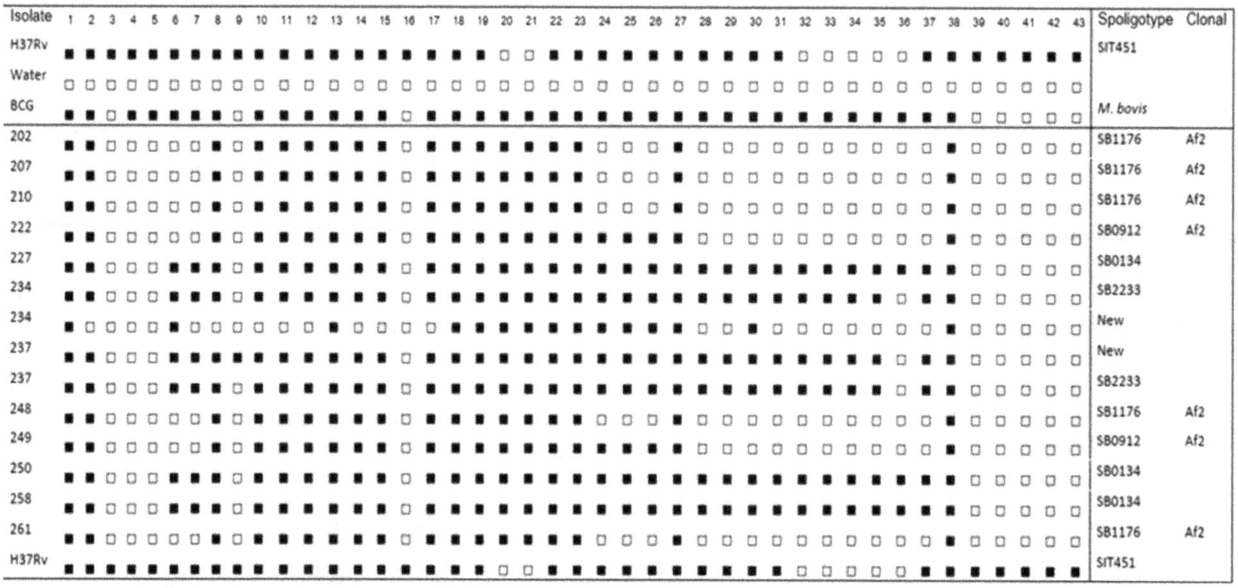

FIGURE 2 | Spoligotype patterns of mycobacterial isolates recovered from tuberculosis lesions in cattle. Four clusters of spoligotype patterns and two new strains of *Mycobacterium bovis* were detected. *Mycobacterium tuberculosis* H37Rv (H37Rv), distilled water (dH$_2$O), and Bacillus Calmette-Guérin (BCG) are known references.

Previous studies reported lower results compared to the present study (14, 19–23). In a similar area, a previous study by Ameni et al. (11) reported an overall prevalence of 13.5%, with a higher (22.2%) proportion among the Holstein breed. In 2013, Ameni et al. (20) again reported a much lower herd prevalence of 9.4% and individual animal prevalence of 1.8%. On the other hand, a study from the eastern part of Ethiopia reported a prevalence of 51.2% at herd level and 20.3% at individual animal level (23). These significant differences could be attributed to the type of dairy farms and animal breeds included in the study.

TABLE 4 | Owners or farm mangers awareness about bTB and bTB mode of transmission among dairy farm owners.

Questions	Yes (%)	No (%)
Know bTB	45 (69.2)	20 (30.8)
Know bTB is zoonotic	27 (41.5)	38 (58.5)
Eat raw meat	54 (83.1)	11 (16.9)
Drink raw milk	56 (86.2)	9 (13.8)
Sharing rooms with animals	57 (87.7)	8 (12.3)
History of TB in a family or workers	9 (13.8)	56 (86.2)

For example, in the study conducted by Ameni et al. (20), the majority of the farms were smallholder farmers at household level and the animals were the Zebu breeds, which are known to be less susceptible to bTB. In the present study, the majority of the animals from commercial farms were crossbreeds between HF and the local Zebu breeds, which are more susceptible to bTB compared to Zebu cattle (11). Another reason for higher prevalence in this study could be explained by the expansion of intensive dairy farms, which together with an absence of control and prevention policies leads to increased morbidity and transmission of bTB.

Based on multivariable logistic regression analysis of the risk factors in the present study, poor farm management condition was significantly associated with bTB positivity at the herd level. This observation was consistent with the results by Kemal et al. (23) from Eastern Ethiopia. Similarly, Mekonnen et al. (22) reported that farm hygiene is one of the risk factors significantly associated with the bTB at herd level. Hygiene is an essential component in the assessment of farm conditions, and it was assessed in terms of the waste disposal, frequency of waste cleaning, and drainage conditions. Farms with poor management conditions may facilitate the persistence of M. bovis infection, creating a conducive environment for easy proliferation and transmission.

In this study, breed of cattle was one of the predictors of bTB positivity. Previous studies reported by Ameni et al. (11) and Vordermeier et al. (24) indicated that Zebu cattle are more resistant to bTB than either crossbreed or HF breed. Other studies from the United Kingdom (25) and the Republic of Ireland (26) demonstrated that HF cattle have significant heritability to susceptibility to bTB. In the study area, as HFs have a higher milk yield, there is a high tendency to replace the Zebu with HF or crossbreed to increase milk production. This, on the other hand, is a serious challenge in terms of bTB transmission and its impact on the absence of bTB control policies.

In the present study, animals from large commercial farms were more likely to be positive for bTB diseases when compared to traditional farms with smaller herds. This is consistent with the type of breeds that are largely found in such setup. In the study area, commercial farms are largely populated by European breeds and crossbreeds. Studies in Eastern Ethiopia also demonstrated that commercial farms are more likely to be positive for bTB (23). In the commercial dairy system, a large number of cattle are kept in an indoor system with poor ventilation, likely facilitating the transmission of infectious pathogens.

Similar to a previous study by Dejene et al. (27), animals with poor BCS were associated with bTB infection. This study did not define the cause-and-effect relationship between BCS and bTB infection. Either animals with poor BCSs are more susceptible to developing clinical bTB or bTB-positive animals develop a poor BCS as a result of being infected with M. bovis, or a combination of both. Clinically, poor body condition is a typical sign that follows M. bovis infection in cattle.

Following the SICCT test, selected cows were humanely slaughtered to assess the gross pathology and take samples for mycobacteria isolation and typing. The result showed that all animals slaughtered were positive for gross TB lesions. The severity of the lesion was higher in the lymph nodes of the thoracic region. This observation is related to the route of infection, which is predominantly a respiratory route especially in dairy cattle kept in intensive dairy farms (28). Thus, the thoracic lymph nodes are affected predominantly as they are draining the lungs. On the other hand, in cattle that are kept on pasture, the digestive tract is the predominant site of infection of M. bovis and gross pathology (11).

In the present study, the spoligotyping result showed that 58.0% of the known strains (registered on the M.bovis.org) belong to the African 2 (AF2) clonal complex. The AF2 complex is known by the deletion of spacers from 3 to 7 in the spoligotype signatures. These strains of M. bovis are known by localized distribution in Eastern African countries including Ethiopia, Uganda, Burundi, and Tanzania (29). The SB1176 strain, which is grouped under AF2 clonal complex, was the dominant M. bovis clonal complex in the study area. Consistently, previous studies in a similar study area also reported that SB1176 was the dominant one (30). In the present study, all the known strains of M. bovis isolates were clustered. This shows that there is an active M. bovis transmission between farms in the study area.

Based on the questionnaire survey about the awareness of the farm owners and/or managers regarding bTB and its zoonotic transmission, a significant number of the respondents did not know the zoonotic importance of bTB. Additionally, the respondents reported that the practice of eating raw meat, drinking raw milk, and their workers sharing the same house with their cattle was very high. Previous studies (14, 23) have also demonstrated a gap in the awareness of the farm owners in this regard. We have observed that all the farms including the commercial and mixed farms sell raw milk/unpasteurized milk to the locals and/or to the milk distributors who collect milk from farms and then transport to Addis Ababa, except one dairy farm that has its own milk and dairy product processing facility. On the other hand, in addition to drinking raw or unpasteurized milk, yogurt, which is prepared from unpasteurized milk, is one of the dairy products being highly consumed in the area. This shows that there is a high zoonotic potential for M. bovis in the study area. Increasing the awareness of the farmers on the zoonotic importance of bTB and its method of transmission is recommended.

The main limitations of the study include not testing of more than 30 animals per farm due to the lack of willingness of the farmers to allow more animals to get tested. For the same reason, the small numbers of selected animals for postmortem examination because the farmers were not able to sell their animals even if they were told the animals were bTB positive. However, this study covers a wide area of subjects in bTB including the epidemiology, awareness of farmers toward the zoonotic importance of bTB, and the cluster of isolates indicating the active transmission of *M. bovis* in the study area. This information could be used by policymakers working on the control and prevention of bTB.

CONCLUSION

The result of this study showed a high prevalence of bTB in the Addis Ababa milkshed and low level of consciousness of the owners on its transmission to humans. Therefore, launching of control measures of bTB and creation of public awareness on its zoonotic transmission and its prevention measures are required.

ETHICS STATEMENT

The study obtained ethical approved from the Armauer Hansen Research Institute (AHRI) Ethics Review Committee (Ref P018/17), from the Ethiopian National Research Ethics Review Committee (Ref 310/253/2017), the Queen Mary University of London Research Ethics Committee, London UK (Ref

16/YH/0410); and by the Aklilu Lemma Institute of Pathobiology (ALIPB), Addis Ababa University (Ref ALIPB/IRB/011/2017/18). Written informed consent was obtained from all the owners of the farms.

AUTHOR CONTRIBUTIONS

BT and GA conceived the study. BT, AZ, MB, AM, and GA contributed to the study design and development of laboratory assays. BT, AZ, MZ, MG, MT, FI, MB, DJ, HM, MA, TB, BG, AM, and GA contributed to the implementation of the study and data acquisition. BT did statistical analyses, wrote the first draft of the manuscript, and had final responsibility for the decision to submit for publication. All authors reviewed the final draft and agreed with its content and conclusions.

ACKNOWLEDGMENTS

We thank all the members of the field and laboratory teams at AHRI and ALIPB; Mr. Getinet Abebe, Mr. Befikadu Assefa, Mr. Mengistu Mulu, Mr. Lemma Terfasa, and Mr. Tadesse Regassa for assistance with fieldwork and postmortem examination; and Mrs. Sofia Yimam, Mr. Selfu Girma, and Dr. Assegedech Sirak for assistance with histopathology and AFB examination. Finally, we would like to acknowledge Mr. Andargachew Abeje for developing the study area map and our drivers Mr. Elias Mulugeta, Mr. Yitbarek Getachew, and Mr. Assefa Mijena.

REFERENCES

1. Fitzgerald SD, Kaneene JB. Wildlife reservoirs of bovine tuberculosis worldwide: hosts, pathology, surveillance, and control. *Vet Pathol.* (2013) 50:488–99. doi: 10.1177/0300985812467472
2. Cosivi O, Grange JM, Daborn CJ, Raviglione MC, Fujikura T, Cousins D, et al. Zoonotic tuberculosis due to *Mycobacterium bovis* in developing countries. *Emerg Infect Dis.* (1998) 4:59–70. doi: 10.3201/eid0401.980108
3. WHO. *Global Tuberculosis Report 2019.* France: World Health Organization (2019).
4. OIE. *Bovine Tuberculosis.* Paris: World Organization for Animal Health (2019).
5. Thornton PK. Livestock production: recent trends, future prospects. *Philos Trans R Soc Lond B Biol Sci.* (2010) 365:2853–67. doi: 10.1098/rstb.2010.0134
6. Cousins D. Mycobacterium bovis infection and control in domestic livestock. *Revue Scientifique et Technique-Office International des Epizooties.* (2001) 20:71–85. doi: 10.20506/rst.20.1.1263
7. ECA. *Eradication, Control and Monitoring Programmes to Contain Animal Diseases.* Luxembourg: European Court of Auditors (2016).
8. UNDP-Ethiopia. *Transforming Ethiopia's Livestock Sector.* Addis Ababa: United Nations Development Programme (UNDP) (2017).
9. CIA. *Africa: Ethiopia-The World Fact Book-Central Intelligence Agency.* Washington, DC: Central Intelligence Agency (2020).
10. CSA. *Federal Democratic Republic of Ethiopia, Agricultural Sample Survey.* Addis Ababa: CSA (2009).
11. Ameni G, Aseffa A, Engers H, Young D, Gordon S, Hewinson G, et al. High prevalence and increased severity of pathology of bovine tuberculosis in Holsteins compared to zebu breeds under field cattle
12. husbandry in central Ethiopia. *Clin Vaccine Immunol.* (2007) 14:1356–61. doi: 10.1128/CVI.00205-07
12. Berg S, Firdessa R, Habtamu M, Gadisa E, Mengistu A, Yamuah L, et al. The burden of mycobacterial disease in ethiopian cattle: implications for public health. *PLoS ONE.* (2009) 4:e5068. doi: 10.1371/journal.pone.0005068
13. Nicholson MJ, Butterworth MH. *A Guide to Condition Scoring of Zebu Cattle.* Addis Ababa: International Livestock Centre for Africa (1986).
14. Ameni G, Amenu K, Tibbo M. Bovine tuberculosis: prevalence and risk factor assessment in cattle and cattle owners in Wuchale-Jida, Central Ethiopia. *J Appl Res Vet Med.* (2003) 1:17–26. Available online at: https://hdl.handle.net/10568/32984
15. World Organization for Animal Health. *Terrestrial Manual: Bovine Tuberculosis.* Paris: World Organization for Animal Health (2009).
16. Corner LA. Post mortem diagnosis of *Mycobacterium bovis* infection in cattle. *Vet Microbiol.* (1994) 40:53–63. doi: 10.1016/0378-1135(94)90046-9
17. OIE. Bovine tuberculosis. In: *Manual of Diagnostic Tests and Vaccines for Terrestrial Animals. Part 2, Section 2.3. Chapter 2.3.3.* (2010).
18. Kamerbeek J, Schouls L, Kolk A, van Agterveld M, van Soolingen D, Kuijper S, et al. Simultaneous detection and strain differentiation of *Mycobacterium tuberculosis* for diagnosis and epidemiology. *J Clin Microbiol.* (1997) 35:907–14. doi: 10.1128/JCM.35.4.907-914.1997
19. Firdessa R, Tschopp R, Wubete A, Sombo M, Hailu E, Erenso G, et al. High prevalence of bovine tuberculosis in dairy cattle in central Ethiopia: implications for the dairy industry and public health. *PLoS ONE.* (2012) 7:e52851. doi: 10.1371/journal.pone.0052851
20. Ameni G, Tadesse K, Hailu E, Deresse Y, Medhin G, Aseffa A, et al. Transmission of *Mycobacterium tuberculosis* between Farmers

and Cattle in Central Ethiopia. *PLoS ONE.* (2013) 8:e76891. doi: 10.1371/journal.pone.0076891

21. Gumi B, Schelling E, Firdessa R, Aseffa A, Tschopp R, Yamuah L, et al. Prevalence of bovine tuberculosis in pastoral cattle herds in the Oromia region, southern Ethiopia. Trop Anim Health Prod. (2011) 43:1081–7. doi: 10.1007/s11250-010-9777-x

22. Mekonnen GA, Conlan AJK, Berg S, Ayele BT, Alemu A, Guta S, et al. Prevalence of bovine tuberculosis and its associated risk factors in the emerging dairy belts of regional cities in Ethiopia. *Prev Vet Med.* (2019) 168:81–9. doi: 10.1016/j.prevetmed.2019.04.010

23. Kemal J, Sibhat B, Abraham A, Terefe Y, Tulu KT, Welay K, et al. Bovine tuberculosis in eastern Ethiopia: prevalence, risk factors and its public health importance. *BMC Infect Dis.* (2019) 19:39. doi: 10.1186/s12879-018-3628-1

24. Vordermeier M, Ameni G, Berg S, Bishop R, Robertson BD, Aseffa A, et al. The influence of cattle breed on susceptibility to bovine tuberculosis in Ethiopia. *Comp Immunol Microbiol Infect Dis.* (2012) 35:227–32. doi: 10.1016/j.cimid.2012.01.003

25. Brotherstone S, White IM, Coffey M, Downs SH, Mitchell AP, Clifton-Hadley RS, et al. Evidence of genetic resistance of cattle to infection with *Mycobacterium bovis*. *J Dairy Sci.* (2010) 93:1234–42. doi: 10.3168/jds.2009-2609

26. Bermingham ML, More SJ, Good M, Cromie AR, Higgins IM, Brotherstone S, et al. Genetics of tuberculosis in Irish Holstein-Friesian dairy herds. *J Dairy Sci.* (2009) 92:3447–56. doi: 10.3168/jds.2008-1848

27. Dejene SW, Heitkönig IM, Prins HH, Lemma FA, Mekonnen DA, Alemu ZE, et al. Risk factors for bovine tuberculosis (bTB) in cattle in Ethiopia. *PLoS ONE.* (2016) 11:e0159083. doi: 10.1371/journal.pone.01 59083

28. Tulu B, Martineau HM, Zewude A, Desta F, Jolliffe DA, Abebe M, et al. Cellular and cytokine responses in the granulomas of asymptomatic cattle naturally infected with *Mycobacterium bovis* in Ethiopia. *Infect Immun.* (2020) 88:e00507-20. doi: 10.1128/IAI. 00507-20

29. Berg S, Garcia-Pelayo MC, Müller B, Hailu E, Asiimwe B, Kremer K, et al. African 2, a clonal complex of *Mycobacterium bovis* epidemiologically important in East Africa. *J Bacteriol.* (2011) 193:670–8. doi: 10.1128/JB.00750-10

30. Ameni G, Desta F, Firdessa R. Molecular typing of *Mycobacterium bovis* isolated from tuberculosis lesions of cattle in north eastern Ethiopia. *Vet Rec.* (2010) 167:138–41. doi: 10.1136/ vr.b4881

5

A NanoLuc Luciferase Reporter Pseudorabies Virus for Live Imaging and Quantification of Viral Infection

Yalin Wang[1†], Hongxia Wu[1†], Bing Wang[1†], Hansong Qi[1], Zhao Jin[2], Hua-Ji Qiu[1*] and Yuan Sun[1*]

[1] State Key Laboratory of Veterinary Biotechnology, Harbin Veterinary Research Institute, Chinese Academy of Agricultural Sciences, Harbin, China, [2] College of Life Science and Agriculture Forestry, Qiqihar University, Qiqihar, China

*Correspondence:
Yuan Sun
sunyuan@caas.cn
Hua-Ji Qiu
qiuhuaji@caas.cn

[†] These authors have contributed equally to this work

Pseudorabies (PR), also known as Aujeszky's disease, is an acute infectious disease of pigs, resulting in significant economic losses to the pig industry in many countries. Since 2011, PR outbreaks have occurred in many Bartha-K61-vaccinated pig farms in China. The emerging pseudorabies virus (PRV) variants possess higher pathogenicity in pigs and mice than the strains isolated before. Here, a recombinant PRV (rPRVTJ-NLuc) stably expressing the NanoLuc (NLuc) luciferase fusion with the red fluorescent protein (DsRed) was constructed to trace viral replication and spread in mice. Moreover, both DsRed and NLuc luciferases were stably expressed in the infected cells, and there was no significant difference between wild-type and recombinant viruses in both growth kinetics and pathogenicity. Seven-week-old BALB/c mice were infected with 10^3 50% tissue culture infective dose rPRVTJ-NLuc and subjected to daily imaging. The mice infected with rPRVTJ-NLuc displayed robust bioluminescence that started 4 days postinfection (dpi), bioluminescence signal increased over time, peaked at 5 dpi, remained detectable for at least 6 dpi, and disappeared at 7 dpi, meanwhile, the increased flux accompanied by the spread of the virus from the injection site to the superior respiratory tract. However, the signal was also observed in the spinal cord, trigeminal ganglion, and partial region of the brain from separated tissues, not in living mice. Our results depicted a new approach to rapidly access the replication and pathogenicity of emerging PRVs in mice.

Keywords: pseudorabies virus, NanoLuc luciferase, *in vivo*, image, mouse

INTRODUCTION

Pseudorabies (PR), a devastating disease in the pig industry worldwide, is characterized by neurological signs, respiratory signs, high morbidity, and mortality of piglets, whereas older pigs mostly exhibit respiratory and reproductive diseases (1). Pseudorabies virus (PRV) is the causative agent of the acute infectious PR in swine. Due to control efforts and strict implementation of national eradication programs, PR has been eradicated from domestic pigs in North America and several European countries. However, the disease is sporadic in many other countries, including China (2). In late 2011, there was a PR outbreak on many large pig farms where piglets were vaccinated with Bartha-K61vaccine, and quickly the disease occurred in six provinces in China. The mortality rate of infected piglets was from 10 to 50%, which caused great economic loss (3). Moreover, about 57.8% of 5,033 serum samples isolated during the year 2013 to 2016 were positive for PRV gE antibody, so PRV variant strains were still prevalent in China (4). The PRV variants shared 97.1–99.9% nucleotide (nt) and 96.6–99.5% amino acid (aa) homology with PRV reference strains, and they belonged to different clades (3). Mutation of glycoproteins C and D of PRV variants led to the escape from Bartha-K61 vaccine-induced immunity (5), so gE/gI/TK-deleted PRV variant strains as a substitute for Bartha-K61 vaccine were used in China to control PR at present. Except for the immunogenicity change, the pathogenicity of PRV variant strains enhanced compared with the classic strain in both pigs and mice; however, it is not clear about the mechanism of enhanced pathogenicity to its hosts (6).

Fluorescent proteins or luciferase-tagged viruses have been widely used in the researches of viral infection and replication mechanisms (7–9). Reporters that have luminescence properties possess greater advantages in some areas of virological research due to higher signal–noise ratio and sensitivity compared with fluorescent proteins (10). Many studies have demonstrated several significant advantages of investigating viral pathogenesis with imaging. Bioluminescence imaging (BLI) is a powerful alternative, enabling rapid measurements of viral load and tissue distribution (11–14). Spatial and temporal progression of infection can be quantified, and viral replication and dissemination in the animals can be identified (15). The traditional approaches for viral pathogenicity studies require the killing of animals at diverse time points for the determination of viral titers in excised organs and tissues, whereas BLI does not (16). In addition, BLI can identify unexpected sites or patterns of viral infection that could be missed if organs are not collected or if entire organs are not analyzed for viral titers (14). This approach has been exploited in multiple viruses, including dengue virus, herpes simplex virus type 1, Sindbis virus, influenza virus, and Sendai virus (12, 14, 15, 17, 18).

Here, we generated a recombinant PRV (rPRVTJ-NLuc) stably expressing the engineered luciferase variant NanoLuc and red fluorescent protein DsRed. NLuc is a 19-kDa luciferase engineered from the deep-sea shrimp that possesses ~150-fold greater specific activity than firefly luciferase (19, 20). The reporter gene of NLuc that fused with DsRed was inserted immediately downstream of the US9 gene. The replication dynamics of the recombinant PRV is similar to PRVTJ. Moreover, rPRVTJ-NLuc possesses pathogenicity and lethality indistinguishable from those of PRVTJ in mice. These results demonstrated that the recombinant PRV was not attenuated both in vitro and in vivo. Furthermore, we reported the visualization of PRV infection in mice. These data suggest that imaging of the recombinant PRV can be used to rapidly assess the replication and pathogenicity characteristics of emerging PRVs; these will provide a reference for control PR caused by PRV variants.

MATERIALS AND METHODS
Cells, Viruses, and Plasmids
The PRVTJ strain (GenBank accession number: KJ789182.1) was isolated from a pig farm outbreak in Tianjin of China, propagated in PK-15 cells, and stored at −70°C. PK-15 and Vero cells were maintained at 37°C with 5% carbon dioxide (CO_2) in Dulbecco's modified Eagle medium (DMEM, Thermo-Fisher Scientific, Carlsbad, CA, United States) supplemented with 10%

fetal bovine serum (Gibco, Grand Island, NY, United States). Both cell lines were obtained from the China Center for Type Culture Collection (Wuhan, China).

The left and right homologous arms (flanking the PRV US9 gene, named as L and R) of transfer vector were amplified by using primer pairs P1S/P1R and P2S/P2R. The NLuc gene was amplified with primers P4S/P4R from pNL2.1 vector (Promega, Madison, WI) and inserted into the DsRed expressing vector pDsRed2-C1 (Clontech, USA) through EcoRI site firstly, and then, the inserted fragment together with CMV promoter and polyA terminator was amplified by PCR with primers P3S/P3R. The resulting L arm, R arm, and exogenous gene were amplified; 100–300 ng of DNA template was used per reaction for overlap PCR; the long DNA segment was cloned into blunt T-vector and sequenced to make sure to get the target sequence. Then, the large DNA segment was amplified, purified, and ligated into the pOK12 vector (Novagene, USA) between the KpnI and XhoI DNA restriction enzyme sites to get the recombinant vector pOK-NLuc-DsRed using T4 DNA ligase (Thermo Scientific, USA).

Transfection, Virus Rescue, and Plaque Purification
The genomic DNA of PRVTJ was extracted using the phenol–chloroform extraction method. Vero cells seeded in six-well culture plates were co-transfected with 1-µg pOK-DsRed-NLuc plasmid and 1-µg genomic DNA of PRVTJ strain using 4 µl of the X-tremeGENE HP DNA transfection reagent (Roche, USA) according to the manufacturer's instructions. The first generation recombinant viruses were collected at 2–3 days after transfection.

For plaque purification, PK-15 cells seeded in six-well cell culture plates were infected with 10-fold serially diluted rPRVTJ-NLuc strain from 10^{-1} to 10^{-5} for 1 h at 37°C in a 5% CO_2 incubator; then, the supernatant was removed; cells were covered with 1% agarose gel and incubated for 2 days till clear cytopathic effect with red fluorescent of DsRed protein formed. Marked plaques were picked by pushing the 200-µl tip through the overlay agarose, and this was diluted in 1-ml DMEM for the next generation of plaque purification. A total of five generations of plaque purification were performed to obtain the purified recombinant viruses.

Virus Titration and One-Step Growth Assay
The viral titer was determined by 50% cell culture infectious dose ($TCID_{50}$). In brief, PK-15 cells seeded in 96-well plates were infected with 10-fold serially diluted viruses (10^{-2} to 10^{-8}) and cultured at 37°C in a 5% CO_2 incubator for 72 h. The number of wells with red fluorescence was counted, and the viral titers were calculated using the Reed & Muench method (21).

One-step growth kinetic of rPRVTJ-NLuc was compared with PRVTJ. The monolayers of PK-15 cells in the 24-well cell culture plates were infected with rPRVTJ-NLuc or PRVTJ at a multiplicity of infection (MOI) of 10 for 1 h at 37°C. Extracellular viruses were inactivated by low-PH treatment (22); supernatant and cells were harvested at different time points (12-h interval) till 60-h post-infection; three repeat samples were harvested at each time point and stored at −80°C. After the sample returned to room temperate, the cellular debris was removed by centrifugation, and the $TCID_{50}$ of supernatant was detected on PK-15 cells. Average values and standard deviations of the three independent experiments were calculated.

Polymerase Chain Reaction

Genomic DNA was extracted from PK-15 cells infected with rPRVTJ-NLuc or PRVTJ at an MOI of 1 for 12 h using the Tissue DNA Kit (Omega). The primer pairs P5S/P5R, P6S/P6R, and P7S/P7R that were complementary to the glycoprotein B (gB), glyco-protein I (gI), NLuc luciferase, and DsRed fluorescent protein genes are listed in **Table 1**. The amplification was conducted in a total volume of 50 µl containing 25 µl of 2× PrimeSTAR buffer (TaKaRa, Japan), 3 µl of DNA, 9.5 µl of sterilized water, and 1.0 mM for each primer. The reaction was heated at 95°C for 5 min, followed by 35 cycles of 98°C for 10 s, 58°C for 30 s, and 72°C for 2 min, with a final elongation step of 72°C for 10 min. The PCR product was analyzed using 1.0% agarose gel electrophoresis.

Western Blot Assay

The monolayers of PK-15 cells in the 6-well cell culture plates were infected with rPRVTJ-NLuc, rPRVTJ-DsRed, or PRVTJ A at an MOI of 1 at 37°C for 24 h. The total protein of cells was collected after adding an NP40 lysis buffer containing 1% phenylmethylsulfonyl fluoride (Solarbio, Beijing, China) prot, separated by sodium dodecyl sulfate-polyacrylamide gel electrophoresis, and transferred onto nitrocellulose membranes. The membranes were blocked with 5% skim milk for 2 h at 37°C and incubated at room temperature for 2 h with specific mouse anti-gD, an anti-gB monoclonal antibody (a gift of Jing Zhao, State Key Laboratory of Veterinary Biotechnology, Harbin Veterinary Research Institute, Chinese Academy of Agricultural Sciences, Harbin, China) and anti-DsRed polyclonal antibody (Solarbio, Beijing, China). The membranes were washed with phosphate-buffered saline (PBS) with Tween buffer for three times and incubated with DyLight 800 goat anti-mouse IgG (1:8,000) (Thermo Fisher Scientific) at 37°C for 45 min; the membranes were washed for another three times, then visualized and analyzed with an Odyssey infrared imaging system (LI-COR Biosciences, Lincoln, NE, USA).

Luciferase Assay

PK-15 cells seeded in 96-well cell culture plates were infected with 10-fold serially diluted rPRVTJ-NLuc strain from 10^0 to 10^{-5} at 37°C in a 5% CO_2 incubator for 12 h. The supernatants were removed, and cells were washed once with PBS before cell culture lysis buffer (Promega) was added. Cell lysates were assayed for luminescence activity with the Nano-Glo Assay System (Promega), and luminescence was detected with TD-20/20 luminometer (Turner Designs).

Infection of Mice With rPRVTJ-NLuc or PRVTJ and Tissue Collection

All the mice were handled according to the Guide for the Care and Use of Laboratory Animals of Harbin Veterinary Research Institute (HVRI), Chinese Academy of Agricultural Sciences,

TABLE 1 | Sequences of oligonucleotides used in PCR.

Fragments	Primers	Sequences of primers (5'-3')	Length (bp)
L arm	P1S	GGTGCCTGCTGTACTACGTGTACGA GCCCTGCATC	1274
	P1R	CTACACGTGCCTGGCGACGATGCC	
R arm	P2S	CGAGCGAGCGAGCGAACGGGAG	1023
	P2R	CTAGGAGATGGTACATCGCGGGGCGC GCTCGCG	
CMV-DsRed -polyA	P3S	TAGATAACTGATCATAATCAGCCATACCA	1486
	P3R	CGCCGTTTAAACGCAGTGAAAAAAATGCTTTA	
NLuc	P4S	GTCTTCACACTCGAAGATTTC	513
	P4R	TTACGCCAGAATGCGTTCGCAC	
gB	P5S	GGGGTTGGACAGGAAGGACACCA	198
	P5R	AACCAGCTGCACGCGCTCAA	
gI	P6S	TGGCTCTGCGTGCTGTGCTC	343
	P6R	CATTCGTCACTTCCGGTTTC	
DsRed	P7S	ATGGCCTCCTCCGAGAACG	747
	P7R	TTATCTAGATCCGGTGGAACCCG	

China. Two mice experiments were made in this work: one for the pathogen detection and another one for the live imaging test. For the pathogen detection, 35 6-week-old specific-pathogen-free (SPF) female BALB/c mice were used in this study. The mice were randomly allocated into seven groups, five mice in one box. Mice of groups 1, 2, and 3 were injected intramuscularly (i.m.) with 10^4, 10^3, or 10^2 $TCID_{50}$ of PRV TJ strain in 100-µl DMEM, respectively. Groups 4, 5, and 6 were injected i.m. with 10^4, 10^3, or 10^2 $TCID_{50}$ rPRVTJ-NLuc in 100 µl of DMEM, respectively. Group 7 was the mock-inoculations (medium only) in parallel. Mice were scored daily for symptoms of PRV infection using the following three-point system adapted from the protocol previously described (23). All the mice in the infected and control groups were anesthetized by CO_2 before euthanasia, using the broken-neck method at 7 dpi. Fresh tissues from the heart, liver, spleen, lungs, kidneys, brain, spinal cord, and trigeminal ganglion of mice were collected, one part of the samples was fixed in buffered formalin for hematoxylin and eosin assay, and 100 mg of another part of the samples was stored at −80°C for DNA extraction. Total DNA was extracted using Tissue DNA Kit (Omega) according to the manufacturer's instructions and stored at −20°C for quantitative PCR (qPCR) analysis.

Real-Time PCR (Quantitative PCR)

Real-time PCR (qPCR) was used to quantitatively analyze the viral loading in the brain, heart, liver, spleen, lung, kidney, spinal cord, and trigeminal ganglion using the reported method of Meng (24). Briefly, viral genomic DNA was amplified using the gI gene-specific primer PRV-F1 (5'-GCC GAG TAC CTC TGC C-3'), PRV-R1 (5'-CGA GAC GAA CAG CCG-3'), and TaqMan probes HEX-PRV-Var (HEX-5'-CCG CGT GCA CCA CGA AGC CT-3'-BHQ1); each sample was done in triplicate, deionized water as the negative control.

Pathology and Histopathology

The samples were fixed in buffered formalin and embedded in paraffin wax. Tissue sections were prepared and stained with hematoxylin and eosin assay for histopathological examinations.

In vivo Imaging

For the live imaging test, a total of 30 7-week-old SPF female BALB/c mice were separated into six groups for PRV infection, five mice in each group, and another five mice were injected with DMEM as control. Mice were infected with 10^3 TCID$_{50}$ rPRVTJ-NLuc or PRVTJ by three different inoculation routes: inoculated intraperitoneally (i.p.) (in the lower abdominal region), i.m. (in the right hind leg muscles), or subcutaneously (s.c.) (in the back of the neck). *In vivo* imaging was performed from 3 to 7 dpi with a 24-h interval using the BLI system of the LB 983 NightOWL II (Berthold, Germany) equipped with a cooled slow-scan CCD camera and driven by the IndiGo^{TM} software (version 2.0.5.0, Berthold). At each time point, five mice in each group per day were anesthetized with isoflurane (Burbank, CA 91502, USA) and injected with 100 μl of Nano-Glo reagent (Promega) (diluted 1:20 in PBS) *via* the tail vein. Flux measurements were acquired from regions of interest automatically gated to the signal contours, keeping the mice at 37°C during the whole progress. All the mice in the infected and control groups were anesthetized by CO_2 before euthanasia, using the broken-neck method after imaging the experiment. All data in composite images utilized the same scale.

Statistics

Data represent means ± standard deviations ($n \geq 3$). The comparison between groups was performed by a Student's *t*-test with a two-tailed analysis. Data are considered significant when $P < 0.05$.

RESULTS

Generation and Characterization of the Recombinant Pseudorabies Virus Expressing NanoLuc

PRV genome is characterized by two unique regions (U$_L$ and U$_S$), and the U$_S$ region flanked by internal and terminal repeat sequences. As reported, the noncoding interval sequence between U$_S$9 open reading frame and U$_S$2 open reading frame in the U$_S$ regions is long enough to tolerate large exogenous genes (25). A single cassette of NLuc fused with the DsRed was designed immediately downstream of the US9 gene of the PRV TJ genome (**Figure 1A**). The transfer vector pOK-DsRed-NLuc with two 1.5-kb homologous arms and PRVTJ genomic DNA were co-transfected into Vero cells, and the first generation of recombinant virus was collected at 2–3 days after transfection when the cytopathic effect formed on the Vero cells. We obtained the purified virus through five rounds of plaque purification. The plaque morphology of rPRVTJ-NLuc had no significant difference from its parental virus (**Figure 1B**). We confirmed that the chimeric NLuc cassette was inserted immediately into the downstream of the US9 gene of PRVTJ using corresponding specific primers by PCR and sequencing. The stability of the

reporter genes, NLuc, and DsRed, was also tested by following amplification and serial passages in PK-15 cells (P1 to P20) (**Figure 1D**). These results indicated there were gB and gI genes in the genome backbone of the recombinant PRV, which was the same as its parental strain. Also, the reporter genes could exist in the backbone simultaneously and stably, which were detected in the following passages. The expression of DsRed and viral protein was checked by Western blot using antibody target DsRed, gD, and gB proteins. The same bands of gB and gD presented in the samples of rPRVTJ-NLuc, rPRVTJ-DsRed, and PRVTJ infected groups; meanwhile, the band of DsRed protein of rPRVTJ-NLuc was larger than rPRVTJ-DsRed due to NLuc fused with it (**Figure 1E**).

We compared the growth kinetics of rPRVTJ-NLuc with the parental strain PRVTJ in PK-15 cells. The titers of rPRVTJ-NLuc in the culture supernatant had no significant difference with those of PRVTJ during 60-h post-infection (hpi), suggesting that the growth properties of rPRVTJ-NLuc were similar to those of PRVTJ (**Figure 1C**). To examine the relationship between NLuc expression level and rPRVTJ-NLuc infection, the correlation between the input of rPRVTJ-NLuc and NLuc luciferase activities was evaluated. PK-15 cells were infected with rPRVTJ-NLuc with different amounts of input virus: ranging from 10^0 to 10^5 TCID$_{50}$/ml. NLuc luciferase activities were measured at 12 hpi. The activities of luciferase in supernatants increased over time, and the yield of luminescent flux was directly correlated with viral titers ($R^2 = 0.96$) (**Figures 1F,G**). The result demonstrated that the luminescent flux could represent the titer of the recombinant PRV in the infected cell.

rPRVTJ-NLuc Possesses Similar Pathogenicity to PRVTJ in Mice

To monitor symptoms and organ lesions preferably, mice were infected with 10^4, 10^3, or 10^2 TCID$_{50}$ PRVTJ or rPRVTJ-NLuc *via* the i.m. route. Clinical signs, including pruritus, anxiety, rolling, and scratching of the injection site, were recorded every day throughout the experiment. The mice infected with 10^4 TCID$_{50}$ viruses (groups 1 and 4) began showing clinical signs around 72 hpi. The mice infected with 10^3 TCID$_{50}$ viruses (groups 2 and 5) showed similar symptoms but delayed. The mice infected with 10^2 TCID$_{50}$ doses of viruses (groups 3 and 6) showed barely clinical symptoms. No difference was observed in the clinical performance of mice injected with the same dose of PRVTJ and rPRVTJ-NLuc (**Table 2**). Mice infected with 10^4, 10^3, or 10^2 TCID$_{50}$ of PRVTJ or rPRVTJ-NLuc lost body weight and led to die in a dose-dependent manner (**Figures 2A, B**). The mice infected with the same dose of PRVTJ or rPRVTJ-NLuc exhibited similar weight loss and mortality. These results demonstrated that the clinical symptoms of the recombinant PRV did not change after the insertion of the reporter genes.

Next, we determined whether the fatal clinical outcome and distinct pathology of the mice that were infected could be attributed to viral replication in specific tissues. Various tissues, as listed earlier, were collected after euthanasia for qPCR analysis to determine PRV DNA loads. As shown in **Figure 2C**, the virus could be detected in the brain, kidney, spinal cord, and

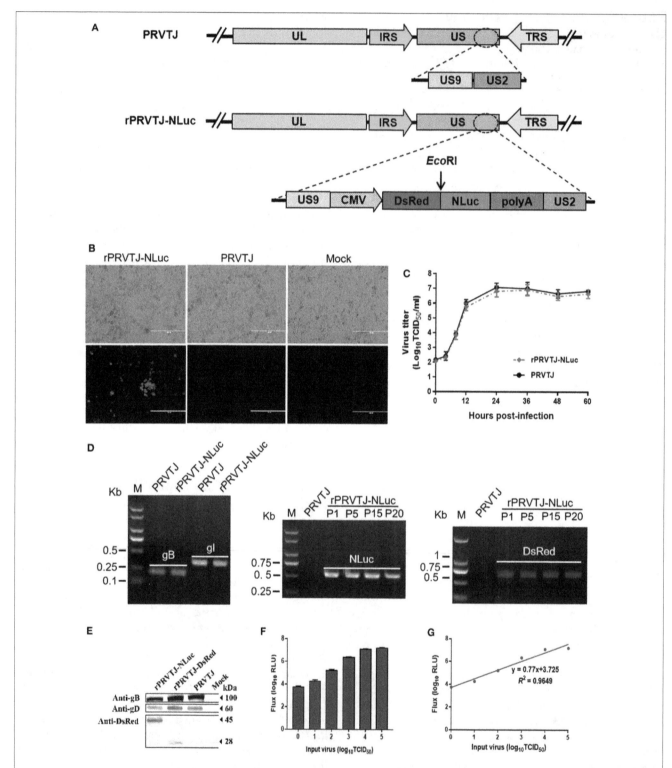

FIGURE 1 | Generation and characterization of the recombinant PRV expressing NLuc luciferase. **(A)** Schematic representation of NLuc and DsRed cassette inserting immediately downstream of the *US9* gene. **(B)** Recombinant PRV can form plaques and express DsRed in the PRV-infected PK-15 cells. Original magnification ×200; bar, 400 µm. **(C)** One-step growth curve of rPRVTJ-NLuc. **(D)** Identify of rPRVTJ-NLuc by PCR. Left panel, verification of the *gB*, *gI* gene in the genome of rPRVTJ-NLuc, and PRVTJ. Middle panel and right panel, identification of the NLuc and DsRed reporter genes in different passages in infected PK-15 cells, respectively. **(E)** Expression of NLuc fused with DsRed in rPRVTJ-NLuc-infected cells was detected by Western blot, the DsRed expression of rPRVTJ-DsRed as control; moreover, viral protein gD and gB of all PRV strains were also detected using anti-gD and anti-gB monoclonal antibodies, normal cells as mock. **(F)** Average luciferase activity of the recombinant PRV in the PK-15 cells at 12 hpi with defined amounts of input virus (*n* = 5). **(G)** Correlation curve between titers of virus and luciferase activities using Pearson's correlation coefficient.

TABLE 2 | Clinical signs score of the mice infected with rPRVTJ-NLuc or PRVTJ.

Virus	Dose (TCID$_{50}$)	Days post-infection						
		1	2	3	4	5	6	7
PRVTJ	10^4	0	0	11 ± 1	-	-	-	-
	10^3	0	0	6.6 ± 0.55	-	-	-	-
	10^2	0	0	4 ± 0.71	7.25 ± 0.5	4 ± 1	2 ± 1	2 ± 0
rPRVTJ-NLuc	10^4	0	0	9.75 ± 0.96	-	-	-	-
	10^3	0	0	4.5 ± 1	10 ± 1.73	5 ± 0	-	-
	10^2	0	0	3 ± 0.71	5.8 ± 0.84	2.6 ± 0.89	2 ± 1	3 ± 0
DMEM	100 µl	0	0	0	0	0	0	0

Extended scoring systems for clinical signs. Clinical signs were recorded every day, incorporating 4 parameters such as:pruritus, anxiety, rolling and scratching of the injection site, each parameter was scored from 0 = no clinical symptom; 1 = mild symptoms, such as subtle neurological symptoms, untidy hair and minor depression; 2 = common symptoms, such as pruritus, rolling and scratching the injection site; 3 = severe symptoms, such as severe pruritus, self-mutilate even acute death. The results are expressed as mean value ± s.d. (n = 5) of total value of 4 parameters. -, death.

trigeminal ganglion of peracute death mice infected with 10^4 or 10^3 TCID$_{50}$ PRVs groups (groups 1, 2, 4, and 5). No virus was detected in the 10^2 TCID$_{50}$ groups (groups 3 and 6), as well as the control group (group 7). PRV replication was detected principally in kidneys, brain, spinal cord, and trigeminal ganglion tissues after i.m. injection, but there was no significant difference in PRV DNA loads between rPRVTJ-NLuc and PRVTJ infected groups, which was consistent with the clinical signs score and pathological analysis, indicating that the replication and spread properties of rPRVTJ-NLuc were similar to those of the parental strain.

Histopathological examination of several tissues (brain, lungs, and kidneys) was performed to check the difference between the mice infected with PRVTJ and rPRVTJ-NLuc (**Figure 2D**), and tissue samples were taken from three mice in each group at the humane endpoint. Firstly, there were local hemorrhage, degeneration, necrosis of partial neuron, Purkinje cell, and glial cell proliferation in the brain of both PRV infected groups. The lungs of the PRV-infected groups showed congestion, the proliferation of alveolar epithelial cells, and a few lymphocytes infiltration. There were degeneration and necrosis of renal tubular epithelial cells in the kidneys of the PRV infected groups. Secondly, it is noteworthy that low-dose PRV infection induces significant histopathological changes in the central nervous system (CNS) of mice as well. The histopathological changes of these mice organs infected with PRVTJ or rPRVTJ-NLuc did not differ on every dosage. Finally, the heart, liver, and spleen of all the PRV-infected mice and all the mice infected with 10^2 TCID$_{50}$ (groups 3 and 6) PRV had no histopathological changes. Collectively, these data indicated that the insertion of NLuc into the PRV genome did not influence histopathological changes of PRV-infected mice.

In summary, there is no difference in clinical symptoms, replication, spread, and histopathology between the mice infected with rPRVTJ-NLuc and its parental virus. So, the insertion of NLuc into the PRV genome was stable, and the recombinant

rPRVTJ-NLuc could be used as a tool to study the pathogenicity of PRVTJ.

In vivo Imaging of rPRVTJ-NLuc Showed the Viral Replication and Dissemination in Mice

BLI has been exploited in multiple viruses, including dengue virus, herpes simplex virus type 1, Sindbis virus, and Sendai virus (15, 17, 18). Here, we used rPRVTJ-NLuc to visualize PRV replication and spread in mice. Seven-week-old BALB/c mice were infected with 10^3 TCID$_{50}$ rPRVTJ-NLuc and subjected to daily imaging (**Figure 3A**). Bioluminescence was detected as early as 4 dpi at the site of injection. Luminescent flux increased throughout infection and peaked on day 6, then waning. The enhanced signal could be detected when rPRVTJ-NLuc spread from the injection site to the superior respiratory tract.

To get better *in vivo* images, mice were infected with rPRVTJ-NLuc and PRVTJ by three different inoculation routes. Mice were infected with 10^3 TCID$_{50}$ viruses *via* inoculated i.p. (in the lower abdominal region), i.m. (in the right hind leg muscles), or s.c. (in the back of the neck). As expected, mice infected with rPRVTJ-NLuc displayed robust bioluminescence, which started 4 dpi, increased over time, peaked at 5 dpi, remained detectable for at least 6 dpi (**Figure 3B**), and disappeared at 7 dpi when the virus was cleared after a sublethal infection. All mice inoculated viruses *via* i.m. route showed severe clinical symptoms at 4 dpi, pruritus, rolling, and scratching the injection site, and all died at 5 dpi. This result illustrated that the i.m. route may more easily cause peracute death. Real-time imaging of the same mouse over time from each group revealed viral load and dissemination from the injection site to the spinal cord and CNS.

To confirm the local tissues scattering bioluminescence, selected mice were killed, and their organs were immediately removed. Isolated organs were placed in a furimazine bath, and BLI was undertaken. Signals of the spinal cord, trigeminal ganglion, and a partial region of the brain were observed (**Figure 3C**). There were robust bioluminescence signals in the spinal cord, brain, and trigeminal ganglion based on the flux of each excised organs (**Figure 3C**). These results were consistent with the viral distribution in diverse organs of mice infected with rPRVTJ-NLuc, which possessed the ability to visualize a pathogenic infection in mice.

DISCUSSION

Since late 2011, there were PR-like outbreaks in a large number of vaccinated pig farms in China (26). It is found that the PRV variant strain and the classical strain belong to different phylogenetic branches. In our previous study, the epidemic strain exhibited enhanced pathogenicity in mice and pigs (6). The reemergence of the PRV outbreak resulted in huge economic losses to the pig industry in China, so the ability that can quickly assess the pathogenicity of the epidemic strains and its susceptibility to antiviral interventions was urgently required.

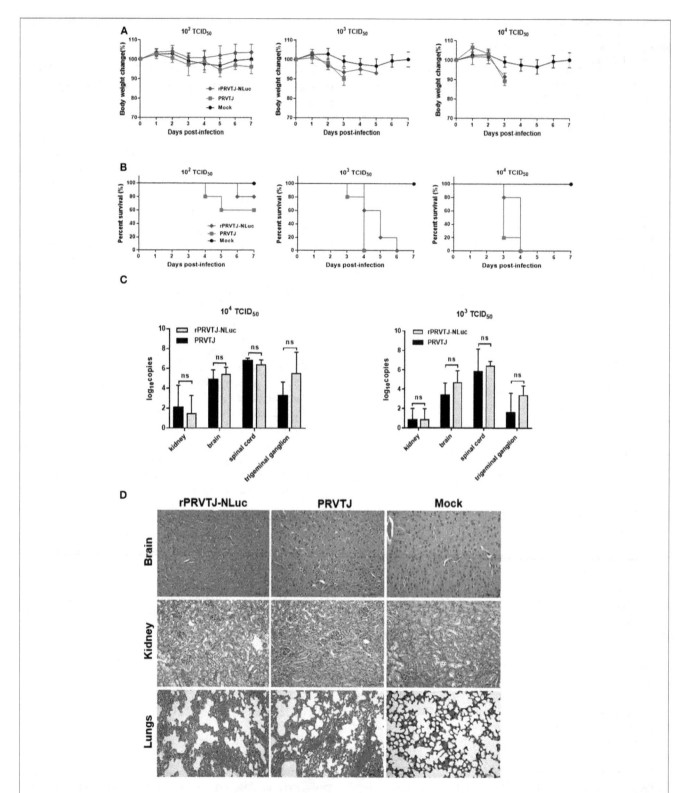

FIGURE 2 | Pathogenicity of recombinant PRV compared with PRVTJ in mice. Six-week-old SPF BALB/c mice were injected intramuscularly with 10^4, 10^3, or 10^2 $TCID_{50}$ of rPRVTJ-NLuc or PRVTJ. **(A)** Average body weights of the infected mice ($n = 5$) at 7 dpi. **(B)** Survival rates of mice infected indicated a dose of viruses. **(C)** Viral DNA copies in different tissue. All the mock-infected and PRV-infected mice were euthanized and subjected to dissection at a moribund stage or 7 dpi. Specific tissues were collected from the mice infected with 10^4 or 10^3 $TCID_{50}$ rPRVTJ-NLuc or PRVTJ and tested by qPCR. **(D)** Histopathological changes in diverse organs of mice infected with rPRVTJ-NLuc or PRVTJ; bar = $100\,\mu m$.

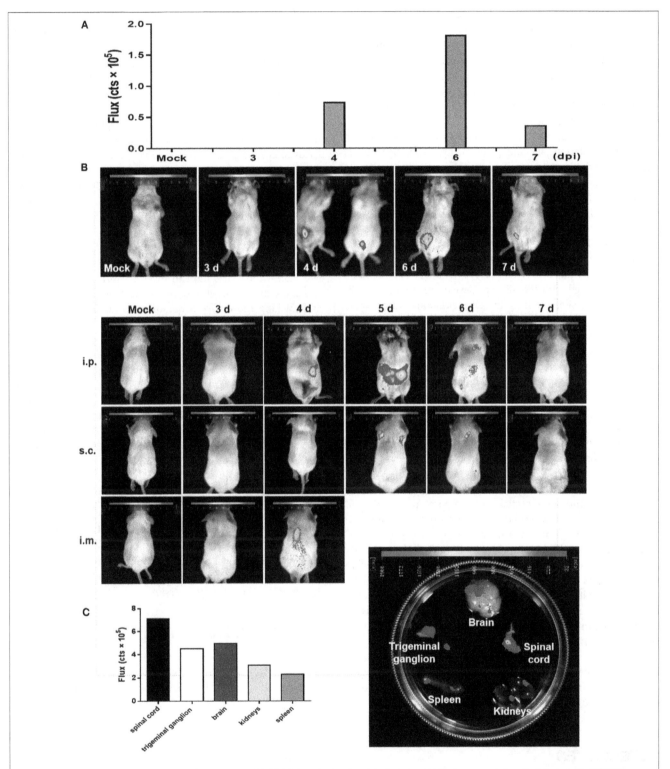

FIGURE 3 | *In vivo* imaging of a PRV reporter in a mouse model. **(A)** Noninvasive imaging detected robust bioluminescence in the mice infected with 10^3 $TCID_{50}$ rPRVTJ-NLuc or PRVTJ and analyzed for bioluminescence at indicated time points. **(B)** Longitudinal *in vivo* imaging of rPRVTJ-NLuc in mice showed viral replication and dissemination. Mice were inoculated intraperitoneally, subcutaneously, or intramuscularly with 10^3 $TCID_{50}$ rPRVTJ-NLuc and PRVTJ. *In vivo* imaging was performed every day from 3 dpi at the indicated time points. **(C)** *In situ* localization of NLuc luciferase activity in the excised organs of mice infected with the recombinant PRV. Seven-week-old SPF BALB/c mice were i.p. inoculated with 10^3 $TCID_{50}$ rPRVTJ-NLuc and killed at 4 dpi. Organs were dissected out and placed separately in a substrate bath. Bioluminescent images were taken 10 min later, and the representative image shows the distribution of luminescent activity in the specimen (right). Quantification of the luminescent activity in the excised organs. After an exposure time of 30 s, a region of interest was manually defined, and the luminescent activity was calculated by the IndiGo™ software (left). All the images of the mice shown in the figure were one representation of five repeats.

In this study, we constructed a recombinant PRV stably expressing the NLuc luciferase fusion with red fluorescent protein DsRed. The double-labeled strategy is convenient for *in vitro* screening of the recombinant virus with DsRed and the *in vivo* imaging with NLuc luciferase. There was no difference in the growth properties of rPRVTJ-NLuc and PRVTJ. Moreover, the recombinant rPRVTJ-NLuc possessed pathogenicity and lethality in mice indistinguishable from those of PRVTJ.

The infection of PRV in rodents routinely shows severe clinical manifestations, including pretty itchy, frantically clawing, and biting of the inoculation site, even self-mutilation and acute death eventually (27). To monitor the symptoms and organ lesions preferably, we infected mice with a lower dosage, 10^4, 10^3, or 10^2 TCID$_{50}$ PRVTJ, or rPRVTJ-NLuc *via* i.m. route. Similar symptoms were found in mice infected with 10^4 or 10^3 TCID$_{50}$ PRVTJ or rPRVTJ-NLuc; the groups of 10^2 TCID$_{50}$ viruses and control were no symptomatic; all these results were the same as Brittle reported. Previous studies demonstrated that mice infected with PRV-Becker develop severe pruritus in the inoculation site, resulting in self-mutilation and peracute death with no detectable behavioral CNS pathology and no obvious pathological changes in the brain. Merely, the peripheral nervous system (dorsal root ganglia and trigeminal ganglia) has significant pathological changes (2, 28). Nevertheless, we detected the replication of the virus and inflammatory pathological changes in CNS tissue and kidneys of mice; maybe, these explained why PRVTJ has higher pathogenicity than the classic PRV strains.

The sensitivity and noninvasive longitudinal measurements enable the monitoring of PRV infection and clearance of a lower-dose infection of rPRVTJ-NLuc in mice (**Figures 3A,B**). Actually, 6-week-old mice were tended to death because of PRV infection. To obtain continuously spatial and temporal progression of PRV infection, the 7-week-old mice were used to perform *in vivo* imaging. In a mouse inoculated i.p. with the dose of 10^3 TCID$_{50}$, the infection began primarily in i.p. injection site. By 6 dpi, the bioluminescence signal decreased and appeared in the position of the spinal cord, indicating the spread of the virus to the CNS. We confirmed the infection of the spinal cord by imaging of excised organs and qPCR (**Figure 3C**), showing stronger bioluminescence and higher virus load in the spinal cord than *in vivo* image. The infection continued to be cleared and was undetectable at 7 dpi. This longitudinal measurement course could detect the dynamics of PRV by *in vivo* imaging and elucidate mechanisms of viral dissemination in a mouse model. It is compelling that a series of reporter virus expressing

the NLuc luciferase has the potential to assess the pathogenicity and properties of viral replication and *in vivo* dissemination of diverse PRV stains. Thus, this strategy should be widely applicable to any PRV isolate and will be useful to rapidly access the replication and pathogenicity characteristics of emerging PRV strains.

Although the BLI potentially offers significant advantages over other traditional virological methods, it also has a few disadvantages, e.g., the attenuation of the signal by hair and organ pigmentation, overlapping signals, and the attenuation of signals due to organ depth from the surface. Bioluminescence was not detected in the brain in any of our experiments of whole-body imaging, which is most probably due to the signal attenuation caused by the skull of mice. We confirmed the bioluminescence signal in the brain and trigeminal ganglion by imaging of excised organs. The result is consistent with detectable viral distribution in diverse tissues. Therefore, these data show that although bioluminescence is promising, precise viral tracking and the exact quantification of viral titers require combinations of these methodologies.

In summary, the recombinant PRV stably expressing NLuc luciferase is shown to be a potential tool for studying the pathogenicity mechanism of the PRV variant. We further showed that the recombinant PRV could be applied to study the infection mechanisms of PRVTJ strain by BLI. In further studies, the reporter virus will be used in the research of pathogenicity mechanism diversity of PRV variants and classic strains.

AUTHOR CONTRIBUTIONS

YS and H-JQ designed research. YW and HW performed experiments. BW wrote the manuscript. The authors YW, HW, and BW have the equal contribution for this work and all authors reviewed the manuscript. All authors contributed to the article and approved the submitted version.

ACKNOWLEDGMENTS

We thank HQ, ZJ, and employees of the Research Institute for Biological Safety Problems for their assistance in the present study.

REFERENCES

1. Verpoest S, Cay B, Favoreel H, De Regge N. Age-dependent differences in pseudorabies virus neuropathogenesis and associated cytokine expression. *J Virol.* 91:JVI.02058-16. doi: 10.1128/JVI.02058-16

2. Sun Y, Luo Y, Wang CH, Yuan J, Li N, Song K, et al. Control of swine pseudorabies in China: opportunities and limitations. *Vet Microbiol.* (2016) 183:119–24. doi: 10.1016/j.vetmic.2015.12.008

3. An TQ, Peng JM, Tian ZJ, Zhao HY, Li N, Liu YM, et al. Pseudorabies virus

variant in Bartha-K61-Vaccinated pigs, China, 2012. *Emerg Infect Dis.* (2013) 19:1749–55. doi: 10.3201/eid1911.130177

4. Gu J, Hu D, Peng T, Wang Y, Ma Z, Liu Z, et al. Epidemiological investigation of pseudorabies in Shandong Province from 2013 to 2016. *Transbound Emerg Dis.* (2018) 65:890–8. doi: 10.1111/tbed.12827

5. Ren JL, Wang HB, Zhou L, Ge XN, Guo X, Han J, et al. Glycoproteins C and D of PRV strain HB1201 contribute individually to the escape from bartha-K61 vaccine-induced immunity. *Front Microbiol.* (2020) 11:323. doi: 10.3389/fmicb.2020.00323

6. Luo Y, Li N, Cong X, Wang CH, Du M, Li L, et al. Pathogenicity and genomic characterization of a pseudorabies virus variant isolated from Bartha-K61-

vaccinated swine population in China. *Vet Microbiol.* (2014) 174:107–15. doi: 10.1016/j.vetmic.2014.09.003

7. Hoenen T, Groseth A, Callison J, Takada A, Feldmann H. A novel Ebola virus expressing luciferase allows for rapid and quantitative testing of antivirals. *Antiviral Res.* (2013) 99:207–13. doi: 10.1016/j.antiviral.2013.05.017

8. Hogue IB, Bosse JB, Engel EA, Scherer J, Hu JR, Del Rio T, et al. Fluorescent protein approaches in alpha herpesvirus research. *Viruses.* (2015) 7:5933–61. doi: 10.3390/v7112915

9. Anindita PD, Sasaki M, Nobori H, Sato A, Carr M, Ito N, et al. Generation of recombinant rabies viruses encoding NanoLuc luciferase for antiviral activity assays. *Virus Res.* (2016) 215:121–8. doi: 10.1016/j.virusres.2016.02.002

10. Rameix-Welti MA, Le Goffic R, Herve PL, Sourimant J, Remot A, Riffault S, et al. Visualizing the replication of respiratory syncytial virus in cells and in living mice. *Nat Commun.* (2014) 5:5104. doi: 10.1038/ncomms6104

11. Schoggins JW, Dorner M, Feulner M, Imanaka N, Murphy MY, Ploss A, et al. Dengue reporter viruses reveal viral dynamics in interferon receptor-deficient mice and sensitivity to interferon effectors in vitro. *Proc Natl Acad Sci USA.* (2012) 109:14610–5. doi: 10.1073/pnas.1212379109

12. Tran V, Moser LA, Poole DS, Mehle A. Highly sensitive real-time in vivo imaging of an influenza reporter virus reveals dynamics of replication and spread. *J Virol.* (2013) 87:13321–13329. doi: 10.1128/JVI.02381-13

13. Pan W, Dong Z, Li F, Meng W, Feng L, Niu X, et al. Visualizing influenza virus infection in living mice. *Nat Commun.* (2013) 4:2369. doi: 10.1038/ncomms3369

14. Karlsson EA, Meliopoulos VA, Savage C, Livingston B, Mehle A, Schultz-Cherry S. Visualizing real-time influenza virus infection, transmission and protection in ferrets. *Nat Commun.* (2015) 6:6378. doi: 10.1038/ncomms7378

15. Cook SH, Griffin DE. Luciferase imaging of a neurotropic viral infection in intact animals. *J Virol.* (2003) 77:5333–8. doi: 10.1128/JVI.77.9.5333-5338.2003

16. Luker KE, Hutchens M, Schultz T, Pekosz A, Luker GD. Bioluminescence imaging of vaccinia virus: effects of interferon on viral replication and spread. *Virology.* (2005) 341:284–300. doi: 10.1016/j.virol.2005.06.049

17. Luker GD, Bardill JP, Prior JL, Pica CM, Piwnica-Worms D, Leib DA. Noninvasive bioluminescence imaging of herpes simplex virus type 1 infection and therapy in living mice. *J Virol.* (2002) 76:12149–61. doi: 10.1128/JVI.76.23.12149-12161.2002

18. Burke CW, Mason JN, Surman SL, Jones BG, Dalloneau E, Hurwitz JL, et al. Illumination of parainfluenza virus infection and transmission in living animals reveals a tissue-specific dichotomy. *PLoS Pathog.* (2011) 7:e1002134. doi: 10.1371/journal.ppat.1002134

19. Hall MP, Unch J, Binkowski BF, Valley MP, Butler BL, Wood MG, et al. Engineered luciferase reporter from a deep sea shrimp utilizing a novel imidazopyrazinone substrate. *ACS Chem Biol.* (2012) 7:1848–57. doi: 10.1021/cb3002478

20. England CG, Ehlerding EB, Cai W. NanoLuc: A small luciferase is brightening up the field of bioluminescence. *Bioconjug Chem.* (2016) 27:1175–87. doi: 10.1021/acs.bioconjchem.6b00112

21. Reed LJ, Muench H. A simple method of estimating fifty percent endpoints. *AM J EPIDEMIOL.* (1938) 27:493–7. doi: 10.1093/oxfordjournals.aje.a118408

22. Mettenleiter T. Glycoprotein gIII deletion mutants of pseudorabies virus are impaired in virus entry. *Virology.* (1989) 171:623–5. doi: 10.1016/0042-6822(89)90635-1

23. Wang J, Guo R, Qiao Y, Xu M, Wang Z, Liu Y, et al. An inactivated gE-deleted pseudorabies vaccine provides complete clinical protection and reduces virus shedding against challenge by a Chinese pseudorabies variant. *BMC Vet Res.* (2016) 12:277. doi: 10.1186/s12917-016-0897-z

24. Meng XY, Luo Y, Liu Y, Shao L, Sun Y, Li Y, et al. A triplex real-time PCR for differential detection of classical, variant and Bartha-K61 vaccine strains of pseudorabies virus. *Arch Virol.* (2016) 161:2425–30. doi: 10.1007/s00705-016-2925-5

25. Tang YD, Liu JT, Fang QQ, Wang TY, Sun MX, An TX, et al. Recombinant pseudorabies virus (PRV) expressing firefly Luciferase effectively screened for CRISPR/Cas9 single guide RNAs and antiviral compounds. *Viruses.* (2016) 8:90. doi: 10.3390/v8040090

26. Tong W, Liu F, Zheng H, Liang C, Zhou YJ, Jiang YF, et al. Emergence of a

Pseudorabies virus variant with increased virulence to piglets. *Vet Microbiol.* (2015) 181:236–40. doi: 10.1016/j.vetmic.2015.09.021

27. Brittle EE, Reynolds AE, Enquist LW. Two modes of pseudorabies virus neuroinvasion and lethality in mice. *J Virol.* (2004) 78:12951–63. doi: 10.1128/JVI.78.23.12951-12963.2004

6

Epidemiology and Associated Risk Factors for Brucellosis in Small Ruminants Kept at Institutional Livestock Farms in Punjab, Pakistan

Qudrat Ullah [1,2,3†], Tariq Jamil [1,4*†], Falk Melzer [1], Muhammad Saqib [5*],
Muhammad Hammad Hussain [6], Muhammad Aamir Aslam [7], Huma Jamil [3],
Muhammad Amjad Iqbal [8], Usman Tahir [9], Shakeeb Ullah [2], Zafar Iqbal Qureshi [3],
Stefan Schwarz [4] and Heinrich Neubauer [1]

[1] Institute of Bacterial Infections and Zoonoses, Friedrich-Loeffler-Institut, Jena, Germany, [2] Faculty of Veterinary and Animal Sciences, Gomal University, Dera Ismail Khan, Pakistan, [3] Department of Theriogenology, Faculty of Veterinary Science, University of Agriculture, Faisalabad, Pakistan, [4] Institute of Microbiology and Epizootics, Freie Universität, Berlin, Germany, [5] Department of Clinical Medicine and Surgery, Faculty of Veterinary Science, University of Agriculture, Faisalabad, Pakistan, [6] Independent Researcher, Bardia, NSW, Australia, [7] Institute of Microbiology, Faculty of Veterinary Science, University of Agriculture, Faisalabad, Pakistan, [8] Veterinary Research Institute, Lahore, Pakistan, [9] Livestock and Dairy Development, Government of Punjab, Lahore, Pakistan

*Correspondence:
Tariq Jamil
tariq.jamil@fli.de
Muhammad Saqib
drsaqib_vet@hotmail.com

†These authors have contributed
equally to this work

Brucellosis is reportedly endemic in ruminants in Pakistan. Both *Brucella abortus* and *B. melitensis* infections have been documented in domestic animals and humans in the country. This study aimed to identify the burden of anti-*Brucella* antibodies in small ruminants as well as associated potential risk factors with its occurrence at nine institutional livestock farms in Punjab, Pakistan. The sera collected from equal number of sheep and goats (500 from each species) were screened by indirect-ELISA for anti-smooth-*Brucella* antibodies followed by a serial detection by real-time PCR. Overall, 5.1% (51/1000) seropositivity was registered corresponding to 5% (25/500) prevalence in goats and 5.2% (26/500) in sheep. *Brucella*-DNA could not be detected in any of the tested sera by real-time PCR. Multiple logistic regression model indicated that farm location (OR 34.05), >4 years of age (OR 2.88), with history of reproductive disorders (OR 2.69), and with BCS of ≤3 (OR 12.37) were more likely to test positive for brucellosis at these farms. A routine screening, stringent biosecurity, and quarantine measures are warranted for monitoring and eradication of the infection. Similarly, isolation and molecular investigation of the etiologic agent(s) are needed to understand the relationship of epidemiology and out-breaks of brucellosis in the country.

Keywords: sheep, goats, brucellosis, risk factors, Pakistan

INTRODUCTION

Brucellosis is a bacterial zoonosis with worldwide distribution, which is caused by bacteria of the genus *Brucella*. This genus comprises; *B. melitensis, B. abortus, B. suis, B. canis, B. ovis,* and *B. neotome* (classical *Brucella* species), *B. ceti* and *B. pinipedialis* from marine mammals, *B. microti* from voles, *B. inopinata* from human females, *B. papionis* from baboons and recently *B. vulpis* from red foxes (1–6). Based upon host preference; *B. abortus* predominantly infects bovines, *B. melitensis* small ruminants, *B. canis* dogs, *B. suis* pigs, and *B. ovis* rams, however, infection in non-prefered hosts is transmissible (7–9). In developing countries, a higher prevalence rate is observed where it causes abortion and retention of fetal membranes (10). The infection may stay undiagnosed due to its asymptomatic form and the infected animals may conceive subsequently, but remain carriers for their life. The infection is of economic importance, especially in developing countries (11). Direct or indirect contact with infected animals and consumption of contaminated raw milk and products are the main routes of transmission, respectively, in animals and humans (12). Brucellosis is an established occupational health hazard (13–16). Diagnosis remains a challenge and is based primarily on serology [e.g., Rose Bengal Test (RBT) and Milk Ring Test (MRT)]. Molecular detection of *Brucella*-DNA (e.g., PCR) in clinical/biological samples, is coupled with serology to identify the etiology precisely where necessary. The bacterial isolation

is a gold standard for the diagnosis, but requires specific growth conditions. Moreover, owing to fastidious nature of the organism (*B. abortus* for one), the turn-around-time for the samples is beyond a week. Vaccination is recommended but practiced mostly in elite herds in developing countries including in Pakistan (17). Treatment of brucellosis in ruminants is also not very popular in the country hence, test and slaughter/culling policy remains a sole solution for eradication of the infection in farm animals.

Pakistan is an agriculture-based country in south-Asia, where livestock plays a vital role in the national economy. The total livestock population in the country is 142.8 millions, where small ruminants (sheep and goat) share 80.27 million heads (18). In the past, brucellosis has been reported in both large and small ruminants in Punjab, Pakistan (19–23). This study was aimed to ascertain the current status of brucellosis in small ruminants at institutional livestock farms located in Punjab. Additionally,

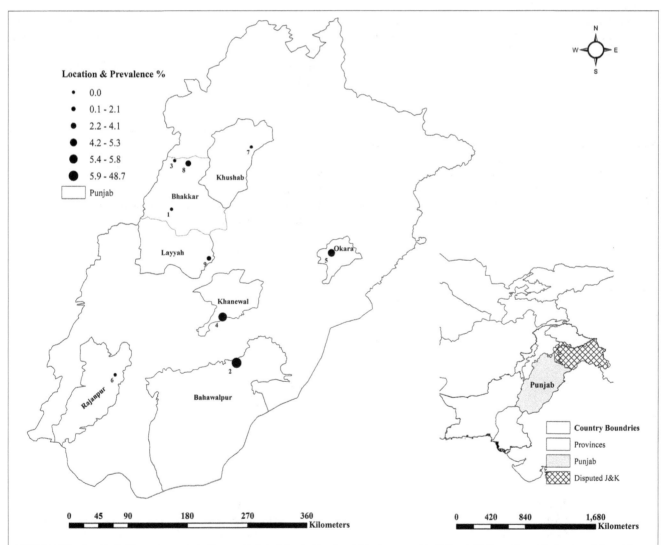

FIGURE 1 | Frontiers Media SA remains neutral with regard to jurisdictional claims in published maps and institutional affiliations. Gegraphical representation of the small ruminant farms tested for brucellosis in Punjab, Pakistan.

we determined the risk factors associated with the occurrence of the disease.

MATERIALS AND METHODS

A total of 1,000 sera (500 each from sheep and goats) were collected from nine different institutional livestock farms maintained under the Livestock and Dairy Development Department (L&DD), Government of Punjab, Lahore, Pakistan (**Figure 1**) (24). The sample size was calculated for an estimated disease prevalence of 50% at a 95% confidence interval, and 5% desired absolute precision (**Table 1**) (25). A minimum of 384 samples from each species were required by this method. The sample size was further inflated to accommodate for the potential losses during the transportation. The final sample size was proportionally allocated to each farm according to the population of the animals at each farm. Available identification record was used at each farm, to randomly select animals by using a random number generator and to collect the animal level data. Individual animals were restrained and blood was collected in a 9 mL vacutainer tube without anticoagulant through the jugular vein. No animals were harmed during this process. The animals had no prior history of brucellosis vaccination.

Sera were screened by ID Screen® Brucellosis Serum Indirect Multi-species (IDVet, Grabels, France), an indirect-ELISA for detection of anti-smooth-lipopolysaccharide (LPS) (*B. abortus, B. melitensis,* and *B. suis*). The samples were tested at the National Reference Laboratory (NRL) for brucellosis, Friedrich-Loeffler-Institut (FLI), Jena, Germany as per manufacturer's recommendations. DNA was extracted from sera by using the High Pure Template Kit (Roche, Rotkreuz, Switzerland) and molecular detection was serially done by real-time PCR as described by Probert et al. (26). The DNA extraction was run along with *E. coli* controls. The real-time PCR was run along with *B. abortus* (ATCC 23448) and *B. melitensis* (ATCC 23456) as

positive controls. In tandem with positive controls, nuclease-free water was run as negative control (NTC).

Brucellosis prevalence at species level was calculated by dividing the number of positive animals (numerator) by the total number of animals sampled (denominator). The statistical analysis was performed in two parts. In the first part, univariate and multivariate analysis were conducted to determine the association of the risk factors with the seroprevalence. The univariate analysis was conducted for farm related and animal level variables. Seroprevalence of brucellosis was considered as an outcome or dependent variable while biological plausible variables [e.g., farm location, species, sex, age/parity status, breed, history of reproductive disorders, and body condition score (BCS)] were considered as explanatory or independent variables. A $p \leq 0.05$ was considered as a level of significance. A backward stepwise approach was used for the binary logistic regression analysis (27). Nagelkerke R^2 (NR^2) and Hosmer and Lemeshow test (HLT) were used to assess the model-fitness. The statistical analysis was conducted using the IBM SPSS Statistics (IBM Corporation, Armonk, New York, USA).

The second part of statistical analysis was performed using R software and each of the variable was tested one by one alone in a mixed effect model approach with "farm" variable as random factor and using "lmer" function from lme4 package, and logistic binary model function (28). The results of these models showed that five variables were significantly associated with seroprevalence of brucellosis, i.e., species, age, parity status, reproductive disorders, and body condition score (see **Table 4**). To check if any of these variables showing significance association were confounded, all the five variables were tested in one single model and stepwise backward regression was performed (i.e., least significant variables were taken out in the next model). After running the model, collinearity and confounding behavior was tested by determining variance inflation factor using "vif" function from "car" package. Those variables were taken out of the model which showed high p-value and high variance

TABLE 1 | Seroprevalence in small ruminants of Punjab, Pakistan.

Farm[a]	Goats[b]		Sheep[c]		Total	
	Pos./Tested	Prev.%(95% CI)	Pos./Tested	Prev.%(95% CI)	Pos./Tested	Prev.%(95% CI)
1	0/0	-	0/41	0 (0–8.6)	0/41	0 (0–8.6)
2	0/0	-	18/37	48.7 (31.9–65.6)	18/37	48.7 (31.9–65.6)
3	0/0	-	0/22	0 (0–15.4)	0/22	0 (0–15.4)
4	13/203	6.4 (3.5–10.7)	1/40	2.5 (0.1–13.2)	14/243	5.8 (3.2–9.5)
5	7/44	15.9 (6.6–30.1)	0/88	0 (0–4.1)	7/132	5.3 (2.2–10.6)
6	0/43	0 (0–8.2)	0/9	0 (0–33.6)	0/52	0 (0–6.8)
7	0/0	-	0/45	0 (0–7.9)	0/45	0 (0–7.9)
8	0/0	-	6/145	4.1 (1.5–8.8)	6/145	4.1 (1.5–8.8)
9	6/210	2.9 (1.1–6.1)	0/73	0 (0–4.9)	6/283	2.1 (0.8–4.6)
Total	26/500	5.2 (3.4–7.5)	25/500	5 (3.3–7.3)	51/1,000	5.1 (3.8–6.7)

[a]The seroprevalence varied significantly among sampled farms; $\chi^2 = 159.281$, $p < 0.001$.
[b]The seroprevalence in sheep varied significantly among sampled farms; $\chi^2 = 163.790$, $p < 0.001$.
[c]The seroprevalence in goats varied significantly among sampled farms; $\chi^2 = 15.530$, $p = 0.001$.

TABLE 2 | Univariable analysis of the seroprevalence of brucellosis in small ruminants sampled from nine institutional livestock farms of Punjab, Pakistan.

Variable	Category	Pos. / tested	Prev. % (95% CI)	Odds ratio	95% CI	p-value*
Farm	Farm 2	18/37	48.7 (31.9–65.6)	25.7	12.84–55.52	<0.001
	Others	33/963	3.4 (2.4–4.8)	Ref	-	
Species	Sheep	26/500	5.2 (3.4–7.5)	1.042	0.593–1.831	0.886
	Goats	25/500	5 (3.3–7.3)	Ref	-	
Sex	Females	47/893	5.3 (3.9–6.9)	1.43	0.51–4.05	0.5
	Males	4/107	3.7 (1–9.3)	Ref	-	
Age	Above 4Y	35/440	7.9 (5.6–10.9)	2.94	1.60–5.38	<0.001
	Below 4Y	16/560	2.9 (1.6–4.6)	Ref	-	
Parity Status	Multiparous	40/594	6.7 (4.9–9.1)	2.59	1.31–5.12	0.006
	Nulli/Primi	11/406	2.7 (1.4–4.8)	Ref	-	
Breeds	Buchi	18/37	48.7 (31.9–65.6)	26.7	12.84–55.52	<0.001
	Others	33/963	3.4 (2.4–4.8)	Ref	-	
Reproductive disorders	Yes	25/178	14.0 (9.3–20.0)	5.00	2.81–8.89	<0.001
	No	26/822	3.2 (2.1–4.6)	Ref	-	
BCS	<underline<>3	34/172	19.8 (14.1–26.5)	11.74	6.39–21.62	<0.001
	>3	17/828	2.1 (1.2–3.3)	Ref	-	

*Statistical value of significance: $p \leq 0.05$.

inflation factor. In the next model if the *p*-value and variance inflation factor of the other remaining variables changed by a factor of 20%, then the taken-out variable was considered to be confounded with other variables. The maps were generated by using ArcGIS version 10.5.1 (ESRI, Redlands, CA, USA).

RESULTS

Anti-*Brucella* antibodies were detected in 51 (5.1%, CI 3.8–6.7) samples from sheep and goats. The farm-herd based and univariate analysis showed the seroprevalence almost identical in goats (5.2%) and sheep (5.0%), $p = 0.886$ (**Tables 1, 2**). Seropositive animals were detected at the five of nine sampled farms, and the prevalence varied from 2.1% (Farm 9) to 48.7% (Farm 2), $p < 0.001$. In goats, the highest seroprevalence was recorded in the small ruminants at Farm 5 (15.9%) and the lowest at the Farm 9 (2.9%), $p = 0.001$. In sheep, the seropositivity ranged from 2.5% (Farm 4) to 48.7% (Farm 2), $p < 0.001$ (**Figure 1**). None of the samples contained *Brucella* DNA as confirmed by negative real-time PCR results.

The univariable analysis indicated that sheep at Farm 2 were significantly ($p < 0.001$) more likely to test positive for anti-*Brucella* antibodies (OR 25.7, CI 12.84–55.52). In females, the seropositivity (5.3%) and odds for testing positive (OR 1.43, 0.51–4.05) were higher as compared to males (3.7%), $p = 0.5$. The small ruminants; above 4 years of age (7.9%, OR 2.94 CI 1.60–5.38), of multiparous status (6.7%, OR 2.59 CI 1.31–5.12), belonging to Buchi breed (48.7%, OR 26.7 CI 12.84–55.52), with history of reproductive disorders (13.6%, OR 3.19

CI 1.29–7.95) and having BCS ≤3 (19.8%, OR 11.74 CI 6.39–21.62) were found significantly ($p < 0.05$) more likely to test seropositive (**Table 2**).

The multivariable analysis indicated that small ruminants; kept at Farm 2 (OR 34.05 CI 13.47–86.10), above 4 years of age (OR 2.88 CI 1.39–5.94), with history of reproductive disorders (OR 2.69 CI 1.33–5.42), and BCS ≤3 (OR 12.37 CI 5.98–25.57) were significantly ($p < 0.01$) more likely to test positive for anti-*Brucella* antibodies (**Table 3**). The values of Nagelkerke R^2 (0.407) and Hosmer and Lemeshow test (Ci-square value; $\chi 2 = 3.092$, $p = 0.543$) indicated that it was a reasonable model to predict seroprevalence of brucellosis at the sampled farms.

In the second part of statistical analysis, using mixed effects model approach while testing each variable one by one in each model, the following were significant, i.e., species, age, parity status, reproductive disorders, and body condition score while sex and breed were non-significant (**Table 4**). Using backward regression analysis, testing all these five significant variables together, species and body condition score were found significant while age, parity status, and reproductive disorders were non-significant, with age showing least significant *p*-value (0.82) and high vif value (3.50) (**Table 5**). Variable "age" was taken out in the next model, and species, parity status, and body condition score were significant while reproductive disorders was non-significant (0.33) in this model and all variables showed lower vif values. Variable "reproductive disorders" was taken out in the next model, and all the remaining three variables (i.e., species, parity status, and body condition score) were significant and displayed low vif values. Low vif values in the last model pointed out that all the three variables were not confounded (**Table 5**).

TABLE 3 | Multivariable analysis of the seroprevalence of brucellosis in small ruminants sampled from nine institutional livestock farms of Punjab, Pakistan.

Variable	Exposure variable	Comparison	OR	95%CI	p-value*
Farm	Farm 2	Others	34.05	13.47–86.10	<0.001
Age group	>4 years	<4 years	2.88	1.39–5.94	0.004
Reproductive disorders	Yes	No	2.69	1.33–5.42	0.006
BCS	<underline<>3	> 3	12.37	5.98–25.57	<0.001

Model Fit: Nagelkerke R^2 = 0.407, Hosmer and Lemeshow Test (χ^2 = 3.092, p = 0.543).
*Statistical value of significance: p ≤ 0.05.

TABLE 4 | Each independent variable was tested separately in Mixed effect logistic regression model with farm as random factor.

Dependent variable	Model Sr. No	Independent variable	Estimate	z-value	p-value*
Brucella-iELISA outcome	1	Species	−2.546	−2.903	0.003
	2	Age	0.4379	2.563	0.01
	3	Sex	−0.1153	−0.203	0.83
	4	Parity	−1.1371	−3.033	0.002
	5	Breed	−0.1660	−0.995	0.31
	6	Reproductive disorder	0.3344	2.814	0.004
	7	BCS	−2.8795	−7.739	1e−14

*Statistical value of significance: p ≤ 0.05.

TABLE 5 | Stepwise backward regression models with starting model containing five independent variables and farm as random factor*.

Dependent variable	Model Sr. No	Independent variables tested together in one model	p-values*	Variance inflation factor (vif) value
Brucella-iELISA outcome	1	Species	0.003	1.01
		Age	0.82	3.50
		Parity status	0.16	3.44
		Reproductive disorders	0.35	1.07
		BCS	6.63e−14	1.06
	2	Species	0.003	1.01
		Parity status	0.005	1.09
		Reproductive disorders	0.33	1.06
		BCS	5.48e−14	1.04
	3	Species	0.002	1.01
		Parity status	0.001	1.03
		BCS	1.83e−14	1.04

*Variable showing least significance and high variance inflation factor (vif) value were taken out in next model; (Statistical value of significance: p ≤ 0.05).

DISCUSSION

Brucellosis remains an endemic infection in livestock in Pakistan (17, 29). Serology is a preferred and handy choice for diagnosis of brucellosis. ELISA is a sensitive test and is useful for diagnostic screening on larger scale but is unable to differentiate precisely between vaccinated and infected animals (30, 31). Molecular biological tests e.g., PCR, focus on the presence of DNA in the sample and are potentially able to differentiate the vaccine and field strains of *Brucella* (32). Real-time PCR can even detect and differentiate at lower amounts of DNA in a clinical sample

when compared to conventional PCR. However, it requires the presence of bacterial DNA in the sample, which may not be present at every time during and after an infection and might be affected by laboratory procedures (33). Hence, a proper validation process is needed for every test. We used indirect-ELISA as a single screening test and real-time PCR for confirmation of the etiology.

Among variables, the odds for testing positive varied significantly depending upon the farm location and were significantly higher in the animals kept at Farm 2 (**Tables 1, 3**). These findings are supported by previous reports (20, 22, 34).

This could be related to the environmental factors including herd management system at these farms. Furthermore, small ruminants had a close contact with bovines at Farms (2, 5, 6, 7, and 8), where brucellosis was reported previously (21, 23, 35). Moreover, common grazing and watering areas, use of brucellosis positive males for breeding and introduction of new animals without testing could be the factors responsible for brucellosis incidence at these locations (36, 37).

Age (>4 years) and parity status (multiparous) were found significantly associated ($p < 0.05$) with higher odds as compared to younger (<4 years) and null/primiparous (≤ 1 parturited) animals, respectively. Furthermore, age was also found significantly associated ($p < 0.05$) with seroprevalence (OR 2.88) by multivariate analysis (**Table 3**). A similar trend was reported in both sheep and goats with significant association (21, 38), non-significant association (22), and without determination of association (39, 40). This may be ascribed to increased frequency of contact with other animals with respect to age, higher coital chances, and sexual maturity as compared to younger animals (12, 41).

Reproductive disorders showed significant association (OR 2.69, $p = 0.006$) with brucellosis in the current study (**Tables 2, 3**). It is understandable as late abortion and retention of fetal membranes are characteristic signs of brucellosis. These findings are supported by similar results reported previously by others investigators (19, 34, 42). However, a non-significant association ($p > 0.05$) in sheep has also been documented (22). Furthermore, animals having BCS ≤ 3, were more likely to test positive (OR 12.37, $p < 0.001$) in our study which is concordance with findings of Ethiopian workers (43). A possible reason could be the higher susceptibility of animals already infected with brucellosis to other infections or the loss in BCS caused by the brucellosis itself.

CONCLUSION AND RECOMMENDATIONS

In conclusion, we found anti-*Brucella* antibodies in sheep and goats at these livestock farms in Punjab, Pakistan. Farm location, age, and species of the animals, history of reproductive disorders and BCS were found to play a significant role for brucellosis seropositivity in these animals. Although vaccination is recommended and treatment is possible for brucellosis, they are not considered safe for human health, hence regular screening and culling of the reactor animals remain the only choice to monitor and eradicate brucellosis. Introduction of the new stock at these farms should be carried out only after screening and quarantine. Furthermore, farm workers should be advised to adopt protection measures as a routine. Abortion at these farms should not go unnoticed and must be investigated to confirm its cause to adopt recommended control measures. If abortions occur, disinfection of the area should be ensured along with strict biosecurity measures to restrict chances of dissemination of infection through the dogs, cats, other domestic animals, visitors, and farm equipment/supply movement. Standardization and validation of the diagnostic tests are required based on the local conditions. Isolation and molecular investigations of the etiological agents might be helpful for future understanding of the epidemiology of the infection and the relationship of the outbreaks.

AUTHOR CONTRIBUTIONS

QU and TJ: Conceptualization. FM and MS: methodology. MH and MA: formal analysis. TJ and QU: investigation. UT, MI, and QU: data curation. TJ: writing-original draft preparation. SU, ZQ, HJ, SS, and HN: writing-review and editing. All authors contributed to the article and approved the submitted version.

ACKNOWLEDGMENTS

Authors are thankful to Higher Education Commission (HEC)-Pakistan to support the stay of QU under the project International Research Support Program (IRSP) and TJ under the project 90% Overseas Scholarship Scheme at Friedrich-Loeffler-Institut (FLI), Jena, Germany. Authors would also like to thank the Livestock and Dairy Development (L&DD), Government of Punjab, Pakistan for their cooperation in the provision of samples. The agencies had no role in designing, performing, and publication of the results.

REFERENCES

1. Garrity GM, Bell JA, Lilburn TG. *Taxonomic Outline of the Prokaryotes. Bergey's Manual of Systematic Bacteriology*. New York, NY: Springer-Verlag (2004). p. 55.

2. Foster G, Osterman BS, Godfroid J, Jacques I, Cloeckaert A. *Brucella ceti* sp nov and *Brucella pinnipedialis* sp nov for *Brucella* strains with cetaceans and seals as their preferred hosts. *Int J Syst Evol Micr.* (2007) 57:2688–93. doi: 10.1099/ijs.0.6 5269-0

3. Scholz HC, Hubalek Z, Sedlacek I, Vergnaud G, Tomaso H, Al Dahouk S, et al. *Brucella microti* sp. nov., isolated from the common vole *Microtus arvalis. Int J Syst Evol Micr.* (2008) 58:375–82. doi: 10.1099/ijs.0.6 5356-0

4. Scholz HC, Nöckler K, Göllner C, Bahn P, Vergnaud G, Tomaso H, et al. *Brucella inopinata sp.* nov., isolated from a breast implant infection. *Int J Syst Evol Micr.* (2010) 60:801–8. doi: 10.1099/ijs.0.011148-0

5. Whatmore AM, Davison N, Cloeckaert A, Al Dahouk S, Zygmunt MS, Brew SD, et al. *Brucella papionis* sp. nova, isolated from baboons (*Papio* spp.). *Int J Syst Evol Micr.* (2014) 64:4120–8. doi: 10.1099/ijs.0.065482-0

6. Scholz HC, Revilla-Fernandez S, Dahouk SA, Hammerl JA, Zygmunt MS, Cloeckaert A, et al. *Brucella vulpis* sp nov., isolated from mandibular lymph nodes of red foxes (*Vulpes vulpes*). *Int J Syst Evol Micr.* (2016) 66:2090–8. doi: 10.1099/ijsem.0.000998

7. Saleem MZ, Akhtar R, Aslam A, Rashid MI, Chaudhry ZI, Manzoor MA, et al. Evidence of *Brucella abortus* in non-preferred caprine and ovine hosts by real-time PCR assay. *Pak J Zool.* (2019) 51:1187–9. doi: 10.17582/journal.pjz/2019.51.3.sc3

8. Jamil T, Melzer F, Khan I, Iqbal M, Saqib M, Hussain MH, et al. Serological and molecular investigation of *Brucella* species in dogs in Pakistan. *Pathogens.* (2019) 8:294. doi: 10.3390/pathogens8040294

9. Saeed U, Ali S, Khan TM, El-Adawy H, Melzer F, Khan AU, et al. Seroepidemiology and the molecular detection of animal brucellosis in Punjab Pakistan. *Microorganisms*. (2019) 7:449. doi: 10.3390/microorganisms7100449

10. Corbel MJ. *Brucellosis in Humans and Animals*. Geneva: World Health Organization (2006).

11. McDermott J, Grace D, Zinsstag J. Economics of brucellosis impact and control in low-income countries. *Rev Sci Tech*. (2013) 32:249–61. doi: 10.20506/rst.32.1.2197

12. Gul S, Khan A. Epidemiology and epizootology of brucellosis: a review. *Pak Vet J*. (2007) 27:145–51.

13. Ali S, Ali Q, Neubauer H, Melzer F, Elschner M, Khan I, et al. Seroprevalence and risk factors associated with brucellosis as a professional hazard in Pakistan. *Foodborne Pathog Dis*. (2013) 10:500–5. doi: 10.1089/fpd.2012.1360

14. Asif M, Waheed U, Farooq M, Ali T, Khan QM. Frequency of brucellosis in high risk human groups in Pakistan detected through Polymerase Chain Reaction and its comparison with conventional slide agglutination test. *Int J Agric Biol*. (2014) 16:986–90.

15. Mukhtar F. Brucellosis in a high risk occupational group: seroprevalence and analysis of risk factors. *J Pak Med Assoc*. (2010) 60:1031.

16. Mukhtar F, Kokab F. *Brucella* serology in abattoir workers. *J Ayub Med Coll Abbottabad*. (2008) 20:57–61.

17. Nawaz G, Malik MN, Mushtaq MH, Ahmad FM, Shah AA, Iqbal F, et al. Surveillance of brucellosis in livestock in rural communities of Punjab, Pakistan. *Pak J Agric Res*. (2016) 29:392–8.

18. Anonymous. *Economic Survey of Pakistan: Chapter: Livestock Population of Pakistan*. Pakistan Bureue of Statistics (2006).

19. Arshad M, Munir M, Iqbal K, Abbas R, Rasool M, Khalil N. Sero-prevalence of brucellosis in goats from public and private livestock farms in Pakistan. *Online J Vet Res*. (2011) 15:297–304.

20. Gul ST, Khan A, Ahmad M, Rizvi F, Shahzad A, Hussain I. Epidemiology of brucellosis at different livestock farms in the Punjab Pakistan. *Pak Vet J*. (2015) 35:309–14.

21. Gul ST, Khan A, Rizvi F, Hussain I. Sero-prevalence of brucellosis in food animals in the Punjab Pakistan. *Pak Vet J*. (2014) 34:454–8.

22. Iqbal Z, Jamil H, Qureshi ZI, Saqib M, Lodhi LA, Waqas MS, et al. Seroprevalence of ovine brucellosis by modified Rose Bengal test and ELISA in southern Punjab Pakistan. *Pak Vet J*. (2013) 33:455–7.

23. Jamil T, Melzer F, Saqib M, Shahzad A, Khan KK, Hammad HM, et al. Serological and molecular detection of bovine brucellosis at institutional livestock farms in Punjab, Pakistan. *Int J Environ Res Public Health*. (2020) 7:1412. doi: 10.3390/ijerph17041412

24. Ullah Q, El-Adawy H, Jamil T, Jamil H, Qureshi ZI, Saqib M, et al. Serological and molecular Investigation of *Coxiella burnetii* in small ruminants and ticks in Punjab, Pakistan. *Int J Environ Res Public Health*. (2019) 16:4271. doi: 10.3390/ijerph16214271

25. Thrusfield M. *Veterinary Epidemiology*. Oxford: Wiley (2013).

26. Probert WS, Schrader KN, Khuong NY, Bystrom SL, Graves MH. Real-time multiplex PCR assay for detection of *Brucella* spp. *B. abortus* and *B. melitensis J Clin Microbiol*. (2004) 42:1290–3. doi: 10.1128/JCM.42.3.1290-1293.2004

27. Bursac Z, Gauss CH, Williams DK, Hosmer DW. Purposeful selection of variables in logistic regression. *Source Code Biol Med*. (2008) 3:17. doi: 10.1186/1751-0473-3-17

28. The R Core Team. *R: A Language and Environment for Statistical Computing* Vienna: R Foundation for Statistical Computing (2018).

29. Farooq U, Fatima Z, Afzal M, Anwar Z, Jahangir M. Sero-prevalence of brucellosis in bovines at farms under different management conditions. *British J Dairy Sci*. (2011) 2:35–9.

30. Nielsen K, Yu W. Serological diagnosis of brucellosis. *Prilozi*. (2010) 31:65–89.

31. Uzal FA, Carrasco AE, Echaide S, Nielsen K, Robles CA. Evaluation of an indirect ELISA for the diagnosis of bovine brucellosis. *J Vet Diagn Invest*. (1995) 7:473–5. doi: 10.1177/104063879500700408

32. López-Goñi D, García-Yoldi CM, Marín MJ, de Miguel PM, Muñoz JM, Blasco I, et al. Evaluation of a Multiplex PCR Assay (Bruce-ladder) for molecular typing of all *Brucella* species, including the vaccine strains. *J Clin Microbiol*. (2008) 46:3484. doi: 10.1128/JCM.00837-08

33. Jamil T, Melzer F, Njeru J, El-Adawy H, Neubauer H, Wareth G. *Brucella abortus*: current research and future trends. *Curr Clin Microbiol Rep*. (2017) 4:1. doi: 10.1007/s40588-017-0052-z

34. Naeem KN, Kamran J, Ullah A. Seroprevalence and risk factors associated with Crimean-Congo haemorrhagic fever and brucellosis in people and livestock in Baluchistan and Khyber Pakhtunkhwa Provinces Pakistan. In: *Proceedings of South Asia Regional One Health Symposium* (Paro) (2013). p. 50–1.

35. Nasir AA, Parveen Z, Shah MA, Rashid M. Seroprevalence of brucellosis in animals at government and private livestock farms in Punjab. *Pak Vet J*. (2004) 24:144–6.

36. Ullah S, Jamil T, Mushtaq M, Saleem M. Prevalence of brucellosis among camels in district Muzaffargarh Pakistan. *J Infec Mol Biol*. (2015) 3:52–6. doi: 10.14737/journal.jimb/2015/3.2.52.56

37. Cárdenas L, Peña M, Melo O, Casal J. Risk factors for new bovine brucellosis infections in Colombian herds. *BMC Vet Res*. (2019) 15:81. doi: 10.1186/s12917-019-1825-9

38. Ali S, Akbar A, Shafee M, Tahira B, Muhammed A, Ullah N. Sero-epidemiological study of brucellosis in small ruminants and associated human beings in district Quetta Balochistan. *Pure Appl Microbiol*. (2017) 6:797–804. doi: 10.19045/bspab.2017.60084

39. Ghani M, Siraj M, Zeb A, Naeem M. Sero-epidemiological study of brucellosis among goats and sheep at Pshawar district. *Asian-Australas J Anim Sci*. (1995) 8:489–94. doi: 10.5713/ajas.1995.489

40. Hussain MA, Nazir S, Rajput IR, Khan IZ, Rehman M-u-, Hayat S. Study on seroprevalence of brucellosis in caprine in Kohat (Khyber Pakhtoon Khwa). *Lasbela Uni J Sci Tech*. (2014) 3:14–20.

41. Abubakar M, Mansoor M, Arshed MJ. Bovine brucellosis: old and new concepts with Pakistan perspective. *Pak Vet J*. (2012) 32:147–55.

42. Khan AQ, Haleem SK, Shafiq M, Khan NA, ur Rahman S. Seropositivity of brucellosis in human and livestock in Tribal-Kurram agency of Pakistan indicates cross circulation. *Wetchasan Sattawaphaet Thai J Vet Med*. (2017) 47:349–55.

43. Tsegay A, Tuli G, Kassa T, Kebede N. Seroprevalence and risk factors of brucellosis in small ruminants slaughtered at Debre Ziet and Modjo export abattoirs, Ethiopia. *J Infect Dev Ctries*. (2015) 9:373–80. doi: 10.3855/jidc.4993

7

Control and Prevention of Epizootic Lymphangitis in Mules: An Integrated Community-Based Intervention, Bahir Dar, Ethiopia

Bojia E. Duguma[1]*, Tewodros Tesfaye[1], Asmamaw Kassaye[1], Anteneh Kassa[1] and Stephen J. Blakeway[2]

[1] The Donkey Sanctuary-Ethiopia Office, Addis Ababa, Ethiopia, [2] Director, International Department, The Donkey Sanctuary, Sidmouth, United Kingdom

*Correspondence:
Bojia E. Duguma
dugumabojia@gmail.com

From 2010 to 2017, as part of a wider animal welfare program, The Donkey Sanctuary piloted an integrated, community-based model for the control and prevention of epizootic lymphangitis (EZL) in cart mules in Bahir Dar, Ethiopia. Stakeholders included muleteers, service providers, and transport and animal health regulatory authorities. Interventions included muleteer education, wound prevention, harness improvement, animal health professional training, treatment of early EZL cases, euthanasia for advanced cases, and review of transport services and traffic guidelines. The project followed a participatory project management cycle and used participatory learning and action tools to facilitate stakeholder engagement and ownership. Participatory and classical epidemiology tools were employed to raise and align stakeholder understanding about EZL for effective control and prevention and to evaluate the progress impact of the model through annual prevalence surveys. During the intervention, the annual prevalence of EZL reduced from 23.9% (102/430) (95%CI: 19.8%–27.0%) in 2010 to 5.9% (58/981) (95% CI: 4.4%–7.4%) in 2017, and wound prevalence from 44.3% in 2011 to 22.2% in 2017; trends in the reduction of the prevalence maintained in the face of a mule population that increased from 430 in 2010 to ~1,500 in 2017. While non-governmental organization (NGO)-led interventions can facilitate change by trialing new approaches and accessing new skills and resources, sustainable change requires community ownership and strengthening of service provision systems. To this effect, the project raised muleteer competence in mule husbandry and EZL prevention strategies; strengthened veterinary competence; facilitated more mule-friendly traffic, transport, and waste disposal guidelines and practices; supported mule-community bylaws to control EZL; and established a supportive network between stakeholders including trusting relationships between muleteers and veterinary services. To advance the intervention model in other endemic areas, we recommend elucidation of local epidemiological factors with other stakeholders prior to the intervention, early engagement with veterinary and transport service regulatory authorities, early development of bylaws, exploration of compensation or insurance mechanisms to support euthanasia of advanced cases, and additional social, economic, and epidemiological investigations. In line with the OIE Working Equid Welfare Standards, we suggest that integrated community-based interventions are useful approaches to the control and prevention of infectious diseases.

Keywords: epizootic lymphangitis, Bahir Dar Ethiopia, EZL prevention and control, mule, community-based animal health care

INTRODUCTION

This article reports on a working mule welfare project (the project) that ran from 2010 to 2017 and focused on the control and prevention of wounds and the disease epizootic lymphangitis (EZL) in Bahir Dar, Amhara Region, as an indicator of the success of a more extensive participatory, community-based donkey and mule welfare program in Ethiopia facilitated by The Donkey Sanctuary (TDS), a United Kingdom-based donkey and mule welfare charity.

Around 13.3 million working equids provide essential services in Ethiopia (1). Their contribution to the economy remains generally under-recognized, and services available to the sector are therefore generally poor (2–4).

Around 380,000 of these working equids are mules, with ~140,000 living in the Amhara Region where ~56,000 power carts (1). The Amhara Region also has one of Ethiopia's largest populations of working donkeys. Mule numbers in Bahir Dar, capital of the Amhara Region, are increasing, from 430 in 2010 to around 1,500 in 2017, alongside increasing development and a human population in Ethiopia that doubled between 1995 and 2019 (5).

All mules in Bahir Dar power carts. They transport building materials (timber, stone, and cement) and agricultural goods (seeds, fertilizers, pesticides, and harvested produce) to and from markets, grain and flour to and from grinding mills, water where there is no piped supply, solid waste to municipal dumps, and people (6, 7).

Mules represent a significant investment, make a substantial (sometimes the only) financial contribution to muleteer household economies (6, 8), and provide valuable low-carbon community services, thereby serving the Sustainable Development Goals (9). Yet lack of knowledge; poor husbandry; harness wounds; lameness; colic; infectious diseases such as EZL, African horse sickness, tetanus, strangles, and parasites; and a lack of relevant support services all compromise welfare and productivity (7, 8, 10–14). On average, a mule affected with EZL in Gondar, Amhara, is estimated to cost its owner around ETB 6,000 per year (~GBP 100, July 2021) in lost production (15).

EZL is the most visible and prevalent of the infectious diseases affecting equids in Ethiopia (16–21). In endemic areas, emaciated, abandoned horses and mules with the running sores of advanced EZL can be seen standing in the middle of busy roads where the breezes from passing vehicles provide some respite from flies. Welfare assessment, using the Hand (22–25), identified mule–muleteer–societal relationships,

wounds, and EZL as the main welfare challenges to be addressed in this project. Lameness and nutrition would also be addressed tangentially.

EZL is primarily a chronic contagious disease of equids (17, 18, 20, 26), with horses being most susceptible, donkeys least susceptible, and mules in between. The causal agent is *Histoplasma capsulatum* var. *farciminosum* (HCF), a dimorphic fungus (one that can exist in both unicellular (yeast) and filamentous (mycelial or mold) states) which can live independently in soil, making eradication difficult. It is endemic to Ethiopia (27), particularly in the hot, humid upland areas between 1,500 and 2,800 m above sea level (20).

Control of EZL is challenging, with no completely satisfactory treatment (26). Spread between equids is thought to be facilitated by the presence of open wounds, close contact, flies, and poor work, hygiene, or husbandry practices (28). Treatment requires continuing owner compliance. Early identification and intensive follow-up are critical for successful therapy (17, 29). The more advanced the disease, the more guarded the outcome (30, 31). Tincture of iodine (2%) can be used topically, and sodium or potassium iodide can be parenterally administered via drinking water or feed, although lengthy treatment can lead to iodine toxicity. All are available in Ethiopia. The antifungal drug amphotericin B is generally impractical for working equids because of the specialized treatment protocols, potential side effects, and requirement for close monitoring (32). There is no readily available commercial vaccine for prevention, although an attenuated vaccine and a killed formalized vaccine are reported to have been used for its control in some endemic areas of west Asia (27, 33). Currently, therefore, the only viable means of prevention and control of EZL involves close collaboration between mule-using communities, veterinary services, and regulatory authorities, with cases caught early and intractable cases humanely euthanized.

The TDS program in the Amhara Region followed a strategic review with a move from direct veterinary intervention services to community-based approaches measured against welfare outcomes that could better deal with the technical, social, and economic complexities of donkey and mule welfare including the multifactorial nature of a disease such as EZL (34). It drew on lessons from community-based animal healthcare (35, 36) and participatory epidemiology (37, 38) including the global eradication of rinderpest in cattle (39–41).

In summary, the project trialed a community-based approach to understanding and improving cart mule welfare, in a location where wounds and EZL were the most visible welfare challenges with the explicit intention of exploring sustainability.

TABLE 1 | Number of mules sampled for annual cross-sectional survey of EZL and wounds, 2010–2017 (baseline and implementation surveys).

Survey year	Number of mules sampled	Survey method
2010[a]	430	Census survey
2011	623	Census survey
2012	1,128	Census survey
2013	1,266	Census survey
2014	NA[b]	No survey conducted
2015	394	Sample survey
2016	1,436	Census survey
2017	981	Sample survey

[a] The project baseline survey. [b] NA—not applicable.

METHODS

Materials

Project Study Area

The study was conducted in cart-pulling mules of Bahir Dar city, located next to Lake Tana, source of the Blue Nile, in the Amhara Region, northwestern Ethiopia, at an altitude of 1,820 m above sea level. The average annual rainfall is 1,416 mm. The short rainy season is in March and April, and the long rainy season is from June to September. Bahir Dar has a borderline tropical savannah climate with an average low temperature of 11.7°C and an average high temperature of 26.7°C. The mean relative humidity of Bahir Dar is 58.4% (42).

Project Study Population

The Bahir Dar City Administration provided a mule population estimate of around 500 mules for 2010 at the start of the project. The mule cart sector was informal, mules were not registered nor licensed, and there was little formal engagement between the municipality and sector, so the estimate was based on little data. The baseline survey which aimed for a full census found 430 mules. This number had risen to nearly 1,500 by the end of the project. During the project, the municipality based its annual mule population estimates on project census surveys, rather than its usual general annual estimate of animals in the city. Official full census surveys are conducted every 10 years in Ethiopia. Annual mule numbers are presented in **Table 1**, and the survey methodology is explained in Section Annual cross-sectional surveys: prevalence of EZL and wounds.

Cart mule demographics were fluid. Almost every mule had a dedicated handler (muleteer) who chased work across the city independently, and there appeared to be no stable groupings of mules. Owners with multiple mules generally rent them out in long-term arrangements with the muleteer responsible for almost all aspects of husbandry; and cart mule associations appeared to be loose affiliations. As mule population increased alongside diversification of work opportunities, competition also increased with larger numbers of mules accumulating at collection sites.

Nevertheless, the muleteer community was self-aware. Apart from business risks, EZL was its greatest threat, and many muleteers were aware of the disease and its status across the population. Muleteers were initially wary of the project, but once they understood the project's approach and intentions, most became more trusting. Mules are only kept to work, and working mules are visible, so key informants from within the muleteer community played an essential role in the project's success, helping project staff to find muleteers with mules affected by EZL including in the outer reaches of the city, both during the intervention and the annual surveys.

Project Study Framework

TDS identified the cart mules of Bahir Dar as a target project for two strategic reasons. First, the welfare of cart mules with wounds and EZL is visibly compromised. Second, the visibility of these mules in a regional capital helped raise awareness about working animals more generally and so fed into the awareness-raising and advocacy strand of TDS's broader strategy.

The project followed a participatory project management cycle (PPMC) which allows flexibility, accumulation of learning through review points, and the ability to amend plans and activities in agreement with other stakeholders (43, 44). The cycle can be described as stakeholders identifying and defining the problem together, then planning together, then implementing together, and then monitoring and reviewing together, before starting the cycle again by planning the next stage together, taking into consideration lessons learnt in the previous cycles. Awareness of the need for an exit strategy is explicit from the start, so additional cycles aim increasingly to hand over aspects of the work, while focusing on specific areas of challenge. Also explicit is the need to reduce external contributions to the project over time. This is shown schematically in **Figure 1**.

While TDS identified EZL in mules in Bahir Dar as a social, economic, and animal health and welfare problem, it then needed to involve other stakeholders for the project to work.

Stakeholder Analysis

Stakeholder analysis started by talking with obvious stakeholders such as mule owners and users (muleteers), veterinary service providers, and regulatory officials. TDS then used interviews and stakeholder analysis (45) with these individuals and emerging key informants to understand the wider range of stakeholders, their areas of interest and influence, and the roles they might play in making the project a success.

Epidemiology

The application of epidemiology and epidemiological tools served two main roles during this EZL control and prevention project: to engage all stakeholders with an agreed understanding about EZL prevention and control based on both local knowledge and published articles; and to provide a reliable methodology for annual EZL prevalence surveys for project monitoring and evaluation.

Case Definition and Diagnosis of EZL

The case definition for EZL in this study was a working mule in Bahir Dar with a diagnosis of EZL based on clinical examination with confirmation through direct microscopy.

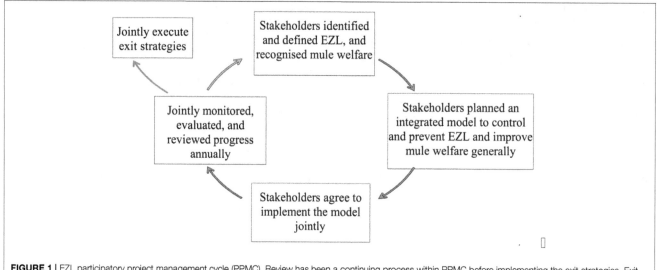

FIGURE 1 | EZL participatory project management cycle (PPMC). Review has been a continuing process within PPMC before implementing the exit strategies. Exit strategies can happen at different times for different components of the project.

The clinical examination protocol for EZL involved inspection of the entire skin surface for ulcerative wounds or suppurative spreading dermatitis and lymphangitis and palpation along the lymphatic vessels and lymph nodes for the presence of nodules. Cases were characterized as advanced by the presence of button-type ulcers or nodules, cording or thickening of lymphatic vessels, or functional abnormalities such as lameness, dyspnea, or visual impairment.

Swab samples from any suspect lesions, including ulcerating harness-related lesions, bit sores, or ocular discharge, and aspirates of nodules along the lymphatic vessels or lymph nodes were collected for direct microscopy. Direct microscopic examination of samples was conducted in collaboration with the Bahir Dar Regional Veterinary Laboratory. Both Gram's and Giemsa stains were applied to examine for pleomorphic yeast-like cells with a halo appearance under the oil immersions lens (29).

Annual Cross-Sectional Surveys: Prevalence of EZL and Wounds

A baseline survey to assess general welfare, including prevalence of EZL and wounds, was conducted by the TDS staff in 2010 before making a final commitment to implement the project. This was a full census survey aiming to reach every mule and involved clinical examination of mules for EZL, open wounds, harness fit and quality, lameness, sex, age [estimate based on dentition (46)], and body condition score [BCS, using a five-level scoring methodology (47)] as potential risk factors for EZL. General observations were also made regarding commodities being transported, working practices, and mule–muleteer relationships. The project monitoring and evaluation strategy was to resurvey mules each year to assess the effectiveness of its protocol by measuring annual change in EZL and wound prevalence. In view of the growth and demographic complexity of the mule sector and because the project was about general welfare as well as

EZL, the preferred strategy was to continue with full census surveys, to reach all mules, sample each mule for EZL, and check for open wounds, collect accurate population data, and check general welfare across the growing population of working mules. Resampling of mules was avoided by registering muleteer names during the exercise and marking each mule on the forehead with permanent red ink.

Surveys were conducted by a team composed of veterinarians from Bahir Dar Clinic and Bahir Dar Regional Veterinary Laboratory and TDS staff. To meet the primary objective of controlling EZL, every effort was made to ensure inclusion of each and every mule working, at rest, grazing, left at home, or abandoned for the success and progress impact of the intervention model. Muleteers increasingly assisted in the process as they became more aware that every case is a potential source of infection and needs to be reported as soon as discovered. Other key informants, including the Kebele administration, were also involved in the organization of the census survey. Surveys took place during the month of May when EZL cases are higher and were completed over 2 to 3 weeks.

For reasons outside project control, there was no survey in 2014, and full census surveys were not possible in 2015 and 2017. In 2015, the sample size was calculated based on the 21% prevalence published in a previous Ethiopian study of EZL prevalence in cart mules (17). Assuming 21% prevalence with 95% confidence level, 80% power of test, 5% precision and an estimated population size of 1,400 mules required a minimum sample number of 380 (48), and the project sampled 394 mules. In 2017, because prevalence had risen in 2016, the project reduced the margin of error, assumed prevalence of 50%, precision level of 3% and, with an estimated population of 1,500 mules, calculated a minimum sample number of 889, and 981 mules were sampled (49). Mule selection in 2015 and 2017 used systematic random sampling where every other mule was sampled, and planning together with key informants from the mule community ensured sampling of mules across the full geographic and demographic range in and around Bahir Dar.

Stakeholder Contributions and Ownership of the Interventions

For project success, all stakeholders needed to reach a common understanding about EZL and what they could do to minimize or prevent it.

With the use of two participatory epidemiology approaches, key informant interviews, and focused group discussions (FGDs), factors associated with EZL were explored using a range of participatory exercises. The purpose of these exercises was to build engagement; to respect and understand local perceptions; and to check that these aligned generally with published epidemiology on EZL. These exercises aimed to allow stakeholders, whatever their level of education or literacy, to contribute their knowledge and experience, share in the analysis, and take ownership of the prevention and control strategy.

The key informant interviews and FGDs were conducted primarily by the TDS program staff. Themes and results were shared with the wider community in subsequent meetings and training sessions through narrative, reporting of ranking results, and map building (37, 50, 51).

Key Informant Interviews

Individual, semi-structured, face-to-face interviews were conducted with 12 key informants. These included five experienced muleteers, one municipality officer, two animal health professionals, two traffic police officers, one senior livestock officer, and one manager of a private waste collection business. Each interview involved a set of questions to open wider conversations that allowed interviewees to add ideas that might not have occurred to the interviewer.

Questions explored the socioeconomic impact of EZL on cart mules in Bahir Dar; factors predisposing to EZL; challenges to controlling and preventing EZL; the roles of the different institutions and associations; and what should be done about EZL.

FGDs

Five FGDs were held to explore muleteer perceptions about EZL and its epidemiology. Participation criteria were agreed with stakeholders such that all participants were experienced muleteers, were members of cart mule associations, and had some form of social responsibility in the community as well as passion and willingness to participate. Muleteers new to the carting business in Bahir Dar who lacked background about EZL and its impact on the city and children driving carts for their older relatives were therefore excluded.

Around 30 mule-related associations were registered with the Bahir Dar municipality, but some were short term, for example, as part of a small microfinance scheme, and were no longer functional. Participants in the FGDs came from the eight most active associations based on the large size of membership, longer years of establishment, integrity of their bylaws, and diverse work type and geographic locations. Despite being members of an association, muleteers work independently, and FGDs were

mixed depending on when different muleteers had the time to join a session. Location and timing of FGDs were dictated by the muleteers and their daily schedules.

Topics were explored in the FGDs with the help of participatory learning and action (PLA) tools (50, 51), which allow participants to represent their worlds, their knowledge, and their experience, in a variety of ways including diagrams, pictures, and maps. The discussions between participants as they create the representations, the representations themselves, and the detailed discussion afterwards are all equally important parts of the process. PLA tools help ensure that all participants contribute, even the quietest ones. When facilitated well, the process holds attention beyond that of a general discussion, allowing every point to be fully examined.

The topics explored (and the PLA tools used) were as follows:

- *Socioeconomic impacts of EZL* (brainstorming and discussion);
- *Predisposing factors to EZL*: identify (brainstorming) and rank and discuss (simple ranking);
- *Pairwise ranking*: using the top risk factors identified in the previous exercise, compare and rank these risk factors in pairs;
- *Seasonal calendars*: draw a line that represents your working year; mark the four main seasons—Tseday, Bega, Belg, and Kiremt; add in other major events in the year, e.g., types of work that may vary during the year, and times of the year when EZL cases are lowest and highest; and explain and discuss; and
- *Mapping Bahir Dar from a mule perspective*: participants worked on a map of the city showing collection sites including feeding and watering points, parking, markets, construction sites, and grain mills, adding other meeting sites of importance and marking routes used to move through the city while discussing the challenges they faced (participatory mapping).

Planning and Implementation

Once the various stakeholders had established a common understanding about the problem, TDS facilitated a series of consultative workshops to agree on a collective implementation plan.

Workshops started with a summary of project progress to date (as in Sections Project study framework–Epidemiology) and then used a problem tree exercise (52) to explore root causes and intervention points.

These meetings helped identify key intervention activities, reach an agreement on how the work should be monitored and evaluated, assign roles and responsibilities, and reach an agreement on other implementation modalities and a timeline. The idea of an exit strategy for TDS involvement was introduced from the start to provide focus.

Facilitated learning including practical training—for all stakeholders (including TDS) but most actively for muleteers, harness makers, and animal health professionals—was a central theme, as was ensuring availability of treatment for treatable cases and euthanasia for incurable cases. Other activities aimed at changing attitudes, behaviors, and practice regarding mule transport within the municipality transport officials and traffic police.

The project started with an official public launch. Stakeholders needed to commit to being part of the "project team" before the official launch to help build trust, to reinforce that the project could only succeed as a joint effort, and to mitigate against groups dropping out.

Education of Muleteers

Muleteer education was practical and participatory. It targeted all muleteers and responded to points raised by all stakeholders including the muleteers themselves. TDS was involved with the local veterinary staff in improving muleteer understanding and practical knowledge of mule behavior and handling; improving general mule care and management; and reducing wounds and improving hygiene and segregation practices around EZL. Transport officials and traffic police worked together with muleteers on traffic-related education.

Specifics included herd health and EZL prevention (where herd can mean all the mules in Bahir Dar or a subset, such as those belonging to one muleteer, or all members of a cart mule association, if they can be managed in any way separate from other mules); use of improved harness (saddle, bits, and straps made of natural materials) and implications of sharing harness; daily mule checks for early identification of all health problems including wounds and EZL; early treatment including how to engage with veterinary services; principles and practice of wound management (including application of tincture of iodine); case segregation while housing, feeding, and being at collection sites; understanding the concept of euthanasia and how it supports control and prevention of EZL; and safe road use including knowledge of road safety regulations and good communication while driving.

Mule welfare training modules were initially developed and delivered monthly by TDS staff and then through training delegates selected by their cart mule associations who provided training to other muleteers, including new muleteers outside their own association. The treatment protocol for active EZL cases required muleteers to clean wounds and apply tincture of iodine initially under the direct supervision of an animal health professional. This training support was later taken over by local animal health professionals. Harness training was facilitated by TDS harness specialists (animal health assistants trained by TDS international harness specialists). Road safety training was facilitated by local traffic police officers.

Training of Harness Makers

Almost all cart mule wounds were related to poor harnessing practice, and the project therefore needed to address this. It developed, tested, and piloted improved saddle prototypes, humane bits, and canvas straps. Training was provided to 12 harness makers stationed at two locations in Bahir Dar on the making, fitting, repair, and maintenance of this harness. TDS initially supplied the raw materials, e.g., wood, canvas, and the bit-making tools, during the prototype and testing phase.

Training of Animal Health Professionals

Local animal health professional staff included veterinary surgeons (6-year university training), BVScs (Bachelors of Veterinary Science, 3-year university training), and animal health assistants (3-year technical college training) at the public veterinary clinics in central Bahir Dar, Meshanti, Zanzelima, Gonbat, and Tis-Abay. Except central Bahir Dar with six to eight veterinary staff, other public veterinary clinics were health posts with one to two veterinary staff. There were also around seven or eight private animal health practitioners across Bahir Dar. Turnover among veterinary staff in public clinics, particularly the small health posts, was high, although some interested individuals remained engaged with the project even after promotion.

Before the project, muleteers were not taking mules with EZL to veterinary clinics for two reasons: because the animal health staff lacked competence in EZL diagnostics, treatment, and euthanasia (and equid medicine generally) and because clinics lacked the necessary drugs.

TDS therefore trained the animal health professionals and equipped the public veterinary clinics with tincture of iodine (2%) and potassium iodide.

Animal health professional training was prepared in four modules: mule behavior and handling; EZL diagnosis, treatment, and euthanasia; EZL epidemiology and herd health; and community facilitation skills and equine husbandry. Each module was delivered as a Continuing Professional Development (CPD) course and followed up with more informal practical hands-on training in the field at veterinary clinics.

Once the project was established, veterinarians with competence to train others (see Section Monitoring and evaluation of the project), including in communication skills, were selected for Training of Trainer (ToT) training so that they could continue to train muleteers and deliver further CPD training to other animal health professionals as necessary. Trainees were followed monthly by the TDS team up until 2015 and semiannually thereafter. The project targeted all animal health professionals for training.

Treatment of Early EZL Cases and Euthanasia of Advanced Cases

Treatment and euthanasia were critical elements of the intervention to contain spread of EZL because untreated or abandoned EZL mule cases remain a source of infection for other mules in Bahir Dar.

Cases were classified as early, established, advanced, and untreatable (recommended for euthanasia). Treatable cases were treated by incision of nodules when present, application of tincture of iodine, and administration of parenteral iodides (potassium iodide, Ubiche) in drinking water (30). Length of treatment increased the more severe the case classification. For the detailed procedure and outcome, please refer to Supplementary Section of the manuscript.

Euthanasia was performed using intravenous injection of barbiturates (Pentoject® 200 mg/ml solution, pentobarbital sodium 20% w/v, XVD132, Animalcare Limited, UK).

TABLE 2 | The Donkey Sanctuary general competence framework for trainees.

Competence level	Description and assessment process
Starter	All trainees start at this level to acknowledge and encourage interest. No real knowledge or experience but with active interest.
Becoming independent	Acknowledgement of starting actively along training journey. An active trainee, a reflective learner, with good attitude and regular attendance.
Independent	A trainee who has continued to show competence in what was taught and to demonstrate reflective practice, for at least 6 months after completing the formal training. Assessed by the TDS staff through practical follow-up field work.
Trainer	Independent practitioner in a primary area of competence, with additional independent competence following Training of Trainers (ToT) training. Identified for ToT training by demonstrating good communication skills, an interest in helping others to learn, strong reflective practice, and an interest and enthusiasm for becoming a trainer, and who has then reached independent level in training practice (assessed by the same competence framework).

Monitoring and Evaluation of the Project

Progress indicators for each aspect of the project were identified and agreed on by all stakeholders. Annually repeated cross-sectional surveys were conducted to assess prevalence of EZL and wounds as key indicators for the success of the project (see Sections Project study population and Annual cross-sectional surveys: prevalence of EZL and wounds).

Training was assessed using the TDS four-level general competence framework for trainees: starter, becoming independent, independent, and trainer (see **Table 2**).

Field reports were prepared monthly, project progress reports were prepared quarterly, and project evaluation reports were prepared annually. All stakeholders took part in consultative review workshops. External evaluations were conducted by Amhara Region regulatory signatories (Bureau of Livestock Agency and Bureau of Finance and Economics) midterm and at the end of the 5-year project agreement between TDS and the Government.

Project Exit Strategy

The project started with a 5-year agreement between TDS and the regional bureaus. The project aimed to find an approach to improving mule welfare, including reducing prevalence of EZL, that could be owned and sustained locally with a minimum of external input. Reflective learning among all stakeholder groups, including TDS, would be a central part of the work. TDS envisaged gradually reducing its involvement over further project cycles, while continuing to help refine the approach

and institutionalize key components such as cart mule business, training, and animal welfare standards.

This would involve empowering communities, mainstreaming best practices into the relevant sectors, recognizing EZL as a notifiable disease by the Bahir Dar municipality, transforming the local veterinary clinics to handle EZL cases and euthanize advanced cases by the regional livestock agency, formalizing and regulating mule-powered transport by the transport sector, supplying improved harness by local harness makers, formulating local community bylaws among the cart muleteers, and ideally encouraging institutions and organizations such as veterinary schools, the Ethiopian Veterinary Association, or the Ethiopian Animal Health Assistant Association to review their curricula, strengthen communication and community-engagement practices, and offer equine CPD training.

Gradually refining and reducing involvement over time was the project's exit strategy—a tailing out rather than an abrupt end. However, this was not possible for reasons outside project control.

Statistical Analysis

Information obtained from key informants was captured using facilitator notes and summarized into thematic areas and presented as a narrative. Results of FGDs obtained using different tools were presented in a map and a table.

Statistical analysis for annual prevalence study was carried out with STATA software version 11, using the chi-square statistical test, with the significance test set at a p-value $<$ 0.05. Mule demographics and prevalence studies were presented using proportions.

To examine the statistical significance for the persistence of the prevalence reduction, one-way ANOVA trend analysis was executed for prevalence reduction of both EZL and wounds across the years.

RESULTS

Demography—Survey of Mules and Muleteers

Owners sourced mules from local livestock markets around Bahir Dar including Yigodi, Merawi, and Bahir Dar central market. These mules are likely to have come through more distant markets in Este, Debre Tabor, and Adet, which are part of an equine trade network originating from South Wollo that extends across Central, Southern, and Western Ethiopia.

Mule transport is currently considered an informal economic activity and is unlicensed. Training and support services are limited, with no training available in mule handling, husbandry, or business management.

The major items transported by cart mules in Bahir Dar included construction supplies (56.6%) such as wood, stone, cement, gravel, and sacks of sand to meet the demand for Bahir City expansion; agricultural produce from nearby farms to markets (27.3%); and other commodities for sale and household use (16.1%) including water and flour.

TABLE 3 | Age structure of working mules in Bahir Dar in 2010 (number (N) and %), from baseline data.

Mules < 5 years N (%)	Mules 5–10 years N (%)	Mules > 10 years N (%)
47 (11)	241 (56)	142 (33)

Table 3 presents the age structure of the mule population of Bahir Dar in 2010 (extracted from 2010 baseline survey data), showing that 52% of mules were male and 48% of mules were female.

As part of the baseline, the TDS team assessed the working condition of mules to be generally poor. Almost all carts and harnesses and harnessing systems were poor. All drivers use a stick or whip to drive mules. Mules work throughout the day; there was no shifting practice unlike cart horses in other areas of Ethiopia. They stay loaded without feed and water at collection sites for an extended period particularly on non-market days. Cart owners work with an EZL case until the disease advances to affect the mule's ability to work, for example, by its impact on locomotion or its respiratory system, and finally, they abandon the mule.

Study Framework: Results of the PPMC Approach

Results of the PPMC approach with its collaborative working and flexible review points showed themselves in various ways.

Muleteers at the start mistrusted TDS and the veterinary services, used traditional treatments, and avoided outside interference. However, when they understood that the project was genuine about working with them and saw the potential benefits, they engaged with the veterinary service, with muleteers starting to accept euthanasia. Stakeholders took their own initiatives within the project structure: some cart mule associations introduced EZL bylaws; transport officers and traffic police in consultation with the cart mule associations developed mule-friendly improvements in traffic regulations supported with information bulletins put out through municipality media channels; and traffic police reported reduced numbers of road traffic accidents involving cart mules as the project progressed.

Stakeholder Analysis

Active involvement of diverse stakeholders is a central aspect of a community-based approach. The full list of stakeholders engaged with this project are listed in **Box 1**, grouped by affiliation.

Epidemiology
Case Definition and Diagnosis of EZL

The case definition for EZL provided a common understanding of the disease for diagnosis and training. It was observed consistently during the study that intact and non-staining yeast cells of HCF were common in early cases of EZL, and disintegrated yeast cells with deep-staining dotted granules were more common in relatively advanced cases (see **Figures 2A,B**).

BOX 1 | Project stakeholders by affiliation.

Project stakeholders
Muleteers
Muleteers in general
Delegates from eight of the most active of the 30 cart mule associations
Private sector
Cart and harness makers
Private animal health professionals/clinics
Licensed solid waste management cooperatives
Bahir Dar city administration
Animal health professionals from Bahir Dar clinics and subclinics
Bahir Dar city municipality
Transport officers (make regulations)
Traffic police (enforce regulations)
Solid waste management staff
Amhara regional bureaus
Livestock Agency
Regional Livestock Officer
Lab technicians from Bahir Dar Regional Laboratory
Bureau of Transport
Bureau of Finance and Economics
Regional NGO desk
The Donkey Sanctuary employees
Animal health professionals: veterinarians and allied professionals including harness specialists
Social science staff
Education specialists

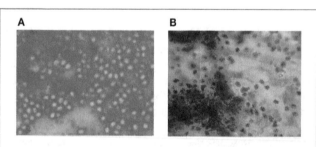

FIGURE 2 | Photomicrographs of *Histoplasma capsulatum* var. *farciminosum* yeast cells showing intact nonstaining yeast cells sampled from an early case **(A)** and disintegrated yeast cells with deep-staining dotted granules from an advanced case **(B)**.

These observations have not been reported in other studies and are therefore of note.

The case definition provided the basis for the annual prevalence surveys. The results from the prevalence survey are presented in **Table 4**.

Epidemiology: Annual Change in Prevalence of EZL in Bahir Dar

As shown in **Table 4**, the prevalence of EZL reduced from 23.9 to 5.9% during the course of the project. The prevalence of wounds reduced from 44.3 to 22.2%. The greatest changes came in the first 2 years of the project, with the prevalence of EZL reducing faster than that of wounds. After year 3, the improvements plateaued, with rises in 2015 for wounds and in 2016 for EZL as the

TABLE 4 | Prevalence of EZL in cart mules in Bahir Dar from baseline and annual prevalence surveys.

Year	Test positive	Prevalence (%)	95% CI (%)	Total tested sample
2010	102	23.9%	19.8%–28.0%	430
Total (baseline)	102			430
2011	79	12.7%	10.0%–15.3%	622
2012	54	4.8%	3.5%–6.0%	1,128
2013	75	5.9%	4.6%–7.2%	1,266
2014	NA[a]	NA	NA	NA
2015	23	5.8%	3.5%–8.2%	394
2016	144	10.0%	8.5%–11.6%	1,436
2017	58	5.9%	4.4%–7.4%	981
Total (project)	433			5,827

[a]NA—Data not available.

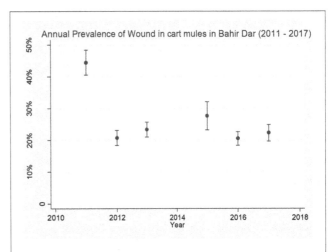

FIGURE 4 | Annual prevalence of open wounds in cart mules in Bahir Dar from 2010 to 2017 [NB: Error bars represent 95% confidence interval around wound prevalence value].

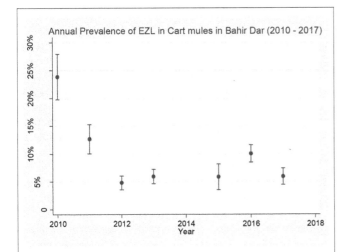

FIGURE 3 | Annual prevalence of EZL in cart mules in Bahir Dar from 2010 to 2017 [NB: Error bars represent 95% confidence interval around EZL prevalence value].

project tested handing more responsibility to private veterinary clinics. Despite this, trend analysis showed that the prevalence reductions in both EZL and wounds over the whole duration of the project were statistically significant ($\chi^2 = 26.57$; $p < 0.001$). Results from the baseline survey in 2010 and the subsequent annual surveys for the prevalence of EZL and wounds during the intervention period from 2011 to 2017 are presented in **Figures 3, 4**. No data were available for 2014 for reasons external to the project.

The prevalence reduction difference from 2010 to 2017 was 18.0% for EZL and 22.1% for wounds. The prevalence reduction trend analysis for both EZL and wound was statistically significant ($\chi^2 = 39.02$; $p < 0.001$). Wound data for 2010 were excluded because open wounds and healed wounds had not been put into different categories. An observation during the annual surveys was that while almost all the open wounds continued to originate from poor harnessing, the severity of wounds was reducing with fewer extensive or infected wounds or discharging abscesses, compared to the baseline stage.

Stakeholder Contributions

Key Informant Interviews

Individual key informant interviews gave insight about how informants understood EZL and related matters, with agreement about the following general themes.

All key informants believed that mules arrive from external markets free of EZL and only become infected in Bahir Dar. Informants agreed that EZL has a devastating socioeconomic effect, and follow-up discussions explored the cost of the mule (~ETB 10,000 = ~GBP 165) compared to the cost of treatment (~ETB 1,000 for early cases). Besides its socioeconomic impact on cart mule business, abandoned mules were a public concern contributing to a poor image of the city. Traffic police complained that abandoned EZL cases were sources of car accidents at various occasions, and an abandoned mule could be a cause of more than one accident over time, particularly at night. Waste collectors believed that terminally sick mules could easily be transported to disposal sites and killed there as it was tiresome to deal with a dead body elsewhere in the city. They suggested for a coordinated effort of stakeholders. Animal health professionals complained about the lack of treatment options and required updated skill sets in all equine practice, not just EZL as a single disease entity. Cart mule association delegates explained how EZL is a real worry to their business. They complained that new owners are a risk because they do not know how to identify, manage, and prevent EZL. They requested that regulatory authorities formalize and develop the sector. There was general agreement that the predisposing factors were wounds mainly from ill-fitting harnessing, poor hygiene, and lack of segregation practices; the main challenges for control are lack of an agreed-upon sound treatment protocol, poor harnessing practice, lack of awareness, lack of mule movement

TABLE 5 | Pairwise ranking of the predisposing factors identified by experienced muleteers during focused group discussions.

Predisposing factors of EZL	Proximity to EZL case (PE)	Owner's lack of experience (OE)	Fly season (FS)	Open wound (OW)	Poor harness (PH)	Poor hoof care (HC)	Working condition (WC)
Proximity to EZL case (PE)[a]		PE	PE	OW	PE	PE	PE
Owner's lack of experience (OE)			OE	OW	OE	OE	OE
Fly season (FS)				OW	FS	FS	FS
Open wound (OW)					OW	OW	OW
Poor harness (PH)						PH	PH
Poor hoof care (HC)							HC
Working condition (WC)[b]							
Total	OW	PE	OE	FS	PH	HC	WC
Rank (score[c])	1st (6)	2nd (5)	3rd (4)	3rd (4)	4th (2)	5th (1)	6th (0)

[a] Proximity at work, feeding, water, grazing, and housing. [b] Types of work engaged such as transporting construction, logs, and flour. [c] Score = number of other factors considered more important than during the individual pairwise comparisons.

control, and the business being informal and owned mainly by a resource-poor class of community and illiterate people; and EZL could be prevented easily through collaboration of relevant sectors including prevention of wounds, segregation of cases, and removal of abandoned EZL mule. Transport officers believed that in the long term, EZL will not be a problem in Bahir Dar because the cart mule work will soon be replaced by motorized vehicles.

FGDs

The results from the individual exercises used in the FGDs are presented below.

Socio-economic impacts of EZL (brainstorming and discussion). Muleteers compared the impact of EZL with the impact of other key endemic diseases that affect their cart mules, specifically colic, African horse sickness, and EZL. They described the negative socioeconomic impact of each on the business: colic occurs rarely and kills only one animal at a time, and it can be prevented; African horse sickness is a risk to other mules but comes once in several years and yet kills some mules while other mules recover; EZL is also a risk to other mules, occurs throughout the year, and has no reliable treatment option, and most EZL cases eventually die.

Predisposing Factors to EZL (Brainstorming, Card Ranking, and Pairwise Ranking). Muleteers identified the main predisposing factors for EZL as open wounds, proximity to another mule affected by EZL, owners' lack of knowledge and experience to prevent EZL, fly season, poor harnessing practice, hoof care, and working conditions.

These factors were then debated in more detail using pairwise ranking in which each factor is compared individually to all the others in turn. A summary of the result is presented in **Table 5**.

Participating muleteers ranked open wounds as the most important factor affecting spread of EZL, followed by proximity to other mules affected by EZL; next were owner's lack of experience and fly season, which were of equal importance; then poor harness was more important than poor hoof care practice; and work type was the least important factor.

Seasonal Calendar. The owners concluded that mules get the disease throughout the year; however, new cases were observed more after the long rainy season during the months of September and October, remain low during the dry seasons, and rise again following the small rainy season in April and May of the year.

Participatory Mapping. Key informants identified cart mule entry points to Bahir Dar, as well as movement and distribution. They located mule pathways and sites where cart mules come together such as markets, construction sites, flour mills, water points, grazing fields, healthcare units, and large group housing sites. The owners worked together to map these using referring points, which were translated onto a Google Map (see **Figure 5**).

The key informants summarized that cart mules were free to work anywhere in the city, be it markets, construction, or other working sites. There was no restriction of movement for an EZL case until it is abandoned. An abandoned EZL case still had access to socialize with apparently normal mules at feeding and water points, other collection sites, or grazing areas. Abandoned cases stay alive for months, and that is when they remain the source of infection for other mules.

Results of Implementation
Education of Muleteers

Table 6 shows the numbers of muleteers who attended structured, subject-based workshops which aimed to raise animal welfare awareness and change behaviors. The subject areas were mule behavior, handling, and care; mule harnessing practice and road traffic rules; wound management, including application of tincture of iodine; and EZL, i.e., detection and reporting, prevention measures, and euthanasia.

Examples of how education activities improved the mule-health-related practices of muleteers included increased number of equine cases visiting the public vet clinic; adoption of project EZL treatment protocols with wound management using application of tincture of iodine and gradual acceptance of euthanasia; segregation of infected and non-affected mules at collection and grazing sites; disinfection of harness materials; greater vigilance in reporting suspected cases of EZL as a

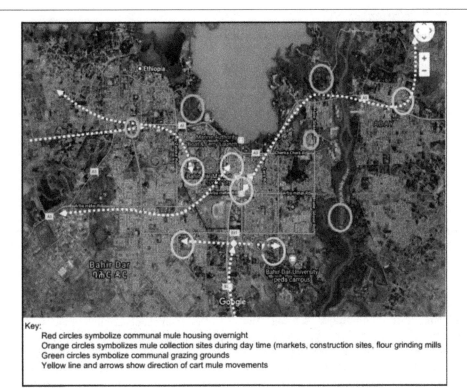

FIGURE 5 | Cart mule movement dynamics and gathering sites in Bahir Dar.

TABLE 6 | Numbers of muleteers attending different training sessions.

Subject/Year	Mule behavior, handling, and care	Mule harnessing practice; road traffic rules	Wound management, including application of tincture of iodine	EZL: detection and reporting, prevention measures, and euthanasia
2011	870	300	169	370
2012	627	624	124	227
2013	580	552	116	380
2014	600	178	73	410
2015	420	164	107	320
2016	280	388	45	187

notifiable disease; and increased use of cart and animal fitted reflectors when driving at night. In general, the muleteers understood that the success and benefit of the intervention relied on shared responsibility, with each taking responsibility not only for their own mule but also for the herd.

Competence levels of individual muleteers are not reported because individual follow-up was difficult, and competence assessment was therefore based on feedback at meetings, field observations at working sites, and observation of changes in practice. Based on these observations, the majority of muleteers were in the "becoming independent" and "independent" category, apart from a few exceptional muleteers who took it upon themselves to mentor others.

Owners with EZL cases were more immediately attentive and engaged than those who had apparently EZL-free mules, but as the intervention progressed, some owners with advanced EZL cases became reluctant to attend the training or treatment clinics because they feared pressure for euthanasia.

The results of the awareness-raising training sessions with traffic police, transport officers, waste collectors, and other municipality development agents came through their changing, more constructive relationships with the muleteers.

Other events, such as World Animal Day, which was observed every year during the first week of October and promoted animal welfare more widely, demonstrated the growth in confidence of project stakeholders who were able

TABLE 7 | Trainings provided for animal healthcare professionals and number of attendees.

Subject/year	Mule behavior, handling, and care	EZL diagnosis, treatment, and euthanasia	EZL epidemiology and principles of herd health	Community facilitation skills and equine husbandry
2011	24	24	24	18
2012	21	18	18	20
2013	21	13	15	18
2014	16	16	14	16
2015	6	6 (4 ToT[a])	8 (4 ToT[a])	
2016			11	11

[a]ToT—trainers' training was provided at a later stage so that new staff can be trained by the local veterinarians.

Training of Harness Makers

Of the 12 harness makers, eight successfully completed the training and were producing improved prototypes of saddle and humane bits and straps. During the intervention period, the harness makers produced 584 improved cart saddles, 430 humane bits, and 893 canvas straps and collars, which were exchanged with poor traditional types.

Training of Animal Health Professionals

Attendance at training sessions for local animal health professionals is presented in **Table 7**. The training was intensive in terms of time and tasks. Mule behavior training was particularly challenging for trainees, most of whom had no experience in working professionally with mules. For various reasons, some veterinarians were irregular in attendance. Most veterinarians demanded incentives for the follow-up treatments. The owners' pressure to get his mule healed and TDS commitment to invest in the treatment were boosters for the success of the training and treatment. Despite the challenges mentioned above, all clinic veterinary staff achieved independent competence during the course of the project, assessed through long-term clinic follow-up. Two veterinarians from Bahir Dar clinic and two from animal health posts excelled in their competence as trainees and then trainers and played an important role in ongoing project success.

Treatment of Early Cases and Euthanasia of Advanced Cases

Treatment and euthanasia were critical components of the project to remove cases from the herd. For the euthanasia protocol, please see the **Supplementary Materials** section. Before the project, euthanasia was rarely done and had not been considered as a disease control practice in the area. Constraints were lack of drugs and a system for the disposal of carcasses as well as difficulty to get owners' consent without any compensation.

In piloting this model, TDS made drugs available, trained professionals, and raised public awareness in the perceptions and value of euthanasia. The Bahir Dar City municipality cooperated in the provision of trailers, disposal sites, and organizing associations working on city sanitation for disposal of euthanized mules. Getting owners' consent to euthanize mules with poor EZL prognosis was the inherent challenge throughout the intervention. Nevertheless, a total of 123 mules were euthanized during the period of the project.

Development of cart mule association bylaws helped reinforce good practice among members and influenced non-members through peer association. The Bahir Dar municipality also, for the first time, developed a range of bylaws relating to working equids; however, this came toward the end of the project period, and no mechanism for effective enforcement was developed before the project ended.

Evaluation of the Project by Signatories

The project was originally signed for 5 years with the intention of piloting a community-based system to control and prevent EZL. The Amhara Regional Livestock Agency, the Bahir Dar City Administration, and Regional Bureau of Transport, all regulated and coordinated by the NGO desk of the Regional Bureau of Finance and Economics, jointly conducted midterm and final evaluations.

The midterm evaluation focused on stakeholder commitment, coordination mechanisms, and testing the impact on the prevalence of EZL. Finding a dramatic reduction in the prevalence of EZL opened the eyes of many stakeholders, particularly the muleteers, animal health professionals, and traffic police.

The final evaluation focused greater emphasis on drawing conclusions about best practice and sustainability. The evaluating team reflected that the project impact was significant and obvious to the general public in Bahir Dar. The most publicly noticeable change was avoidance of abandoned EZL-affected mules in the middle of roads in Bahir Dar city, a prime tourist destination in Ethiopia. The practice of abandoning a mule at the end of its working life to continue to suffer in pain and die of deprivation of food and water is visibly cruel, is a public worry, and portrays a bad image for the city. All parties witnessed and shared success stories: the livestock agency witnessed the treatment success and training modalities for its animal health professionals; the municipality witnessed and appreciated the value of coordination in transforming livelihoods of muleteers; and the traffic police officers witnessed a persistent reduction of cart-mule-associated road traffic accidents.

A learning point was the time needed to establish a community-based project and engage stakeholders. One 2-year project extension was completed to strengthen the intervention, but for reasons beyond its control, the project then ended.

Outcome of Project Exit Strategy

The objective of an exit strategy is for the project as an entity to end its input, leaving behind a self-sustaining positive impact.

The benefits of the euthanasia program to mule herd health and the mechanism of operation have been recognized in Bahir Dar. A bylaw was established to sustain the change and control and prevent EZL. The articles contained in the bylaw require notification of an EZL case to the nearest traffic police or public veterinary clinic within 48 h, segregation of an EZL case, euthanasia of a terminally sick EZL case, prevention of wound, and registration of new muleteers as they join the business. The Bahir Dar city administration mainstreamed the disposal mechanism of dead mules alongside solid waste.

The traffic regulations mainstreamed animal-powered transport systems into the Bahir Dar traffic public awareness-raising program to minimalize road traffic accidents. Subjects promoted include use of reflectors; improved harness and mule health and welfare; a minimum muleteer age; and skill and knowledge of driving to prevent road traffic accidents.

Trust has been established between Bahir Dar public veterinary clinic service providers and muleteers for the treatment of early cases and euthanasia of terminally sick cases.

However, the long-term sustainability of the EZL project relies on many factors including further formalization of animal-powered transport into the city/regional development program alongside recognition that it is not about to be replaced by mechanized transport and transformation of animal healthcare delivery to include equine medicine and welfare. Also the low status of the sector, the low level of formal education among muleteers with limited alternative livelihood options, the current informal nature of the business, and the influx of new mules into the city remain challenges to sustainability.

DISCUSSION

Overview

The TDS tested a community-based model for the control and prevention of EZL and wounds in cart mules in Bahir Dar as part of a wider donkey and mule welfare program in the Amhara Region of Ethiopia. The focus of the project was identified following a welfare assessment using the 'Hand' tool. Previous studies in Bahir Dar (13, 53) and across multiple countries (54) reported lameness as the most common problem facing working equids. This assessment identified mule–muleteer–societal relationships, wounds, and EZL as the most serious challenges facing mules in Bahir Dar with lameness, nutrition, and abandonment at end of life as additional problems.

The lack of a reliable treatment or a commercially available vaccine limits options for EZL control and prevention. As a result, EZL poses a threat to mule cart businesses and to mule

welfare and is the commonest cause of mule abandonment in Bahir Dar. Mules that can no longer pull carts for whatever reason are left to die of thirst and starvation, are often associated with traffic accidents (18, 27, 31), and present a poor image of the city.

TDS recognized that most working equine welfare problems are a result of poor management practices, lack of an affordable healthcare model, and underlying socioeconomic factors and that an effective and lasting solution to EZL control and prevention required involvement of all the relevant stakeholders, including muleteers, service providers, and policy makers, and the interplay of participatory and classical epidemiology. The project built on lessons from previous unsuccessful attempts to control EZL through treatment-only interventions in Bahir Dar and elsewhere (30, 33). TDS identified EZL as a visible indicator of poor welfare for cart mules in Bahir Dar and therefore also of wider program success.

With the ratification of the OIE Working Equid Welfare Standards, the project saw itself as modeling an approach to how these standards might be implemented and therefore increase interest in the outcomes of the work.

Impact

With a drop in prevalence of EZL from 23.9% (102/430) in 2010 to 5.9% (58/981) in 2017 and of open wounds from 44.3% in 2011 to 22.2% in 2017, the project suggests that prevalence of wounds and EZL can be significantly reduced in working mules through a community-based intervention as described. These drops in prevalence were associated with improved owner husbandry and handling of mules, improved cart and harness design, more mule-friendly municipal traffic practices, more trusting relationships between mule owners and local veterinary staff, improved equine medical competence among local veterinary staff, treatments provided for EZL, reduced abandonment of sick animals, mule community bylaws relating to EZL control put in place, and a means for animals with advanced incurable EZL to be humanely euthanized.

EZL prevalence in 2010 was within the range reported across Ethiopia in cart horses (16, 55), which varied from 39.1% in Mojo to 21.1% in Nazret, and was comparable to reports from Ejaji and Bako where prevalence was 21% in cart mules (17). Prevalence of wounds in 2010 was also comparable to previous reports in Bahir Dar and the adjacent town of Adet (8, 56), where most wounds were also associated with poor harnessing practice (10). Prevalence of EZL in 2017 in Bahir Dar was below any previously published reports of EZL prevalence in working equids in an EZL endemic area of Ethiopia. This reduction in EZL prevalence over the course of the project was significant. The authors are not aware of any other published reports of projects intended to control and prevent EZL in similar or indeed any other circumstances.

The drop in EZL and wound prevalence took place within the first 2 years and over the first 3 years of the project, respectively. These reduced prevalence rates were maintained in the face of year-on-year rises in the population of working mules. It is possible that part of the reduction in prevalence was due to a dilution effect from newly arrived mules, but this factor would not explain the consistent sustained reduction. Equally, the arrival of new mules occurred alongside an increase in mule use and busier collection points, factors that could facilitate an increased rate of EZL spread. During World War II, it was the collection and mixing of horses that challenged the control of EZL (27). With the annually increasing population, we believe that if it were not for the control imposed by the project, the prevalence could have worsened. The rise in the prevalence of EZL in 2016 after a trial in 2015 to hand treatment responsibility to private veterinarians showed how quickly prevalence can rise and highlighted the lack of an economic model for effective private veterinary services in Bahir Dar.

The move in Ethiopia to delineate public and private roles in veterinary services is still in its infancy and beyond the project's scope, but this holds out hope for the future (57). Future projects might help facilitate herd health veterinary service models, possibly with well-established cart mule associations as the herd, whereby instead of being paid for individual treatments, veterinarians are paid collectively against reduction in incidence and prevalence for all association mules.

Possible factors constraining further reductions in prevalence of EZL include the dynamic and unregulated nature of the cart mule business in Bahir Dar with changing demographics; new muleteers with limited experience of wound management and EZL control; mixing of mules during the course of their work, feeding, watering, and general husbandry' unregulated movement around the city of known EZL cases; treatment factors including the investment in time needed; the financial investment in the mule making it difficult for muleteers to accept euthanasia; and the lack of an enabling regulatory framework. Further demographic research on the mule population would have provided rich data but was not possible within the resources of the project. From a welfare point of view, the failure to reduce wound prevalence below 20% was disturbing; however, there was an observed reduction in wound severity during the annual surveys.

In EZL endemic areas, dealing rapidly with EZL cases which act as potential sources of infection, through treatment of treatable cases or euthanasia of untreatable cases, is vital for effective control and prevention. In the project, TDS supplied medicines, equipment, and euthanasia drugs and used each treatment as an opportunity to build competence of animal health professionals. Treatment outcomes were comparable to previously published reports (30, 31, 33, 58, 59).

Epidemiology

The application of epidemiology and epidemiological tools served two roles in this project. First was to corroborate existing knowledge, take forward understanding about EZL, and inform the work. Second was to engage stakeholders so that they understood and took ownership of the steps needed to control and prevent the disease. The project used both participatory and classical epidemiology methods.

Although elucidating causal relationships between EZL and wounds or other associated factors was not an objective of the study, it was important to corroborate potential risk factors associated with EZL as mentioned in the literature including open wounds, hygiene, and collection site practice (17, 27, 60). Using participatory epidemiology tools, we found that muleteers already recognized proximity to an EZL case in a population (including abandoned mules), open wounds, poor harnessing, new owners with limited experience, poor hoof care, poor working conditions, and fly season as predisposing factors to EZL (**Table 5**).

Key informants claimed that mules get EZL throughout the year, with new cases being more common following a rainy season (30). However, the project observed the highest numbers of new EZL cases just before the long rainy season, after which untreatable cases were abandoned and die, and the cycle continues. Possible reasons for this include that during the rainy season, economic activities like construction will be reduced, which affects muleteers' income, affecting their expenditure on the care of mules.

The project was not able to explore potential clustering effects of mules temporarily gathered at a given working station. Mules mix fairly flexibly at daytime collection sites, grazing areas, and communal housing sites (see map in **Figure 4**); EZL-affected individuals are not quarantined; most mules in Bahir Dar work all day with no shift system; owners with more than one mule are generally renting them out. So clustering was considered unlikely to affect results significantly. Nevertheless, ideally, the project would have explored mule demographics in greater detail epidemiologically, socially, and economically.

Community-Based Approach and Sustainability

The project provides an example of how NGO-led interventions can test new models for change through better access to targeted funding, skill sets, and resources. However, ownership by the local community is needed to make the change last.

In this project, the community-based approach and participatory methods were essential to success by empowering stakeholders, increasing engagement, ensuring local ownership, and building bridges and common understanding between different stakeholder groups. The results of the project are similar to the successes of other community-based animal healthcare initiatives (35, 36, 61).

Encouraging signs of growing stakeholder ownership included development of bylaws and guidelines and use of media to transmit information. The public launch of the project and yearly follow-up events such as World Animal Day proved beneficial in creating a sense of teamwork among the stakeholders and also worked as awareness-raising and advocacy tools.

The successes of the project were achieved despite working animals having no mention in Ethiopia's federal 5-year Growth and Transformation Plans and there being no animal welfare legislation, poor equine health and welfare practices, and little recognition of the valuable social services provided by mules and muleteers. The achievements in shifting viewpoints, particularly among the regulatory authorities, were therefore significant.

Sustaining project impact may require policy changes such as more flexible approaches to pharmaceuticals and equipment procurement by the veterinary regulatory authorities to allow government clinics to respond better to local healthcare priorities or more effective regulation of public and private veterinary roles to allow development of more effective service models.

The sustainability challenges facing the project are common to all donor veterinary projects, and not unique to community-based projects nor to NGO-led projects. The global campaign to eradicate rinderpest took decades and many different approaches, and the current campaign to eradicate peste des petits ruminants is also a long-term campaign. Empowering local veterinary services and involving communities are common to stories of success.

The project responds to a recently published work by Gizaw et al. (62), which assessed veterinary service delivery in Ethiopia, by demonstrating a model for development of services that can work for marginalized mule–muleteer communities in urban settings. The work by Gizaw et al. and this project highlight the need for a study of appropriate veterinary service design and community facilitation skills within the curricula of veterinary training institutes to ensure animal health and welfare professionals' awareness of the different approaches that can be used to achieve improved health and welfare for animals, particularly in resource-poor or otherwise marginalized communities. While holistic socioeconomic transformation of the mule sector will take time, the project has shown what is possible and can act as a seed for change.

Cost-Effectiveness and Carbon Benefits

The ~ETB 10,000 (~GBP 165) cost of a mule in Bahir Dar reported by muleteers compared to the ~ETB 1,000 cost of EZL treatment if caught early gives a sense of scale to the recent (2021) estimates by Molla et al. (15), in their study of the economic costs of EZL in cart mules and horses in two urban locations in the Amhara Region, with an average annual animal level loss of ETB 6,587 per cart animal per year averaged out between EZL-affected and EZL-unaffected animals.

Using the above figures with mule numbers in Bahir Dar and reduction in EZL prevalence, together with project costs, allows estimation of the cost-benefit. Figures are not presented for this project because they are broad approximations, but they do suggest that there should be a cost-benefit for repeating this work where there are working mules in EZL endemic areas, that the approach could be institutionalized sustainably within public/private veterinary services in Ethiopia (63, 64), and that as the confidence of muleteers and other stakeholders grew, they might realize the benefits of investing in the improvements, including veterinary treatments. Future projects would do well to include economic analysis into their work from the start through collaboration with socioeconomists, ideally from local institutes.

It is also worth noting that Molla et al. (15) did not specifically include additional potential benefits that might accrue to the project from reduced wounds and increased work efficiency from improved communication between mules,

muleteers, and municipality. Nor do they include potential carbon/climate/ecosphere-related benefits.

High-welfare mules, working safely and efficiently, are an effective low carbon form or transport, particularly for short distances (65). Throughout the project, transport officials in Bahir Dar held to the idea that mule transport will be replaced by motorized, currently fossil-fuel powered, vehicles, even in the face of year-on-year increases in mule numbers. Nevertheless, they also, for the first time, introduced municipal bylaws to facilitate more efficient, high-welfare mule transport. This demonstrates that community-based projects might play a part in establishing an environment conducive to low-carbon transportation.

Study Limitations and Challenges

In this study, the socioeconomic conditions and demographic volatility of working mules made follow-up of individual new cases problematic and unaffordable, particularly as EZL and wounds are generally protracted conditions requiring complex interventions. Elucidation of causal relationships between associated risk factors was not pursued as a project priority. To do this within the constraints of such a project would face ethical challenges.

The challenge of exploring clustering effects has been discussed above alongside the desirability for future projects to explore other epidemiological, social, and economic aspects of the cart mule sector, possibly through using a cross-disciplinary team with involvement from local institutes.

Sampling was challenging because of the dynamic nature of the mule population. The plan was to do a full census every year; however, this was not possible in some years. For sample surveys in 2015 and 2017, to reduce the duration of work disruption for muleteers and to ensure representation, mules were mostly examined at their working stations. At times, this posed challenges to the practicality of our systematic random sampling strategy of sampling every other mule (e.g., in a work station where we found only one mule). While there is a possibility that this might introduce sampling bias, we went beyond calculated sample size to minimize this possibility. The risk that vets drawn toward EZL cases despite the sampling methodology might overestimate EZL prevalence was also a possibility.

Unlike most towns, in Bahir Dar, equine power transport is limited to cart mules (6). With increasing urbanization and a high unemployment rate, rapidly growing cart mule numbers presented a challenge to the project as mostly inexperienced new muleteers with new mules arrived. Nevertheless, established muleteers, trained animal health professionals, and traffic police officers took responsibility to engage with new arrivals, and EZL and wound prevalence reductions remained comparatively low.

While muleteers in Bahir Dar are all male, this is not the case elsewhere in Ethiopia. There appears to be a more even balance of female and male equine owners in rift valley towns near Ziway where EZL is also present. In future projects, it would be useful to explore similarities and differences between male and female muleteers.

While case definitions for the different stages of EZL may seem clear to animal health professionals, all treatment protocols require the compliance of muleteers, each of whose social and economic circumstances are different. Some with advanced case of EZL chose to move to the periphery of the town and work outside normal hours to continue making money from their infected mule in the face of social disapproval. Future projects might want to consider compensation or insurance schemes to improve compliance and help reduce prevalence still further; however, these need to be carefully designed and run, both with stakeholder involvement, if they are to be effective. If the status and economic security of the cart mule sector were to rise, these options might become more feasible and acceptable.

The continuing belief by planners and regulators that cart mules will be replaced by motor transport has held back the development of animal-powered transport despite its social value. The project has helped break down this prejudice slightly, but ideally, animal-powered transport should be included in government development plans. Similarly, a lack of understanding about animal welfare presents a challenge to improving the efficiency and effectiveness of the sector.

Applicability and Replicability

The project is applicable not only to other cities in Ethiopia with endemic EZL but also to animal healthcare challenges in other circumstances, including other countries with EZL (62). Successful replication requires recognition of the time needed to build the project on a secure foundation of stakeholder engagement from community to regulatory level. This includes establishing a common understanding of the epidemiology prior to the intervention and close engagement with veterinary and transport service regulatory bodies. Specifically for EZL, early development of community-level and municipality bylaws would be helpful and a compensation or insurance mechanism to facilitate euthanasia of advanced cases would be worth exploring.

CONCLUSIONS

The project achieved its aim of demonstrating an affordable sustainable approach to improving mule welfare with a reduction in EZL and wounds in cart mules in Bahir Dar between 2010 and 2017 despite rapidly changing mule demographics.

Every step was manageable within existing local institutions, with locally available resources, and economic considerations suggest it could be affordable. Although, for reasons outside its control, the project could not go far enough in embedding

the processes, much of the routine work was already being handed over.

To replicate the intervention in other endemic areas, we recommend engaging with stakeholders and establishing the epidemiology at the start, developing bylaws, and exploring an insurance or compensation mechanism for euthanasia cases.

Participatory methodologies were essential for engaging stakeholders and empowering communities, and the lessons learnt show the value of a community-based approach to infectious disease control alongside wider human and animal welfare benefits, particularly in resource-poor or otherwise marginalized communities.

With the OIE Working Equid Welfare Standards now adopted internationally, the authors suggest that integrated community-based interventions are a useful approach to EZL control and prevention in endemic areas within wider working equid welfare improvement programs.

AUTHOR CONTRIBUTIONS

BD and SB designed and supervised the study. TT, AKassaye, and AKassa implemented the programme on the ground. BD, SB, and AKassaye wrote up the study. All authors contributed to the article and approved the submitted version.

ACKNOWLEDGMENTS

We would like to thank all the project stakeholders who showed what is possible when people work in collaboration; The Donkey Sanctuary field team in Ethiopia who delivered the program, of which this project was a part; Sally Price, who trained the local team on community-based participatory approaches; Chris Garrett, who did the same in developing practical harness competence; Joe Anzuino, for supporting the veterinary aspect; Angie Garner, for facilitating the availability of supplies; and The Donkey Sanctuary who funded the work through the generosity of its supporters. We would also like to acknowledge the enormous contribution made by the reviewers who gave generously of their time to help strengthen and refine this article.

REFERENCES

1. CSA (Central Statistics Agency). Agricultural Sample Survey 2020/21. Statistical Bulletin 589, Vol. 2 Report on Livestock and Livestock Characteristics (Private Peasant Holdings). (2021). Addis Ababa: Central Statistical Agency (CSA).

2. Behnke R, Fitaweke M.The contribution of livestock to the Ethiopian economy - Part II, IGAD LPI Working Paper N° 2–11, Djibouti(2011). p. 20-22. Available online at: https://core.ac.uk/download/pdf/132642443.pdf-

3. Ochieng F, Alemayahu M, Smith D. *Improving the productivity of donkeys in Ethiopia*. In: Responding to the Increasing Global Demand for

Animal Products: Programme and Summaries 4, London, DFID (2004). p. 93–94. Available online at: https://assets.publishing.service.gov.uk/media/57a08cb6e5274a31e00013b2/R7350j.pdf

4. Temesgen Z, Sitota T. The welfare issues of working equine in Ethiopia: a review. *Europ J Biol Sci.* (2019) 11:82–90. Available online at: https://www.idosi.org/ejbs/11(3)19/3.pdf

5. World Bank 2019. Population total – Ethiopia (1995-2019). Available online at: https://data.worldbank.org/indicator/SP.POP.TOTL?end=2019&locations=ET&start=1995. Retrieved May 29, 2021.

6. Bekele H, Teshome W, Nahom W, Legesse G. *Socioeconomic impact of epizootic lymphangitis in cart mules in Bahir Dar city, North West Ethiopia*

(Conference presentation). Proceedings of the 7th international colloquium on working equids (July 2014), Royal Holloway, University of London, United Kingdom (2014). Available online at: https://www.researchgate.net/publication/302499290_7th-colloquium-on-working-equids-proceedings

7. Fentie G, Teka F, Fikadu A, Ayalew N, Tsegalem A. Injuries in donkeys and mules: causes, welfare problems and management practices in Amhara Region, Northern Ethiopia. *Am-Euras J Sci Res*. (2014) 9:98–104. doi: 10.5829/idosi.aejsr.2014.9.4.21802

8. Dressie D, Temesgen W, Yenew M. Study On Welfare Assessment of Cart Pulling Mule in Bahir Dar Town, Northwest Ethiopia. *Rep Opinion*. (2017) 9:73–86. http://www.dx.doi.org/10.7537/marsroj090717.12

9. Perry B. We must tie equine welfare to international development. *Veterinary Record*. (2017) 181:600. doi: 10.1136/vr.j5561

10. Meselu D, Abebe R, Mekibib B. Prevalence of epizootic lymphangitis and bodily distribution of lesions in cart-mules in Bahir Dar town, northwest Ethiopia. *J Vet Sci Technol*. (2018) 9:1–4. doi: 10.4172/2157-7579.1000509

11. Solomon T, Mussie HM, Fanaye S. Assessment of carting equine welfare and management practice in Bahir Dar town. *Int J Adv Res Biol Sci*. (2016) 3:100–112. Available online at: https://ijarbs.com/pdfcopy/dec2016/ijarbs13.pdf

12. Mulualem T, Mekonnen A, Wudu T. Seroprevalence and risk factors of African Horse Sickness in mules and donkeys in selected sites of West Amhara Region, Ethiopia. *Afr J Microbiol Res*. (2012) 6:4146–51. doi: 10.5897/AJMR11.1475

13. Ali A, Orion S, Tesfaye T, Zambriski JA. The prevalence of lameness and associated risk factors in cart mules in Bahir Dar, Ethiopia. *Trop Anim Health Prod*. (2016) 48:1483–9. doi: 10.1007/s11250-016-1121-7

14. Takele B, Nibret E. Prevalence of gastrointestinal helminthes of donkeys and mules in and around Bahir Dar, Ethiopia. *Ethiop Vet J*. (2013) 17:13–30. doi: 10.4314/evj.v17i1.2

15. Molla AM, Fentahun T, Jemberu WT. Estimating the economic impact and assessing owners' knowledge and practices of epizootic lymphangitis in equine cart animals in Central and South Gondar Zones, Amhara Region, Ethiopia. *Front Vet Sci*. (2021) 8:673442. doi: 10.3389/fvets.2021.673442

16. Amenil G, Siyoum F. Study on histoplasmosis (epizootic lymphangitis) in cart-horses in Ethiopia. *J Vet Sci*. (2002) 3:135–40. doi: 10.4142/jvs.2002.3.2.135

17. Ameni G, Terefe W, A. cross-sectional study of epizootic lymphangitis in cart-mules in Western Ethiopia. *Prev Vet Med*. (2004) 66:93–9. doi: 10.1016/j.prevetmed.2004.09.008

18. Ameni G. Epidemiology of equine histoplasmosis (epizootic lymphangitis) in carthorses in Ethiopia. *Vet J*. (2006) 172:160–65. doi: 10.1016/j.tvjl.2005.02.025

19. Ameni G. Pathology and clinical manifestation of epizootic lymphangitis in cart mules in Ethiopia. *J Equine Sci*. (2007) 18:1–4. doi: 10.1294/jes.18.1

20. Endebu B, Roger F. Comparative studies on the occurrence and distribution of Epizootic lymphangitis and Ulcerative lymphangitis in Ethiopia. *Int J Appl Res Vet Med*. (2003) 1:219–222. Available online at: http://www.jarvm.com/articles/Vol1Iss3/Endebu.htm

21. Scantlebury CE, Zerfu A, Pinchbeck GP, Reed K, Gebreab F, Aklilu N, et al. Participatory appraisal of the impact of Epizootic lymphangitis in Ethiopia. *Prev Vet Med*. (2015) 120:265–76. doi: 10.1016/j.prevetmed.2015.03.012

22. Blakeway S. The multi-dimensional donkey in landscapes of donkey-human interaction. *Relat Beyond Anthropocentrism*. (2014) 2:59–77. doi: 10.7358/rela-2014-001-blak

23. Cousquer G. Promoting pack mule welfare on expedition. *Prof Mountaineer*. (2015) 9:14–6. Available online at: https://www.travindy.com/2015/12/pack-mule-welfare-abuses-in-mountain-tourism/

24. Cousquer G. *Knowing the mule: Faring well in Moroccan mountain tourism*. (PhD thesis), University of Edinburgh, Edinburgh. (2018).

25. Blakeway S, Cousquer GO. *Donkeys and mules and tourism*. In N. Carr & D. M. Broom (Eds.), Tourism and animal welfare (2018). p. 126–3. Wallingford: CAB International. doi: 10.1079/9781786391858.0126

26. Scantlebury C, Reed K. *Epizootic lymphangitis*. In: Infectious Diseases of the Horse, Ed: TS Mair & RE Hutchinson, Equine Veterinary Journal Ltd, Ely, Cambridge shire, United Kingdom (2009). p. 397–406.

27. Al-Ani F. Epizootic lymphangitis in horses: a review of literature. *Rev Sci Tech Off Int Epiz*. (1999) 18:691–699. doi: 10.20506/rst.18.3.1186

28. Taboada J. Epizootic lymphangitis. In: Kahn CM, Line S, Aiello SE, editors. *The Merck veterinary manual*. Whitehouse Station, NJ: Merck and Co. (2018). Available online at: https://www.msdvetmanual.com/generalizedconditions/fungal-infections/epizootic-lymphangitis. (accessed 29 May 2021).

29. Carter GR, Chengappa MM, Claus W, Rikihisa Y. *Essentials of Veterinary Bacteriology and Mycology*. (4th ed.). Philadelphia : Lea & Febiger (1991). p. 284.

30. Getachew A. Clinical trial of iodides combined with ancillary treatment on Epizootic lymphangitis in cart horses at Debre Zeit and Akaki towns. *Faculty Vet Med*. (2004)

31. Mekonnen N, Makonnen E, Aklilu N, Ameni G. Evaluation of berries of Phytolacca dodecandra for growth inhibition of Histoplasma capsulatum var. farciminosum and treatment of cases of epizootic lymphangitis in Ethiopia. *Asian Pacific J Trop Biomed*. (2012) 2:505-510. doi: 10.1016/S2221-1691(12)60086-0

32. Jones K. Epizootic lymphangitis: the impact on subsistence economies and animal welfare. *Vet J*. (2006) 172:402–4. doi: 10.1016/j.tvjl.2006.06.003

33. Tagesu A. Review on equine Epizootic lymphangitis and its impact in Ethiopia. *J Vet Med Res*. (2017) 4:1–8. Available online at: https://www.jscimedcentral.com/VeterinaryMedicine/veterinarymedicine-4-1087.pdf

34. Gardiner A. Veterinary anthropology explored. *Vet Rec*. (2016) 178:575–6. doi: 10.1136/vr.i2888

35. Catley A, Blakeway S, Leyland T. Community-based animal healthcare: a practical guide to improving primary veterinary services (2002). p. 368.

36. Catley A, Leyland T. Community participation and the delivery of veterinary services in Africa. *Prev Vet Med*. (2001) 49:95–113. doi: 10.1016/s0167-5877(01)00171-4

37. Catley A, Alders RG, Wood JL. Participatory epidemiology: approaches, methods, experiences. *Vet J*. (2012) 191:151–60. doi: 10.1016/j.tvjl.2011.03.010

38. Alders RG, Ali SN, Ameri AA, Bagnol B, Cooper TL, Gozali A, et al. Participatory Epidemiology: principles, practice, utility, and lessons learnt. *Front Vet Sci*. (2020) 7:532763. doi: 10.3389/fvets.2020.532763

39. Mariner J, Roeder P. Admassu, B. Community participation and the global eradication of rinderpest. *PLA Notes*. (2002) 45:29–33. Available online at: https://www.iied.org/pla-45-community-based-animal-healthcare

40. Mariner JC, House JA, Mebus CA, Sollod AE, Chibeu D, Jones BA, et al. Rinderpest eradication: appropriate technology and social innovations. *Science*. (2012) 337:1309–12. doi: 10.1126/science.1223805

41. Roeder P, Mariner J, Kock R. Rinderpest: the veterinary perspective on eradication. *Philos Trans R Soc Lond B Biol Sci*. (2013) 368:20120139. doi: 10.1098/rstb.2012.0139

42. Samy A, Ibrahim MG, Mahmod WE, Fujii M, Eltawil A, Daoud W. Statistical assessment of rainfall characteristics in Upper Blue Nile Basin over the period from 1953 to 2014. *Water*. (2019) 11:468. doi: 10.3390/w11030468

43. Hart T, Burgess R., Beukes O, Hart C. (2005). Reducing pitfalls in agricultural development projects: a case for the Participatory Project Management Cycle (PPMC). *S Afr J Agric Ext*. (2005) 34:104–21. Accessed online at: https://www.ajol.info/index.php/sajae/article/view/3681

44. Hart T, Burgess R., Hart C. A participatory project management cycle: can it add value to agricultural development? *S Afr J Agric Ext*. (2005) 34:201–20. Available online at: https://www.ajol.info/index.php/sajae/article/view/3670

45. Brouwer JH, Hiemstra W, Martin P. Using stakeholder and power analysis and BCPs in multi-stakeholder processes. *PLA Notes*. (2012) 65:184–92. Available online at: https://pubs.iied.org/g03412

46. Michael T, Matthew T, Wilbur L. *A systematic approach to estimating the age of a horse*. In: AAEP – Proceedings, (1999). p. 45. Available online at: https://www.dentalage.co.uk/wp-content/uploads/2014/09/martin_mt_1993_daa_horses.pdf

47. The Donkey Sanctuary. *Body Scoring*. In: The Clinical Companion of the Donkey. 1st Edition, Linda Evans and Michael Crane (eds), The Donkey Sanctuary, UK (2018). p. 258.

48. Fowler FJ. *Survey research methods*. 4th ed. Thousand Oaks, CA: SAGE. (2009). doi: 10.4135/9781452230184

49. Thrusfield M, Christley R, Brown H, Diggle P, French N, Howe K.et al. Veterinary Epidemiology, 4th Ed. (2018). John Wiley & Sons Ltd. doi: 10.1002/9781118280249

50. IIED 1994. RRA Notes 20: Livestock. Available online at: https://www.iied.org/rra-notes-20-livestock

51. IIED 2013. PLA Notes. Available online at: https://www.iied.org/participatory-learning-action-pla

52. ODI. Planning tools: Problem Tree Analysis (2009). Available online at: https://odi.org/en/publications/planning-tools-problem-tree-analysis/. (accessed June 25, 2021)

53. Meseret B, Mersha C, Tewodros T, Anteneh K, Bekele M, Nahom W. Lameness and associated risk factors in cart mules in Northwestern Ethiopia. *Global Veterinaria.* (2014) 12:869–77. Available online at: https://www.idosi.org/gv/gv12(6)14/21.pdf

54. Pritchard JC, Lindberg AC, Main DC, Whay HR. Assessment of the welfare of working horses, mules and donkeys, using health and behaviour parameters. *Prev Vet Med.* (2005) 69:265–83. doi: 10.1016/j.prevetmed.2005.02.002

55. Hadush B, Michaelay M, Menghistu H, Abebe N, Genzebu AT, Bitsue HK et al. al. Epidemiology of epizootic lymphangitis of carthorses in northern Ethiopia using conventional diagnostic methods and nested polymerase chain reaction. *BMC Vet Res.* (2020) 16:375. doi: 10.1186/s12917-020-02582-2

56. Seyoum A, Birhan G,Tesfaye T. (2015). Prevalence of work related wound and associated risk factors in cart mules of Adet town, North-Western Ethiopia. *Am-Euras J Sci Res.* (2015) 10:264–71.

57. Gizaw, S and Berhanu, D. Public-private partnerships (PPPs) for veterinary service delivery in Ethiopia (2019). Nairobi, Kenya: ILRI. Available online at: https://www.ilri.org/publications/public-private-partnerships-ppps-veterinary-service-delivery-ethiopia. (accessed July 7, 2021).

58. Worku T, Wagaw N, Hailu B. *Epizootic lymphangitis in cart mules: a community-based clinical trial in Bahir Dar, north-west Ethiopia.* In: The 6th International Colloquium on Working Equids: Learning from Others. London: The Brooke (2010). p. 256–61.

59. Hadush B, Ameni G, Medhin G. Equine histoplasmosis: treatment trial in cart horses in Central Ethiopia. *Trop Anim Health Prod.* (2008) 40:407–11.

60. Radostits OM, Gay CC, Hinchcliff KW, Constable PD. *Veterinary Medicine: A Textbook of the Diseases of Cattle.* Horses, Sheep, Pigs and Goats (10th Edition). London, Elsevier Saunders. (2007).

61. Waziri MI, Yunusa KB. The concept and methods of community participation in animal and human disease surveillance. *Res Square.* (2020). doi: 10.21203/rs.3.rs-22448/v1

62. Gizaw S, Woldehanna M, Anteneh H, Ayledo G, Awol F, Gebreyohannes G, et al. Animal health service delivery in crop-livestock and pastoral systems in Ethiopia. *Front Vet Sci.* (2021) 8:601878. doi: 10.3389/fvets.2021.601878

63. Leonard, D. (ed.) *Africa's Changing Markets for Health and Veterinary Services: The New Institutional Issues.* Macmillan Press, London; St. Martin's Press, New York. (2000)

64. Leonard, D. Structural Reform of the Veterinary Profession in Africa and the New Institutional Economics

65. Valette D. Invisible Workers: The Economic Contributions of Working Donkeys, Horses and Mules to Livelihoods. The Brooke (2015). Available online at: https://www.thebrooke.org/sites/default/files/Advocacy%20and%20policy/Invisible-workers-report.pdf

8

Genetic Characterization of Feline Parvovirus Isolate Fe–P2 in Korean Cat and Serological Evidence on its Infection in Wild Leopard Cat and Asian Badger

Young Ji Kim [1,2†], Sun-Woo Yoon [1,3†], Jin Ho Jang [4,5], Dae Gwin Jeong [1,3], Beom Jun Lee [2] and Hye Kwon Kim [6*]*

[1] *Infectious Disease Research Center, Korea Research Institute of Bioscience and Biotechnology, Daejeon, South Korea,*
[2] *College of Veterinary Medicine, Chungbuk National University, Chungju, South Korea,* [3] *College of Bioscience, University of Science and Technology, Daejeon, South Korea,* [4] *Department of Wildlife Disease, College of Veterinary Science, Jeju National University, Jeju, South Korea,* [5] *Chungnam Wild Animal Rescue Center, Kongju National University, Yesan, South Korea,*
[6] *Department of Microbiology, College of Natural Science, Chungbuk National University, Cheongju, South Korea*

Correspondence:
Beom Jun Lee
beomjun@chungbuk.ac.kr
Hye Kwon Kim
khk1329@chungbuk.ac.kr

[†] *These authors have contributed equally to this work*

Feline parvovirus (FPV) is a small, non-enveloped, single-stranded DNA virus that infects cats. We recently isolated a feline parvovirus Fe–P2 strain from a dead stray cat in Iksan, 2017. Its partial genomic sequence (4,643 bases) was obtained, and phylogenetic analysis based on the VP2 nucleotide sequence showed that the FPV Fe-P2 strain was closely related to the FPV isolate Gigucheon in cat, 2017 (MN400978). In addition, we performed a serum neutralization (SN) test with the FPV isolates in various mammalian sera. These were from raccoon dog, water deer, Eurasian otter, Korean hare, leopard cat, and Asian badger, which were kindly provided by Chungnam Wild Animal Rescue Center. Notably, serological evidence of its infection was found in Asian badger, *Meles leucurus* (2/2) and leopard cat, *Prionailurus bengalensis* (5/8) through SN tests, whereas there was no evidence in raccoon dog, water deer, Eurasian otter, and Korean hare based on the collected sera in this study. These findings might provide partial evidence for the possible circulation of FPV or its related viruses among wild leopard cat and Asian badger in Korea. There should be additional study to confirm this through direct detection of FPVs in the related animal samples.

Keywords: feline parvovirus, feline panleukopenia, leopard cat, Asian badger, serum neutralization

INTRODUCTION

Feline parvovirus (FPV) is a single-stranded DNA virus which is a variant of *Carnivore protoparvovirus 1*, belonging to the genus *Protoparvovirus* within the family *Parvoviridae*. A range of serious condition (often lethal disease, inducing vomiting, enteritis, diarrhea, and acute lymphopenia) in young animal is closely involved the *Carnivore protoparvovirus 1*.

FPV is the main causative agent for feline panleukopenia, which can also be caused by canine parvovirus (CPV) variants, CPV-2a, 2b, and 2c (1, 2). CPV-2 can only infect dogs, whereas its variant can infect cats (1, 3). Thus, parvovirus members of *Carnivore protoparvovirus 1* might be one of the host range variants (4). Also, mink enteritis virus (MEV) and raccoon parvovirus (RaPV) are included in that.

FPV can infect not only domestic cats, but also other species such as raccoons, foxes, and minks (5). Previous findings have reported the detection of FPV-sequences in tissues of the African wild cat and in feces of both cheetahs and honey badgers (6). In Italy, FPV was detected in red foxes (*Vulpes vulpes*) (2.8%, 7/252) and Eurasian badgers (*Meles meles*) (10%, 1/10), and in Portugal, parvovirus DNA was detected in Egyptian mongoose (57.8%), red fox (78.9%), and stone marten (75%) (7, 8). Although FPV can infect diverse animal species, it is difficult to confirm the FPV-infection cases due to the genetic similarity and cross-reactivity between FPV and CPV (3).

The parvovirus contains two open reading frames. One is the codes for non-structural proteins (NS1 and NS2) and the other is the codes for structural viral proteins (VP1 and VP2). Several amino acid changes in the structural protein VP2, its major capsid protein, were associated with host specificity and antigenic properties for the parvovirus (9–11). Based on VP2 gene analysis, there were three genetic clusters (G1, G2, and G3) of FPV around the world. In Korea, FPVs belonging to both the G1 and G2 clusters were found (12). In Korea, 2% of 200 cats were FPV-positive in Seoul (11). To date there has been no study about the possible interspecies transmission of FPV among wild mammals in Korea.

In this study, a recent feline parvovirus Fe-P2 strain was isolated from a fecal swab from a stray cat carcass found in Iksan, 2017. Using this isolate, its genomic sequence was obtained, and serum neutralization (SN) tests were performed with various sera from several wild mammals

rescued by the Chungnam Wild Animal Rescue Center between 2016 and 2018. Through these experiments, this study provide evidence for the possible interspecies transmission of FPV (or its related viruses) among wild carnivores in Korea.

MATERIALS AND METHODS

Virus Isolation

A fecal swab was collected from a dead stray cat found in Iksan, Korea, 2017. The swab was transported to the lab with virus transport medium (Noble Bio. Co., Ltd., Hwasung, Korea). The transport medium containing the fecal swab was centrifuged at 3,000 g for 20 min at 4°C, and the supernatant was filtered through a 0.22 μm syringe filter, MF-Millipore™ Membrane Filter (Merck, Darmstadt, Germany). The filtered supernatant was inoculated on the monolayer of CRFK cells and incubated for 1 h, followed by phosphate buffered saline (PBS) washing. The inoculated cells were further incubated for 7 d with DMEM, supplemented with 2.5% fetal bovine serum (FBS) and cytopathic effect (CPE) was observed after two blind passages (**Figure 1A**). After freezing and thawing, the supernatant was aliquoted for further testing.

Polymerase Chain Reaction and Sequencing

DNA was extracted from the virus stock using QIAamp DNA Mini Kit (QIAGEN, Hilden, Germany). First, PCR targeting VP2 was performed by using primer sets: 555-F† 5′-CAGGA AGATATCCAGAAGGA-3′ and 555-R[†] 5′-GGTGCTAGTTG ATATGTAATAAACA-3′ (13).

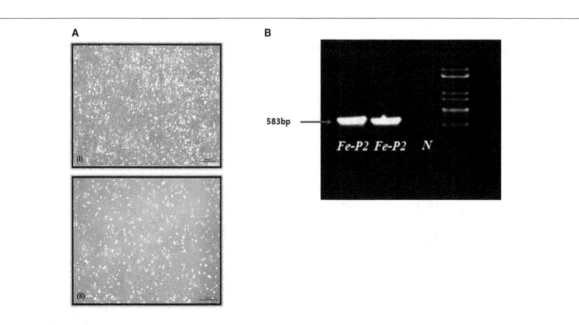

FIGURE 1 | (A) Cytopathogenic effect of feline parvovirus (FPV) Fe-P2 on cell culture. (7 days); (i) Uninfected cell control, (ii) CRFK infected with FPV Fe-P2, **(B)** Screening of clinical samples by PCR assay using CPV-2a and b primers. A single DNA amplicon of 583 bp is shown after using the CPV-2a and b primer pair, Fe-P2, FPV isolate; N, negative control.

A PCR 583 bp amplicon (**Figure 1B**) was obtained and further sequenced by Cosmogenetech, Seoul, Korea. Genomic sequencing was performed using the designed primers based on the reference FPV genomic sequence (MN683826) and PCR-positive sequences. Primer information is presented in **Table 1**.

Genetic Analysis

Phylogenetic analysis based on the nucleotide sequences showed that the detected feline parvoviruses belonged to the genera Protoparvovirus. The obtained genomic sequences of the FPV Fe-P2 strain were further analyzed with related sequences from GenBank using BioEdit (14) and MEGA version 7.0 (15) tools. Phylogenetic trees based on the genomic sequences and VP2 were drawn with the maximum likelihood method, with 1,000 replicates of bootstrap sampling and using the Kimura 2-parameter model using MEGA version 7.0. Genomic sequence data generated in this study have been deposited in GenBank under the accession number MN683826.

Serum Neutralization Test

A total of 109 sera from wild mammals, including raccoon dog, water deer, Eurasian otter, Korean hare, leopard cat, and Asian badger, were obtained from rescued wild animals from the Chungnam Wild Animal Rescue Center. The information on the animal species and collection dates is presented in **Table 2**.

For the SN test, the sera samples were first inactivated at 56°C for 30 min. The inactivated sera were two-fold diluted from an initial dilution of 1:10 with DMEM in 96 well-plates. The diluted sera were then mixed with the same volume of FPV Fe–P2 isolate in 200 Tissue Culture Infective Dose (TCID$_{50}$)/50 μl. The mixture was incubated for an hour at 37°C and 100 μl of that were transferred to the CRFK monolayers with 5% FBS in a 96 well-cell culture plate, followed by incubation at 37°C for 4–5 days. Then, the plates were examined for CPE.

RESULTS

Genetic Characterization of the Feline Parvovirus Fe–P2

The partial genomic sequence of 4,643 bases of FPV Fe–P2 strain was obtained in this study. Two main open reading frames (ORFs) encoding VP1 and VP2 were deposited as complete coding sequences. As a determinant of the host range of parvoviruses, it appears to be the minority amino acids of the capsid protein that determine the ability of the virus to replicate in different hosts (3). The host-specific amino acid position in VP2; 80, 93, 103, 297, 300, 305, 323, 564, and 568 (6) were compared with other FPVs and CPVs. All the amino acids were well-conserved among FPVs including the Fe–P2 strain, although these differed from CPV-2a, 2b, and 2c strains (**Table 3**). The partial genomic sequence-based phylogenetic tree was drawn with other strains of *Carnivore protoparvovirus 1* (**Figure 2A**). Based on the phylogenetic relationship, it is suggested that the FPV Fe–P2 strain was not related to the recently reported FPV from wild raccoon dogs (GenBank Accession No. MF069445 and MF069447) in Canada (16). Phylogenetic analysis based on the VP2 nucleotide sequence showed that the FPV Fe–P2 strain

TABLE 1 | Primers used for genotyping and sequence analysis.

Primer	Sequence (5′ → 3′)	Sense	Position (Fe–P2)
555-F[a]	CAGGAAGATATCCAGAAGGA	+	3,841–3,860
555-R[a]	GGTGCTAGTTGATATGTAATAAACA	–	4,423–4,399
FPVin-F4	GGCAATTGCTCCCGTATT	+	2,465–2,482
FPVin-R4	AGCCATGTTTCCTTTAACTGCAG	–	2,915–2,893
FPV-F3	CAGAATCTGCTACTCAGCC	+	3,085–3,103
FPV-R5	ACCAACCACCCACACCAT	–	4,823–4,806
NSF-1	CTGGCAACCAGTATACTG	+	115–132
NSR-1	GCTTGTGCTATGGCTTGAGC	–	1,357–1,338

[a]*Primers for amplification of the 583 bp products represent a parvovirus-specific VP2 gene (6).*

TABLE 2 | Wild animal sera information for the serum neutralization test.

Animal species*	Collected year	No. of sera
Raccoon dog (*Nyctereutes procyonoides koreensis*)	2016–2018	96
Asian badger (*Meles leucurus*)	2016–2017	2
European Otter (*Lutra lutra*)	2018	1
Leopard cat (*Prionailurus bengalensis*)	2018	8
Korean hare (*Lepus coreanus*)	2017	1
Water deer (*Hydropotes inermis*)	2018	1
	Total sera	109

A total of six mammalian species: Asian badger (Meles leucurus), leopard cat (Prionailurus bengalensis), water deer (Hydropotes inermis), Eurasian otter (Lutra lutra), raccoon dog (Nyctereutes procyonoides koreensis), and Korean hare (Lepus coreanus).

belonged to the G1 cluster (**Figure 2B**). The FPV Fe–P2 in this study was closely related to a feline-specific FPV strain (GenBank Accession No. MN400978), which was reported previously in Korea (**Figure 2B**), showing 99.16% sequence identity.

Serum Neutralizing Antibodies Against FPV Fe-P2 in Leopard Cat and Asian Badger

In the result of the SN test against FPV Fe-P2 with a total of 109 sera from wild mammals (section Serum Neutralization Test), the neutralizing antibodies were evident in the sera of Asian badgers and wild leopard cats, showing SN titer, 80–1,280 (**Table 4**). Five out of eight leopard cats and all the Asian badgers (two samples) were seropositive with the SN test. The other wild mammals, including 96 Raccoon dogs, one water deer, one Eurasian otter, and one Korean hare did not have SN titers more than 20 against FPV Fe–P2. The SN titers in Asian badger were 80 and 320, while that in leopard cats were between 80 and 1,280.

DISCUSSION

FPV-infected cats older than 6 weeks develop symptoms from subclinical level to sudden death within 12 h (5). FPV-infectious disease is characterized by severe panleukopenia and enteritis, which is also associated with high mortality and morbidity (3, 5, 17). Multiple, epizootic outbreaks of FPV infection in most unvaccinated cats were reported in Australia between 2014 and

TABLE 3 | Amino acids positions for host-specificity between dogs and cats.

Virus strain	Accession number	Amino acid VP2								
		80	93	103	297	300	305	323	564	568
Feline parvovirus Fe-P2*	MN683826*	K	K	V	S	A	D	D	N	S
Feline parvovirus (FPV)	HQ184189	K	K	V	S	A	D	D	N	S
	AB054226	K	K	V	S	A	D	D	N	S
	KP081409	K	K	V	S	A	D	D	N	S
	KJ415112	K	K	V	S	A	D	D	N	S
Canine parvovirus (CPV)-2a	EU009201	R	N	A	A	G	Y	N	S	R
	KT156829	R	N	A	A	G	Y	N	S	R
Canine parvovirus (CPV)-2b	FJ977077	R	N	A	A	G	Y	N	S	R
	EF599097	R	N	A	A	G	Y	N	S	R
	EU009206	R	N	A	A	G	Y	N	S	R
Canine parvovirus (CPV)-2c(a)	EF599098	R	N	A	A	D	Y	N	S	R

*The partial genomic sequence of 4,643 bases from Feline Parvovirus Fe-P2 (MN683826).

2018 (2). In Korea, FPV infection was found in 2% of cats in Seoul (11), and FPVs belonging to the G1 and G2 clusters were circulating (12). In this study, an FPV isolate Fe-P2 from 2017 was included in the G1 cluster, and amino acids of the VP2 protein indicate that the isolate would have the same host specificity as other FPVs. Observing no close relationship with recent novel strains of FPV from wild raccoon dogs in Canada (16), the FPV isolate Fe–P2 in this study might be one of the strains circulating in Korea. In addition, the amino acids positions for host-specificity of Fe–P2 strain were the same as other feline parvoviruses rather than canine parvoviruses. There were no apparent genetic differences between Fe-P2 strain and other FPVs. Although there should be additional screening on the prevailing FPV genotypes in Korea, we used this isolate to screen the serological evidence of FPV infection in wild animals.

As we can collect sera of six wild animals from the Chungnam Wild Animal Rescue Center, we tried to screen SN antibodies using the recent FPV isolate, Fe-P2 in this study. As expected, no SN antibodies were observed in Korean hare and water deer, which could be regarded as negative controls for the SN test in this study. Notably, two wild mammals, leopard cat and Asian badger were seropositive in the SN test using the FPV isolate Fe-P2 with 109 sera of wild mammals from Korea. The SN titers were notable due to relatively high titers, 80 and 1,280 in leopard cats and 80 and 320 in Asian badgers.

Parvoviruses have shown consistently evolution over many years at a faster rate than other DNA viruses. Also, a variety of wild animals have increasingly detected as parvoviruses hosts (8). FPV has been known to infect other species like raccoon dogs, foxes, minks, African wild cats, cheetahs, and honey badgers (5, 6). Furthermore, FPV was still frequently found in wild animals like otters, minks, and martens (18, 19). The FPV-positive rate in Canadian otters was almost 30%. Hence, it was suggested that otters might be a principal maintenance host for FPV enabling viral persistence and serving as a source for other susceptible species (18). In this study, the serum from otter had SN titer

<20 in the SN test against FPV Fe-P2 strain. However, since only one otter sample was tested, there may be a possibility for FPV infection in the species, additional screening would provide more detailed information.

In this study, five out of eight leopard cats were seropositive against the FPV Fe-P2 strain, which may indicate they were infected by FPV previously. This is not surprising as FPV had already been detected in leopard cats in Taiwan and Vietnam (20, 21). However, seropositive Asian badgers (two samples) in the SN test against FPV Fe-P2 strain, were identified in this study for the first time. While FPV was detected in honey badger (*Mellivora capensis*) in South Africa (6), in this study we report the serological evidence of FPV infection in Asian badgers (*Meles leucurus*), which belong to a different subfamily that had never been reported before. Thus, this study might provide partial evidence for the possible circulation of FPV or its related viruses among wild leopard cat and Asian badger in Korea.

As a variant of *Carnivore protoparvovirus 1*, FPV had wide range of host animals. Evidence for FPV infection in a diverse range of wild mammals indicated that FPV has been circulating not only in cats but also in other mammals, with sporadic interspecies transmission. In this study, we could suggest Asian badgers and wild leopard cats as potential hosts for FPV infection in Korea. However, conventional parvoviruses may have observed cross-reactivity through high virus-neutralizing (VN) antibodies titers between FPV and CPV (22), thus we cannot exclude the possible infection of CPVs in those animals. There should be additional study to confirm this through direct detection of FPVs in the related animal samples. Therefore, it would be more feasible that there was serological evidence of FPV or its related viruses in Asian badgers and wild leopard cats in Korea.

Thus, FPV and its related viruses may circulate in the wild life hosts. The leopard cats and Asian badgers in this study were

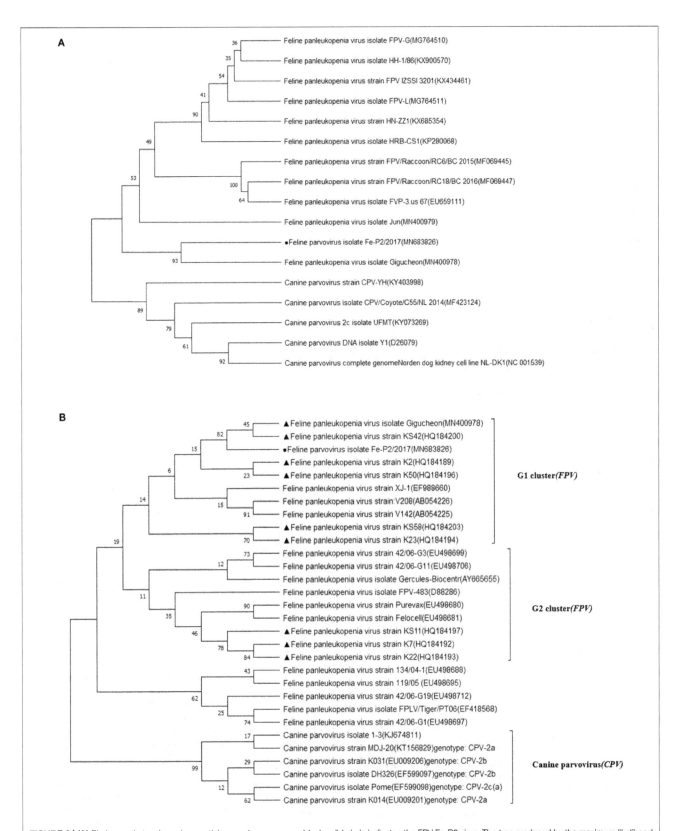

FIGURE 2 | (A) Phylogenetic tree based on partial genomic sequences; black solid circle indicates the FPV Fe-P2 virus. The tree produced by the maximum likelihood method using MEGA 7.0 software shows the phylogenetic relationship between the 5 canine parvovirus strains and 12 feline parvoviruses. **(B)** Phylogenetic tree based on VP2 nucleotide sequences; black solid circle indicates the Fe-P2 virus, and black solid triangles indicate viruses isolated in Korea. The tree produced by the maximum likelihood method using MEGA 7.0 software shows the phylogenetic relationship between the 6 canine parvovirus strains and 24 feline parvoviruses.

TABLE 4 | Serum neutralization test results.

Animal species	Year	SN-positive/total sera*	SN titer of the positive
Raccoon dog (*Nyctereutes procyonoides koreensis*)	2016–2018	0/96	<20
Leopard cat (*Prionailurus bengalensis*)	2016–2018	5/8	80, 1,280, 1,280, 1,280, 1,280
Asian badger (*Meles leucurus*)	2016–2017	2/2	80, 320
Korean hare (*Lepus coreanus*)	2017	0/1	<20
Water deer (*Hydropotes inermis*)	2018	0/1	<20
European otter (*Lutra lutra*)	2018 Total (sera)	0/1 7/109	<20

Five out of eight leopard cats and two Asian badgers were seropositive with the SN test.

rescued animals from human populated regions, which means that they were near human habitat. Therefore, a vaccination or a control policy against FPV and its related viruses should be considered not only for household cats, but also for wild animals.

AUTHOR CONTRIBUTIONS

HK and JJ: conceptualization. YK and S-WY: methodology. JJ: resources. DJ: data curation. YK and HK: writing—original draft preparation. BL, S-WY, and DJ: writing—review and editing. BL and S-WY: supervision. HK and DJ: funding acquisition. All authors contributed to the article and approved the submitted version.

REFERENCES

1. Truyen U, Parrish CR. Canine and feline host range of canine parvovirus and feline panleukopenia virus: distinct host cell tropisms of each virus *in vitro* and *in vivo*. *J Virol*. (1992) 66:5399–408. doi: 10.1128/JVI.66.9.5399-5408.1992
2. Jenkins E, Davis C, Carrai M, Ward MP, O'Keeffe S, van Boeijen M, et al. Feline parvovirus seroprevalence is high in domestic cats from disease outbreak and non-outbreak regions in Australia. *Viruses*. (2020) 12:320. doi: 10.3390/v12030320
3. Steinel A, Parrish CR, Bloom ME, Truyen U. Parvovirus infections in wild carnivores. *J Wildlife Dis*. (2001) 37:594–607. doi: 10.7589/0090-3558-37.3.594
4. Parrish CR. Emergence, natural history and variation of canine, mink, feline parvoviruses. *Adv Virus Res*. (1990) 38:403–502. doi: 10.1016/S0065-3527(08)60867-2
5. Stuetzer B, Hartmann K. Feline parvovirus infection and associated diseases. *Vet J*. (2014) 201:150–5. doi: 10.1016/j.tvjl.2014.05.027
6. Steinel A, Munson L, van Vuuren M, Truyen U. Genetic characterization of feline parvovirus sequences from various carnivores. *J. Gen*. (2000) 81:345–50. doi: 10.1099/0022-1317-81-2-345
7. Duarte MD, Henriques AM, Barros SC, Fagulha T, Mendonça P, Carvalho P, et al. Snapshot of viral infections in wild carnivores reveals ubiquity of parvoviruses and susceptibility of Egyptian mongoose to feline panleukopenia virus. *PLoS One*. (2013) 8:e59399. doi: 10.1371/journal.pone.0059399
8. Ndiana LA, Lanave G, Desario C, Berjaoui S, Alfano F, Puglia I, et al. Circulation of diverse protoparvoviruses in wild carnivores, Italy. *Transbound Emerg Dis*. (2020). doi: 10.1111/tbed.13917
9. Decaro N, Desario C, Miccolupo A, Campolo N, Parisi A, Marella V, et al. Genetic analysis of feline panleukopenia viruses from cats with gastroenteritis. *J. Gen*. (2008) 89:2290–8. doi: 10.1099/vir.0.2008/001503-0
10. Truyen U, Gruenberg A, Chang SF, Obermaier B, Veijalainen P, Parrish CR. Evolution of the feline-subgroup parvoviruses and the control of canine host range *in vivo*. *J Virol*. (1995) 69:4702–10. doi: 10.1128/JVI.69.8.4702-4710.1995

11. Kim SG, Lee KI, Kim HJ, Park HM. Prevalence of feline panleukopenia virus in stray and household cats in Seoul, Korea. *J Vet Clin*. (2013) 30:333–8.
12. An DJ, Jeong W, Jeoung HY, Yoon SH, Kim HJ, Park JY, et al. Phylogenetic analysis of feline panleukopenia virus (FPLV) strains in Korean cats. *Res Vet Sci*. (2011) 90:1637. doi: 10.1016/j.rvsc.2010.05.010
13. Buonavoglia C, Martella V, Pratelli A, Tempesta M, Cavalli A, Buonavoglia D, et al. Evidence for evolution of canine parvovirus type 2 in Italy. *J Gen Virol*. (2001) 82:3021–5. doi: 10.1099/0022-1317-82-12-3021
14. Hall TA. BioEdit: a user friendly biological sequence alignment editor and analysis program for windows 95/98/NT. *Nucleic Acids Symp Ser*. (1999) 41:95–8.
15. Kumar S, Stecher G, Tamura K. MEGA7: Molecular Evolutionary Genetics Analysis version 7.0 for bigger datasets. *Mol Biol Evol*. (2016) 33:1870–4. doi: 10.1093/molbev/msw054
16. Canuti M, Britton AP, Graham SM, Lang AS. Epidemiology and molecular characterization of protoparvoviruses infecting wild raccoons (Procyon lotor) in British Columbia, Canada. *Virus Res*. (2017) 242:85–9. doi: 10.1016/j.virusres.2017.09.015
17. Barker IK, Povey RC, Voigt DR. Response of mink, skunk, red fox and raccoon to inoculation with mink virus enteritis, feline panleukopenia and canine parvovirus and prevalence of antibody to parvovirus in wild carnivores in Ontario. *Can J Comp Med*. (1983) 47:188–97.
18. Canuti M, Todd M, Monteiro P, Van Osch K, Weir R, Schwantje H, et al. Ecology and infection dynamics of multi-host amdoparvoviral and protoparvoviral carnivore pathogens. *Pathogens*. (2020) 9:124. doi: 10.3390/pathogens9020124
19. Viscardi M, Santoro M, Clausi MT, Cozzolino L, Decaro N, Colaianni ML, et al. Molecular detection and characterization of carnivore parvoviruses in free-ranging Eurasian otters (*Lutra lutra*) insouthern Italy. *Transbound. Emerg. Dis*. (2019) 66:1864–72. doi: 10.1111/tbed.13212

20. Chen CC, Chang AM, Wada T, Chen MT, Tu YS. Distribution of Carnivore protoparvovirus 1 in freeliving leopard cats (*Prionailurus bengalensis chinensis*) and its association with domestic carnivores in Taiwan. *PLoS One.* (2019) 14:e0221990. doi: 10.1371/journal.pone.0221990

21. Ikeda Y, Miyazawa T, Nakamura K, Naito R, Inoshima Y, Tung KC, et al. Serosurvey for selected virus infections of wild carnivores in Taiwan and Vietnam. *J Wildl Dis.* (1999) 35:578–81. doi: 10.7589/0090-3558-35.3.578

22. Nakamura K, Ikeda Y, Miyazawa T, Tohya Y, Takahashi E, Mochizuki M. Characterisation of cross-reactivity of virus neutralising antibodies induced by feline panleukopenia virus and canine parvoviruses. *Res Vet Sci.* (2001) 71:219–22. doi: 10.1053/rvsc.2001.0492

23. Hueffer K, Parker JS, Weichert WS, Geisel RE, Sgro JY, Parrish CR. The natural host range shift and subsequent evolution of canine parvovirus resulted from virus specific binding to the canine transferrin receptor. *J Virol.* (2003) 77:1718–26. doi: 10.1128/JVI.77.3.1718-1726.2003

9

Emergence and Phylogenetic Analysis of a Getah Virus Isolated in Southern China

Tongwei Ren, Qingrong Mo, Yuxu Wang, Hao Wang, Zuorong Nong, Jinglong Wang, Chenxia Niu, Chang Liu, Ying Chen, Kang Ouyang, Weijian Huang and Zuzhang Wei*

Laboratory of Animal Infectious Diseases and Molecular Immunology, College of Animal Science and Technology, Guangxi University, Nanning, China

*Correspondence:
Zuzhang Wei
zuzhangwei@gxu.edu.cn

Getah virus (GETV) has caused many outbreaks in animals in recent years. Monitoring of the virus and its related diseases is crucial to control the transmission of the virus. In the summer of 2018, we conducted routine tests on clinical samples from different pig farms in Guangxi province, South China, and isolated and characterized a GETV strain, named GX201808. Cytopathic effects were observed in BHK-21 cells inoculated with GX201808. The expression of E2 protein of GETV could be detected in virus-infected cells by indirect immunofluorescence assays. Electron microscopic analysis showed that the virus particles were spherical and ~70 nm in diameter with featured surface fibers. The multistep growth curves showed the virus propagated well in the BHK-21 cells. Molecular genetic analysis revealed that GX201808 belongs to Group 3, represented by Kochi-01-2005 isolated in Japan in 2005, and it clustered closely with the recently reported Chinese strains isolated from pigs, cattle, and foxes. A comparison of the identities of nucleotides and amino acids in the coding regions demonstrated that the GX201808 showed the highest amino acid identity (99.6%) with the HuN1 strain, a highly pathogenic isolate resulting in an outbreak of GETV infection in swine herds in Hunan province in 2017. In the present study, GETV was identified and isolated for the first time in Guangxi province of southern China, suggesting that future surveillance of this virus should be strengthened.

Keywords: genetic analysis, phylogenetic analysis, isolation, emergence, Getah virus

INTRODUCTION

Getah virus (GETV) is an enveloped, single-stranded positive-sense RNA virus. GETV is a member of the genus *Alphavirus* in the family *Togaviridae*, which are transmitted mostly by various mosquito species (1). The virus comprises a genome of ~11.7 kb containing a 5′-untranslated region (UTR), two large open reading frames (ORFs), a 3′-UTR, and a poly-A tail (2). The ORF1 is situated at the 5′-end of the genome and encodes non-structural polyproteins (nsP1 to nsP4). The ORF2 is located at the 3′-end of the genome and encodes structural polyproteins that are transcribed into five structural proteins, namely, C, E3, E2, 6K, and E1, respectively (3, 4).

GETV has been shown to be distributed widely in the Asiatic, Australia, and Eurasian regions since the prototype GETV strain (MM2021) was first isolated from mosquitoes in Malaysia in 1955

(5–10). Sero-epizootiologic investigations showed that the virus is present in pigs, horses, goats, cattle, boars, and other animals including humans (9, 11–14), suggesting that the host range of the virus has expanded broadly. GETV infections can cause fever, rashes, and edema of the hindlegs in horses (15), fetal death and reproductive disorders in pigs (16) as well as fever,

TABLE 1 | Detailed information on the GETV strains in this study.

Strain	GenBank number	Year	Host	Country
MM2021	AF339484	1955	*C. gelidus*	Malaysia
Sagiyama virus	AB032553	1956	Mosquito	Japan
M1	EU015061	1956	*Culex* sp.	China
MI-110-C2	LC079087	1978	*Equus caballus*	Japan
MI-110-C1	LC079086	1978	*Equus caballus*	Japan
LEIV 17741 MPR	EF631999	2000	*Culex* sp.	Mongolia
LEIV 16275 Mag	EF631998	2000	Mongolia	Russia
HB0234	EU015062	2002	*Culex tritaeniorhynchus* Giles	China
South Korea	AY702913	2004	Swine	South Korea
YN0540	EU015063	2005	*Armigeres subalbatus*	China
Kochi/01/2005	AB859822	2005	*Sus scrofa*	Japan
HNJZ-S1	KY363862	2011	Pig	China
YN12031	KY434327	2012	*Armigeres subalbatus*	China
YN12042	KY450683	2012	*Culex tritaeniorhynchus* Giles	China
SC1210	LC107870	2012	*Armigeres subalbatus*	China
12IH26	LC152056	2012	*Culex tritaeniorhynchu*	Japan
14-I-605-C2	LC079089	2014	*Equus caballus*	Japan
14-I-605-C1	LC079088	2014	*Equus caballus*	Japan
HNJZ-S2	KY363863	2015	Pig	China
15-I-752	LC212972	2015	*Equus caballus*	Japan
15-I-1105	LC212973	2015	*Sus scrofa domesticus*	Japan
HNNY-1	MG865966	2016	Pig	China
HNNY-2	MG865967	2016	Pig	China
GETV-V1	KY399029	2016	Pig	China
16-I-676	LC223132	2016	*Equus caballus*	Japan
16-I-674	LC223131	2016	*Equus caballus*	Japan
16-I-599	LC223130	2016	*Equus caballus*	Japan
HNPDS-2	MG865969	2017	Pig	China
HNPDS-1	MG865968	2017	Pig	China
AH9192	MG865965	2017	Pig	China
JL17/08	MG869691	2017	Mosquito	China
JL1707	MH722255	2017	Mosquito	China
HuN1	MF741771	2017	Porcine	China
SD17/09	MH106780	2017	Fox	China
JL1808	MH722256	2018	Cattle	China
SC201807	MK693225	2018	Pig	China
GETV-GDFS2-2018	MT086508	2018	Pig	China

anorexia, depression, neurologic symptoms, and death in foxes (17). GETV infections in horses and pigs have been reported several times in Japan since the 1970's (18–21), and the outbreak of GETV infections in horses were reported in 1990 in India (22). In China, GETV is widely distributed in 15 provinces ranging from the southwest to northern areas of China since it was first identified from mosquitos in Hainan province, and it has caused several outbreaks in animals in recent years (2, 7, 17, 23–28). In 2017, an outbreak of GETV infection was reported in swine herds in Hunan province, China, resulting in the death of ~200 piglets and reproductive disorders of more than 150 pregnant sows (25). Lethal infections in blue foxes caused by GETV were also reported in Shandong province, East China (17). The latest GETV outbreak in racehorses occurred in Guangdong province, South China, in 2018 (27). Recently, serum samples from beef cattle showing sudden onset of fever have occurred in GETV-positive animals (26).

In this study, we conducted routine tests on clinical samples for GETV in samples from different farms in Guangxi province, South China, in 2018. A GETV strain was isolated from the serum of a GETV-positive animal. The virus was genetically closely related to recently isolated strains, HuN1, SD17/09, and JL1808 from different animals in Hunan, Shandong, and Jilin province, respectively, indicating a potential national emergence of this virus.

MATERIALS AND METHODS

Cell Culture and Antibody Production

Baby hamster kidney cells (BHK-21; ATCC CCL10) were cultured in modified Eagle's medium (MEM) supplemented with 10% fetal bovine serum (FBS) as described in our previous study (29). To generate the E2 antibody against GETV, the E2 coding region was amplified by RT-PCR using forward primer (5'-CGGGATCCAGTGTGACGGAACACTT-3') and reverse primer (5'-CCGGAATTCGGCATGCGCTCGTGGCGCGCA-3'). The forward and reverse primers carried the EcoR I and BamH I restriction sites, respectively. Thermal cycling conditions were 94°C for 3 min, followed by 30 cycles of 94°C for 30 s, 60°C for 30 s, 72°C for 90 s, and a final elongation step at 72°C for 10 min. The E2 PCR produced were double digested with the EcoR I and BamH I and then ligated into similarly digested pET-32a (+) expression vector (Novagen), resulting in plasmid pET32a-E2 and BL21 (DE3). *Escherichia coli* cells were transformed with pET32a-E2 and then induced by 1 mM IPTG for 4 h. A HIS binding kit (Novagen) was then used to purify the recombinant E2 protein. New Zealand white rabbits were injected with the purified recombinant E2 protein to generate a polyclonal antibody against the GETV E2 protein. Affinity chromatography with protein A was used to purify the polyclonal antibody (anti-GETV-E2 PcAb).

Sample Collection, Viral RNA Extraction, and GETV Detection

Three hundred fifty field samples (sera) were collected from clinically diseased pigs in Guangxi province, South China. Viral RNA from 200 μl of each sample was extracted using the

Prep Body Fluid Viral DNA/RNA Mini Prep kit (Axygen AXY) according to the manufacturer's instructions. The extracted RNA was then used for cDNA synthesis using M-MLV reverse transcriptase with random hexamers (Takara Bio, Inc., Dalian, China) according to the manufacturer's instructions. RT-PCR was then performed to detect GETV using primers as described in a previous study (23). Thermal cycling involved initially heating at 94°C for 3 min, followed by 35 cycles of 94°C for 30 s, 55°C for 30 s, and 72°C for 60 s, with a final extension step at 72°C for 10 min.

Virus Isolation

The PBS-diluted GETV-positive sera were filtered through 0.22-μm filters (Millipore, Billerica, MA, USA) and plated onto BHK-21 cell monolayers seeded in a six-well plate. After 1 h of incubation at 37°C, the cells were washed twice with PBS and maintained in MEM supplemented with 2% FBS (Gibco) in a 5% CO_2 incubator. The cells were observed on a daily basis for the presence of cytopathic effects (CPE). The supernatants (200 μl) were subsequently used for serial passages into BHK-21 cells. The third passage (P3) identified the presence of the virus by

RT-PCR and indirect immunofluorescence assays (IFAs) using a polyclonal antibody against GETV E2 protein. The isolates were plaque purified three times and then used for complete genome sequencing.

Plaque Assay

Viral plaque assays were performed using BHK-21 cells grown in six-well plates. Viral samples were serially 10-fold diluted in MEM. Samples, 200 μl, of each dilution were inoculated onto monolayers of BHK-21 cells and incubated for 1 h. The cells were then overlaid with a mixture of MEM containing 1% low-melting agarose (Cambrex, Rockland, ME, USA) and 2% FBS and incubated at 37°C for 3 days in 5% CO_2. After careful removal of the medium, the cells were stained with 3–4 ml of staining solution consisting of 0.5% crystal violet and 25% formaldehyde solution for 15 min, and visible plaques were observed.

Growth Curve

Viral growth kinetics were determined using BHK-21 cells as described previously (23). Briefly, BHK-21 cells in six-well plates were inoculated with GETV (P3) at a multiplicity of infection

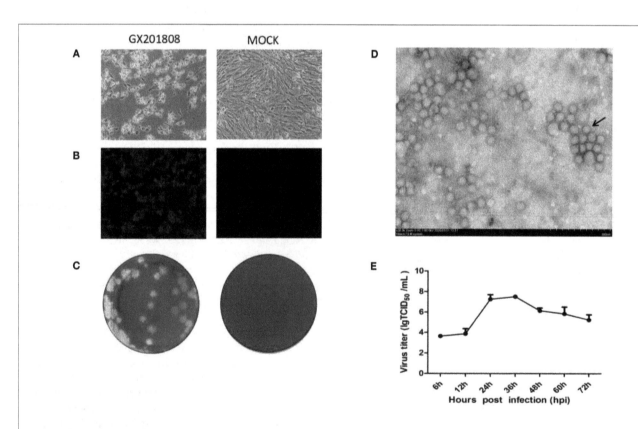

FIGURE 1 | Isolation and identification of the Getah virus (GETV) GX201808 strain grown in baby hamster kidney (BHK-21) cells. (A) Cytopathic effects (CPEs) in BHK-21 cells infected with the GETV GX201808 strain. Mock-infected and virus-infected BHK-21 cells were observed at 36 hpi. (B) GETV GX201808 strain was identified in infected BHK-21 cells using immunofluorescence assay (IFA) at 24 hpi. The infected BHK-21 cells were fixed and stained using an anti-GETV-E2 PcAb against the GETV E2 protein and goat anti-rabbit H&L IgG. Images were taken using a 20x objective. (C) Plaque morphology of GETV GX201808 on BHK-21 cells. Monolayers of BHK-21 cells in six-well plates were infected with GETV GX201808. The cell monolayers were overlaid with 1% agarose and stained with crystal violet at 48 hpi. (D) Electron microscopic examination of morphology of GETV particles. BHK-21 cells were infected with GETV GX201808, and the precipitated viruses from the supernatants were processed for electron microscopy. (E) The growth of GETV GX201808 at a multiplicity of infection (MOI) of 1 on BHK-21 cells. The viral titers were determined as $TCID_{50}$, and the values obtained were the means of three independent experiments.

(MOI) of 0.1. After 1 h of incubation at 37°C, the BHK-21 cells were washed twice with PBS. Two hundred microliters of BHK-21 cell supernatants were harvested at 6, 12, 24, 36, 48, and 72 hpi and stored at −70°C until use. The virus titers ($TCID_{50}$) for each time point were assessed using BHK-21 cells and calculated according to the Reed–Muench method. The growth curves were determined after measuring the mean titers of three independent measurements at each time point.

Indirect Immunofluorescence Assay

The expression of viral proteins in GETV-infected BHK-21 cell was tested by IFAs. BHK-21 cell monolayers were inoculated with passaged viruses at one MOI. Twenty-four hours post-inoculation, the infected cells were washed twice with PBS, followed by fixation in cold acetone at −4°C for 30 min. The cells were washed five times with PBS and then blocked with 1% BSA (fraction V bovine serum albumin; Roche, Mannheim, Germany), which was diluted in PBS, for 30 min at room temperature. After being washed with PBS, the cells were incubated with primary anti-GETV-E2 PcAb (1:100) for 1 h at room temperature. Then the cells were washed with PBS five times followed by incubation with goat anti-rabbit IgG (H + L; Alexa (Fluor® 488, Abcam) for 1 h at 37°C. The cells were subsequently washed five times with PBS. Finally, images were captured using an inverted fluorescence microscope (Nikon, Tokyo, Japan).

Preparation of Virus Particles and Electron Microscopy

BHK-21 cell monolayers were inoculated with the virus at one MOI. At 24 hpi, 30 ml of supernatant from the infected cells was harvested and filtered through 0.22-μm filters (Millipore, Billerica, MA, USA) and then mixed with 7.5 ml of 50% PEG-8000 to a final 10% concentration. The mixture was gently stirred at 4°C overnight and then centrifuged at 12,000 rpm at 4°C for 2 h. After careful removal of the supernatants, the precipitated viruses were re-suspended in 1 ml of TBS. The virus–TBS mixture was stirred at 4°C for 30 min for being negatively stained and was visualized by transmission electron microscopy (TEM).

Complete Genome Determination

The viral genomic RNA was extracted from BHK-21 cells infected with GETV and then reversed transcribed into cDNA using M-MLV reverse transcriptase (TaKaRa, Dalian, China) according to the manufacturer's instructions. PCR was performed using TaKaRa LA Taq (TaKaRa, Dalian, China) to amplify the complete genomic sequence using the previously published PCR primers (23). The reaction conditions were 94°C for 3 min, followed by 30 cycles of 94°C for 30 s, 60°C for 30 s, 72°C for 90 s, and a final elongation step at 72°C for 10 min. The positive amplicons were purified using an E.Z.N.A.TM Gel Extraction kit (OMEGA, USA) and then inserted into a pMD18-T vector (TaKaRa, Dalian, China) for nucleotide sequencing in both directions using universal primers T7 and SP6. The genomic sequence of GETV was assembled using the SeqMan program of DNAstar software, version 7.0 (DNASTAR Inc., Madison, WI, USA).

Sequence Alignments and Phylogenetic Analysis

Differences in sequence of this isolate and all other GETV strains available from GenBank were analyzed using the MegAlign program with DNAstar 7.0 software. The information regarding

TABLE 2 | Nucleotide and amino acid sequences and identity analysis of GX201808 and the other GETV strains.

Strains	GX201808 (%)				
	Complete genome	Non-structural polyprotein		Structural polyprotein	
	nt	nt	aa	nt	aa
MM2021		94.6	97.4		
Sagiyama virus	96.9	96.5	98.0	97.1	99.1
M1	97.6	97.4	98.2	97.6	98.9
Sagiyama virus Original		96.6	98.3		
MI-110-C1	98.1	98.2	99.2	98.0	99.5
MI-110-C2	98.1	98.2	99.3	98.0	99.4
LEIV16275 Mag	97.1	97.0	98.8	97.1	99.3
HB0234	97.5	97.4	98.9	97.4	98.9
Getah virus South Korea	97.8	97.9	99.2	97.7	99.4
Kochi-01-2005	99.0	99.0	99.4	97.4	99.2
YN0540	97.5	97.6	99.2	97.4	99.2
LEIV 17741 MPR	98.1	98.3	99.3	98.0	99.2
HNJZ-S1	97.4	97.5	99.3	97.3	99.0
121H26	97.4	97.5	99.2	97.2	99.1
SC1210	97.4	97.3	99.0	97.4	99.2
YN12031	95.9	95.9	98.0	95.9	98.6
YN12042	97.4	97.4	99.1	97.3	99.1
14-I-605-C1	97.3	97.4	99.2	97.2	99.1
14-I-605-C2	97.3	97.4	99.2	97.2	99.1
15-I-752	97.3	97.4	99.2	97.2	99.1
15-I-1105	97.3	97.4	99.1	97.2	99.0
HNJZ-S2	97.4	97.5	99.1	97.2	99.1
16-I-599	97.3	97.4	99.1	97.2	98.9
16-I-674	97.3	97.4	99.1	97.2	99.0
16-I-676	97.3	97.4	99.1	97.1	98.9
GETV-V1	97.4	97.4	99.0	97.4	99.1
HNNY-1	97.4	97.5	99.3	97.4	99.1
HNNY-2	97.4	97.5	99.3	97.3	99.1
AH9192	97.3	97.1	98.7	97.3	99.0
HNPDS-1	97.4	97.5	99.3	97.4	99.1
HNPDS-2	97.4	97.4	99.3	97.4	99.1
HuN1	99.3	99.4	99.6	99.2	99.4
JL1707	97.4	97.4	98.9	97.3	99.0
JL1708	97.4	97.4	99.1	97.3	99.1
SD17/09	99.4	99.3	99.6	99.4	99.5
JL1808	99.3	99.3	99.7	99.3	99.6
SC201807	97.3	97.4	99.2	97.2	99.2
GZ201808		97.1	98.7	97.2	99.1
GETV-GDFS2-2018	97.2	97.1	98.9	97.3	99.0

the reference GETV strains is listed in **Table 1**. Phylogenetic analyses were carried out based on the complete genome and E2 gene by MEGA version 6.0 using the maximum likelihood (ML) method with p-distances for nucleotide sequences, and the bootstrap test value was calculated using 1,000 replicates.

RESULTS

Virus Detection, Isolation, and Plaque Purification

Routine tests were conducted on clinical samples collected from different pig farms in Guangxi province of southern China. Of the 350 field samples collected from the clinically diseased pigs in Guangxi province, South China, two serum samples from a swine herd were positive for GETV, as determined by specific RT-PCR (data not shown). One GETV-positive sample (GX201807) was collected from 42 weaning piglets of ~25 days old, which only exhibited fever for 1–2 days in a swine herd in Nanning, Guangxi Province, which has a total piglet population of 307. Another GETV-positive sample (GX201808) was collected from 12 pregnant sows suffering from reproductive disorders in a pig farm located in YuLin, Guangxi Province, which has a total sow population of 196. The GETV-positive sera samples were negative for PRRSV, SVV, PRV, JEV, and CSFV as demonstrated by RT/-PCR (data not shown).

Serum samples, which were GETV positive as determined by PCR, were inoculated into BHK-21 cells for virus isolation. CPE was generated in cells characterized by shrinkage, rounding, and detachment after 48 hpi (**Figure 1A**). The GETV isolates, named as GX201808, were obtained after serial passages and plaque purification in BHK-21 cells. The supernatants of each passage were GETV positive as confirmed by RT-PCR (data not shown). IFA analysis was conducted using an anti-GETV-E2 PcAb to confirm the isolation of the GETV strain. **Figure 1B** shows staining specific for E2, which was evident in GX201808-infected BHK-21 cells. The plaques generated by GETV in BHK-21 cells were regular in shape with distinct edges (**Figure 1C**). No viable particles were isolated in GX201807-inoculated BHK-21 cells, as confirmed by CPE, RT-PCR, and IFA (data no shown).

Electron microscopic examination of precipitated GX201808 strain particles revealed a cluster of typical morphology usually associated with alphaviruses. The virus particles were spherical with an average of 70 nm in diameter and featured surface fibers (**Figure 1D**). The multistep growth curves of the GETV strain was further analyzed using BHK21 cells. As shown in **Figure 1E**, the numbers of GX201808 particles exhibited a gradual increase from 6 hpi and reached a peak titer of ~10^8TCID$_{50}$ at 36 hpi. The titers then decreased slowly, reaching a titer of ~10^5TCID$_{50}$ at 72 hpi. These results revealed that a strain of GETV was successfully isolated when using BHK-21 cells.

Genetic and Phylogenetic Analyses of the Virus

The full-length genome of the GETV strain GX201808 was sequenced and submitted to GenBank under accession

no. MT269657. The entire genome of the GETV strain contained 11,691 bp in length excluding the polyA tail and possessed a typical alphavirus genome organization with 2 main ORFs, ORF1, and ORF2, and short UTRs at the 5'- and 3'-termini. All GETV strains available from GenBank were downloaded for sequence comparison and phylogenetic analysis. The results showed that GX201808 shared 94.9–99.4% sequence identity at the nucleotide level with other strains and the highest identity (99.4%) with strain SD17/09, which was recently isolated from foxes in China. The complete genome of GX201808 strain showed 97.3–99.3% identity with strains isolated from pigs in China, and only 97.6% identity with the strain (M1) first isolated in mosquitoes in China. Sequence comparison at the amino acid level of the GX201808 strain with other reported strains showed the sequence identities ranging from 97.4 to 99.7%, and 98.6 to 99.6% in the non-structural and structural polyproteins, respectively (**Table 2**).

Phylogenetic analysis showed that GETVs were divided into four evolutionary groups. Group I only had the oldest GETV strain (MM2021) isolated in 1963. Two GETVs strains isolated in Japan in 1956 formed Group II. Most of the GETV strains isolated from mosquitoes, pigs, horses, cattle, and other animals, including the strain GX201808 in this study were classified as Group III. Two GETV strains, YN12031 and LEIV/16275/Mag, were classified as Group IV (**Figure 2**).

DISCUSSION

GETV has a widespread geographic distribution, and the host range of the virus is expanding gradually (1, 3). Guangxi province of southern China is located in tropical and subtropical areas of the planet. The tropical and subtropical climates of these regions provide a favorable environment for the reproduction of mosquitoes, which play a key role in the spread of GETV among different hosts (30). The existence of GETV-infected animals and mosquitoes in Hunan, Guangdong, and Yunnan provinces, which are the neighboring provinces located in the east and west of Guangxi province, has meant that they are likely to spread, and they have already been reported (23, 25, 27, 28). In this study, we detected and isolated for the first time in Guangxi province, a GETV strain in pig sera using BHK-21 cells, proving the existence of GETV in this region of China. These GETV-positive samples were collected from weaning piglets exhibiting sudden onset fever or pregnant sows suffering from reproductive disorders.

Recently, an outbreak of GETV infection in swine herds resulted in reproductive disorders of pregnant sows and the death of piglets (25), indicating that this virus may pose a potential threat to swine health. Consistent with the findings of the previous study that reported the isolation of a strain of YN12031 (23), the GETV isolate GX201808 could generate CPE in BHK-21 cells characterized by shrinkage, rounding, and detachment. The virus could produce plaques and grow well in BHK-21 cells. Electron microscopic examination revealed that the virus particles were spherical with an average diameter of 70 nm, and

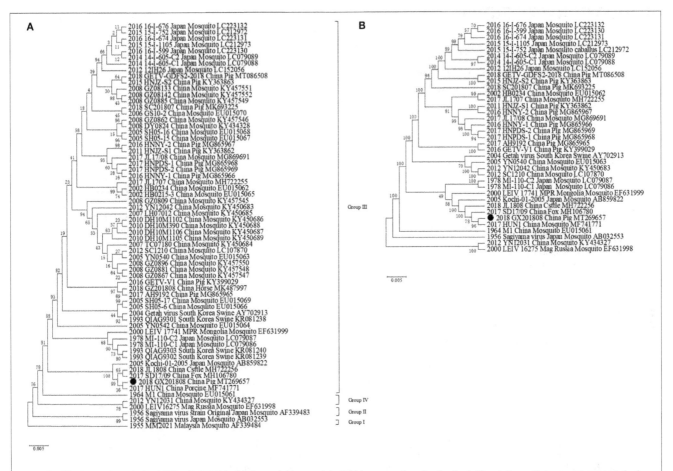

FIGURE 2 | Phylogenetic analysis of GETV GX201808 with the available complete GETV genomes from the GenBank. The phylogenetic trees were generated using the neighbor-joining method implemented in the program MEGA 6.0. Bootstrap values are expressed as a percentage based on 1,000 replications. The strain obtained in this study is indicated by a closed triangle. **(A)** Diagrammatic representation of a tree based on the complete E2 gene nucleotide sequences of GETVs. **(B)** Diagrammatic representation of a tree based on the complete genome sequence of GETV GX201808 and the available complete GETV genomes from the GenBank.

they featured surface fibers, which was consistent with a previous study showing GETV particles display the typical morphology of alphaviruses (23, 31). The expression of E2 in the GX201808-infected cells could be detected by a specific polyclonal antibody raised against the E2 protein of GETV by IFA. This demonstrated that the GETV GX201808 strain was successfully isolated from BHK-21 cells. Viable GETV could not be isolated from BHK-21 cells inoculated with samples of GX201807, and this might be attributed to only a few virus particles in the samples or that the viruses had lost their viability during sample transportation from the pig farms to the laboratory.

It was shown that all the known GETV strains could be grouped into four evolutionary groups (24). The GX201808 strain was clustered in Group III and had the closest relationship with the HuN1 strain, which caused an outbreak of GETV infection in swine herds in Hunan province, China, leading to the death of piglets and reproductive disorders in pregnant pigs in 2017 (25). GX201808 also clustered closely with the recently reported Chinese GETV strains JL1808 and SD17/09 isolated from cattle and foxes, respectively (17, 26). Sequence comparison showed that GX201808 shares high sequence identity at the

nucleotide level with the strains HuN1, SD17/09, and JL1808. Group III, represented by the first Chinese strain (M1) that was isolated in 1964 from mosquitoes, contains most GETV strains appearing in mosquitoes, pigs, horses, cattle, foxes, and other animals and has become the dominant viruses circulating among species (17, 23, 26–28).

An increase of high seroprevalence in pigs in the field was detected, and high virus titers were found in pigs infected experimentally with GETV, indicating that this species might be a natural reservoir and amplifiers of GETV (32–34). It has also been shown that GETV strains can circulate among pigs and horses simultaneously within the same region in Japan in 2015, and these were found to be closely related genetically (32). Recent studies also showed that mosquito-borne swine GETVs might play a role in transmitting GETV to blue foxes, cattle, and horses in different provinces of China (26, 27, 29), indicating that this virus has the potential to spread nationally and expand its host range. In response, we recommend that continuous surveillance of GETV infection in animals should be implemented in order to control the circulation of this potentially dangerous virus.

AUTHOR CONTRIBUTIONS

ZW conceptualized the study. TR and QM took part in the data curation. YW and ZN made the formal analysis. KO, YC, and WH were in charge of the investigation. HW, JW, and CN were in charge of the methodology. ZW was in charge of the project administration, wrote, reviewed, and edited the manuscript.

All authors contributed to the article and approved the submitted version.

ACKNOWLEDGMENTS

The authors would also like to thank Dr. Dev Sooranna of Imperial College London for English language edits of the manuscript.

REFERENCES

1. Weaver SC. Host range, amplification and arboviral disease emergence. *Arch Virol Suppl.* (2005) 2005:33–44. doi: 10.1007/3-211-29981-5_4
2. Zhai YG, Wang HY, Sun XH, Fu SH, Wang HQ, Attoui H, et al. Complete sequence characterization of isolates of getah virus (genus alphavirus, family togaviridae) from China. *J Gen Virol.* (2008) 89:1446–56. doi: 10.1099/vir.0.83607-0
3. Gould EA, Coutard B, Malet H, Morin B, Jamal S, Weaver S, et al. Understanding the alphaviruses: recent research on important emerging pathogens and progress towards their control. *Antiviral Res.* (2010) 87:111–24. doi: 10.1016/j.antiviral.2009.07.007
4. Pfeffer M, Kinney RM, Kaaden OR. The alphavirus 3'-nontranslated region: size heterogeneity and arrangement of repeated sequence elements. *Virology.* (1998) 240:100–8. doi: 10.1006/viro.1997.8907
5. Ksiazek TG, Trosper JH, Cross JH, Basaca-Sevilla V. Isolation of Getah virus from Nueva Ecija Province, Republic of the Philippines. *Trans R Soc Trop Med Hyg.* (1981) 75:312–3. doi: 10.1016/0035-9203(81)90346-1
6. Bryant JE, Crabtree MB, Nam VS, Yen NT, Duc HM, Miller BR. Isolation of arboviruses from mosquitoes collected in northern Vietnam. *Am J Trop Med Hyg.* (2005) 73:470–3. doi: 10.4269/ajtmh.2005.73.470
7. Li XD, Qiu FX, Yang H, Rao YN, Calisher CH. Isolation of Getah virus from mosquitos collected on Hainan Island, China, and results of a serosurvey. *Southeast Asian J Trop Med Public Health.* (1992) 23:730–4.
8. Scherer WF, Funkenbusch M, Buescher EL, Izumit. Sagiyama virus, a new group A arthropod-borne virus from Japan. I. Isolation, immunologic classification, and ecologic observations. *Am J Trop Med Hyg.* (1962) 11:255–68. doi: 10.4269/ajtmh.1962.11.255
9. Kanamitsu M, Taniguchi K, Urasawa S, Ogata T, Wada Y, Wada Y, et al. Geographic distribution of arbovirus antibodies in indigenous human populations in the indo-australian archipelago. *Am J Trop Med Hyg.* (1979) 28:351–63. doi: 10.4269/ajtmh.1979.28.351
10. Gur'ev EL, Gromashevskii VL, Prilipov AG, L'Vov S D. Analysis of the genome of two Getah virus strains (LEIV 16275 Mar and LEIV 17741 MPR) isolated from mosquitoes in the North-Eastern Asia. *Vopr Virusol.* (2008) 53:27–31
11. Sanderson CJ. A serologic survey of queensland cattle for evidence of arbovirus infections. *Am J Trop Med Hyg.* (1969) 18:433–9. doi: 10.4269/ajtmh.1969.18.433
12. Shortridge KF, Mason DK, Watkins KL, Aaskov JG. Serological evidence for the transmission of getah virus in Hong Kong. *Vet Rec.* (1994) 134:527–8. doi: 10.1136/vr.134.20.527
13. Sugiyama I, Shimizu E, Nogami S, Suzuki K, Miura Y, Sentsui H. Serological survey of arthropod-borne viruses among wild boars in Japan. *J Vet Med Sci.* (2009) 71:1059–61. doi: 10.1292/jvms.71.1059
14. Li Y, Fu S, Guo X, Li X, Li M, Wang L, et al. Serological survey of getah virus in domestic animals in yunnan province, China. *Vector Borne Zoonotic Dis.* (2019) 19:59–61. doi: 10.1089/vbz.2018.2273
15. Kamada M, Ando Y, Fukunaga Y, Kumanomido T, Imagawa H, Wada R, et al. Equine Getah virus infection: isolation of the virus from racehorses during an enzootic in Japan. *Am J Trop Med Hyg.* (1980) 29:984–8. doi: 10.4269/ajtmh.1980.29.984
16. Yago K, Hagiwara S, Kawamura H, Narita M. A fatal case in newborn piglets with getah virus infection: isolation of the virus. *Nihon Juigaku Zasshi.* (1987) 49:989–94. doi: 10.1292/jvms1939.49.989
17. Shi N, Li LX, Lu RG, Yan XJ, Liu H. Highly pathogenic swine getah virus in blue foxes, eastern China, 2017. *Emerg Infect Dis.* (2019) 25:1252–4. doi: 10.3201/eid2506.181983
18. Sentsui H, Kono Y. reappearance of getah virus infection among horses in Japan. *Nihon Juigaku Zasshi.* (1985) 47:333–5. doi: 10.1292/jvms1939.47.333
19. Nemoto M, Bannai H, Tsujimura K, Kobayashi M, Kikuchi T, Yamanaka T, et al. Getah virus infection among racehorses, Japan, 2014. *Emerg Infect Dis.* (2015) 21:883–5. doi: 10.3201/eid2105.141975
20. Bannai H, Ochi A, Nemoto M, Tsujimura K, Yamanaka T, Kondo T. A 2015 outbreak of Getah virus infection occurring among Japanese racehorses sequentially to an outbreak in 2014 at the same site. *BMC Vet Res.* (2016) 12:98. doi: 10.1186/s12917-016-0741-5
21. Nemoto M, Bannai H, Ochi A, Niwa H, Murakami S, Tsujimura K, et al. Complete genome sequences of getah virus strains isolated from horses in 2016 in Japan. *Genome Announc.* (2017) 5:17. doi: 10.1128/genomeA.00750-17
22. Brown CM, Timoney PJ. Getah virus infection of Indian horses. *Trop Anim Health Prod.* (1998) 30:241–52. doi: 10.1023/A:1005079229232
23. Li YY, Fu SH, Guo XF, Lei WW, Li XL, Song JD, et al. Identification of a newly isolated getah virus in the china-laos border, China. *Biomed Environ Sci.* (2017) 30:210–4. doi: 10.3967/bes2017.028
24. Li YY, Liu H, Fu SH, Li XL, Guo XF, Li MH, et al. From discovery to spread: the evolution and phylogeny of getah virus. *Infect Genet Evol.* (2017) 55:48–55. doi: 10.1016/j.meegid.2017.08.016
25. Yang T, Li R, Hu Y, Yang L, Zhao D, Du L, et al. An outbreak of getah virus infection among pigs in China, 2017. *Transbound Emerg Dis.* (2018) 65:632–7. doi: 10.1111/tbed.12867
26. Liu H, Zhang X, Li LX, Shi N, Sun XT, Liu Q, et al. First isolation and characterization of Getah virus from cattle in northeastern China. *BMC Vet Res.* (2019) 15:320. doi: 10.1186/s12917-019-2061-z
27. Lu G, Ou J, Ji J, Ren Z, Hu X, Wang C, et al. Emergence of Getah Virus Infection in Horse With Fever in China, (2018). *Front Microbiol.* (2019) 10:1416. doi: 10.3389/fmicb.2019.02601
28. Xing C, Jiang J, Lu Z, Mi S, He B, Tu C, et al. Isolation and characterization of Getah virus from pigs in Guangdong province of China. *Transbound Emerg Dis.* (2020) 67:2249–53. doi: 10.1111/tbed.13567
29. Wang H, Niu C, Nong Z, Quan D, Chen Y, Kang O, et al. Emergence and phylogenetic analysis of a novel Seneca Valley virus strain in the Guangxi Province of China. *Res Vet Sci.* (2020) 130:207–11. doi: 10.1016/j.rvsc.2020.03.020
30. Xia H, Wang Y, Atoni E, Zhang B, Yuan Z. Mosquito-associated viruses in China. *Virol Sin.* (2018) 33:5–20. doi: 10.1007/s12250-018-0002-9
31. Hu T, Zheng Y, Zhang Y, Li G, Qiu W, Yu J, et al. Identification of a novel Getah virus by virus-Discovery-cDNA random amplified polymorphic DNA (RAPD). *BMC Microbiol.* (2012) 12:305. doi: 10.1186/1471-2180-12-305
32. Bannai H, Nemoto M, Niwa H, Murakami S, Tsujimura K, Yamanaka T, et al. Geospatial and temporal associations of getah virus circulation among pigs and horses around the perimeter of outbreaks in Japanese racehorses in 2014 and (2015). *BMC Vet Res.* (2017) 13:187. doi: 10.1186/s12917-017-1112-6
33. Kumanomido T, Wada R, Kanemaru T, Kamada M, Hirasawa K, Akiyama Y. Clinical and virological observations on swine experimentally infected with getah virus. *Vet Microbiol.* (1988) 16:295–301. doi: 10.1016/0378-1135(88)90033-8
34. Hohdatsu T, Ide S, Yamagishi H, Eiguchi Y, Nagano H, Maehara N, et al. Enzyme-linked immunosorbent assay for the serological survey of Getah virus in pigs. *Nihon Juigaku Zasshi.* (1990) 52:835–7. doi: 10.1292/jvms1939.52.835

10

Genetic Variability of 3′-Proximal Region of Genomes of Orf Viruses Isolated from Sheep and Wild Japanese Serows (*Capricornis crispus*) in Japan

Kaori Shimizu [1], Asari Takaiwa [1], Shin-nosuke Takeshima [2], Ayaka Okada [1,3] and Yasuo Inoshima [1,3,4,5]*

[1] Laboratory of Food and Environmental Hygiene, Cooperative Department of Veterinary Medicine, Gifu University, Gifu, Japan, [2] Department of Food and Nutrition, Jumonji University, Saitama, Japan, [3] Education and Research Center for Food Animal Health, Gifu University (GeFAH), Gifu, Japan, [4] The United Graduate School of Veterinary Sciences, Gifu University, Gifu, Japan, [5] Joint Graduate School of Veterinary Sciences, Gifu University, Gifu, Japan

*Correspondence:
Yasuo Inoshima
inoshima@gifu-u.ac.jp

Orf virus is a prototype species of the genus *Parapoxvirus*, subfamily *Chordopoxvirinae*, family *Poxviridae*. Japanese orf viruses, infecting sheep and wild Japanese serows (*Capricornis crispus*), have been considered to be genetically closely related based on the sequence identities of the open reading frames (ORFs) 11, 20, and 132 in their genomes. However, since the genome size of orf viruses is about 140 kbp long, genetic variation among Japanese orf viruses remains unclear. In this study, we analyzed the sequences of ORFs 117, 119, 125, and 127 located in the 3′-proximal region of the viral genome using two strains from sheep and three strains from Japanese serows isolated from 1970 to 2007, and compared them with the corresponding sequences of reference orf viruses from other countries. Sequence analysis revealed that ORFs 125 and 127, which encode the inhibitor of apoptosis and viral interleukin (IL)-10, respectively, were highly conserved among the five Japanese orf viruses. However, high genetic variability with deletions or duplications was observed in ORFs 117 and 119, which encode granulocyte macrophage colony-stimulating factor and IL-2 inhibition factor (GIF), and inducer of cell apoptosis, respectively, in one strain from sheep and two strains from Japanese serows. Our results suggest that genetic variability exists in Japanese orf viruses even in the same host species. This is the first report of genetic variability of orf viruses in Japan.

Keywords: genetic variability, Japanese serows, nucleotide sequence, orf virus, sheep

INTRODUCTION

Orf virus is a prototype species of the genus *Parapoxvirus*, subfamily *Chordopoxvirinae*, family *Poxviridae* (1). Orf virus has a linear double-stranded DNA genome (134–139 kbp) with high GC content (~63–64%) and encodes 132 putative gene products (2). Orf virus is the causative agent of orf disease, also known as contagious pustular dermatitis, contagious ecthyma, or scabby mouth mainly in sheep and goats, and can be transmitted to humans (3). In Japan, the first reports of orf virus infections in sheep and wild Japanese serows (*Capricornis crispus*) were published in

1952 (4) and 1979 (5), respectively. Previously, we have reported nucleotide sequence homology in three open reading frames (ORFs) 11, 20, and 132 among 13 orf viruses isolated or polymerase chain reaction (PCR)-detected from sheep and wild Japanese serows (6). These ORFs encode viral envelope (7), virus interferon resistance (8), and viral vascular endothelial growth factor (VEGF) (9), respectively. The amino acid sequences derived from ORFs 11 and 20 were identical among the 13 orf viruses, and only one amino acid substitution was found in ORF 132 in an orf virus isolated from sheep (6). Therefore, the three viral genes of Japanese orf viruses are highly conserved. However, since only a part of the whole genome (∼140 kbp) has been sequenced so far, the degree of genetic variation in other regions remains unclear.

To explore genetic differences between Japanese orf viruses, we conducted next-generation sequencing (NGS) of some strains of these orf viruses. However, whole genome sequences were not obtained, due to the large number of unmapped reads in the 3′-proximal region of viral genome (**Figure 1**). We hypothesized that the 3′-proximal region of a viral genome has genetic variation. Thus, in the present study, we characterized four ORFs 117, 119, 125, and 127, which are located in the 3′-proximal region of the viral genome. ORFs 117, 119, 125, and 127 encode granulocyte macrophage colony-stimulating factor and interleukin 2 (IL-2) inhibition factor (GIF) (11), inducer of cell apoptosis (12), inhibitor of apoptosis (13, 14), and viral IL-10 (15), respectively.

MATERIALS AND METHODS

Viruses

For epidemiologic and genetic characteristics of Japanese orf virus, five Japanese strains isolated from 1970 to 2007 were used. Two strains of Iwate (16) and HIS (17) were isolated from sheep and three strains of S-1 (18), R-1 (19), and GE (6) were isolated from wild Japanese serows (**Table 1**). Viruses were propagated in fetal lamb lung cells (kindly provided by Dr. H. Sentsui, Nihon University, Japan) at 37°C in Dulbecco's modified Eagle's medium (Wako, Osaka, Japan) supplemented with 10% fetal bovine serum (PAA Laboratories, Pasching, Austria).

Whole Genome Re-sequencing and Assembly

Total DNA extracted from virus-infected cells using a DNeasy Blood and Tissue Kit (Qiagen, Hilden, Germany) were used for constructing the libraries using Nextera XT DNA sample Prep Kit (Illumina, San Diego, CA, USA), and sequenced using an Illumina MiSeq (Illumina). Obtained short read sequences collected in FASTQ files were aligned to the orf virus strain NZ2 (DQ184476) as the reference genome using Burrows–Wheeler transformation (BWA) ver 0.7.12-r103 software (25) and constructed binary version of the sequence alignment/map (bam) file using SAM tools ver. 0.1.19-96b5f2294a software (26).

Abbreviations: GIF, granulocyte-macrophage colony-stimulating factor and IL-2 inhibition factor; IL-2, interleukin 2; ORF, open reading frame; PCR, polymerase chain reaction; VEGF, vascular endothelial growth factor.

Analysis of ORF

DNA was extracted from virus-infected cells using a DNeasy Blood and Tissue Kit (Qiagen) according to the manufacturer's instructions. Four different PCRs were carried out with GoTaq Hot Start Green Master Mix (Promega, Madison, WI, USA) using Veriti thermal cycler (Applied Biosystems, Foster City, CA, USA). The PCR conditions and analyzed ORFs are provided in **Supplementary Table S1** and **Figure 1**, respectively. PCR products were purified using NucleoSpin Gel and PCR Clean-up (Macherey-Nagel, Duren, Germany), and the nucleotide sequences were determined by direct sequencing using a BigDye Terminator Cycle Sequencing Kit v3.1 (Applied Biosystems, Foster City, CA, USA). Sequence analysis was carried out using the software Genetyx-Win version 13 (Genetyx, Tokyo, Japan), and phylogenetic analysis was performed using the MEGA7 program (27). Phylogenetic trees were constructed using maximum likelihood methods, and the reliability of the branches was evaluated by 1,000 replicates. Sequence and phylogenetic analyses were compared with the reference orf viruses (**Table 1**).

RESULTS

NGS was performed using total DNA extracted from the concentrated virus. However, whole genome sequences were not obtained, possibly due to the large number of deletion in the 3′-proximal region of viral genome (**Figure 1**).

Specific PCR products of 799 bp for ORF 117 and 537–652 bp for ORF 119 were obtained from the four strains (Iwate, HIS, S-1, and GE) and from all five Japanese orf viruses, respectively. High genomic variability was seen in ORFs 117 and 119 in Japanese orf viruses. In ORF 117, 96.6–100% nucleotide identity was observed among four strains. Surprisingly, R-1 strain from Japanese serow completely lacked ORF 117 (**Figure 2A**). Partial deletion in ORF 117 was also observed in the amino acid sequences in reference orf virus strain NA1/11 isolated from sheep in China. In ORF 119, deletions were observed in the first half of the amino acid sequences in S-1 and R-1 strains as well as the reference Chinese NA1/11 strain (**Figure 2B**). Two and 12 amino acid deletion was observed in HIS and three reference strains from sheep and goat (NZ2, IA82, and YX), respectively. In the Iwate strain, 10 amino acids were found to be duplicated.

Specific PCR products of 522 and 561 bp were obtained for ORFs 125 and 127 from all of five Japanese orf viruses. Amino acid sequences derived from these ORFs from four Japanese orf viruses (Iwate, S-1, R-1, and GE) were found to be 100% identical. The sequence from HIS strain revealed only two and seven amino acid substitutions in ORFs 125 and 127, respectively (**Supplementary Tables S2, S3**). The sequences of ORFs 125 and 127 were highly conserved among Japanese orf viruses. In the phylogenetic analysis, there were mainly two branches, and all Japanese orf viruses were classified into the same group (**Figure 3**). Our results indicate that Japanese orf viruses are closer to the IA82 and NZ2 strains isolated in the United States and New Zealand, respectively, than other reference strains. Sequences obtained in this study were

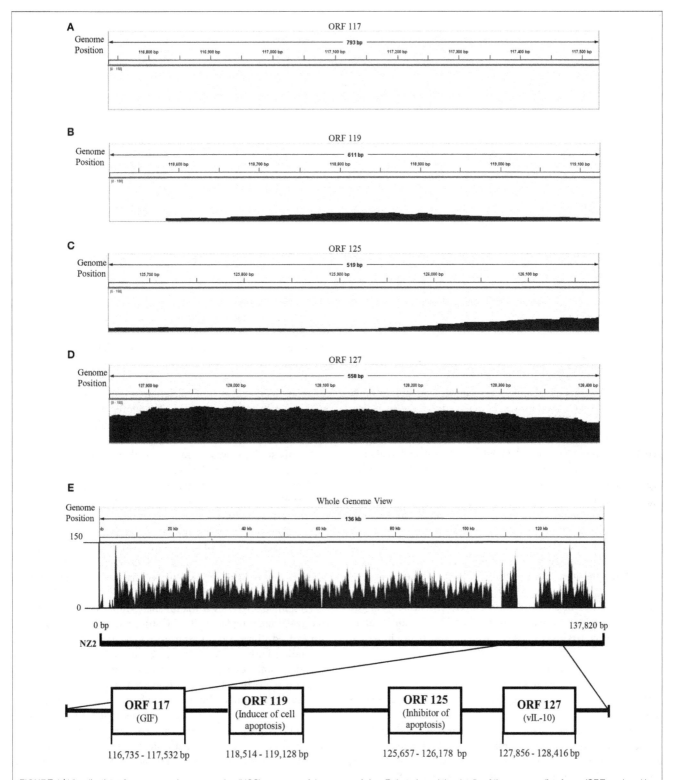

FIGURE 1 | Visualization of next-generation sequencing (NGS) coverage of Japanese orf virus R-1 strain and the details of the open reading frame (ORF) analyzed in this study. NZ2 strain (GenBank accession no. DQ184476) was used as the reference strain. Binary version of the sequence alignment/map (bam) file was loaded onto the Integrated Genome Viewer (IGV) (10). The vertical axis shows the number of reads mapping to each location of the genome. Zoomed view of ORF 117 **(A)**, ORF 119 **(B)**, ORF 125 **(C)**, and ORF 127 **(D)**. Whole genome view **(E)**.

TABLE 1 | Japanese and reference orf viruses used in this study.

Strain	Host	Year of isolation	Country	Deposited and reference accession no.[a]				References
				ORF 111–119	ORF 125	ORF 127	Complete genome	
Iwate	Sheep	1970	Japan	LC487906	LC476578	LC476583		(16, 20, 21)
HIS	Sheep	2004	Japan	LC476574	LC476579	LC476584		(17, 21)
S-1	Japanese serow	1985	Japan	LC476575	LC476580	LC476585		(18, 20, 21)
R-1	Japanese serow	1999	Japan	LC476576	LC476581	LC476586		(19, 20)
GE	Japanese serow	2007	Japan	LC476577	LC476582	LC476587		(6)
NZ2	Sheep	1982	New Zealand				DQ184476	(2)
IA82	Sheep	1982	USA				AY386263	(22)
SA00	Goat	2000	USA				AY386264	(22)
NA1/11	Sheep	2011	China				KF234407	(23)
GO	Goat	2012	China				KP010354	(24)
YX	Goat	2012	China				KP010353	(24)

[a]ORF, open reading frame.

submitted to DDBJ/EMBL/GenBank, and the accession numbers are given in **Table 1**.

DISCUSSION

In this study, we carried out ORF sequence analysis for five Japanese orf viruses, and our results revealed that the sequences of ORFs 125 and 127 were highly conserved. However, high genomic variability was seen in ORFs 117 and 119. Observed genetic variability was found to be the 3′-proximal region of Japanese orf viruses. To the best of our knowledge, this is the first report on the genetic variability of Japanese orf viruses.

In the phylogenetic analysis of ORF 125, Japanese orf viruses isolated from Japanese serows were classified into a group isolated from sheep. It has been reported that analyses of the phylogenetic tree of 47 ORFs including ORF 125 were found to assist in easily distinguishing between goat- and sheep-originated orf viruses (24). These results indicate a possibility that sheep orf virus may have infected Japanese serows. Furthermore, analyses of the phylogenetic tree of ORFs 125 and 127 clearly showed that the Japanese orf viruses were closer to IA82 and NZ2 strains than to other reference strains. In Japan, sheep are frequently imported from the United States and New Zealand for improved growth and to encourage breeding (28). Therefore, it is possible that these orf viruses came along with the imported animals and were introduced into breeding sheep and wild Japanese serows in Japan.

Our results showed genetic variability in ORFs 117 and 119 in the Japanese orf viruses, suggesting that there is heterogeneity even in viruses infected with the same host species. In addition, deletions in ORF 119 were observed in Japanese (HIS, S-1, and R-1) and reference (NZ2, IA82, NA1/11, and YX) strains. Based on the previous comparative analysis, it is presumed that genes in the central region of the orf virus genome are more conserved, whereas those in the terminal region show remarkably high variability (29). Notably, this variability is accompanied by a high frequency of gene recombination and nucleotide deletions

(23). The genetic analysis of ORFs 117 and 119 may help to characterize or differentiate strains that are otherwise shown to be identical by the envelope coding genes (30). A previous study demonstrated that viruses with high deletion in ORFs 114–120 showed low virulence in animal inoculation experiments and that genomic deletions attenuate virulence (24). At present, the relationship between the deletion of ORF 117 and virulence in the R-1 strain is unknown. Therefore, there is a need to analyze the correlation between genetic variability and virulence in more detail.

In this study, it was revealed that there were differences in conservation and variability among ORFs. Viral IL-10 encoded by ORF 127 shares remarkable similarity to mammalian IL-10. Mammalian IL-10 is highly conserved across all mammalian species (15). IL-10 is a multifunctional cytokine that has suppressive effects on inflammation, antiviral responses. Orf virus produces viral IL-10 by itself and avoids host's inflammatory and immune response by it (31). This suggests that viral IL-10 encoded by ORF 127 might require high conservation in orf virus. On the other hand, GIF encoded by ORF 117 does not resemble any known mammalian granulocyte-macrophage colony–stimulating factor (GM-CSF)- or IL-2-binding proteins, and indeed, there are no reports of any other protein capable of binding both GM-CSF and IL-2. In addition, human GM-CSF does not respond in sheep cells due to its inability to bind to ovine receptor (32). Therefore, GIF was thought to have evolved a unique binding specificity in sheep, the natural host of the orf virus (33). This suggests that GIF encoded by ORF 117 is gene whose necessity changes depending on the host species. It is thought that differences in necessity of gene may affect conservation and variability of the gene encoded by ORFs.

Japanese serows are wild animals and a natural monument that is endemic in Japan (34). Japanese serows are often witnessed in mountain villages and can come into contact with livestock sheep. There have been reports that a single strain of orf virus caused outbreak of proliferative dermatitis in various ruminant species at a zoo (35). Orf virus from Japanese serows can be

A

```
GE      1:MACLMVFLAVLALCGSVHSAQWIGERDFCTAHAQDVFARLQVWMRIDRNVTAADNSSACALAIETPPSNFDADVYVAAAGINVSVSAINCGFFNMRQVET 100
S-1     1:.................................................................................................... 100
R-1     0:---------------------------------------------------------------------------------------------------- 0
Iwate   1:.................................................................................................... 100
HIS     1:....R............................................................................................... 100
NZ2     1:....R............................................................................................... 100
IA82    1:....R............................................................................................... 100
SA00    1:....R.....F.................M..............................N.....................................S... 100
NA1/11  1:....R.....F.................M.....................----------------------T............................ 77
GO      1:....R.....F.................M...........V..........N.............................................S... 100
YX      1:...IR.....F.................M...........V..........N.............................................S... 100

GE    101:TYNTARRQMYVYMDSWDPWALDDPQPLFSQEYENETLPYLLEVLELARLYIRVGCTVPGEQPFEVIPGIDYPHTGMEFLQHVLRPNRRFAPAKLHMDLEV 200
S-1   101:.................................................................................................... 200
R-1     0:---------------------------------------------------------------------------------------------------- 0
Iwate 101:........................L..................C...........................C............................ 200
HIS   101:.................VI................................................................................. 200
NZ2   101:.................VI................................................................................. 200
IA82  101:.................M................................................................................. 200
SA00  101:..D.........T....V.............................T.........S......................................... 200
NA1/11 78:............T....V.............................T.........S......................................... 177
GO    101:............T....V.............................T.........S......................................... 200
YX    101:..D.........T....V.............................T.........S......................................... 200

GE    201:DHRCVSAVHVKAFLQDACSARKARTPLYFAGHGCNHPDRRPKNPVPRPQHVSSPISRKCSMQTAR                                    265
S-1   201:................................................................                                    265
R-1     0:----------------------------------------------------------------                                    0
Iwate 201:........................................S......L..F..........                                       265
HIS   201:................................................................                                    265
NZ2   201:................................................................                                    265
IA82  201:................................................................                                    265
SA00  201:.Y......Y......................S...............M...L.....                                           265
NA1/11 178:......I....................................................                                        242
GO    201:...............................S...............M...L.....                                           265
YX    201:.Y.............................S...............M...L.....                                           265
```

B

```
GE      1:MDSRRLALAVAFGGVLASMTQRRRLASLIASIGQRLMGGDGMRRVAVRLIDQLMAGPPDINDEAFQREIRVGVGELFQALHRVVE----------QARRE 90
S-1     1:-----------------------------..................................................-----------.....  61
R-1     1:-----------------------...........................................................-----------.....  65
Iwate   1:........................................................................................LFQALHRVVE..... 100
HIS     1:.........................................................................N......--...-----------..... 88
NZ2     1:.........................................................................N......--...-----------..... 88
IA82    1:..............................................................................--...-----------..... 88
SA00    1:.................................................................D..............................T... 90
NA1/11  1:--------------------.............................................D..............................T... 70
GO      1:.................................................................D.............................. 90
YX      1:.................................................................D.....---------...-----------..... 78

GE     91:KYFEVCGAGNDADAPVVEMDTAAAPPQPQPQPAPFVVTPQNAFMFVPQGSHVHVDESVDPFFGMSPSIFGRDLPLQPPEELLSDYDPLMSQAGEPPSPRSPC 190
S-1    62:.................................................................................................... 161
R-1    66:.................................................................................................... 165
Iwate 101:.................................................................................................... 200
HIS    89:..................................................................................P................. 188
NZ2    89:...........................L......................................................P................. 188
IA82   89:.......................................................................................H............ 188
SA00   91:.......S.......S......L....LAI..........S...................I...................................... 190
NA1/11 71:.........G.......................V....S...................F...................................... 170
GO     91:.......S.............LAI..........S...................I...................................... 190
YX     79:.......S.............LAI..........S...................I...................................... 178

GE    191:EADLWCFETLGDSDSD                                                                                     206
S-1   162:................                                                                                     177
R-1   166:................                                                                                     181
Iwate 201:................                                                                                     216
HIS   189:................                                                                                     204
NZ2   189:................                                                                                     204
IA82  189:................                                                                                     204
SA00  191:..........N.....                                                                                     206
NA1/11 171:...............                                                                                     186
GO    191:..........N...AS                                                                                     206
YX    179:..........N...AS                                                                                     194
```

FIGURE 2 | Alignment of the amino acid sequences derived from ORF 117 **(A)** and ORF 119 **(B)**. Amino acids identical to GE strain at the given positions are represented by dots. R-1 strain completely lacked ORF 117. In ORF 119, deletions were observed in the first half of the nucleotide sequences in S-1 and R-1 strains. In the box, duplicate in Iwate strain is shown.

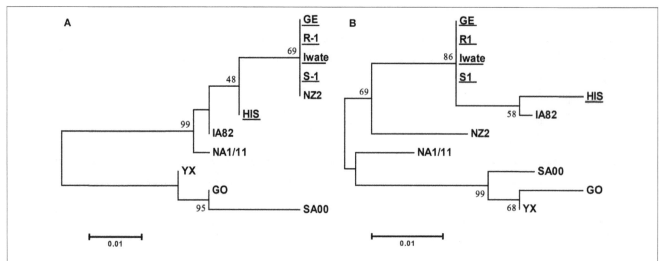

FIGURE 3 | Phylogenetic tree based on deduced amino acid sequences derived from ORF 125 **(A)** and ORF 127 **(B)**. Strains used in this study are underlined. The percentage bootstrap values calculated from 1,000 replicates are indicated above the internal nodes.

spread to sheep or farmers, or orf virus from sheep can be spread to Japanese serows. It is important to know the characteristics of Japanese orf viruses in order to reduce the spread risk.

We tried NGS analysis, but it was unsuccessful. NGS results indicated the 3'-proximal region of the genome of Japanese orf viruses has genetic variation. Our results obtained by Sanger sequencing for variable region of Japanese orf viruses may be useful for understanding the characteristics of these viruses. However, we analyzed the limited region of the viral genomes, and sequencing other regions using improved methods for NGS might be required to better understand the characteristics of Japanese orf viruses.

AUTHOR CONTRIBUTIONS

KS and YI analyzed all data and were major contributors in writing the manuscript. KS, AT, ST, and AO performed the nucleotide/amino acid sequencing and phylogenetic analysis. All authors read and approved the final manuscript.

ACKNOWLEDGMENTS

We would like to acknowledge Dr. Hiroshi Sentsui (Nihon University, Japan) for providing fetal lamb lung cells.

REFERENCES

1. Skinner MA, Buller RM, Damon IK, Lefkowitz EJ, McFadden G, McInnes CJ, et al. Poxviridae. In: King AMQ, Adams MJ, Carstens EB, Lefkowitz EJ, editors. *Virus Taxonomy: Ninth Report of the International Committee on Taxonomy of Viruses.* New York, NY: Elsevier Academic Press (2012). p. 291–309. doi: 10.1016/B978-0-12-384684-6.00028-8

2. Mercer AA, Ueda N, Friederichs SM, Hofmann K, Fraser KM, Bateman T, et al. Comparative analysis of genome sequences of three isolates of Orf virus reveals unexpected sequence variation. *Virus Res.* (2006) 116:146–58. doi: 10.1016/j.virusres.2005.09.011

3. Knowles, DP. Poxviridae. In: MacLachlan NJ, Dubovi EJ, editors. *Fenner's Veterinary Virology.* 4th ed. Amsterdam: Elsevier Academic Press. (2011) p. 151–65. doi: 10.1016/B978-0-12-375158-4.00007-9

4. Asakawa Y, Imaizum K, Tajima Y, Endo, M. Studies on a contagious ecthyma-like disease observed among the sheep. *Jpn J Med Sci Biol.* (1952) 5:475–86. doi: 10.7883/yoken1952.5.475

5. Kumagai T, Shimizu M, Ito Y, Yamamoto S, Ito T, Ohyama S, et al. Contagious pustular dermatitis of Japanese serows in Akita Prefecture. In: *Proceeding of the 87th Meeting of the Japanese Society of Veterinary Science.* Kanagawa. (1979).

6. Inoshima Y, Ito M, Ishiguro, N. Spatial and temporal genetic homogeneity of orf viruses infecting Japanese serows (*Capricornis crispus*). *J Vet Med Sci.* (2010) 72:701–7. doi: 10.1292/jvms.09-0467

7. Inoshima Y, Morooka A, Sentsui, H. Detection and diagnosis of parapoxvirus by the polymerase chain reaction. *J Virol Methods.* (2000) 84:201–8. doi: 10.1016/S0166-0934(99)00144-5

8. McInnes CJ, Wood AR, Mercer, AA. Orf virus encodes a homolog of the vaccinia virus interferon-resistance gene E3L. *Virus Genes.* (1998) 17:107–15.

9. Lyttle DJ, Fraser KM, Fleming SB, Mercer AA, Robinson, AJ. Homologs of vascular endothelial growth factor are encoded by the poxvirus orf virus. *J Virol.* (1994) 68:84–92. doi: 10.1128/JVI.68.1.84-92.1994

10. *The Integrative Genomics Viewer.* Available online at: http://software.broadinstitute.org/software/igv/ (accessed 7 January, 2020).

11. McInnes CJ, Deane D, Haig D, Percival A, Thomson J, Wood AR. Glycosylation, disulfide bond formation, and the presence of a WSXWS-like motif in the orf virus GIF protein are critical for maintaining the integrity of binding to ovine granulocyte–macrophage colony-stimulating factor and interleukin-2. *J Virol.* (2005) 79:11205–13. doi: 10.1128/JVI.79.17.11205-11213.2005

12. Li W, Chen H, Deng H, Kuang Z, Long M, Chen D, et al. Orf virus encoded protein ORFV119 induces cell apoptosis through the extrinsic and intrinsic pathways. *Front Microbiol.* (2018) 9:1056. doi: 10.3389/fmicb.2018.01056

13. Westphal D, Ledgerwood EC, Hibma MH, Fleming SB, Whelan EM, Mercer AA. A novel Bcl-2-like inhibitor of apoptosis is encoded by the parapoxvirus ORF virus. *J Virol.* (2007) 81:7178–88. doi: 10.1128/JVI.00404-07

14. Westphal D, Ledgerwood EC, Tyndall JD, Hibma MH, Ueda N, Fleming SB, et al. The orf virus inhibitor of apoptosis functions in a Bcl-2-like manner, binding and neutralizing a set of BH3-only proteins and active Bax. *Apoptosis*. (2009) 14:1317–30. doi: 10.1007/s10495-009-0403-1

15. Fleming SB, McCaughan CA, Andrews AE, Nash AD, Mercer, AA. A homolog of interleukin-10 is encoded by the poxvirus orf virus. *J Virol*. (1997) 71:4857–61. doi: 10.1128/JVI.71.6.4857-4861.1997

16. Kumagai T, Shimizu M, Ito Y, Konno S, Nakagawa N, Sato K, et al. Contagious pustular dermatitis of sheep. In: *Proceeding of the 71st Meeting of the Japanese Society of Veterinary Science*. Tokyo. (1971).

17. Kano Y, Inoshima Y, Shibahara T, Ishikawa Y, Kadota K, Ohashi S, et al. Isolation and characterization of a parapoxvirus from sheep with papular stomatitis. *JARQ*. (2005) 39:197–203. doi: 10.6090/jarq.39.197

18. Suzuki T, Minamoto N, Sugiyama M, Kinjo T, Suzuki Y, Sugimura M, et al. Isolation and antibody prevalence of a parapoxvirus in wild Japanese serows (*Capricornis crispus*). *J Wildl Dis*. (1993) 29:384–9. doi: 10.7589/0090-3558-29.3.384

19. Inoshima Y, Murakami K, Wu D, Sentsui H. Characterization of parapoxviruses circulating among wild Japanese serows (*Capricornis crispus*). *Microbiol Immunol*. (2002) 46:583–7. doi: 10.1111/j.1348-0421.2002.tb02738.x

20. Inoshima Y, Murakami K, Yokoyama T, Sentsui, H. Genetic heterogeneity among parapoxviruses isolated from sheep, cattle and Japanese serows (*Capricornis crispus*). *J Gen Virol*. (2001) 82:1215–20. doi: 10.1099/0022-1317-82-5-1215

21. Inoshima Y, Ishiguro, N. Molecular and biological characterization of vascular endothelial growth factor of parapoxviruses isolated from wild Japanese serows (*Capricornis crispus*). *Vet Microbiol*. (2010) 6:63–71. doi: 10.1016/j.vetmic.2009.07.024

22. Delhon G, Tulman ER, Afonso CL, Lu Z, de la Concha-Bermejillo A, Lehmkuhl HD, et al. Genomes of the parapoxviruses ORF virus and bovine papular stomatitis virus. *J Virol*. (2006) 78:168–77. doi: 10.1128/JVI.78.1.168-177.2004

23. Li W, Hao W, Peng Y, Duan C, Tong C, Song D, et al. Comparative genomic sequence analysis of Chinese orf virus strain NA1/11 with other parapoxviruses. *Arch Virol*. (2015) 160:253–66. doi: 10.1007/s00705-014-2274-1

24. Chi X, Zeng X, Li W, Hao W, Li M, Huang X, et al. Genome analysis of orf virus isolates from goats in the Fujian province of southern China. *Front Microbiol*. (2015) 6:1135. doi: 10.3389/fmicb.2015.01135

25. Li H, Durbin R. Fast and accurate long-read alignment with Burrows-Wheeler transform. *Bioinformatics*. (2010) 26:589–95. doi: 10.1093/bioinformatics/btp698

26. Li H, Handsaker B, Wysoker A, Fennell T, Ruan J, Homer N, et al. The Sequence Alignment/Map format and SAMtools. *Bioinformatics*. (2009) 25:2078–9. doi: 10.1093/bioinformatics/btp352

27. Kumar S, Stecher G, Tamura K. MEGA7: molecular evolutionary genetics analysis version 7.0 for bigger datasets. *Mol Biol Evol*. (2016) 33:1870–4. doi: 10.1093/molbev/msw054

28. *Animal Quarantine Annual Report*. Available online at: http://www.maff.go.jp/aqs/tokei/toukeinen.html. (accessed 7January 2020).

29. Rziha HJ, Bauer B, Adam KH, Röttgen M, Cottone R, Henkel M, et al. Relatedness and heterogeneity at the near-terminal end of the genome of a parapoxvirus bovis 1 strain (B177) compared with parapoxvirus ovis (Orf virus). *J Gen Virol*. (2003) 84:1111–6. doi: 10.1099/vir.0.18850-0

30. Hosamani M, Bhanuprakash V, Scagliarini A, Singh, RK. Comparative sequence analysis of major envelope protein gene (B2L) of Indian orf viruses isolated from sheep and goats. *Vet Microbiol*. (2006) 116:317–24. doi: 10.1016/j.vetmic.2006.04.028

31. Haig DM, McInnes, CJ. Immunity and counter-immunity during infection with the parapoxvirus orf virus. *Virus Res*. (2002) 88:3–16. doi: 10.1016/S0168-1702(02)00117-X

32. McInnes CJ, Haig, DM. Cloning and expression of a cDNA encoding ovine granulocyte-macrophage colony-stimulating factor. *Gene*. (1991) 105:275–9. doi: 10.1016/0378-1119(91)90163-6

33. Fleming SB, Wise LM, Mercer, AA. Molecular genetic analysis of orf virus: a poxvirus that has adapted to skin. *Viruses*. (2015) 23:1505–39. doi: 10.3390/v7031505

34. Ohdachi SD, Ishibashi Y, Iwasa MA, Fukui D, Saitoh T. *The Wild Mammals of Japan. 2th edn*. Kyoto: Shoukadoh Book Sellers (2015) p. 314–7.

35. Guo J, Rasmussen J, Wünschmann A, de La Concha-Bermejillo A. Genetic characterization of orf viruses isolated from various ruminant species of a zoo. *Vet Microbiol*. (2004) 99:81–92. doi: 10.1016/j.vetmic.2003.11.010

11

Laboratory Diagnosis of a NZ7-like Orf Virus Infection and Pathogen Genetic Characterization, Particularly in the *VEGF* Gene

Yongzhong Yu [1*†], Xuyang Duan [1†], Yuanyuan Liu [1], Jinzhu Ma [1], Baifen Song [1], Zhengxing Lian [2*] and Yudong Cui [1*]

[1] College of Biological Science and Technology, Heilongjiang Bayi Agricultural University, Daqing, China, [2] College of Animal Science and Technology, China Agricultural University, Beijing, China

*Correspondence:
Yongzhong Yu
yyz1968@126.com
Zhengxing Lian
lianzhx@cau.edu.cn
Yudong Cui
1016856109@qq.com

† These authors have contributed equally to this work

Orf is a widespread contagious epithelial viral disease found particularly in most sheep breeding countries in the world. Recently, an orf virus (ORFV) strain OV-HLJ05 was isolated from an outbreak in northeast China. Three genes of interest including ORFV011 (B2L), ORFV059 (F1L), and ORFV132 (VEGF) of ORFV, were recruited to identify and genetically characterize this newly isolated virus. Amino acid (aa) sequence compared with the ORFV references listed in GenBank, both B2L and F1L of OV-HLJ05 showed less microheterogeneity from their references. In contrast, the VEGF gene was included in the NZ7-VEGF like group as previously considered by Mercer in 2002. Unexpectedly, further multiple VEGF matches were made, using 34 published sequences from China and India, resulting in 27 strains of the NZ7 members. Based on Karki's report in 2020, NZ7-VEGF like viruses are emerging more and more frequently in these two countries, damaging the Asian sheep industry. Obvious heterogeneity with the NZ2, insertion of two oligopeptides TATI(L)QVVVAI(L) and SSSS(S) motif were found in the NZ7-like VEGF protein. These VEGFs are divided mainly into two types and a significant increase in the number of hydrogen bonds within the NZ7-like VEGF dimers was observed. The NZ7-like ORFV apparently favors the goat as a host and an emphasis on this in future epidemiological and pathological studies should be considered, focusing on the NZ7-like virus.

Keywords: orf virus, isolation, identification, genetic characterization, VEGF genotype

INTRODUCTION

Orf is an animal pustular dermatitis and an epitheliotrophic contagious disease directly caused by the orf virus (ORFV) with a worldwide distribution (1, 2). This viral skin disease commonly affects sheep, goats, and some other ruminants and has a zoonotic potential in humans who are exposed to a contaminated workplace (3–6). Clinically, orf disease progresses from erythema to macule, papule, and vesicle formation and then from pustules to thick scabs. Severely affected animals may lose weight and become more susceptible to secondary bacterial infections (7). Prolonged infection and increased severity are associated with often severe secondary bacterial infection. More usually, minor staphylococcal infection is a frequent occurrence, but mortality rates can be over 5% in infected herds (8). Higher mortality occurs frequently in lambs or kids during the lactation period due to dehydration and starvation, as the pain and distortion of the lips and mouth reduces sucking (8, 9). Because orf has serious economic and environmental impacts in most sheep-feeding countries in the world, it is important to characterize the pathogen of any outbreak in breeding livestock. It is also especially important to determine regional ORFV strains, to predict the risk of outbreak in affected developing countries such as India and China, to improve prevention and control management.

ORFV is a prototype member of genus *Parapoxvirus* (PPV) with a G+C content about 64 percent in the genome (10). The virus has a linear double-stranded closed DNA of nearly 150 kbp in genome length containing 130 to 132 putative genes, with 88 genes conserved in PPVs (1, 10). These genes are responsible for viral replication and the composition of the fixed asset in the center of the genome, while two highly variable regions are located in the closed terminal ends of the viral genome, which encode proteins required for viral invasion (11) or immune evasion (12).

At present there are abundant ORFV isolate sequences published in GenBank, with some full length genome data available, with six of them extensively researched previously such as ORFV-NZ2 (10, 13), ORFV-NZ7 (14, 15), ORFV-SA00, and ORFV-IA82 (16), ORFV-D$_{1701}$ (11), a human biopsy-derived virus ORFV-B029 (partial genome) (17) and eight new ORFV strains from China including ORFV-NA1/11 (18); ORFV-GO, -NP, -YX, and -SJ1 (19); NA17 (*Accession number:MG674916*) (20), Shanxi (*Accession number:AEN14425*) and Fujian-XP (*Accession number:AIZ05258*). These strains may provide many references for evaluating an emerging pathogen from any orf epidemic.

For more accurate diagnosis of orf in the lab, both conventional PCR and real-time PCR methods are used for higher specificity and sensitivity in the detection of viral ORFV pathogens. These techniques have been developed based on the major membrane glycoprotein gene *B2L* (ORFV011) (6, 21, 22) or on the DNA polymerase gene (23). Generally, *B2L* with conserved quality in different PPV species is used as a common and precise marker for examining a virus with its genetic stability, such as ORFV, bovine popular stomatitis virus (BPSV), pseudocowpox virus (PCPV) and parapoxvirus of red deer in New Zealand (PVNZ) (21). Parapox virus can therefore be confirmed by the *B2L* gene on a molecular level in the laboratory, because GenBank can provide abundant *B2L* reference information for researchers (24). Though the *B2L* gene is adopted for the genetic phylogenetic investigation of ORFV (25–28), *B2L* gene data alone is not sufficient to confirm a viral species.

The secondary gene of interest for pathogen investigation is the *F1L* gene (ORFV059) that encodes an envelope protein to exploit a subtle interaction between virus and host, then initiates viral invasion by binding to heparan-sulfate sensors outside the host cells (29). *The* F1L protein, as the main immunogenic protein of ORFV, is transcribed in the mid-late stage of the viral infection period and can bind to glycosaminoglycan (GAG) on the mammalian cell (30). Several functional regional and amino acid motifs are also found in F1L proteins, including a proline-rich region (PRR) and KGD motif, unique motifs in ORFV, and some conservative motifs such as GAG, D/ExD, and Cx3C among

the *Poxviridae* family, which are apparent in sequence alignment of ORFVs (31).

The ORFV132 gene has been of interest because it encodes a vascular endothelial growth factor (VEGF) of ORFV which has a direct responsibility for the extensive vascular hyperplastic lesions (32). As a result, the ORFV132 gene is expressed early during infection of ORFV (15); but it has not been found in other poxviruses. The *VEGF* gene therefore plays a unique role in virulence analysis, although it is not the only virulence factor that has been identified. The *VEGF* genes among PPVs show numerous variants which can share only 41 to 61% amino acid sequence identity (16). For ORFVs, two genotype groups were classed by the NZ2- and NZ7-VEGF like genes which show little DNA homology to each other, whereas the flanking sequences are over 98% homologous (15). The reported sequence variations might reflect the genetic drift of the *VEGF* gene although the rate of drift seems greater than generally seen in poxvirus genes (33). More recently, Karki et al., reported that the majority of Indian ORFV isolates showed 78.4 to 99.3% amino acid identity with each other in the VEGF gene, even like the NZ7-like VEGF (34). Given that different ORFV isolates from the world show these two genotypes in VEGF, this study places the emphasis on the regional distribution of VEGF genotype, to explain its genetic characteristics and clinical features related to the environment and species.

This paper reports on a new ORFV isolate from the northeast of China. Genetic studies of three genes mentioned above and the VEGF molecular structure observation with high resolution have been performed following the virological identification.

MATERIALS AND METHODS
Clinical Case and Virus Isolation

During an outbreak in the autumn of 2017, a local farmer reported that five young Boer goats were found to be affected by a contagious skin disease with obvious lesions in the oral cavity or lips, but lesion material had only been collected from a 6-month-old kid, that died in an isolation area.

In this flock of over 200 Boer goats, there were no other domestic mammals. The sheep pen was simple, with only guardrails and a roof and sanitary conditions were poor. It was speculated that the outbreak may have been related to stock bought in from other provinces in China several months ago. According to the farmer, none of the animals in this flock had been given orf vaccine before this outbreak but they had been treated with externally applied agents such as gentian violet. The majority of affected animals had recovered spontaneously except the single death.

For virus isolation, Madin-Darby bovine kidney (MDBK) and human keratinocyte cell line (HaCaT) cells (both of these cells are cryopreserved in liquid nitrogen in our laboratory) were cultured separately in DMEM containing 10% fetal bovine serum (FBS), 100 U/mL penicillin and 100 μg/mL streptomycin at 37°C with 5% CO_2 (35). As per Yu's protocol, a confluent monolayer of MDBK cells were inoculated with some viral supernatant (36). When 70 to 80% cytopathic effect (CPE) was reached, the cells were harvested followed by freezing at

−80°C. The virions were further purified by sucrose gradient ultra-centrifugation. A major virus band was obtained after centrifugation of virus infected MDBK cells in the 32–36% sucrose gradient. Electron microscopy (EM) investigation was completed by negative staining.

EM for Ultrastructural Analyses

The viral samples were assayed immediately as described by Yu et al. (36). Lead citrate was used to make the contrast background, to distinguish ORFV virion with outline geometrical characters and some surface structures.

Immunofluorescence Microscopy

Cells were fixed with 4% paraformaldehyde for 20 min, then incubated in PBS containing 0.2% Triton-X100 for permeabilizing. After three washes in PBS, the cells were incubated with 1% bovine serum albumin (BSA) solution for 30 min. The fixed cells were incubated with 2E4 monoclonal antibody (mAb) (anti-B2L) (hybridoma cells of 2E4 mAb are cryopreserved in liquid nitrogen in our laboratory) for 1 h at 37°C. After three washes with PBS, secondary antibodies were introduced to bind 2E4 mAb at a 1:500 dilution in PBS for 30 min. Anti-mouse Ig conjugated with fluorescein isothiocyanate (FITC) (Sigma-Aldrich) was used as the secondary antibody and images were taken using a Leica fluorescence microscope.

DNA Clone, Sequencing, and Phylogenetic Analysis

Viral DNA was prepared based on commercial kits protocols for polymerase chain reaction (PCR) amplification. Primers used in this study involving in B2L, F1L, and VEGF genes, were designed referencing the ORFV-NZ2 strain (*Accession number: DQ184476*). In addition, the alternative primers of VEGF gene were designed according to the ORFV-NZ7 strain (*Accession number: S67522*) (**Table 1**). After DNA amplification and purification, the target genes were each inserted into PMD18T vectors and the recombinant plasmids of positive clone were sent to Sangon Biological Engineering Technology and Services Co. Ltd. (China), for sequencing. For genetic relationship analysis of B2L, F1L, and VEGF genes among some reference strains available on GenBank at the amino acid (aa) level, a series of aa composition comparisons of the isolates were conducted using the DNAStar program (DNAStar, Inc. USA). All different source sequences in the world were included in **Table 2** and molecular phylogeny and the genetic relationship of this ORFV strain with others were calculated as referenced by Yu et al. (36).

Homologous Modeling Analyzes on the Present VEGFs

Prediction of the three dimensional structure of the VEGF-variants of ORFVs was modeled using SWISS-MODEL online program (*http://swissmodel.expasy.org*). The structure of the VEGF-variants, including protein subunits A and B, chain A and chain B, were viewed and aligned using the *UCSF Chimera version 1.1.* where the function of Iterative Magic Fit was used for energy minimization and the alignments were manually

optimized. Ramachandran plots for the viral VEGF models were compared to determine if the viral models contained residues that did not conform to acceptable ϕ and/or ψ angles (33).

RESULTS
A Case of Orf

For descriptive epidemiology of this outbreak in Daqing city of Heilongjiang province of China (**Figure 1A**), this case was briefly reported in the materials and methods. Affected animals had visible scars from clinical lesions of contagious ecthyma in their lips and angulus oris. The subject kid had developed severe anabrosic lesions in its mouth region, prior to death (**Figure 1B**). Clinical material such as scabs were gathered from the dead Boer kid for laboratory virus isolation.

ORFV Isolation and Identification

In the laboratory, a sterile suspension was prepared using the clinical material to inoculate MDBK and HaCaT cell monolayers, until the CPE was observed on day 3 or 4. The CPE of infected cells was obvious by their appearance and in contrast, there was no pathological change in the mock infected cells (**Figure 1C**).

The PPV virion with an ovoid shape and spiral crisscross pattern was easily identified by morphological features using EM (**Figure 1D**). Virus particles in ultrathin sections were observed in the cytoplasm of infected cells at 72 h post inoculation (pi) (**Figure 1D**).

Immunofluorescence was used to determine the causative agent responsible for CPE, with the virus recognized by 2E4 mAb during cell infection. The images were taken using a Leica fluorescence microscope (**Figure 1E**).

The target genes in viral DNA samples were detected successfully by PCR. Although all of the target bands appeared, before that there was an interlude during this period. Initially, 3 pairs of synthetic oligonucleotide primers namely B2L-F/R, F1L-F/R, and VEGF-F/R designed according to the NZ2 strain were used for PCRs. Both B2L and F1L were successful but absence of VEGF band was shown. It is not surprising that application of PCR primers (VEGF-F'/R') designed according to the NZ7 strain allows us to detect the VEGF gene. Together, these three bands were corresponding to our expectation with the full-length genes as 1,137, 1,029, and 447 bp, respectively, in a 1.0% agarose gel electrophoresis (**Figure 1F**). The PCR products were purified and cloned for direct sequencing, and sequence analysis confirmed this ORFV isolate, which was named OV-HLJ05.

Genetic Characterization of OV-HLJ05

The three genes *B2L*, *F1L*, and *VEGF* were sequenced to analyze the genetic characterization of OV-HLJ05. Using the Jotun Hein Method in MegAlign program (DNAStar, Inc. USA), a rough outline of the genetic factors of the virus was confirmed.

For the *B2L* gene, a total of twenty-four aa sequences from different sources in the world, including the NZ2 strain (*Accession number: AAA50479, ABA00527*); OV-IA82 (*AAR98106*); OV-SA00(*AAR98236*); OV-D1701 (*ADY76795*); OV-B029 (*AHH34200*); OV-HLJ04 (*KU523790*); and OV-HLJ05 (*MK317955*), were used for alignment in this study. These B2Ls

TABLE 1 | PCR primers designed referencing to the popular strains of ORFV.

Name	Nucleotide	Endonuclease	Reference
B2L-F	CG*GGATCC*ATGTGGCCGTTCTCCTCCATC	*BamH* I	OV-NZ2(*DQ184476*)
B2L-R	CCC*AAGCTT*TTAATTTATTGGCTTGCAGAACTC	*Hind* III	OV-NZ2(*DQ184476*)
F1L-F	CG*GAATCC*ATGGATCCAC CCGAAATCACG	*EcoR* I	OV-NZ2(*DQ184476*)
F1L-R	CCC*AAGCTT*CACACGATGGCCGTGACC	*Hind* III	OV-NZ2(*DQ184476*)
VEGF-F	CGC*GGATCC*ATGAAGTTGCTCGTCGGCATA	*BamH* I	OV-NZ2(*DQ184476*)
VEGF-R	CCC*AAGCTT*CTAGCGGCGTCTTCTGGGCG	*Hind* III	OV-NZ2(*DQ184476*)
VEGF-F'	GC*GGATCC*ATGAAGTTAACAGCTACCATA	*BamH* I	OV-NZ7(*S67522*)
VEGF-R'	CCC*AAGCTT*TCGTCTAGGTTCCCTAGT	*Hind* III	OV-NZ7(*S67522*)

TABLE 2 | Part of VEGF genes published in GenBank recent years were used in this study.

No.	Name of strain or isolate	Country	Host	Collection date	GenBank Accession No.	Target gene
1	OV-SA00▲	USA	Goat	2004	AY386264	VEGF
2	OV-NZ2▲	New Zealand	Sheep	2006	DQ184476	VEGF
3	OV-NZ7▲	New Zealand	Sheep	2016	S67522	VEGF
4	ORFV Mukteswar/09	India	Sheep	2010	GU139358	VEGF
5	Cam/09	India	Camel	2010	GU460373	VEGF
6	ORFV/Mukteswar/59/05/Goat/P51	India	Goat	2018	MF414681	VEGF
7	ORFV/Mukteswar/59/05/Goat/P6	India	Goat	2018	MF414682	VEGF
8	ORFV/Meghalaya/SP45/Goat/2003	India	Goat	2018	MF414683	VEGF
9	ORFV/Shahjahanpur/82/Goat/2004	India	Goat	2018	MF414684	VEGF
10	ORFV/Jalandhar/SP41/Goat/2007	India	Goat	2018	MF414685	VEGF
11	ORFV/Bangalore/89/05/Goat	India	Goat	2018	MF414686	VEGF
12	ORFV/Hyderabad/25/Sheep/2006	India	Sheep	2018	MF414687	VEGF
13	ORFV/Gujarat/SP26/Goat/2006	India	Goat	2018	MF414688	VEGF
14	ORFV/Assam/LK/Goat/2014	India	Goat	2018	MF414689	VEGF
15	ORFV/Bhopal/Goat	India	Goat	2018	MF414690	VEGF
16	NP	China	Goat	2015	KP010355	VEGF
17	NA17	China	Goat	2015	MG674916	VEGF
18	Shanxi	China	Ovis aries	2016	AEN14425	VEGF
19	Fujian-XP	China	Goat	2016	AIZ05258	VEGF
20	NA1/11	China	Sheep	2014	JQ663432	VEGF
21	Xinjiang1	China	Goat	2013	KF666562	VEGF
22	SY17	China	Sheep	2018	MG712417	VEGF
23	OV-HN3/12	China	Sheep	2018	KY053526	VEGF
24	Shihezi2/SHZ2	China	Goat	2013	KF726849	VEGF
25	Shihezi3/SHZ3	China	Goat	2013	KF726850	VEGF
26	DG	China	Goat	2016	KM675376	VEGF
27	YX	China	Goat	2016	KM675382	VEGF
28	XD	China	Goat	2016	KM675377	VEGF
29	FQ	China	Goat	2016	KM675383	VEGF
30	GT	China	Goat	2016	KM675384	VEGF
31	SL	China	Goat	2016	KM675385	VEGF
32	DS	China	Goat	2016	KM675386	VEGF
33	GS	China	Goat	2016	KM675387	VEGF
34	SJ2	China	Goat	2016	KM675388	VEGF
35	GO	China	Goat	2016	KM675380	VEGF
36	SJ1	China	Goat	2016	KM675381	VEGF
37	OV-HLJ05★	China	Goat	2019	MK317956	VEGF

Black pentastar means the orf virus isolate in this paper; Black triangle means the important reference strain.

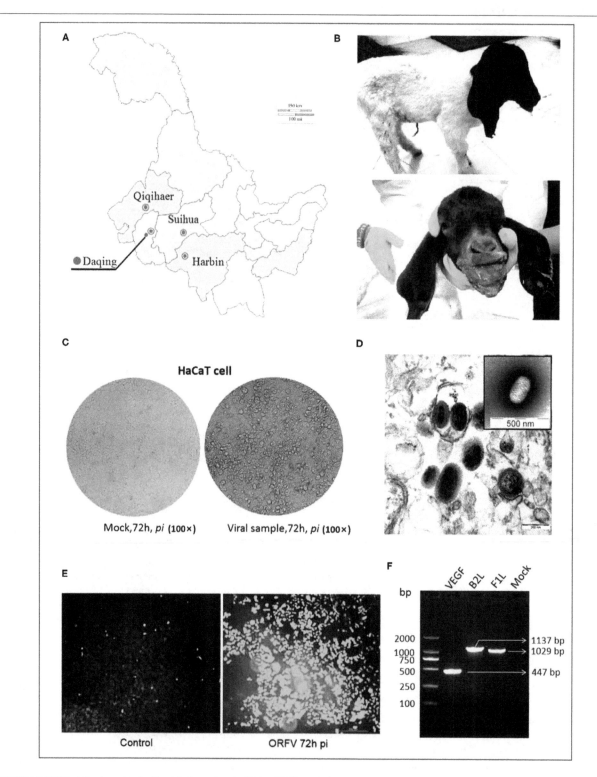

FIGURE 1 | ORFV isolation from an orf outbreak in the northeast of China. **(A)** Picture indicates the geographical location of the outbreak in China, Sep 2017. **(B)** Typical clinical lesions of orf in a Boer goat kid. The severe tumid lesions in his mouth region showed more pejorative anabrosis nidus. **(C)** Cytopathic effect on HaCaT cells infected by ORFV sample. Mock-infected HaCaT cells appeared an ordered fashion after 72 h, while HaCaT cells infected with the supernatants became ragged, appearing rounded and pyknotic, with retraction of the cell membranes from surrounding cells at 72 h *pi* (×200). **(D)** The virions in MDBK cell revealed the typical ovoid shape when observed by electron microscopy. **(E)** The result of the immunofluorescence assay. Anti-B2L monoclonal antibody (mAb) (2E4, 1:200) was used as the primary antibody. **(F)** Amplification of *B2L* gene, *F1L* gene, and *VEGF* gene. Lane 1:DL2000 DNA Marker (bp); Lane 2: *VEGF* gene (447 bp); Lane 3: *B2L* gene (1137 bp); Lane 4: *F1L* gene (1029 bp); Lane 5: Mock.

were employed from the GenBank datasets for aa sequence multiple comparison and revealed that all B2Ls were like each other, sharing 93.1 to 98.4% amino acid identity (**Figure 2A**). It is worth noting that OV-HLJ05 shared 98.4% aa identity with the SA00 strain (*AY386264*) in B2L protein and 97.4% identity with NZ2, so it should be closely related to the SA00 strain genetically.

On comparison of F1L homologs in ORFVs, a total of 18 aa sequences, including NZ2 (*Accession number: ABA00576*), IA82 (*AAR98154*), SA00 (*AAR98284*), B029 (*AHH34248*), Chinese OV-HLJ05 (*MK317957*). and OV-HLJ04 (*MK317958*), FJ-MH2015(*KU199840*), SDLC(*AKL79702*), NP (*AKU76812*), SJ1(*AKU76936*), YX (*AKU76548*), GDQY(*AIY55506*), Jilin(*FJ808075*), Nongan (*JQ271535*), NA1-11(*AHZ33756*), GO (*AKU76680*), Hubei (*KJ619840*), and Xinjiang (*KC291656*), were aligned in batches. This study found that the *F1L* gene was highly conserved as well within the ORFV group, except for the proline rich region with a repetitive character in the N-terminal of F1L protein. In addition, several highly conserved motifs mentioned by Scagliarini et al. (37) and Yogisharadhya et al. (31) such as the GAG motif, KGD (Lys-Gly-Asp) motif, KTR motif, D/ExD motif and a Cx3C motif of interest all remained stable in their basic amino acid composition (**Figure 2B**).

Taken together, the *B2L* gene and the *F1L* gene in all isolates from around the world were relatively conservative in viral genomes.

For the *VEGF* gene, it was also found during the multiple alignment that two clustering groups known as the NZ2- and the NZ7-VEGF like isolates between aa sequences were used in this study. The isolates involved in comparison were ORFV-NZ2 (*DQ184476*), SA00 (*AY386264*), NZ7 (*S67522*), IA82 (*AY386263*), D1701 (*AF106020*), B029 (*KF837136*), NA1/11 (*JQ663432*), NA17(*MG674916*), Shanxi (*AEN14425*), Fujian-XP (*AIZ05258*), GO (*KM675380*), NP (*KM576379*), YX (*KM675382*), and SJ1(*KM675381*). Among them, OV-HLJ05 (*MK317956*) was shown to share 100% identity with the NA17, Shanxi and Fujian-XP strains, which all came from the Jilin, Shanxi and Fujian provinces in China, 94.6% identity with the SA00 strain and 89.2% identity with the NZ7 strain (**Figure 3A**). The phylogenetic tree showed that the OV-HLJ05 has a highly homologous relationship to SA00 compared with NZ7 despite coming from the same group (**Figure 3B**). In contrast, the inconsistent amino acid residues in the NZ7 strain occurred about 16 times, compared with eight times in the SA00 strain (data not shown). According to the current alignments, these two groups formed immediately by the program possessed obvious differences in VEGF sequence length between each other. The NZ7-VEGF like group had approximately 150 more residues, but the NZ2-VEGF like group had about 130 residues. Those additional residues in the NZ7-VEGF like individuals were shown as a TATI(L)QVVVAI(L) motif (IR1) and a SSSSS or SSSS motif (IR2) and they occupied two positions front and back in the protein respectively (**Figure 5A**). Insertion of TATI(L)QVVVAI(L) made the first two cysteine positions move back, but the other eight cysteine residue positions have not been impaired by insertion mutation. Residue substitution mutation on the first cysteine residue position, meant that cysteine was replaced by glycine in some NZ2-VEGF like strains including NZ2, D1701, B029,

and IA82 (**Figure 5A**), but no mutation on this position was observed in the NZ7-VEGF like individuals. In the NZ7-VEGF like individuals like OV-HLJ05, the serine level has been raised because of the additional SSSSS or SSSS motif (**Figure 5**).

In aa composition, the 37 VEGFs published in GenBank including NZ2, NZ7, SA00, and 22 isolates from China and 12 isolates from India showed two separate parts in the phylogenetic tree map (**Table 2**). The percentage of the NZ7-like VEGFs have about 79.4% of all sequences derived from China and India, while only 20.6% of sequences have the NZ2-like VEGFs (**Figure 4**).

Structural Modeling Implied Heterogeneity Between the Current VEGFs

The predicted structures of the VEGF-variants of ORFVs were determined by comparison to the solved crystal structure of subunits A and B of 2gnn.1 (orf Virus NZ2 Variant of VEGF-E in SWISS-MODEL). Homologous modeling showed maximum heterogeneity at loop three (**Figure 5C**) and the contact points of chain A and chain B (**Figure 6**) between the VEGFs. There was more heterogeneity between the NZ2-like VEGFs and the NZ7-like VEGFs, but the essential structure was conservative (**Figure 5**). In addition, the residues involved in dimerization of chain A and chain B of VEGF protein monomer were from $ST^{34}NEW^{37}MRTL^{41}DK^{43}S^{44}G^{45}$ of chain B in the OV-HLJ05 strain, compared with $NT^{24}KGW^{27}SEVL^{31}K^{32}G^{33}S^{34}$ in the NZ2 strain. Among these two motifs, the "TxxWxxxL(x)KSG (GS)" motif was a relatively conservative pattern that was probably responsible for dimerization of chain A and chain B and the motifs **WxxxL**. Another two motifs, **TxxR** in NZ2 and **TxxQ** in NZ7, were responsible for binding VEGFR-2 according to Mercer's report, with x representing any amino acid residue. For the dimerization, H-bonds between chain A and chain B, particularly at the binding site, were labeled in different lengths ranging from 2.7 to 3.4 Å (**Figure 6**).

DISCUSSION

Orf epidemics are common in the world particularly in developing countries such as China, India, and South Africa but this disease has been largely ignored, due to relatively low mortality rates, or spontaneous recovery (38). In this study, a small outbreak of orf involving a suburban livestock farm in northeast China was investigated, where the Boer goat kid presented for evaluation died. The ORFV was suspected to be responsible for this outbreak and it was confirmed and identified in our laboratory.

As a primary subject of study, the B2L protein of ORFV is a F13L homolog of Vaccinia virus (VACV). The F13L is purportedly required for the efficient formation of enveloped VACV virions (39) and contains the variant HKD (His-Lys-Asp) motif of phospholipases and phospholipid synthases (40, 41), leading to a report of associated lipase activity (42). The B2L protein owns the same HKD variant as in F13L which has an NKD pattern, where the His in HKD is substituted by the Asn both in F13L and B2L, while the detailed biochemical lipase function of B2L protein remains unclear. The *B2L* gene is used

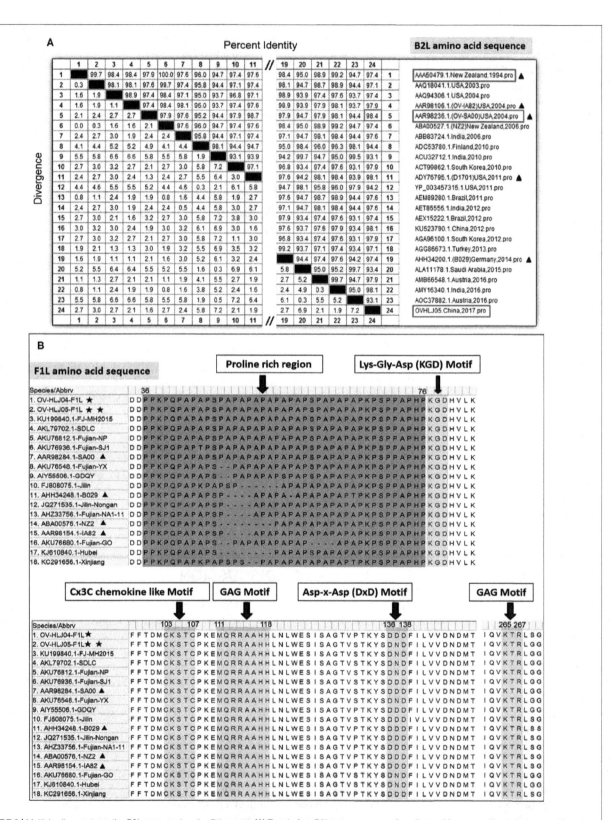

FIGURE 2 | Multiple alignments on the *B2L* genes and on the F1L genes. **(A)** Twenty-four *B2L* gene sequences from the world were used in multiple comparisons and their aa identity was displayed in **(A)**. Black triangles represent five important isolates published previously. Blue boxes represent the isolates which this study investigated. Red boxes represent the maximum among these subjects. **(B)** Fourteen *F1L* gene sequences from China together with NZ2, IA82, SA00, and B029, were used in multiple alignment and the obvious difference was showed at the proline rich regions of N-terminal. Other motifs were essentially conservative (31). One black pentastar indicates the orf virus isolate of previous; Two-black-pentastar indicates the orf virus isolate in this paper.

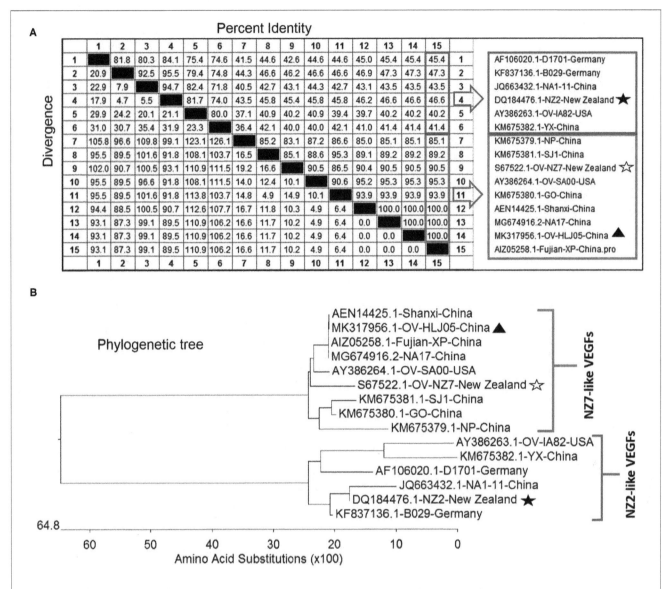

FIGURE 3 | Comparison of different VEGFs with the OV-HLJ05 strain and related sequences published in GenBank. Solid black pentacle denotes the NZ2 strain; hollow black pentacle denotes the NZ7 strain; solid black triangle denotes the OV-HLJ05 strain in this study. **(A)** An alignment of the deduced amino acid sequences of the VEGFs from various sources was generated using MegAlign and Clustal W Method. The aligned sequences are assembled in blue box (low identity to OV-HLJ05) or red box (high identity to OV-HLJ05). **(B)** Predicted evolutionary relationships between the OV-HLJ05 strain and the references in the world mentioned above. They include OV-HLJ05, divided into two groups as the NZ2-like VEGFs (blue half-lattice frame) or the NZ7-like VEGFs (red half-lattice frame).

for phylogenetic analysis of ORFV (25–28) and PCR by *B2L* has been described previously as an available tool to amplify target DNAs within the PPV genus (21). However, merely to investigate molecular characterization of ORFV isolate, information of the *B2L* gene combined with the *F1L* and *VEGF* genes is necessary for understanding of the virus. Comparative analysis resulted in OV-HLJ05 owning an extensive homologous relationship with the SA00 and the NZ7 rather than the NZ2 in these three genes. Unsurprisingly, OV-HLJ05 has some divergence from other candidates in the *B2L* gene product constitution (see **Figure 2A**), but this was not enough to affect their conservative nature due to their over 93% identity.

Another evidence of stability is for the F1L protein. Beside the proline rich regions, during the sequence alignment, the study found the functional motifs, which was mentioned by Yogisharadhya's team (31). The similar quality suggested that the F1L was maintaining its multiple roles with intra- and extra-cellular activity during ORFV infection and the largest heterogeneity between these F1L targets was found to be only located in the proline-rich regions. This event was initiated by the natural deletion or loss of individual proline residues in viral generation, but in fact it hardly impairs F1L's functions (37).

Previously, all VEGFs were shown as only 41 to 61% aa sequence identity among PPVs by Delhon et al. (16). In ORFV,

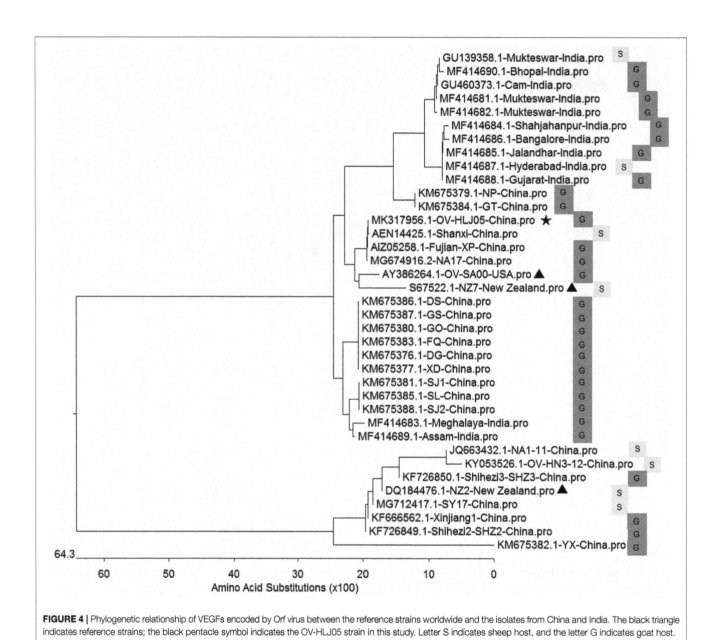

FIGURE 4 | Phylogenetic relationship of VEGFs encoded by Orf virus between the reference strains worldwide and the isolates from China and India. The black triangle indicates reference strains; the black pentacle symbol indicates the OV-HLJ05 strain in this study. Letter S indicates sheep host, and the letter G indicates goat host.

genetic consistency presents a polarized distribution, therefore, two typical genotype groups also known as the NZ2- and the NZ7-like VEGFs were presented by Mercer (33). The VEGFs were used as representatives of the diversity analysis within the ORFVs even though this study did not know the scale and distributed situation of the two groups (14, 15, 33). Genetically, it was possible that the NZ7-like VEGF was acquired by ORFV independently of the NZ2 acquisition event and from a different source. The virus with NZ7 VEGF genotype can be found around the world, particularly in India as described by Karki et al. (34) and in China as shown by the results of this study, so the virus may have been selected by adaptation or from host species from distinct environments. Both these VEGF-like ORFVs can stabilize the inheritance of the genome, with the remaining critical issues studied by epidemiology and pathology.

The data from this study suggested that OV-HLJ05 strain was closer to the SA00 strain at the aa level particularly in the *VEFG* product (**Figures 3A,B**). Except for three Chinese isolates including NA17, Shanxi and Fujian-XP, OV-HLJ05 was found to share 95.3% identity of VEGF with the SA00 strain and to exceed 90.5% identity with the NZ7 (**Figure 3A**). There was increasing evidence that clinical symptoms of the affected kid in this outbreak were similar to reports from Guo et al. (26) with the SA00 strain affecting North American and Texan Boer goat flocks, Hosamani et al. (43), involving the Muk5905 strain in a Mukteswar goat in India, Charles (44) with TZ/BB/13 strain in a Tanzanian goat and Zhang et al. (45) who reported on three strains SDLC, SDTA, and SDJN identified from a Shandong goat in East China, as relevant examples. None of the quoted studies provided any VEGF information.

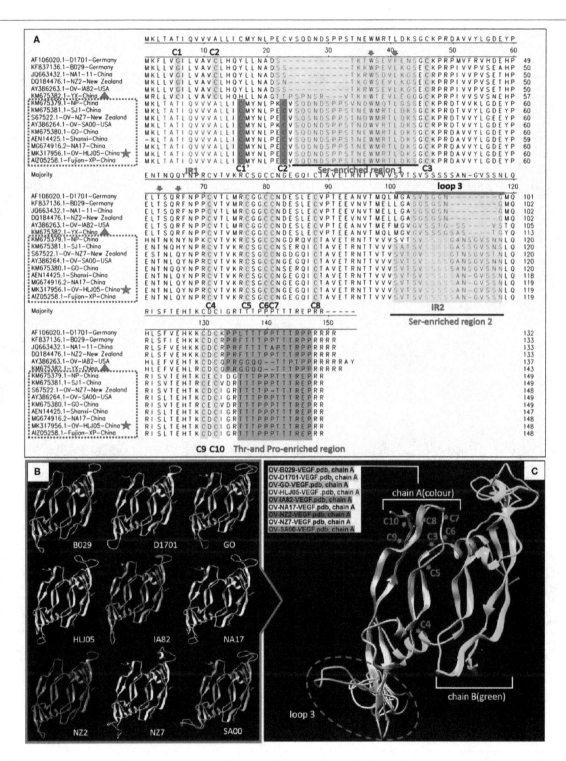

FIGURE 5 | Comparison of amino acid levels between primary and secondary structures of VEGFs. **(A)** Alignment in primary structure of VEGFs. VEGF references of the whole length genome published from GenBank were employed to reflect the structural homology with OV-HLJ05. Important residues matching the consensus of the alignment of the viral VEGFs are shaded in various colors. The two green regions indicate Ser-enriched region I and II; the two yellow regions indicate "insertion mutation" [IRI:TATI(L)QVVVAI(L) motif and IRII:SSSSS or SSSS motif]; the Thr- and Pro-enriched region is shaded in purple (potential O-linked glycosylation sites) (33); two cystine knot motifs C1' and C2' are shaded in red whereas the other constitutionally stable ones (C1 to C10) are shaded in blue color. These include the eight cysteines of the cystine-knot motif (15, 33). Loop3 is indicated by a red line. The red arrows indicate binding site of VEGFR-2 (33); dotted blue frames represent the NZ7-VEGF like members, red pentacles represent OV-HLJ05 and red triangles represent YX from China. **(B)** Ribbon representations of the predicted structures of dimer of selected members of the VEGF family are shown, respectively. **(C)** Superimposed structures by members from **(B)**. On the **(A)** chain, cystine residues (C3 to C10) are labeled by red letters, and the loop3-regions in **(A)** are shown by an oval dotted red frame.

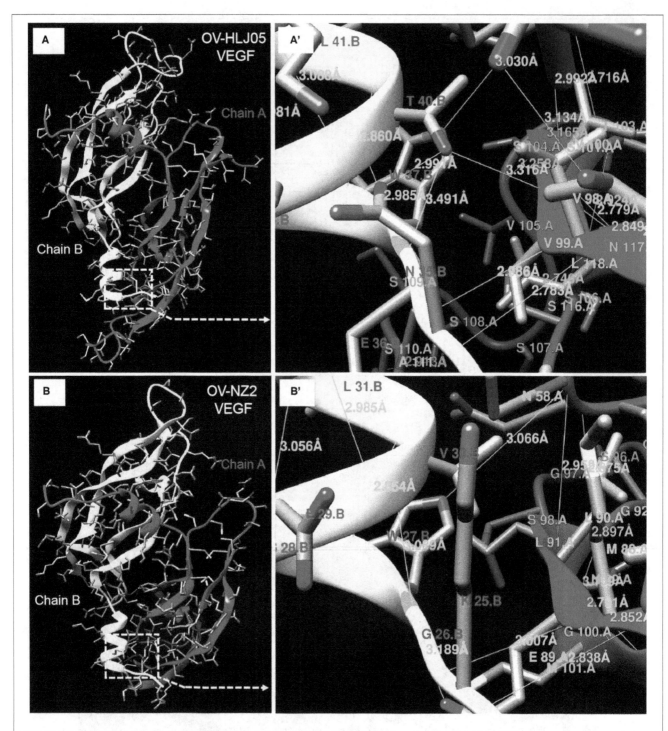

FIGURE 6 | Deeper insight on dimer structures of OV-NZ2 VEGF and OV-HLJ05 VEGF. **(A)** The dimer structure of OV-HLJ05 VEGF is composed of chain A (red) and chain B (yellow). **(A')** showed the enlarged outline of the contact sites of chain A and chain B with more hydrogen bonds. **(B)** The dimer structure of NZ2 VEGF is composed of chain A (also in red) and chain B (also in yellow). **(B')** showed the enlarged outline of the contact sites of chain A and chain B with several hydrogen bonds. The contact parts from **(A',B')** were intuitively compared for finding the inner differences of OV-HLJ05 VEGF and NZ2 VEGF, resulting in distinction on amino acid residue configuration with various hydrogen bond distance in the contact regions.

For investigating the essential divergence between the NZ7-VEGFs and the NZ2-VEGFs, the full length of VEGF primary structures were elaborately arranged in a pool, of course, the region rich in threonine (T) and proline (P) (15) is retained in the C-terminal of all the 33 VEGFs (**Figure 5**). Despite showing little DNA homology to each other, such as insertion of a TATI(L)QVVVAI(L) motif and a SSSS(S) motif; besides deficiency or substitution, whereas the flanking sequences are over 98% homologous. Depending on the huge homologous nature, the PPVs may be favorably characterized and distinguished with the VEGF-like gene (15). Theoretically, despite the surprising extent of sequence variation among the viral VEGFs, key motifs of structural and functional importance were conserved (33). As both NZ2- and NZ7-like VEGFs have been shown to bind and activate VEGFR-2 functionally, then in the short term their clinical manifestations are nearly indistinguishable (46–49) and structural modeling more objectively reflected heterogeneity between the current VEGFs. The dimerization, contribution of residues for chain B binding to chain A was measured and the TxxWxxxL(x)KSG (or GS) motif was shared by these two VEGFs. The significant difference found was the number of hydrogen bonds (**Figure 6**), which implied *in vivo* that their biological activities are not exactly consistent.

An additional discovery during alignment using OV-HLJ05 with the fourteen representative ORFV strains, such as NZ2, NZ7, SA00, IA82, D1701, and B029 and another eight strains from China namely NA1-11, GO, NP, SJ1, YX, NA17, Shanxi and Fujian-XP, showed that the YX strain seemed to be a mid-transition type virus variant between the NZ2 and the NZ7 in VEGF, but currently it still belongs to the NZ2 camp due to the C1 and C2 locations at the N-terminal of protein. This finding is based on observation on the two Ser-enriched regions in VEGF sequences (**Figure 5**).

Genetic evidence on the *VEGF* genes has already been used to explain the ORFV scenario. An extreme example of application for the *VEGF* gene was to generate a recombinant ORFV known as D1701, a *VEGF* deletion mutant, by which the influence of ORFV genes in attenuation and virulence were successfully evaluated (50). Available sequence heterogeneity in the *VEGF* gene is likely to be ubiquitous or show individual features of each ORFV isolate from various geographic areas. This variant OV-HLJ05 genetically appears to be consistent to the Shanxi isolate, Jilin-NA17 isolate and Fujian-XP isolate with 100% identity. This condition suggested that the NZ7-VEGF like strain has spread throughout the mainland of China in recent years mainly due to transportation spread and a similar scenario is also presenting in India (34) (**Figure 5**). Accordingly, most isolates from these two countries have highly homologous VEGF profiles to the NZ7 strain, which seems to favor goats as hosts rather than sheep (**Figure 4**). This issue needs to be clarified worldwide by extensive epidemiological and statistical investigation.

The animal inoculation experiment showed that GO (NZ7 member) had the strongest virulence, second was YX, but NP and SJ1 showed low virulence (19). The outcome of an experiment sometimes was not consistent with the clinical feature. Previously, ORFV isolated from a goat severely affected by orf had not led to similar severe symptoms in susceptible kids (51). Consideration of the virulence determinants of a virus should not neglect the impacts of the host health status, age, and lifestyle. The impact of endogenous and exogenous factors on susceptibility to ORFV for some goats will probably reflect the host's specific susceptibility toward a certain individual strain, but the fact that NZ7-like viruses mostly come from goats suggests that the species factor should not be neglected in the clinical investigation.

In summary, an elaborated investigation can be used to diagnose the genetic characterization, molecular epidemiology and likely emerging pathogenicity of any new ORFV variant in the field and it is vital that developing countries control such any orf endemic initiated by either of these two genotypes.

AUTHOR CONTRIBUTIONS

YY, ZL, and YC conceived and designed the experiments. XD, YL, JM, and BS performed the experiments. YY, XD, and YC analyzed the data. YY and XD wrote the manuscript and prepared the Figures. YY, XD, and YC checked and finalized the manuscript. YY and ZL provided resources. All authors read and approved the final manuscript.

REFERENCES

1. de la Concha-Bermejillo, A. Poxviral diseases. In: Farris R, Mahlow J, Newman E, Nix B, editors. *Health Hazards in Veterinary Practice*, 3rd ed. Schaumburg, IL: American Veterinary Medical Association (1995). p. 55–6.

2. Nadeem M, Curran P, Cooke R, Ryan CA, Connolly K. Orf: contagious pustular dermatitis. *Ir Med J.* (2010) 103:152–3.

3. Al-Salam S, Nowotny N, Sohail MR, Kolodziejek J, Berger TG. Ecthyma contagiosum (orf)-report of a human case from the United Arab Emirates and review of the literature. *J Cutan Pathol.* (2008) 35:603–7. doi: 10.1111/j.1600-0560.2007.00857.x

4. Cargnelutti JF, Masuda EK, Martins M, Diel DG, Rock DL, Weiblen R, et al. Virological and clinico-pathological feathers of orf virus infection in experimentally infected rabbits and mice. *Microb Pathog.* (2011) 50:56–62. doi: 10.1016/j.micpath.201 0.08.004

5. Bodilsen J, Leth S. Orf parapoxvirus can infect humans after relevant exposure. *Ugeskr Laeg.* (2013) 175:1121–2.

6. Caravaglio JV, Khachemoune A. Orf virus infection in humans: a review with a focus on advances in diagnosis and treatment. *J Drugs Dermatol.* (2017) 16:684–9.

7. Gelaye E, Achenbach JE, Jenberie S, Ayelet G, Belay A, Yami M, et al. Molecular characterization of orf virus from sheep and goats in Ethiopia, 2008-2013. *Virol J.* (2016) 13:34. doi: 10.1186/s12985-016-0489-3

8. Lewis C. Update on orf. *Farm Anim Pract.* (1996) 18:376–438. doi: 10.1136/inpract.18.8.376

9. Gokce HI, Genc O, Gokce G. Sero-prevalence of contagious ecthyma in lamb and humans in Kars, Turkey. *Turk J Vet Anim Sci.* (2005) 29:95–101.

10. Mercer AA, Ueda N, Friederichs SM, Hofmann Kay, Frasera KM, BatemanT, et al. Comparative analysis of genome sequences of three isolates of Orf virus reveals unexpected sequence variation. *Virus Res.* (2006) 116:146–58. doi: 10.1016/j.virusres.2005.09.011

11. McGuire MJ, Johnston SA, Sykes KF. Novel immune-modulator identified by a rapid, functional screen of the parapoxvirus ovis (Orf virus) genome. *Proteome Sci.* (2012) 10:4. doi: 10.1186/1477-5956-10-4

12. Hosamani M, Scagliarini A, Bhanuprakash V, McInnes CJ, Singh RK. Orf: an update on current research and future perspectives. *Exp Rev Anti Infect Ther.* (2009) 7:879–93. doi: 10.1586/eri.09.64

13. Robinson AJ, Ellis G, Balassu TC. The genome of orf virus: restriction endonuclease analysis of viral DNA isolated from lesions of orf in sheep. *Arch Virol.* (1982) 71:43–55. doi: 10.1007/BF01315174

14. Robinson AJ, Barns G, Fraser K, Carpenter E, Mercer AA. Conservation and variation in orf virus genomes. *Virology*. (1987) 157:13–23. doi: 10.1016/0042-6822(87)90308-4

15. Lyttle DJ, Fraser KM, Fleming SB, Merce AA, Robinson AJ. Homologs of vascular endothelial growth factor are encoded by the poxvirus orf virus. *J Virol*. (1994) 68:84–92. doi: 10.1128/JVI.68.1.84-92.1994

16. Delhon G, Tulman ER, Afonso CL, de la Concha-Bermejillo A, Lehmkuhl HD, Piccone ME, et al. Genomes of the parapoxviruses Orf virus and bovine papular stomatitis virus. *J Virol*. (2004) 78:168–77. doi: 10.1128/JVI.78.1.168-177.2004

17. Friederichs S, Krebs S, Blum H, Wolf E, Lang H, Buttlar H, et al. Comparative and retrospective molecular analysis of Parapoxvirus (PPV) isolates. *Virus Res*. (2014) 181:11–21. doi: 10.1016/j.virusres.2013.12.015

18. Li W, Hao W, Peng Y, Duan C, Tong C, Song D, et al. Comparative genomic sequence analysis of Chinese orf virus strain NA1/11 with other parapoxviruses. *Arch Virol Jan*. (2015) 160:253–66. doi: 10.1007/s00705-014-2274-1

19. Chi XL, Zeng XC, Li W, Hao WB, Li M, Huang XH, et al. Genome analysis of orf virus isolates from goats in the Fujian Province of southern China. *Front Microbiol*. (2015) 6:1135. doi: 10.3389/fmicb.2015.01135

20. Zhong J, Guan J, Zhou Y, Cui S, Wang Z, Zhou S. Genomic characterization of two orf virus isolates from Jilin province in China. *Virus Genes*. (2019) 55:490–501. doi: 10.1007/s11262-019-01666-y

21. Inoshima Y, Morooka A, Sentsui H. Detection and diagnosis of parapoxvirus by the polymerase chain reaction. *J Virol Methods*. (2000) 84:201–8. doi: 10.1016/S0166-0934(99)00144-5

22. Kottaridi C, Nomikou K, Lelli R, Markoulatos P, Mangana O. Laboratory diagnosis of contagious ecthyma: comparison of different PCR protocols with virus isolation in cell culture. *J Virol Methods*. (2006) 134:119–24. doi: 10.1016/j.jviromet.2005.12.005

23. Bora DP, Venkatesan G, Bhanuprakash V, Balamurugan V, Prabhu M, Siva Sankar MS, et al. Taq man real-time PCR assay based on DNA polymerase gene for rapid detection of orf infection. *J Virol Methods*. (2011) 78:249–52. doi: 10.1016/j.jviromet.2011.09.005

24. Karakas A, Oguzoglu TC, Coskun O, Artuk C, Mert G, Gul HC, et al. First molecular characterization of a Turkish orf virus strain from a human based on a partial B2L sequence. *Arch Virol*. (2013) 58:1105–8. doi: 10.1007/s00705-012-1575-5

25. Guo J, Zhang Z, Edwards JF, Ermel RW, Taylor C Jr., de la Concha-Bermejillo A. Characterization of a North American orf virus isolated from a goat with persistent, proliferative dermatitis. *Virus Res*. (2003) 93:169–79. doi: 10.1016/S0168-1702(03)00095-9

26. Guo J, Rasmussen J, Wünschmann A, de la Concha-Bermejillo A. Genetic characterization of orf viruses isolated from various ruminant species of a zoo. *Vet Microbiol*. (2004) l99:81–92. doi: 10.1016/j.vetmic.2003.11.010

27. Hosamani M, Bhanuprakash V, Scagliarini A, Singh RK. Comparative sequence analysis of major envelope protein gene (B2L) of Indian orf viruses isolated from sheep and goats. *Vet Microbiol*. (2006) 116:317–24. doi: 10.1016/j.vetmic.2006.04.028

28. Chan KW, Lin JW, Lee SH, Liao CJ, Tsai MC, Hsu WL, et al. Identification and phylogenetic analysis of orf virus from goats in Taiwan. *Virus Genes*. (2007) 35:705–12. doi: 10.1007/s11262-007-0144-6

29. Scagliarini A, Gallina L, Dal Pozzo F, Battilani M, Ciulli S, Prosperi S. Heparin binding activity of orf virus F1L protein. *Virus Res*. (2004) 105:107–12. doi: 10.1016/j.virusres.2004.04.018

30. Lin C, Chung C, Heine HG, Chang W. Vaccinia virus envelope H3L proteins binds to cell heparan sulfate and is important for intracellular mature virion morphogenesis and virus infection in vitro and in vivo. *J Virol*. (2000) 74:3353–65. doi: 10.1128/JVI.74.7.3353-3365.2000

31. Yogisharadhya R, Bhanuprakash V, Kumar A, Mondal M, Shivachandra SB. Comparative sequence and structural analysis of Indian orf viruses based on major envelope immuno-dominant protein (F1L), an homologue of pox viral p35/H3 protein. *Gene*. (2018) 15:663. doi: 10.1016/j.gene.2018.04.026

32. Fleming SB, Wise LM, Mercer AA. Molecular genetic analysis of orf virus: a poxvirus that has adapted to skin. *Viruses*. (2015) 7:1505–39. doi: 10.3390/v7031505

33. Mercer AA, Wise LM, Scagliarini A, McInnes CJ, Büttner M, Rzihaet HJ, et al. Vascular endothelial growth factors encoded by Orf virus show surprising sequence variation but have a conserved, functionally relevant structure. *J Gen Virol*. (2002) 83:2845–55. doi: 10.1099/0022-1317-83-11-2845

34. Karki M, Kumar A, Arya S, Venkatesan G. Circulation of orf viruses containing the NZ7-like vascular endothelial growth factor (VEGF-E) gene type in India. *Virus Res*. (2020) 281:197908. doi: 10.1016/j.virusres.2020.197908

35. Zhao K, Song D, He W, Lu H, Zhang B, Li C, et al. Identification and phylogenetic analysis of an orf virus isolated from an outbreak in sheep in the Jilin province of China. *Vet Microbiol*. (2010) 142:408–15. doi: 10.1016/j.vetmic.2009.10.006

36. Yu Y, Tan Q, Zhao W, Zhang X, Ma J, Wu Z, et al. Characterization of an orf virus from an outbreak in Heilongjiang province, China. *Arch Virol*. (2017) 162:3143–9. doi: 10.1007/s00705-017-3426-x

37. Scagliarini A, Ciulli S, Battilani M, Jacoboni I, Montesi F, Casadio R, et al. Characterisation of immunodominant protein encoded by the F1L gene of orf virus strains isolated in Italy. *Arch Virol*. (2002) 147:1989–95. doi: 10.1007/s00705-002-0850-2

38. Scagliarini A, Piovesana S, Turrini F, Savini F, Sithole F, Mccrindle C. Orf in South Africa: endemic but neglected. *Onderstepoort J Vet Res*. (2012) 79:1–8. doi: 10.4102/ojvr.v79i1.499

39. Vliegen I, Yang G, Hruby D, Jordan R, Neyts J. Deletion of the vaccinia virus F13L gene results in a highly attenuated virus that mounts a protective immune response against subsequent vaccinia virus challenge. *Antiviral Res*. (2012) 93:160–6. doi: 10.1016/j.antiviral.2011.11.010

40. Koonin EV. A duplicated catalytic motif in a new superfamily of phosphohydrolases and phospholipid synthases that includes poxvirus envelope proteins. *Trends Biochem Sci*. (1996) 21:242–3. doi: 10.1016/S0968-0004(96)30024-8

41. Ponting CP Kerr ID. A novel family of phospholipase D homologues that includes phospholipid synthases and putative endonucleases: identification of duplicated repeats and potential active site residues. *Protein Sci*. (1996) 5:914–22. doi: 10.1002/pro.5560050513

42. Baek SH, Kwak JY, Lee SH, Lee T, Ryu SH, Uhlinger DJ, et al. Lipase activities of p37, the major envelope protein of vaccinia virus. *J Biol Chem*. (1997) 272:32042–9. doi: 10.1074/jbc.272.51.32042

43. Hosamani M, Yadav S, Kallesh DJ, Mondal B, Bhanuprakash V, Singh K. Isolation and characterization of an Indian orf virus from goats. *Zoonoses Public Health*. (2007) 54:204–8. doi: 10.1111/j.1863-2378.2007.01046.x

44. Charles M. Molecular *Diagnosis and Characterisation of orf Virus in Symptomatic Goats in Coast and Dar es Salaam Regions, Tanzania*. (2015). Available online at: http://hdl.handle.net/123456789/1190

45. Zhang K, XiaoY, Yu M, Liu J, Wang Q, Tao P, et al. Phylogenetic analysis of three orf virus strains isolated from different districts in Shandong Province, East China. *J Vet Med Sci*. (2015) 77:1639–45. doi: 10.1292/jvms.15-0368

46. Meyer M, Clauss M, Lepple-Wienhues A, Waltenberger J, Augustin HG, Ziche M, et al. A novel vascular endothelial growth factor encoded by Orf virus, VEGF-E, mediates angiogenesis via signalling through VEGFR-2 (KDR) but not VEGFR-1 (Flt-1) receptor tyrosine kinases. *EMBO J*. (1999) 18:363–74. doi: 10.1093/emboj/18.2.363

47. Ogawa S, Oku A, Sawano A, Yamaguchi S, Yazaki Y, Shibuya M. A novel type of vascular endothelial growth factor, VEGF-E (NZ-7 VEGF), preferentially utilizes KDR/Flk-1 receptor and carries a potent mitotic activity without heparin-binding domain. *J Biol Chem*. (1998) 273:31273–82. doi: 10.1074/jbc.273.47.31273

48. Wise L, Veikkola T, Mercer A, Savory L, Fleming S, Caesar C, et al. Vascular endothelial growth factor (VEGF)-like protein from orf virus NZ2 bindsto VEGFR-2 and neuropilin-1. *Proc Natl Acad Sci USA*. (1999) 96:3071–6. doi: 10.1073/pnas.96.6.3071

49. Shibuya M. Vascular endothelial growth factor receptor-2: its unique signaling and specific ligand, VEGF-E. *Cancer Sci*. (2003) 94:751–6. doi: 10.1111/j.1349-7006.2003.tb01514.x

50. Rziha HJ, Henkel M, Cottone R, Meyer M, Dehio C, Büttner M. Parapoxviruses: potential alternative vectors for directing the immune response in permissive and non-permissive hosts. *J Biotechnol*. (1999) 73:235–42. doi: 10.1016/S0168-1656(99)00141-8

Serological Cross-Reactivity between *Bovine alphaherpesvirus 2* and *Bovine alphaherpesvirus 1* in a gB-ELISA

Stefano Petrini[1]*, Patricia König[2], Cecilia Righi[1], Carmen Iscaro[1], Ilaria Pierini[1], Cristina Casciari[1], Claudia Pellegrini[1], Paola Gobbi[1], Monica Giammarioli[1] and Gian Mario De Mia[1]

[1] National Reference Laboratory for Infectious Bovine Rhinotracheitis (IBR), Istituto Zooprofilattico Sperimentale Umbria-Marche "Togo Rosati", Perugia, Italy, [2] OIE and National Reference Laboratory for Bovine Herpesvirus Type 1 Infection, Friedrich-Loeffler-Institut, Greifswald, Germany

Correspondence:
Stefano Petrini
s.petrini@izsum.it

In this study, we demonstrated for the first time in Italy, the serological cross-reactivity between *Bovine alphaherpesvirus 2* (BoHV-2) and *Bovine alphaherpesvirus 1* (BoHV-1). Five months after arriving at a performance test station in Central Italy, a 6-month-old calf, which was part of a group of 57 animals, tested positive for BoHV-1 in a commercial gB-ELISA test. It was immediately transferred to the quarantine unit and subjected to clinical observation and serological and virological investigations. During this period, the calf showed no clinical signs. The results from laboratory investigations demonstrated the presence of antibodies via competitive glycoprotein B (gB) ELISAs, indirect BoHV-1 ELISAs, and indirect BoHV-2 ELISAs. Furthermore, the plaque reduction assay provided evidence for the presence of antibodies only for BoHV-2, whereas the virus neutralization test showed negative results for both BoHV-1 and BoHV-5. These findings strongly suggest the occurrence of a serological cross-reactivity between BoHV-2 and BoHV-1. Interference of BoHV-2 antibodies in serological BoHV-1 diagnostics should be considered during routine IBR tests, especially when animals are kept in a performance test station.

Keywords: Calf, BoHV-2, BoHV-1, serological cross-reactivity, performance test station

INTRODUCTION

Bovine alphaherpesvirus 2 (BoHV-2) is a member of the family *Herpesviridae* and belongs to the genus *Simplexvirus* (1). The virus was first isolated from a cattle with skin infection on a farm called Allerton in 1957 in South Africa. The aetiological agent is associated with two different clinical forms, a localized skin disease named bovine mammillitis, bovine herpes mammillitis, or bovine ulcerative mammillitis and a generalized disease called Pseudo-Lumpy Skin Disease (PLSD). BoHV-2 infection has been reported in Africa (South Africa, Kenya, Tanzania, Rwanda-Burundi), Europe, the United States, and Australia (2–5). Recently, the virus was isolated from a clinical case of PLSD in northern Italy (6). However, there are very limited data available on the serological evidence of the virus in Italian cattle farms (7). A serological cross-reactivity has been observed between BoHV-2 and *Bovine alphaherpesvirus 1* (BoHV-1), (5, 8). This phenomenon could lead to severe consequences in BoHV-1 serology, resulting in incorrect diagnosis of BoHV-1, both in areas where there are active control/eradication plans for Infectious Bovine Rhinotracheitis (IBR) and in performance test stations. Moreover, BoHV-2 is similar to BoHV-1 in that it can establish viral latency and be reactivated following an immunosuppressive stimulus, leading to the spread of the virus throughout the herd, causing potential economic losses (9).

In this study, we report, for the first time, the occurrence of serological cross-reactivity between BoHV-2 and BoHV-1 in a calf detained at a performance test station located in Central Italy.

CASE DESCRIPTION

A 6-month-old beef calf (Id. 365/29-04), asymptomatic and seronegative for BoHV-1, was introduced into a performance test station located in Central Italy in October 2018. Following the due protocol for the evaluation of morphological and genetic characteristics, the animal was initially quarantined for 30 days. Two consecutive serum samples were taken 24 days apart. The samples were tested for antibodies against glycoprotein B (gB) of BoHV-1 using a commercial competitive ELISA test (gB-ELISA). They were also tested for neutralizing antibodies against BoHV-1 using virus neutralization (VN) test. The protocol of performance test station does not include investigations against Bovine alphaherpesvirus 2 (BoHV-2). Further, upon testing negative for both the antibodies (gB, VN), the animal was introduced into a group of 56 calves of the same age. These animals were selected from different cattle farms know to be IBR free. Serum and blood samples were taken from all the animals, on a monthly basis, for serological and virological investigations of BoHV-1. The serum samples were tested for the specific antibody via competitive gB-ELISA and VN test. In addition, the EDTA blood samples were used for the detection of BoHV-1 DNA via real-time PCR.

The competitive gB-ELISA test was carried out using the protocol provided by the kit, and the results were expressed according to manufacturer's instructions. VN test and real-time PCR were performed according to the protocols described in the OIE Manual of Diagnostic Tests and Vaccines for Terrestrial Animals (10). All the animals tested negative until February 2019.

In March 2019, the above-mentioned calf (Id. 365/29-04) tested positive in the competitive gB-ELISA test. Although, no clinical IBR symptoms were observed, the animal was immediately placed in quarantine for 30 days. Clinical observations were performed on a daily basis and further serological and virological investigations were carried out. In particular, nasal swabs and EDTA blood samples were collected for virus isolation and real-time PCR, respectively, following the procedures described in the OIE Manual of Diagnostic Tests and Vaccines for Terrestrial Animals (10).

The serum samples were tested for BoHV-1 using different commercial ELISAs: (i) competitive gE-ELISA (A, B, C); (ii) competitive gB-ELISA (D, E), and (iii) indirect-ELISA

(F, G, H, I). Additionally, we also performed plaque reduction assay and VN test against BoHV-1.

In order to assess any serological cross-reactivity with other herpesviruses, the serum samples were tested for antibodies against the following aetiological agents: (i) *Bovine alphaherpesvirus 2* (BoHV-2), (ii) *Bovine gammaherpesvirus 4* (BoHV-4), (iii) *Bubaline alphaherpesvirus 1* (BuHV-1), and (iv) *Bovine alphaherpesvirus 5* (BoHV-5). Different indirect ELISA tests were employed to detect BoHV-2 (L), BoHV-4 (M), and BuHV-1 (N). Further, plaque reduction assay and VN test was performed against BoHV-2 and BoHV-5, respectively. The presence of BoHV-2 genome was surveyed via PCR using blood samples.

The ELISA tests were performed following the protocols provided by the kits and the results were expressed according to manufacturer's instructions. Additionally, for the plaque reduction assay BoHV-1 strain Schönböken and BoHV-2 strain RVB 0064 (Biobank, Friedrich-Loeffler-Institut, Insel Riems, Germany) were adjusted to 25–50 plaque forming units (pfu) per 50 μl. Sera were subjected to one freeze-thaw cycle followed by heat inactivation for 30 min at 56°C. Further, 50 μl of 2-fold serially diluted serum was incubated with the test virus for 24 h at 37°C to enable virus neutralization. The serum-virus suspensions were inoculated onto 1-day old Madin-Darby Bovine Kidney cells (1.25 × 10^5 cells per well). The cells were obtained from the collection of cell lines in veterinary medicine (CCLV, FLI, Insel Riems, Germany), identified by the code MDBK-261. After incubating for 1 h at 37°C, supernatants were removed and replaced with semi-solid overlay medium containing 0.25% methylcellulose (11). Plaque counts were determined 3 days later. Titres were defined as highest dilutions that induced relevant neutralization ($\leq$50% of control values).

The VN test for BoHV-5 was performed on 96-well-tissue culture microtiter plates using the NA67 strain of the virus. Sera were heat-inactivated at 56°C for 30 min. Briefly, 50 μl of each 2-fold serial dilutions were mixed with 50 μl of 100 $TCID_{50}$ of virus in duplicates. The plates were incubated at 37°C and 5% CO_2 for 1 h, and then MDBK cells were seeded at a density of 30,000 cells/well (100 μl). The cells were provided by Biobanking of Veterinary Resources (BVR, Brescia, Italy) and identified by the code BS CL 63. Readings were taken after 72 h, when the cytopathic effect was complete in virus positive control cultures. The titer of each serum was expressed as the highest dilution neutralizing the virus. The BoHV-2 genome was detected using a protocol described by De Giuli et al. (12).

RESULTS

No clinical signs were observed in the calves during the quarantine period. The serological results are shown in **Table 1**. The calf (Id. 365/29-04), tested seropositive in 1 out of 2 competitive gB-ELISAs and in 2 out of 4 indirect-ELISAs. BoHV-2 antibodies were also detected via indirect ELISA. However, no seropositivity was observed in competitive gE-ELISA and indirect BoHV-4 and BuHV-1 ELISAs. Additionally, the plaque reduction assay provided

TABLE 1 | Antibody response obtained from different ELISA tests against BoHV-1, BoHV-2, BoHV-4, and BuHV-1 in the serum sample obtained from a performance station in Central Italy.

ELISA											
BoHV-1									BoHV-2	BoHV-4	BuHV-1
Competitive gE-ELISA			Competitive gB-ELISA		Indirect-ELISA				Indirect-ELISA	Indirect-ELISA	Indirect-ELISA
A	B	C	D	E	F	G	H	I	L	M	N
−	−	−	+	−	+	+	−	−	+	−	−

evidence for a positive result only for BoHV-2, with a mean antibody titer of 1:384, while the VN assay showed no evidence for BoHV-1 and BoHV-5. The virological investigations were consistently negative.

DISCUSSION

In this study, we reported a case of serological cross-reactivity between BoHV-2 and BoHV-1 in a calf detained in a performance test station in Central Italy. BoHV-2 infections have also been described in Africa, Europe, the United States, and Australia (2–4). Several European countries have reported unexplained cases of gB-positive singleton reactors and they were found to be gE-negative (5, 8, 13, 14).

In this report, we have shown that 1 out of 2 commercial competitive gB-ELISAs gave a positive result which was not confirmed by BoHV-1 plaque reduction assay, VN, or competitive gE-ELISA tests. These serological results were inconsistent with immune responses usually developed by a BoHV-1 infected animal (15–17). Antibodies against glycoprotein B of BoHV-1 or neutralizing antibodies appear after 7–14 days post-infection, increase at constant levels, and persist for long periods. In contrast, antibodies against glycoprotein E (gE) appear 30–35 days post-infection and also persist for long periods (18, 19). However, Mars et al., reported that non BoHV-1 related gB-singleton reactors were found to be negative in the gE-ELISA test. Our study showed that, the calf detained at the performance station tested negative for all the three gE-ELISA tests. This was in concordance with the findings of previous studies (5, 8, 13). Increase in gE-reactivity was not detected over a period of 3 months. Seroconversion for gE would be expected in unvaccinated animals within this timespan.

The results obtained in this study could be attributed to non-specific reactivity, as indicated by Beer et al., such as batch variation between ELISA kits, sample quality, or the use of fresh serum (20). However, all of these factors have been taken into consideration in this study. Furthermore, different studies have shown that the seropositivity of some animals in competitive gB-ELISA could be attributed to serological cross-reactivity with other ruminant alphaherpesviruses (5, 8). This antigenic relationship has been demonstrated using different diagnostic tests (5, 21). In particular, the epitopes responsible

for the cross-neutralization are located in the major glycoprotein gB, gC, and gD (22). The gB gene is the most conserved among the major herpesvirus glycoproteins (23, 24). In this context, we investigated potential cross-reactivity of BoHV-1 with the following viruses: *Bovine alphaherpesvirus 2* (BoHV-2), *Bovine gammaherpesvirus 4* (BoHV-4), *Bovine alphaherpesvirus 5* (BoHV-5), and *Bubaline alphaherpesvirus 1* (BuHV-1).

Our results demonstrated that indirect-ELISA detected antibodies against BoHV-2 and this was subsequently confirmed via plaque reduction assay and BoHV-2 neutralization assay. The sanitary protocol of the experimental station, does not efficiently control BoHV-2 infection. Thus, the calf was not serologically checked for this viral infection while entering the experimental station.

It is well-known that reactivation is typical of herpesviruses and generally occurs after an immunosuppressive stimulus (25) or after dexamethasone treatment (9). We speculated that the serological cross-reactivity detected 5 months after arriving resulted from the latency state in a calf passing the first infection, rather than a subclinical primary infection. This hypothesis is also supported by the fact that if a primary infection had occurred after the entrance of the calf into the performance station, other animals had to show clinical signs, and then seroconverted against BoHV-2 as well, consequently some more animals might have been identified by gB-ELISA IBR tests. In addition, BoHV-2 spread might not be efficient in this herd (insect control, no role of milking cluster). Additionally, the performance station benefits from a very high biosecurity level, as it is located in an isolated area and is accessed only by personnel dedicated to the activities of the station. Therefore, an accidental entry of wild-type virus is most unlikely.

Furthermore, as the performance station is equipped with traps for biting flies, BoHV-2 transmission by flies may be excluded. This leads us to conclude that a latent BoHV-2 virus might have been reactivated in the calf as a consequence of an immunosuppressive stimulus, possibly when the animal underwent a change of diet or after its introduction into the performance station group. Unfortunately, as required by performance station regulations, the other animals, all asymptomatic and seronegative to BoHV-1 tests, were separated and sold during the study period. Thus, it was not possible to conduct further investigations on the cohabiting calves. However, the seropositivity ascertained in the calf cannot be attributed to vaccination because (i) the health regulations to regarding access a performance station ban the introduction of animals vaccinated against IBR and (ii) there are no commercially available vaccines against BoHV-2. Moreover, according to their regulations, animals entering a performance station are selected from IBR free herds, for which the practice of vaccination is prohibited. The detection of singleton reactors is crucial for the selection of animals in a performance test station, where animals can be introduced only if antibody negative. Additionally, each animal is checked every month to verify that no latent viral infections are reactivated.

Furthermore, in the context of IBR eradication programs, it is important to accurately identify singleton reactors. As an example, in Italy, where an active plan for the eradication of BoHV-1 in beef cattle breeds is in place (26), 20 gB singleton reactors were evidenced in different regions, during the 2018–2019 campaign (data not shown).

CONCLUSIONS

In conclusion, the present study highlights latent reactivation of BoHV-2 in a calf, which confirmed serological cross-reactivity with different commercial BoHV-1 ELISA tests. This should be carefully taken into consideration, when uncertain interpretation of IBR serology occurs, especially in performance test stations, where accidental contact to vaccine virus or wild type BoHV-1 infection can be reliably ruled out. In fact, animals erroneously considered as positive for BoHV-1, could be eliminated needlessly, which concomitantly means losing an animal of high genetic and economic value. In addition, the cross-serological reactivity may have an economic and social impact on control and eradication programs (trade restrictions, loss of negative status, decline in acceptance).

AUTHOR CONTRIBUTIONS

Experimental conception and design were done by SP. Collection of samples was done by CR. Immunological analyses were done by CP, CC, PG, and IP. Analysis, interpretation was done by SP, PK, CR, CI, and MG. Paper writing and editing were done by SP, PK, and GD. All authors read and approved the final manuscript.

ACKNOWLEDGMENTS

The authors are grateful to Prof. J. P. Teifke from Friedrich-Loeffler-lnstitut, Insel Riems, Germany, for providing the NA67 strain of BoHV-5. A special thanks to Prof. Fernando A. Osorio, School of Veterinary Medicine & Biomedical Sciences, University of Nebraska-Lincoln (USA) for providing a critical review of this manuscript and to Prof. Gigliola Canepa, University of Milan (I), for revising the language of the manuscript.

REFERENCES

1. Herpesviridae, ICTV 9th (2011). Available online at: https://talk.ictvonline.org/ictv-reports/ictv_9th_report/dsdna-viruses-2011/w/dsdna_viruses/91/ (accessed October 08, 2020)
2. Martin WB. Lumpy skin disease and pseudo-lumpy skin disease. In: Ristic M, McIntyre MIM, editors. *Disease of Cattle in the Tropics*, 1st ed. Dordrecht: Springer (1981). p. 167–79. doi: 10.1007/978-94-015-6895-1_13
3. Woods JA, Herring JA, Nettleton PF, Kreuger N, Scott MMF, Reid HW. Isolation of bovine herpesvirus-2 (BHV-2) from a case of pseudo-lumpy skin disease in United Kingdom. *Vet Rec.* (1996) 3:113–4. doi: 10.1136/vr.138.5.113
4. Watanabe TTN, Moeller RB, Crossley BM, Blanchard PC. Outbreaks of bovine herpesvirus 2 infections in calves causing ear and facial skin lesions. *J Vet Diagn Invest.* (2017) 29:686–90. doi: 10.1177/1040638717704480
5. Bottcher J, Boje L, Janowetz B, Alex M, Konig P, Hagg M, et al. Epidemiologically non-feasible singleton reactors at the final stage of BoHV-1 eradication: Serological evidence of BoHV-2 cross reactivity. *Vet Microbiol.* (2012) 159:282–90. doi: 10.1016/j.vetmic.2012.04.017
6. Lelli D, Luini M, Gazzola A, Boccardo A, Sozzi E, Sala G, et al. Pseudo-Lumpy Skin disease (BoHV-2): a case study. *Proceedings XVIII National Congress S.I.Di.L.V.* Matera (2019) p. 38.
7. Castrucci G, Cilli V, Andati HG. A serological survey in cattle to Bovid Herpesvirus 2. *Bollettino dell'Istituto Sieroterapico Milanese.* (1974) 53:645–50.
8. Valas S, Bremaud I, Stourm S, Croise B, Memeteau S, Ngwa-Mbot D, et al. Improvement of eradication program for infectious bovine rhinotracheitis in France inferred by serological monitoring of singleton reactors in certified BoHV-1-free herds. *Prev Vet Med.* (2019) 171:104743. doi: 10.1016/j.prevetmed.2019.104743
9. Castrucci G, Cilli V, Frigeri F, Ferrari M, Ranucci S, Rampichini L. Reactivation of Bovid Herpesvirus 1 and 2 and Parainfluenza-3 virus in calves latently infected. *Comp Immunol Microbiol Infect Dis.* (1983) 6:193–9. doi: 10.1016/0147-9571(83)90010-3
10. Manual of Diagnostic Tests and Vaccines for Terrestial Animals. *Infectious Bovine Rhinotracheitis.* (2018). Available online at: https://www.oie.int/fileadmin/Home/eng/Health_standards/tahm/3.04.11_IBR_IPV.pdf (accessed 27 July, 2020).
11. Rauh I, Weiland F, Fehler F, Keil GM, Mettenleiter TC. Pseudorabies virus mutants lacking the essential glycoprotein gII can be complemented by glycoprotein gI of bovine herpesvirus 1. *J Virol.* (1991) 65:621–31. doi: 10.1128/JVI.65.2.621-631.1991
12. De Giuli L, Magnino S, Vigo PG, Labalestra I, Fabbi M. Development of a polymerase chain reaction and restriction typing assay for the diagnosis of bovine herpesvirus 1, bovine herpesvirus 2 and bovine herpesvirus 4 infections. *J Vet Diagn Invest.* (2002) 14:353–6. doi: 10.1177/104063870201400417
13. Mars MH, Rijsewijk FAM, Maris Veldhuis MA, Hage JJ, van Oirschot JT. Presence of bovine herpesvirus 1 gB-seropositive but gE seronegative Dutch cattle with no apparent virus exposure. *Vet Rec.* (2000) 147:328–31. doi: 10.1136/vr.147.12.328
14. Isa G, Schelp C, Truyen U. Comparative investigation of bovine blood samples in three different ELISA tests. *Berl Munch Tierarztl Wochenschr.* (2003) 116:192–6.
15. Kramps JA, Banks M, Beer M, Kerkhofs P, Perrin M, Wellenberg GJ, et al. Evaluation of tests for antibodies against bovine herpesvirus 1 performed in national reference laboratories in Europe. *Vet Microbiol.* (2004) 102:169–81. doi: 10.1016/j.vetmic.2004.07.003
16. Babiuk LA, van Drunen Littel-van den Hurk S, Tikoo SK. Immunology of bovine herpesvirus 1 infection. *Vet Microbiol.* (1996) 53:31–42. doi: 10.1016/S0378-1135(96)01232-1
17. Konig P, Beer M, Makoschey B, Teifke JP, Polster U, Giesow K, et al. Recombinant virus-expressed bovine cytokines do not improve efficacy of a bovine herpesvirus 1 marker vaccine strain. *Vaccine.* (2003) 22:202–12. doi: 10.1016/S0264-410X(03)00565-6
18. Petrini S, Iscaro C, Righi C. Antibody response to Bovine alphaherpesvirus 1 (BoHV-1) in passively immunized calves. *Viruses.* (2019) 11:23. doi: 10.3390/v11010023
19. Petrini S, Righi C, Iscaro C, Viola G, Gobbi P, Scoccia E, et al. Evaluation of passive immunity induced by immunisation using two inactivated gE-deleted marker vaccines against Infectious Bovine Rhinotracheitis (IBR) in Calves. *Vaccines.* (2020) 8:14. doi: 10.3390/vaccines8010014
20. Beer M, Konig P, Schielke G, Trapp S. Diagnostic markers in the prevention of bovine herpesvirus type 1: possibilities and limitations. *Berl Munch Tierarztl Wochenschr.* (2003) 116:183–91.
21. Martin WB, Castrucci G, Frigeri F, Ferrari M. A serological comparison of some animal herpesviruses. *Comp Immunol Microbiol Infect Dis.* (1990) 13:75–84. doi: 10.1016/0147-9571(90)90519-Y
22. Nixon P, Edwards S, White H. Serological comparisons of antigenically related herpesviruses in cattle, red deer and goats. *Vet Res Commun.* (1988) 12:355–62. doi: 10.1007/BF00343256
23. Engels M, Palatini M, Metzler AE, Probst U, Kihm U, Ackermann M. Interactions of bovine and caprine herpesviruses with the natural

and the foreign hosts. *Vet Microbial.* (1992) 33:69–78. doi: 10.1016/0378-1135(92)90036-S

24. Griffin AM. The nucleotide sequence of the glycoprotein gB gene of infectious laryngotracheitis virus: analysis and evolutionary relationship to the homologous gene from other herpesviruses. *J Gen Virol.* (1991) 72:393–8. doi: 10.1099/0022-1317-72-2-393

25. Martin WB, Scott FMM. Latent infection of cattle with Bovid herpesvirus 2. *Arch Virol.* (1979) 60:51–8. doi: 10.1007/BF01318097

26. Maresca C, Scoccia E, Dettori A, Felici A, Guarcini R, Petrini S, et al. National surveillance plan for infectious bovine rhinotracheitis (IBR) in autochthonous Italian cattle breeds: Results of first year of activity. *Vet Microbiol.* (2018) 219:150–3. doi: 10.1016/j.vetmic.2018.04.013

13

Isolation and Characterization of a Porcine Transmissible Gastroenteritis Coronavirus in Northeast China

Dongwei Yuan [1,2], Zihan Yan [1], Mingyue Li [1], Yi Wang [1], Mingjun Su [1*] and Dongbo Sun [1*]

College of Animal Science and Veterinary Medicine, Heilongjiang Bayi Agricultural University, Daqing, China, [2] Daqing Center of Inspection and Testing for Agricultural Products Ministry of Agriculture, Daqing, China

*Correspondence:
Mingjun Su
mingjunsu@163.com
Dongbo Sun
dongbosun@126.com

Transmissible gastroenteritis virus (TGEV) is a coronavirus (CoV) that is a major pathogenity of viral enteritis and diarrhea in suckling piglets, causing high morbidity and mortality. In this study, a TGEV strain HQ2016 was isolated from northeast China and characterized its genome sequence and pathogenicity. The phylogenetic analysis indicated that the TGEV HQ2016 strain was more similar to the TGEV Purdue cluster than to the Miller cluster. Both recombination and phylogenetic analysis based on each structural and non-structural gene revealed no recombination event in the HQ2016 strain. Experimental infection study using colostrum-deprived newborn piglets successfully showed that the HQ2016 can cause clinical symptoms including anorexia and yellow-to-whitish watery diarrhea, which are characteristics of TGE, in the inoculated piglets 48 h post-inoculation. These results provide valuable information about the evolution of the porcine CoVs.

Keywords: transmissible gastroenteritis virus, virus isolate, phylogenetic analysis, pathogenicity, coronavirus

INTRODUCTION

Coronaviruses (CoVs) are the main etiological agents underlying outbreaks of porcine diarrhea, causing substantial economic losses (1). Transmissible gastroenteritis virus (TGEV) is a member of the family *Coronaviridae* that was first reported in 1946 in the USA (2). Since then, the disease always happened in swine-producing areas of the world (1, 3), and reported many times in China in recent years (4–8). Epidemiological investigations have shown that TGEV is often present in the spring and autumn in the northeast of China, sometimes in mixed infections with other diarrhea virus, and caused viral enteritis and severe diarrhea in all ages of pigs, especially with high mortality in suckling piglets (9, 10).

Transmissible gastroenteritis virus is an enveloped virus with a single-stranded, positive-stranded RNA genome of ~28.5-kb. The genome contains nine open reading frames (ORFs), which encode four structural proteins and five non-structural proteins: the spike glycoprotein (S); envelope protein (E); membrane glycoprotein (M); nucleocapsid protein (N); replicases 1a and 1b; ORF 3a and 3b proteins; and ORF 7 protein. The genes of TGEV are arranged in the order of 5′-rep-S-3a-3b-E-M-N-ORF7-3′ (4–6). The mutation in the spikes protein may be an important indicator for evaluating the tropism and virulence of TGEV. The M protein is the main viral particle membrane protein, which is mainly embedded in the lipid vesicle membrane and is connected to the capsule during assembly of the virus nucleocapsid. The E protein is a transmembrane protein, and the N protein is exists in the viral membrane. The ORF3 is composed of two open frames ORF3a and ORF3b. ORF3a deletion is found in many TGEV strains and PRCV strain. The ORF7 counteracts host-cell defenses and affects the persistence of TGEV, and improves the survival rate of TGEV by negatively regulating the downstream caspase-dependent apoptotic pathways (5, 6, 11, 12).

In this study, we isolated a TGEV from clinical samples collected from farms in northeast China using PK15 cells, characterized its genome based on the whole-genome sequence, and investigated its pathogenicity in colostrum-deprived neonatal pigs in terms of a clinical assessment, viral shedding, virus distribution, histopathological changes, and a mortality analysis. The results suggested that we have isolated porcine enteric coronavirus TGEV HQ2016. The genetic characteristics and pathogenicity of this virus provided valuable information for the evolution of TGEV and will helpful research on the molecular pathogenesis of TGEV.

MATERIALS AND METHODS

Specimen Collection and Screening

In 2016, a total of 50 intestine samples from piglets were collected from eight swine-raising farms in northeast China, in which the piglets showing watery diarrhea and dehydration and as known that all sow without any diarrhea viral vaccine inoculation. The intestinal samples were stored at $-80°C$. The samples were homogenized and diluted with sterile phosphate-buffered saline (PBS). The suspensions were repeatedly frozen and thawed three times, vortexed and clarified by centrifugation at $12,000 \times g$ for 10 min at $4°C$ and the supernatants were filtered through $0.22\,\mu m$ filters (Millipore, Billerica, MA, USA). Semi-nest reverse transcription (RT)-PCR (13) was used to identify the samples positive for TGEV, with two pairs of specific primers (TGEV-N-F: GGTAGTCGTGGTG- CTAATAATGA; TGEV-N-R1: CAGAATGCTAGACACAGATGGAA; TGEV-N-R2: GTT-CTCTTCCAGGTGTGTTTGTT).

Virus Isolation and Plaque Purification

PK15 cells (American Type Culture Collection [ATCC] CCL-33) were cultured in Dulbecco's modified Eagle's medium (DMEM; Hyclone, USA) supplemented with 10% fetal bovine serum (FBS; Bovogen, Australia) at $37°C$ in a 5% CO_2 incubator. Growth medium was removed from confluent monolayer cells; the cells were washed twice with DMEM and inoculated with a mixture of the supernatants of the positive tissue samples and DMEM containing $20\,\mu g/ml$ trypsin (GIBCO, 1:250) at a ratio of 1:1. After adsorption for 60 min at $37°C$, the cells were washed with DMEM, and maintenance medium consisting of DMEM supplemented with $10\,\mu g/ml$ trypsin was added. The inoculated cell cultures were observed for CPE for 3–5 days, harvested, and blindly passaged for five times. The viruses in a CPE positive sample was cloned by repeating plaque purify three times and designated as HQ2016.

Virus Titration With a Median Tissue Culture Infective Dose Assay

PK15 cells were seeded on 96-well plates and cultured overnight. The collected TGEV HQ2016 (passaged for 10 times) was 10-fold serially diluted, and used to inoculate cells, with eight replicates

per dilution. The cells were then cultured continuously at $37°C$ under 5% CO_2. The viral CPE was observed for 5–7 days. Tissue culture infective dose ($TCID_{50}$) was determined with the Reed-Muench method (14) and expressed as $TCID_{50}$ per milliliter.

Indirect Immunofluorescence Assay

PK15 cells (1×10^6) were seeded on six-well plates, cultured overnight, and then infected with TGEV HQ2016 (passaged for 10 times) at a multiplicity of infection (MOI) of 1.0. At 24 h after inoculation, the cells were fixed with 4% paraformaldehyde for 15 min and then per-meabilized with 0.2% Triton X-100 for 15 min. The cells were then blocked with 5% skim milk, and incubated overnight at $4°C$ with a TGEV-specific monoclonal antibody (5E8, supplied by Professor L. Feng, Harbin Veterinary Research Institute of the Chinese Academy of Agricultural Sciences, Harbin, China) diluted 1:1000. The cells were washed three times with PBS and incubated with a secondary antibody (fluorescein-isothiocyanate-conjugated goat anti-mouse IgG antibody, diluted 1:500) for 1 h at $37°C$ and then washed three times with PBS. The stained cells were visualized with fluorescence microscopy (Leica DMi8, Germany).

Electron Microscopic Assay

Supernatants from plaque-purified TGEV HQ2016 (passaged for 8 times) infected cell cultures were concentrated by ultracentrifugation method. The supernatants of the cell cultures were centrifuged first at $6,000 \times g$ for 30 min at $4°C$, and then at $60,000 \times g$ for 2 h at $4°C$. After ultracentrifugation, the samples were negatively stained with 2% ammonium molybdate and adsorbed onto 300-mesh copper net for 2 min. The viral particles were examined with an electron microscope (Hitachi H7500, Tokyo, Japan).

Extraction of Viral RNA and Complete Genome Sequencing

Culture supernatants from plaque-purified TGEV HQ2016 (passaged for 8 times) infected cells were collected and used for preparation of viral RNA. Total RNA was extracted using TRIzol Reagent (Invitrogen, Carlsbad, CA, USA), according to the manufacturer's instructions. The RNA samples were sent to testing company (Shanghai Probe Biotechnology Co., Ltd.) to determined complete genomic sequence with the Illumina high-throughput deep sequencing platform (15).

Sequence Analysis

The sequences of TGEV reference strains used in this study were obtained from GenBank, as shown in **Table 1**. The nucleotide and the amino acid sequences of TGEV HQ2016 strain were compared with the corresponding sequences of the TGEV strains in the GenBank database. The sequence was analyzed using the computer program MEGA version 6.0 (16) and DNASTAR (17). Nucleotide and amino acid sequence identities were determined using the Clustal W program. To determine the relationships between representative TGEV isolates and HQ2016 strain, a phylogenetic tree based on the entire genome was

TABLE 1 | Information of the reference TGEV sequences used in this study in the database.

No.	Isolate	Collected year	Country/Origin	GenBank accession no.
1	SHXB	2013	China	KP202848.1
2	Purdue P115	2009	USA	DQ811788.1
3	PUR46-MAD	–	USA	AJ271965.2
4	WH-1	2011	China	HQ462571.1
5	AYU	2009	China	HM776941.1
6	Puedue	–	USA	NC_038861.1
7	HX	2012	China	KC962433.1
8	HE-1	2016	China	KX083668.31
9	SC-Y	2006	China	DQ443743.1
10	Z	2006	USA	KX900393.1
11	HB	1988	USA	KX900394.1
12	Mex-145	2018	USA	KX900402.1
13	Virulent Purdue	1952	USA	DQ811789.2
14	AHHF	2017	China	KX499468.1
15	TS	2016	China	DQ201447.1
16	JS2012	2012	China	KT696544.1
17	Miller M6	2009	USA	DQ811785.1
18	Attenuated H	2009	China	EU074218.2
19	H16	1973	China	FJ755618.2
20	HQ2016	2016	China	MT576083.1

constructed with the MEGA6.0 software through the neighbor-joining method. The reliability of the neighbor-joining tree was estimated by bootstrap analysis with 1,000 replicates.

Recombination Analysis

We used the RDP4 software, including RDP, Bootscan, and SiScan, for a recombination analysis to detect the probable parental isolates and recombination breakpoints of TGEV HQ2016, with the default settings. The criteria used to detect recombination and identify breakpoints were $P < 10^{-6}$ and a recombination score >0.6 (18).

Pathogenicity of TGEV HQ2016 in Newborn Piglets

We used 12 newborn piglets of both sexes without colostrum, who had not been exposed to TGEV before and no anti-TGEV antibodies. The newborn piglets were randomly allocated to the control group ($n = 6$) or the challenged group ($n = 6$). The piglets were fed a mixture of skim milk powder (Inner Mongolia Yi Li Industrial Group Co., Ltd., China) and warm water. The groups were separated by room and ventilation system within the same facility. After acclimation for 1 day, the six piglets in the control group were orally administered 5 ml of DMEM and used as the uninfected controls. The six piglets in the challenged group were orally administered 5 ml of DMEM containing 5×10^6 TCID$_{50}$ of TGEV HQ2016 (passaged for 10 times). All the piglets were observed every 12 h for clinical signs of vomiting, diarrhea, lethargy, and altered temperature or body condition. Rectal swabs were collected from each piglet every 12 h and fecal consistency was scored. The grading standards for the clinical signs and fecal consistency are shown in **Table 2**. Fecal viral RNA shedding was detected with quantitative RT–PCR (19). The sequences

of the primers used were: forward, 5′-AAACAACAGCAACGC TCTCG-3′; reverse, 5′-ATTGGCAACGAGGTCAGTGT-3′. The piglets in the two groups were sacrificed at 84 h after challenge. At necropsy, fresh samples of duodenum, jejunum, ileum, cecum, and colon were collected and fixed in 10% formalin solution. The fresh samples were stored at −80°C before a viral RNA distribution analysis with quantitative RT-PCR (19), and formalin-fixed samples were used for histopathological and immunohistochemical analyses. The mortality of the newborn piglets in each group was recorded daily.

Statistical Analysis

The data, including the results of the clinical symptoms, fecal scores and viral load in which inoculated and control piglets, were compared among the different groups by one-way repeated measures ANOVA and the least significance difference (LSD). All data were processed and analyzed using SPSS21.0 Data Editor (SPSS Inc., Chicago, IL, USA). The results for the comparisons among groups were considered different if *$P < 0.05$ or **$P < 0.01$.

RESULTS
Virus Isolation and Identification

A total of 50 intestinal samples were collected from eight pig farms in northeast China. The piglets on these farms suffered vomiting and diarrhea. TGEV was detected in 20% of the samples, and the positive samples were from six farms. The supernatants of the TGEV-positive samples were used to inoculate PK15 cells, 6 of 10 positive samples were tested for virus isolation. Of which, three sample become positive CPE after five passages. No CPE was observed in control

TABLE 2 | The grading standard for clinical symptom and feces of piglets.

Scores	0	1	2	3	4
Clinical symptoms	Normal	Slow movement, normal appetite	Lies, spirit languishes, loss of appetite	Difficult to walk, dehydration	Difficulty standing, dehydrated seriously and weight loss
Fecal consistency	Normal	Soft feces	Liquid with solid feces admixture	Watery feces	Watery diarrhea

PK-15 cells (**Figure 1A**). The CPE was characterized by cell fusion, cell rounding and shrinkage, and the detachment of the cells into the medium (**Figures 1B,C**). TGEV antigen was identified in the cytoplasm of the virus inoculated PK-15 cells but not in mock inoculated cells by IFA using TGEV-specific monoclonal antibody (**Figures 1D,E**). Coronavirus-like particles with a diameter of 100 to 120 nm, similar to the size of TGEV were identified in the culture supernatant of the virus inoculated PK-15 cell by negative staining electron microscopy (**Figure 1F**). The virus isolate was designated as TGEV HQ2016 strain hereafter. And then, the titer of TGEV HQ2016 reached $10^{5.25}$ $TCID_{50}/0.1$ ml at passage 10.

Complete Genomic Sequence of TGEV Strain HQ2016

The genomic sequence of TGEV HQ2016 strain, determined with the illumina sequencing, platform was 28,571 nucleotides (nt) long, and the sequence was submitted to GenBank under accession number MT576083, and exhibited the genomic organization typical of all previously reported TGEV sequences, which are arranged in the order of 5'-rep-S-3a-3b-E-M-N-ORF7-3' (4–6). The 5' portion of the genome contains a 303-nt untranslated region (UTR) which includes a potential short AUG-initiated ORF (nt 103–110), beginning with a Kozak sequence (5'-UCUAUGA-3'). The viral RNA-dependent RNA replicase include ORF1a (nt 304–12,357) and ORF1b (nt 12,315–20,357). Structural proteins encoding genes were S (nt 20,354–24,697), E (nt 25,846–26,094), M (nt 26,105–26,893), and N (nt 26,906–28,054), respectively. Non-structural protein encoding genes were ORF3a (nt 24,816–25,031), ORF3b (nt 25,125–25,859), and ORF7 (nt 28,029–28,265), respectively. The 3'end of the genome contains a 275-nt untranslated sequence and a poly(A) tail. The octameric sequence 5'-GGAAGAGC-3' occurs upstream from the poly(A) tail.

Genomic Characteristics

The S gene of TGEV HQ2016 was 4,344-nt in length, predicted to a encode protein of 1,447 amino acids. A site of 6-nt deletion was observed in the S gene of TGEV HQ2016 at nt 1,123–1,128, which causes two amino acids shorter at this site than in strains of Virulent Purdue, AHHF, TS, Miller M6, JS2012, Attenuated H, and H16 (**Figure 2A**). A other site of 3-nt deletion was detected at nt 2,387–2,389 of the S gene in attenuated H, H16, and AHHF, while it was not found in strain TGEV HQ2016 and other strains (**Figure 2A**). In the Virulent Purdue, Miller M6, JS2012, and TS strains, amino acid 585 is serine, whereas in the

TGEV HQ2016, it is alanine (**Figure 3**). Amino acids at 32, 72, 100, 184, 208, 218, 389, 403, 418, 487, 562, 590, 649, 675, 815, 951, 1,109, and 1,234 of TGEV HQ2016 S protein are same to those of the Purdue subgroup strains, especially the three viruses from the United States, and HE-1, HX, AYU, WH-1, SHXB, SC-Y from China, but differ from those of the Miller subgroup strains (**Figure 3**). The structural proteins of E, M and N were 249-nt, 789-nt and 1,149-nt in length and predicted to encode proteins of 82, 262, and 382 amino acids, respectively (**Table 3**), and there was no deletions or insertions compared with other TGEV reference strains.

The replicase genes contained ORF1a and ORF1b, which were 12,054-nt and 8,037-nt in length, predicted to encode proteins of 4,017 amino acids and a protein of 2,680 amino-acid, respectively (**Table 3**). There were a common 43-nt region (nt 12,315–12,357) between ORF1a and ORF1b, and a "slippery site" (5'-UUUAAAC-3', nt 12,322–12,328) which allows the ORF1a translation termination site to be bypassed and an additional ORF, ORF1b to be read. Nucleotide sequence analysis indicated that there were no major deletions or insertions presented in replicase genes both in any Purdue and Miller TGEV strains. ORF3a and 3b of TGEV HQ2016 are 216-nt and 735-nt in length, predicted to encode a protein of 71 amino acid and a protein of 244 amino acid, respectively (**Table 3**). Previous research had demonstrated the presence of two deletions in the TGEV ORF3a/b gene in the Miller subgroup (5), a 16-nt deletion and a 29-nt deletion were observed in the strains of Miller subgroup in this study (**Figure 2B**), but no deletions were detected in the ORF3a/b genes of TGEV HQ2016 and other Purdue strains. The ORF7 gene of TGEV HQ2016 was 237-nt in length and predicted to encode a protein of 78 amino acid, which contains the common PP1c-binding motif 5'-RVIFLVI-3'. No deletions or insertions presented in ORF7 of TGEV HQ2016. The recombination analysis showed that no recombination event has ever occurred in TGEV HQ2016. Complete sequence alignment of 5' and 3'-UTR regions, there was no deletions or insertions were found in strain HQ2016. The ORF initiated by short AUG beginning within the Kozak sequence (TCTATGA) in 5' NTR regions, and the octameric sequence of "GGAAGAGC" at upstream of the 3' end poly(A) tail, which could be found in all strains.

Phylogenetic Tree and Homology Analysis

The complete genomic sequence of TGEV HQ2016 was compared with those of 19 TGEV reference strains. Phylogenetic

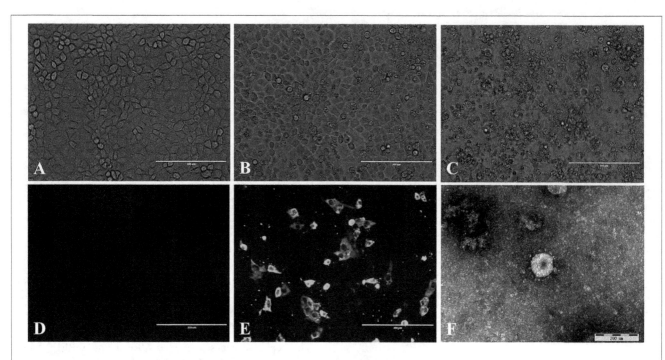

FIGURE 1 | Isolation and identification of the TGEV HQ2016 strain. **(A)** Control (uninfected) PK-15 cells. **(B)** Cytopathic effect (CPE) induced by TGEV HQ2016 after infected 24 h in the PK-15 cell line. **(C)** Cytopathic effect (CPE) induced by TGEV HQ2016 after infected 36 h in the PK-15 cell line. **(D)** IFA identification of control (uninfected) PK15 cells. **(E)** IFA identification of TGEV HQ2016 infected PK15 cells. **(F)** Electron microscopy observation of TGEV HQ2016.

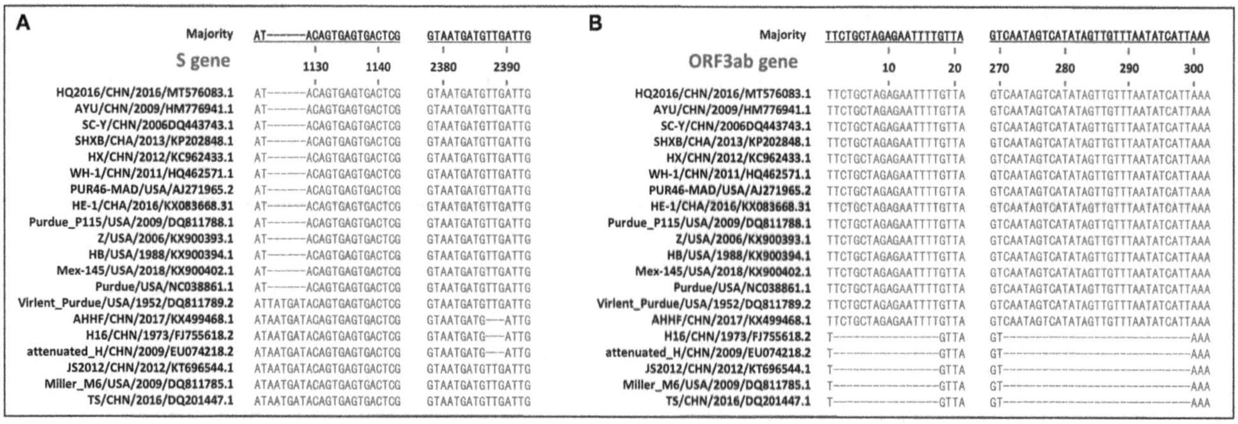

FIGURE 2 | Visualization of genomic deletion regions in the 20 TGEV strains. **(A)** deletion regions of S gene. **(B)** deletion regions of ORF3ab gene.

trees based on the complete genome (**Figure 4**) divided the TGEV strains into the Purdue and Miller genotypes (5). The TGEV HQ2016 strain clustered in the Purdue subgroup, together with SHXB, Purdue, Purdue P115, PUR46-MAD, WH-1, AYU, SC-Y, HX, HE-1, Z, HB, Mex145, Virulent Purdue, and AHHF, whereas the Miller subgroup included TS, JS2012, Miller M6, Attenuated H, and H16. Thus, TGEV strain HQ2016 is closely related to the Purdue strains and more distantly to the Miller strains. The strains of Purdue subgroup appear to share a common ancestor.

To investigate the homology of TGEV HQ2016 with other TGEVs, the nucleotide and predicted amino acid sequences of structural proteins and non-structural proteins were compared (**Table 4**). The results shown that structural proteins (S, E, M, N) and non-structural proteins (replicases 1a and 1b, ORF 3a and 3b, ORF 7) of TGEV HQ2016 shared greater identity with Purdue strains (**Table 4**), identity of predicted amino acid sequence identity in ORF1a was 98.7–100%, in ORF1b was 98.6–100%, in S protein was 97.1–100%, in ORF3a was 88.3–100%, in ORF3b was 97.1–100%, in E protein was 91.5–98.8%, in M

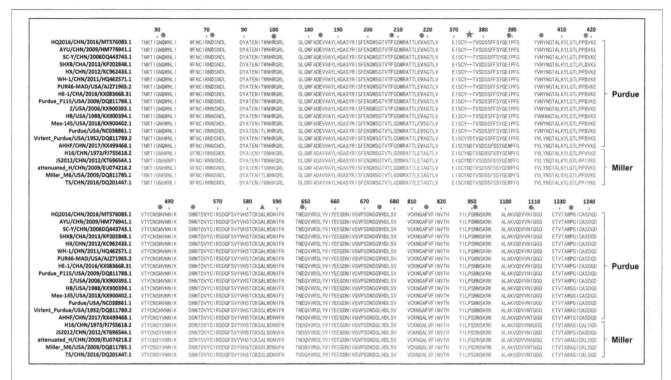

FIGURE 3 | Alignment of partial deduced amino acid sequence of S protein compared with strain TGEV HQ2016. (▲) indicates amino acid 585, (★) indicates 6-nt deletion in the S gene, (●) indicates amino acids of the Purdue subgroup strains include TGEV HQ2016 are different from those of Miller subgroups strains.

protein was 97.3–99.6%, in N protein was 98.2–100%, in ORF7 was 93.6–100%.

Clinical Signs in TGEV HQ2016 Inoculated Piglets

To evaluate the pathogenicity of TGEV HQ2016 in piglets, 12 newborn piglets were used without colostrum. The piglets were active and fleshy before inoculation, with normal fecal consistency. Mild diarrhea and loss of appetite were observed in the piglets of the TGEV HQ2016 inoculated group after 12 h. Severe depression, loss of appetite, vomiting, and yellow and white watery diarrhea appeared in the TGEV HQ2016 inoculated group after 48 h. After 72 h, all the piglets in TGEV HQ2016 inoculated group suffered watery diarrhea and were seriously dehydrated. None of the piglets inoculated with TGEV HQ2016 died within the 84 h of the experimental period, and the control piglets showed no vomiting or diarrhea. The body temperatures, body weight changes, clinical symptoms, and fecal scores of both groups are shown in **Figure 5**. The body temperatures and body weight changes were significantly lower in the piglets of the TGEV HQ2016 inoculated group after 72 h. The clinical symptoms and fecal scores increased continuously for 24 h after TGEV HQ2016 inoculated and differed significantly from those in the control group.

Histopathological Observations

All the piglets were sacrificed after virus challenged 84 h. Pathological changes were mainly observed in the intestinal tracts (jejunum and ileum) of the TGEV-HQ2016-challenged piglets. The whole intestinal tracts, in which yellow watery contents had accumulated, were transparent, thin walled, and gas distended. No lesions were observed in any other organs of the TGEV HQ2016 inoculated piglets or in the organs in the negative control piglets, indicating that the intestinal tract is the target organ of TGEV infection. In a microscopic examination, villus atrophy, degenerate mucosal epithelial cells, and necrosis were observed in both the jejunum and ileum tissues of the TGEV HQ2016 inoculated piglets, but not in those of the control piglets, as shown in **Figure 6**. An immunohistochemical examination showed TGEV antigen in the cytoplasm of the epithelial cells in the atrophied villi of the segments of jejunum and ileum tissues from the piglets inoculated with TGEV HQ2016, but no reactivity in either the jejunal or ileal tissues of the control group, as shown in **Figure 6**.

Viral Loads in Fecal Samples and Intestinal Tissues of TGEV HQ2016 Inoculated Piglets

Because TGEV caused diarrhea and intestinal damage in the newborn piglets, we collected rectal swabs and intestinal samples from them to investigate the viral shedding in the TGEV HQ2016 inoculated piglets. White and yellow watery feces were present in the TGEV HQ2016 inoculated piglets from 48 h after virus challenged. As shown in **Figure 7**, the TGEV viral RNA was detected with quantitative RT-PCR (19). The TGEV levels in the fecal samples were 5–10 $\log_{10}$ RNA copies/g at 12–84 hpi, indicating that TGEV HQ2016 infected and

TABLE 3 | Length of amino acids in the predicted structural and non-structural proteins of TGEV strains.

Strain	ORF1a	ORF1b	S	ORF3a	ORF3b	E	M	N	ORF7
SHXB	4017	2678	1447	71	244	82	262	382	78
Purdue P115	4017	2678	1447	71	244	82	262	382	78
PUR46-MAD	4017	2678	1447	71	244	82	262	382	78
WH-1	4017	2678	1447	71	244	82	262	382	78
AYU	4017	2678	1447	71	244	82	262	382	78
Purdue	4017	2678	1447	71	244	82	262	382	78
HX	4017	2678	1447	71	244	82	262	382	78
HE-1	4017	2678	1447	71	244	82	262	382	78
SC-Y	4017	2678	1447	71	244	82	262	382	78
Z	4017	2678	1447	71	244	82	262	382	78
HB	4017	2678	1447	71	244	82	262	382	78
Mex145	4017	2678	1447	71	244	82	262	382	78
Virulent Purdue	4017	2678	1449	71	244	82	262	382	78
AHHF	4017	2678	1448	71	244	82	262	382	78
TS	4017	2678	1449	65	244	82	262	382	78
JS2012	4017	2678	1449	65	244	82	262	382	78
Miller M6	4017	2678	1449	65	244	82	262	382	78
Attenuated H	4017	2678	1448	65	244	82	262	382	78
H16	4017	2678	1448	65	244	82	262	382	78
HQ2016	4017	2678	1447	71	244	82	262	382	78

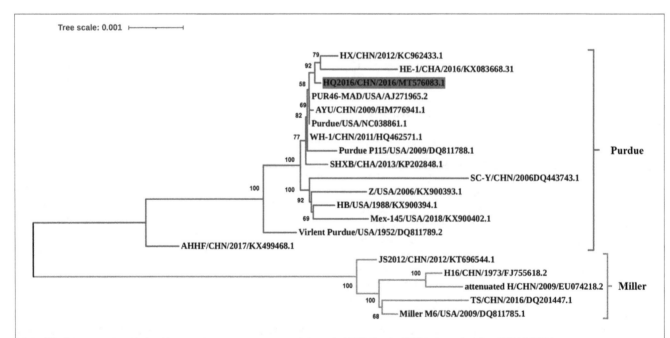

FIGURE 4 | Phylogenetic analysis of the complete genome sequences of the strain HQ2016, other TGEV reference strains. TGEV HQ2016 belongs to the Purdue cluster of TGEV, not the Miller cluster. Complete genome were aligned used Clustal W program which have trimed both 3′ and 5′ ends gaps between TGEV genomes Phylogenetic tree was constructed using the neighbor-joining method with the MEGA 6.0 program. The optimal tree with the sum of branch length = 0.02540989 is shown. The percentage of replicate trees in which the associated taxa clustered together in the bootstrap test (1,000 replicates) are shown next to the branches. The tree is drawn to scale, with branch lengths in the same units as those of the evolutionary distances used to infer the phylogenetic tree. The evolutionary distances were computed using the Tajima-Nei method.

reproduced in these challenged piglets. At the end of the challenge experiment, samples of duodenum, jejunum, ileum, caecum, and colon were collected for viral RNA detection. At 84 hpi, the viral level was highest in the jejunum (7.21 ± 0.11 $\log_{10}$ RNA copies/g), and then (in decreasing order) in the ileum (6.51 ± 0.31 $\log_{10}$ RNA copies/g), cecum (6.28 ± 0.39

TABLE 4 | Nucleotide and amino acid sequence identities (%) of TGEV HQ2016 strain compared with other 19 TGEV strains.

	ORF1a	ORF1b	S	ORF3a	ORF3b	E	M	N	ORF7
SHXB	99.9/99.9	100.0/100.0	100.0/100.0	100.0/100.0	99.9/99.6	99.2/97.6	99.7/99.2	99.9/99.7	99.3/97.4
Purdue P115	99.9/99.9	100.0/100.0	99.9/99.9	100.0/100.0	99.9/99.6	99.6/98.8	99.9/99.6	99.9/99.7	100.0/100.0
PUR46-MAD	100.0/100.0	100.0/100.0	100.0/100.0	100.0/100.0	100.0/100.0	99.6/98.8	99.9/99.6	100.0/100.0	100.0/100.0
WH-1	100.0/100.0	100.0/100.0	100.0/100.0	100.0/100.0	99.9/99.6	99.6/98.8	99.9/99.6	100.0/100.0	100.0/100.0
AYU	99.9/99.9	100.0/100.0	100.0/100.0	100.0/100.0	100.0/100.0	99.6/98.8	99.7/99.2	100.0/100.0	100.0/100.0
Purdue	100.0/100.0	100.0/100.0	100.0/100.0	100.0/100.0	100.0/100.0	99.6/98.8	99.9/99.6	100.0/100.0	100.0/100.0
HX	99.9/99.9	100.0/100.0	99.9/99.9	100.0/100.0	100.0/100.0	99.6/98.8	100.0/100.0	100.0/100.0	100.0/100.0
HE-1	99.9/99.7	99.8/99.7	99.9/99.8	100.0/100.0	100.0/100.0	98.8/98.8	99.5/98.5	99.9/99.7	99.8/98.7
SC-Y	99.5/99.2	99.8/99.8	99.7/99.5	100.0/100.0	99.9/99.6	99.6/98.8	99.7/99.2	99.9/99.7	100.0/100.0
Z	99.9/99.8	99.9/99.9	99.6/99.0	99.1/98.6	99.9/99.6	99.2/98.8	99.7/99.2	99.8/99.7	100.0/100.0
HB	99.9/99.9	100.0/100.0	99.7/99.4	100.0/100.0	99.9/99.6	99.6/98.8	99.7/99.2	100.0/100.0	100.0/100.0
Mex145	99.9/99.8	99.9/99.9	99.7/99.2	99.5/98.6	99.9/99.6	99.2/98.8	99.7/99.2	99.9/99.7	100.0/100.0
Virulent Purdue	99.9/99.7	100.0/100.0	99.5/99.1	99.5/98.6	99.7/99.2	99.2/97.6	99.7/99.2	99.7/99.7	100.0/100.0
AHHF	99.5/99.5	100.0/100.0	98.9/98.6	100.0/100.0	99.9/99.6	99.6/98.8	99.7/99.2	100.0/100.0	100.0/100.0
TS	98.8/98.7	99.0/98.6	98.3/98.1	87.0/89.5	98.5/96.3	98.4/95.1	98.0/96.9	98.1/98.2	96.8/93.6
JS2012	99.0/99.1	99.0/99.7	98.6/98.3	88.0/88.7	98.8/97.1	98.4/95.1	98.2/97.7	98.2/98.4	96.8/93.6
Miller M6	99.0/99.1	99.1/99.6	98.3/97.1	88.0/88.3	98.9/97.5	98.0/93.9	98.2/97.7	98.2/98.4	96.6/93.6
Attenuated H	98.9/98.9	99.0/99.6	98.0/97.7	87.5/88.7	98.8/97.1	96.8/91.5	98.1/97.3	98.1/98.4	96.8/93.6
H16	98.9/98.9	99.0/99.6	98.2/97.9	88.0/88.7	98.9/97.5	97.6/93.9	98.1/97.3	98.2/98.4	96.8/93.6

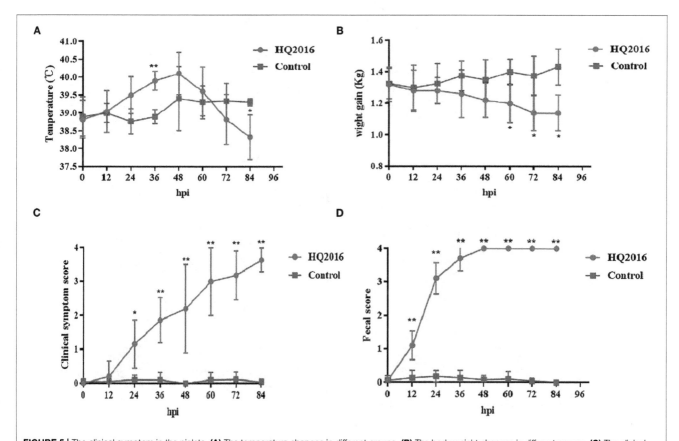

FIGURE 5 | The clinical symptom in the piglets. **(A)** The temperature changes in different groups. **(B)** The body weight changes in different groups. **(C)** The clinical symptom scores in different groups. **(D)** The fecal scores in different groups. Data are shown as mean standard (*$p < 0.05$, **$p < 0.01$).

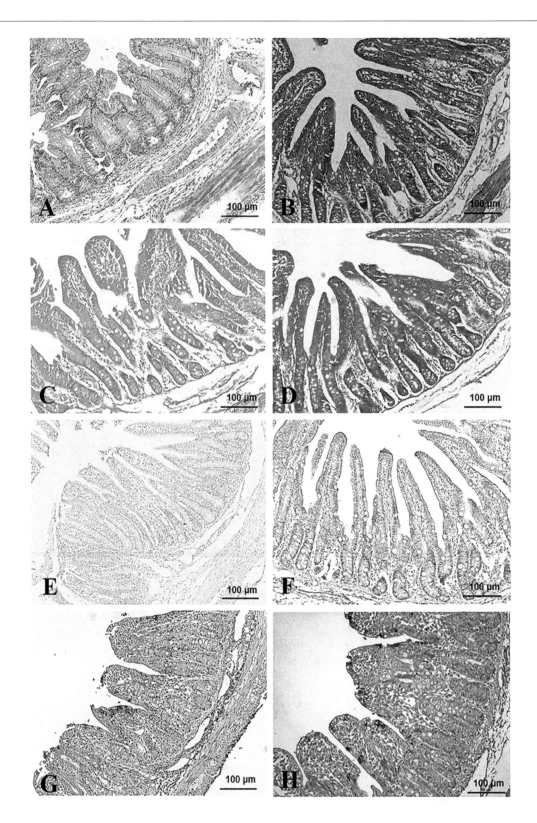

FIGURE 6 | Pathological changes and IHC assays of TGEV HQ2016-inoculated piglets. **(A,B)** H.E staining for jejunum and ileum tissue section of control piglets. **(C,D)** H.E staining for jejunum and ileum tissue section of TGEV HQ2016 challenged piglets. Villus atrophy, degenerate mucosal epithelial cells, and necrosis. **(E,F)** IHC assays for jejunum and ileum tissue section of control piglets. **(G,H)** IHC assays for jejunum and ileum tissue section of TGEV HQ2016 challenged piglets. Positive cells presented in the epithelial cells in the atrophied villi of the segments of jejunal and ileal tissues from the piglets.

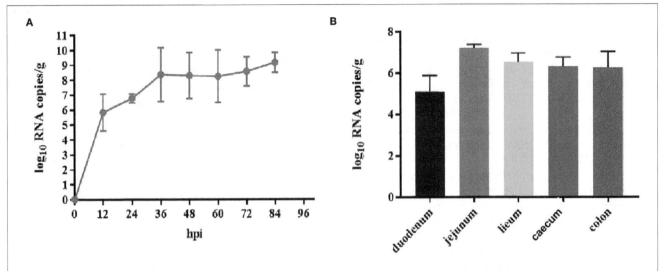

FIGURE 7 | Reproduction of watery diarrhea and viral shedding in newborn piglets inoculated with TGEV HQ2016 via oral feeding. **(A)** Quantification of viral RNA levels of fecal samples of piglets inoculated with TGEV HQ2016. **(B)** Quantification of viral RNA levels in intestine tissues of piglets at 84 h inoculated with TGEV HQ2016.

$\log_{10}$ RNA copies/g), colon (6.23 ± 0.55 $\log_{10}$ RNA copies/g), and duodenum (5.09 ± 0.61 $\log_{10}$ RNA copies/g). These results confirm that TGEV HQ2016 infected the piglets and invaded their intestinal tissues.

DISCUSSION

TGEV is an enteropathic coronavirus that infects pigs, and was first reported in the USA in the 1940s, after which spread throughout the world (1–3). TGEV causes significant diarrhea, vomiting, and dehydration in suckling piglets, with a high mortality rate (10). In recent years, mixed infections of TGEV with other swine diarrhea virus have occurred frequently, causing serious economic losses in the pig industry (1). In this study, a natural strain of TGEV, HQ2016, was successfully isolated from piglets intestinal samples, which collected from swine-raising farms in northeast China. In the farms, sows did not receive any vaccination for preventing diarrhea and piglets developed clinical symptoms including vomiting, diarrhea, rapid weight loss and dehydration. After experimental infection, piglets showed the characteristic clinical symptoms (diarrhea and vomiting) of TGE from 12 h after TGEV HQ2016 inoculated until the end of the experiment. A histopathological analysis showed villous atrophy, together with mucosal epithelial cells degeneration and necrosis, in the jejunum and ileum, and virus-positive cells were present in the villous epithelial cells in the jejunum and ileum by IHC. These results demonstrate that TGEV HQ2016 was replicated and had pathogenicity in enterocyte, is a natural, transmissible, enteric pathogenic porcine coronavirus. Viral nucleic acid of TGEV was detected on rectal swabs as early as 12 h after viral challenge, which indicated that virus infected the intestine and released to intestinal content, as described previously in infections with TGEV (6, 20). At 84 h of TGEV HQ2016 inoculated, we found a high level of viral RNA in jejunum,

ileum, caecum and colon, which is similarity with the report previously (5), but there was no obviously pathological changes and TGEV antigen presence in caecum and colon epithelial cells (which is not shown in the results of this study), this result suggested that caecum and colon contained virus but epithelial cells had not yet been infected. Virus-positive epithelial cells and presence of virus in intestines indicated that TGEV HQ2016 prefers to infect small intestinal epithelial cells and replicate, caused pathological changes in the small intestinal epithelial cells, and then necrotic epithelial cells released the virus into the intestinal contents, and finally excreted through the large intestines. This finding may provide a proof for the study of host cell infection and transmission mechanism in coronavirus.

Traditional TGEVs can be divided into two clusters, the Purdue and Miller groups (4, 5, 7, 12, 21). In this study, we sequenced the entire genome of TGEV HQ2016, and a phylogenetic analysis placed TGEV HQ2016 in the Purdue cluster, indicating that it is more distantly evolutionarily related to the Miller cluster. Additionally, sequence alignment result showed two large deletions in ORF3a/3b that occur in the strains of the Miller cluster are not found in TGEV HQ2016 or the Purdue cluster, this may be considered to a marker of distinguishing the Purdue and Miller cluster of TGEV. Phylogenetic analysis shown that TGEV HQ2016 is closely related to with strains PUR46-MAD, Purdue, WH-1, AYU, which have the same ancestor, and this is consistent with the results of homology comparison. Nucleotide and predicted amino-acid sequence homology comparison shown the structural and non-structural proteins of TGEV HQ2016 is very similar to PUR46-MAD, Purdue, AYU and WH-1. These data suggest that TGEV HQ2016 might be had the same origin with WH-1 and AYU strains in China and more similar with Purdue and PUR46-MAD from USA.

The 5′- and 3′-UTRs of CoVs are critically important for viral replication and transcription (5, 22, 23). The "slippery" heptanucleotide sequence and a pseudoknot structure are both critical for viral RNA synthesis and are involved in ribosomal frame shifting (24). A complete sequence analysis indicated that no deletions or insertions are present in the 5′- or 3′-UTR regions of TGEV HQ2016, and that it contains both the slippery sequence and pseudoknot structure. These sequence data suggest that the replication and transcription mechanisms of TGEV HQ2016 are conserved, as reported previously (5, 21, 25).

CoVs attach to their host cells via the S protein, which is the major immunogenic protein of the virus and stimulate the host to produce antibodies with neutralizing activity (26). There are at least four main antigenic sites on the S protein, designated A, B, C, and D (4, 27, 28). The A/B sites (amino acids 506–706) are the major antigenic sites and have been mapped. Single-amino-acid changes in the S protein might affect its antigenicity or virulence (4–6). A mutation at amino acid 585 in the main major antigenic sites A/B of the S protein of TGEV HQ2016 causes a serine to alanine change, which also occurs in the PUR46-MAD, Purdue, Purdue P115, WH-1, AYU, HX, HE-1, SHXB, SC-Y, Z, HB, Mex145, AHHF, H16, and Attenuated H strains, but not in the JS2012, Miller M6, TS, or Virulent Purdue strains. This mutation may significantly influence receptor binding or the virus interactions with neutralizing antibodies, significantly affecting their antigenicity, this is also considered to be a marker of attenuation (6). There was a 6-nt deletion detected in the TGEV HQ2016 S gene, as in the rest of the Purdue cluster, except for the Virulent Purdue and AHHF strains. A 6-nt deletion (nt 1,123-1,128) in the S gene was considered a trait of the TGEV strains in the Purdue cluster (5). This 6-nt deletion in the S gene was also considered to play a role in viral attenuation (6). The S gene is also a hypervariable region in the TGEV genome, and amino acids 32, 72, 100, 184, 208, 218, 389, 403, 418, 487, 562, 590, 649, 675, 815, 951, 1,109, and 1,234 of TGEV HQ2016 are identical among the viruses in the Purdue cluster, but differ from those in the Miller cluster. These changes of amino acid in S gene may be related to the changes of virus virulence, which needs to be discussed in follow-up research. Except for S gene, ORF3a/3b genes were considered to affect the variation between attenuated and virulent strains (12). However, there are some uncertainties about the effects of deletions in TGEV ORF3a/3b on viral virulence (1, 28–31). In our study, homology analysis shown that HQ2016 and attenuated strains PUR46-MAD (4, 32)

had highly identity. PUR46-MAD was generally considered an attenuated strain of TGEV, which derivative of Purdue P115, and both were derived from the strain virulent Purdue after highly passage in cell culture (4, 12, 25, 32, 33). TGEV HQ2016 used in our infected experiment was only 10th passage in cell culture. Therefore, we think that the virulence of HQ2016 might be reduced by highly passage in cell culture in the future, as previously reported for PUR46-MAD. 6-nt deletion or amino acid mutations in S gene might reduce the virulence of TGEV HQ2016 through the highly passage, this need to be confirmed in future studies. This hypothesis needs to be confirmed in future studies and facilitate the development of an attenuated vaccine for TGEV.

In conclusion, a epidemical strain of TGEV, HQ2016, was isolated from swine-raising farms in northeast China. Typical clinical signs, pathologic alterations and histological changes associated with TGE were observed in piglets inoculated with the TGEV HQ2016 strain. Phylogenetic analysis of whole genome, nucleotide and amino acid sequence homology analysis of the structural proteins and non-structural proteins indicated that TGEV HQ2016 belongs to the Purdue cluster, and it might be had the same origin with WH-1 and AYU strain in China and more similar with Purdue strains from USA. These results provide essential information for further understanding the evolution of TGEV and will facilitate future investigations into the molecular pathogenesis of TGEV.

AUTHOR CONTRIBUTIONS

DY: formal analysis and writing—original draft. ZY: methodology and validation. ML: methodology. YW: data curation. MS: writing and picture editing. DS: supervision. All authors contributed to the article and approved the submitted version.

ACKNOWLEDGMENTS

We also thank International Science Editing for editing the English text of a draft of this manuscript (http://www.internationalscienceediting.com).

REFERENCES

1. Zuniga S, Pascual-Iglesias A, Sanchez CM, Sola I, Enjuanes L. Virulence factors in porcine coronaviruses and vaccine design. *Virus Res.* (2016) 226:142–51. doi: 10.1016/j.virusres.2016.07.003
2. Doyle LP, Hutchings LM. A transmissible gastroenteritis in pigs. *J Am Vet Med Assoc.* (1946) 108:257–9.
3. Xue R, Tian Y, Zhang Y, Zhang M, Tian F, Ma J, et al. Efficacy and immunogenicity of a live *L. acidophilus* expressing SAD epitope of transmissible gastroenteritis virus as an oral vaccine. *Acta Virol.* (2019) 63:301–8. doi: 10.4149/av_2019_310

4. Hu XL, Li NN, Tian ZG, Yin X, Qu LD, Qu JJ. Molecular characterization and phylogenetic analysis of transmissible gastroenteritis virus HX strain isolated from China. *BMC Vet Res.* (2015) 21:72–9. doi: 10.1186/s12917-015-0387-8
5. Zhang X, Zhu YN, Zhu XD, Shi HY, Chen JF, Shi D, et al. Identification of a natural recombinant transmissible gastroenteritis virus between Purdue and Miller clusters in China. *Emerg Microbes Infect.* (2017) 6:e74. doi: 10.1038/emi.2017.62
6. Guo RL, Fan BB, Chang XJ, Zhou JZ, Zhao YX, Shi DY, et al. Characterization and evaluation of the pathogenicity of a natural recombinant transmissible gastroenteritis virus in China. *Virology.* (2020) 545:24–32. doi: 10.1016/j.virol.2020.03.001

7. Li JQ, Cheng J, Lan X, Li XR, Li W, Yin XP, et al. Complete genomic sequence of transmissible gastroenteritis virus TS and 3' end sequence characterization following cell culture. *Virol Sin.* (2010) 25:213–24. doi: 10.1007/s12250-010-3108-2

8. Hou Y, Yue X, Cai X, Wang S, Liu Y, Yuan C, et al. Complete genome of transmissible gastroenteritis virus AYU strain isolated in Shanghai, China. *J Virol.* (2012) 86:11935. doi: 10.1128/JVI.01839-12

9. Zhang X, Zhu Y, Zhu X, Chen J, Shi H, Shi D, et al. ORF3a deletion in field strains of porcine-transmissible gastroenteritis virus in China: a hint of association with porcine respiratory coronavirus. *Transbound Emerg Dis.* (2017) 64:698–702. doi: 10.1111/tbed.12634

10. Xia L, Yang YH, Wang JL, Jing YC, Yang Q. Impact of TGEV infection on the pig small intestine. *J Virol.* (2018) 15:102–9. doi: 10.1186/s12985-018-1012-9

11. Vaughn EM, Halbur PG, Paul PS. Sequence comparison of porcine respiratory coronavirus isolates reveals heterogeneity in the S, 3, and 3-1genes. *J Virol.* (1995) 69:3176–84. doi: 10.1128/JVI.69.5.3176-3184.1995

12. Zhang X, Hasoksuz M, Spiro D, Halpin R, Wang S, Stollar S, et al. Complete genomic sequences, a key residue in the spike protein and deletions in nonstructural protein 3b of US strains of the virulent and attenuated coronaviruses, transmissible gastroenteritis virus and porcine respiratory coronavirus. *Virology.* (2007) 358:424–35. doi: 10.1016/j.virol.2006.08.051

13. Sun B, Li MY, Lin SY, Shen GN, Mao RF, Yan ZH, et al. Establishment and application of semi-nest RT-PCR for detection of transmissible gastroenteritis virus. *Chin Vet Sci.* (2020) 50:556–62. doi: 10.16656/j.issn.1673-4696.2020.0062

14. Reed LJ, Muench HA. Simple method of estimating fifty percent Endpoints. *Am J Hygiene.* (1937) 27:493–7. doi: 10.1093/oxfordjournals.aje.a118408

15. Huang B, Jennison A, Whiley D, McMahon J, Hewitson G, Graham R, et al. Illumina sequencing of clinical samples for virus detection in a public health laboratory. *Sci Rep.* (2019) 9:5409. doi: 10.1038/s41598-019-41830-w

16. Tamura K, Stecher G, Peterson D, Filipski A, Kumar S. MEGA6: molecular evolutionary genetics analysis version 6.0. *Mol Biol Evol.* (2013) 30:2725–9. doi: 10.1093/molbev/mst197

17. Burland TG. DNASTAR's Lasergene sequence analysis software. *Methods Mol Biol.* (2000) 132:71–91. doi: 10.1385/1-59259-192-2:71

18. Martin DP, Murrell B, Golden M, Khoosal A, Muhire B. RDP4: detection and analysis of recombination patterns in virus genomes. *Virus Evol.* (2015) 1:vev003. doi: 10.1093/ve/vev003

19. Yuan DW, Yan ZH, Shen GN, Wang Y, Li MY. Establishment of qRT- PCR for detection of transmissible gastroenteritis virus. *Chin J Vet Sci.* (2020) 40:1913–7. doi: 10.16303/j.cnki.1005-4545.2020.10.04

20. Kim B, Chae C. Experimental infection of piglets with transmissible gastroenteritis virus: a comparison of three strains (Korean, Purdue and Miller). *J Comp Pathol.* (2002) 126:30–7. doi: 10.1053/jcpa.2001.0517

21. Hu WW, Yu QH, Zhu LQ, Liu HF, Zhao SS, Gao Q, et al. Complete genomic sequence of the coronavirus transmissible gastroenteritis virus SHXB isolated in China. *Arch Virol.* (2014) 159:2295–302. doi: 10.1007/s00705-014-2080-9

22. Ritchie DB, Foster DA, Woodside MT. Programmed-1 frameshifting efficiency correlates with RNA pseudoknot conformational plasticity, not resistance to mechanical unfolding. *Proc Natl Acad Sci USA.* (2012) 109:16167–72. doi: 10.1073/pnas.1204114109

23. Sola I, Almazan F, Zuniga S, Luis E. Continuous and discontinuous RNA synthesis in coronaviruses. *Annu ReV Virol.* (2015) 2:265–88. doi: 10.1146/annurev-virology-100114-055218

24. Sanchez CM, Gebauer F, Sune C, Mendez A, Dopazo J, Enjuanes L. Genetic evolution and tropism of transmissible gastroenteritis coronaviruses. *Virology.* (1992) 190:92–105. doi: 10.1016/0042-6822(92)91195-Z

25. Penzes Z, Gonzalez JM, Calvo E, Izeta A, Smerdou C, Mendez A, et al. Complete genome sequence of transmissible gastroenteritis coronavirus PUR46-MAD clone and evolution of the purdue virus cluster. *Virus Genes.* (2001) 23:105–18. doi: 10.1023/A:1011147832586

26. Godet M, Grosclaude J, Delmas B, Laude H. Major receptor-binding and neutralization determinants are located within the same domain of the transmissible gastroenteritis virus (coronavirus) spike protein. *J Virol.* (1994) 68:8008–16. doi: 10.1128/JVI.68.12.8008-8016.1994

27. Brian DA, Baric RS. Coronavirus genome structure and replication. *Curr Top Microbiol Immunol.* (2005) 287:1–30. doi: 10.1007/3-540-26765-4_1

28. Sanchez CM, Pascual-Iglesias A, Sola I, Sonia Zuniga S, Enjuanes L. Minimum determinants of transmissible gastroenteritis virus enteric tropism are located in the N-terminus of spike protein. *Pathogens.* (2019) 9:2. doi: 10.3390/pathogens9010002

29. Balint A, Farsang A, Zadori Z, Hornyak A, Dencso L, Almazan F, et al. Molecular characterization of feline infectious peritonitis virus strain DF-2 and studies of the role of ORF3abc in viral cell tropism. *J Virol.* (2012) 86:6258–67. doi: 10.1128/JVI.00189-12

30. Kim L, Hayes J, Lewis P, Parwani AV, Chang KO, Saif LJ. Molecular characterization and pathogenesis of transmissible gastroenteritis coronavirus (TGEV) and porcine respiratory coronavirus (PRCV) field isolates co-circulating in a swine herd. *Arch Virol.* (2000) 145:1133–47. doi: 10.1007/s007050070114

31. Sola I, Alonso S, Zuniga S, Balasch M, Plana-Duran J, Enjuanes L. Engineering the transmissible gastroenteritis virus genome as an expression vector inducing lactogenic immunity. *J Virol.* (2003) 77:4357–69. doi: 10.1128/JVI.77.7.4357-4369.2003

32. Reguera J, Santiago C, Mudgal G, Ordono D, Enjuanes L, Casasnovas JM. Structural bases of coronavirus attachment to host aminopeptidase N and its inhibition by neutralizing antibodies. *PLoS Pathog.* (2012) 8:e1002859. doi: 10.1371/journal.ppat.1002859

33. Sanchez CM, Izeta A, Sanchez-Morgado JM, Alonso S, Sola I, Balasch M, et al. Targeted recombination demonstrates that the spike gene of transmissible gastroenteritis coronavirus is a determinant of its enteric tropism and virulence. *J Virol.* (1999) 73:7607–18. doi: 10.1128/JVI.73.9.7607-7618.1999

14

Application of Volatilome Analysis to the Diagnosis of Mycobacteria Infection in Livestock

Pablo Rodríguez-Hernández[1], Vicente Rodríguez-Estévez[1], Lourdes Arce[2] and
Jaime Gómez-Laguna[3]*

[1] Department of Animal Production, International Agrifood Campus of Excellence (ceiA3), University of Córdoba, Córdoba,
Spain, [2] Department of Analytical Chemistry, Inst Univ Invest Quim Fina and Nanoquim Inst Univ Invest Quim Fina and
Nanoquim (IUNAN), International Agrifood Campus of Excellence (ceiA3), University of Córdoba, Córdoba, Spain,
[3] Department of Anatomy and Comparative Pathology and Toxicology, International Agrifood Campus of Excellence (ceiA3),
University of Córdoba, Córdoba, Spain

*Correspondence:
Jaime Gómez-Laguna
j.gomez-laguna@uco.es

Volatile organic compounds (VOCs) are small molecular mass metabolites which compose the volatilome, whose analysis has been widely employed in different areas. This innovative approach has emerged in research as a diagnostic alternative to different diseases in human and veterinary medicine, which still present constraints regarding analytical and diagnostic sensitivity. Such is the case of the infection by mycobacteria responsible for tuberculosis and paratuberculosis in livestock. Although eradication and control programs have been partly managed with success in many countries worldwide, the often low sensitivity of the current diagnostic techniques against *Mycobacterium bovis* (as well as other mycobacteria from *Mycobacterium tuberculosis* complex) and *Mycobacterium avium* subsp. *paratuberculosis* together with other hurdles such as low mycobacteria loads in samples, a tedious process of microbiological culture, inhibition by many variables, or intermittent shedding of the mycobacteria highlight the importance of evaluating new techniques that open different options and complement the diagnostic paradigm. In this sense, volatilome analysis stands as a potential option because it fulfills part of the mycobacterial diagnosis requirements. The aim of the present review is to compile the information related to the diagnosis of tuberculosis and paratuberculosis in livestock through the analysis of VOCs by using different biological matrices. The analytical techniques used for the evaluation of VOCs are discussed focusing on the advantages and drawbacks offered compared with the routine diagnostic tools. In addition, the differences described in the literature among *in vivo* and *in vitro* assays, natural and experimental infections, and the use of specific VOCs (targeted analysis) and complete VOC pattern (non-targeted analysis) are highlighted. This review emphasizes how this methodology could be useful in the problematic diagnosis of tuberculosis and paratuberculosis in livestock and poses challenges to be addressed in future research.

Keywords: diagnosis, livestock, mycobacteria, volatilome, veterinary

INTRODUCTION

Analysis of volatile organic compounds (VOCs) is an emerging research area in both human and veterinary medicine (1), which allows a non-invasive, fast, and economic diagnosis as well as identification of new biomarkers as alternative to current diagnostic techniques (2). VOCs are defined as a sub-category of small molecular mass substances within metabolites, which are characterized by its low boiling point and high vapor pressure (3, 4). VOCs are produced into the environment, allowing a direct measuring in the gas phase and offering a minimum sample handling, a non-invasive monitoring, and an easier sampling compared with other metabolites which have to be extracted from biological samples (5, 6). In this context, volatilome (or volatome) is the VOCs' signature produced by an organism (7–10).

The volatilome has a wide variety of uses and applications, such as diagnosis of infectious diseases (11) and neoplasia (12), distinction between vaccinated and non-vaccinated animals (13), monitoring of antibiotic treatment (14), differentiation of diet composition (15, 16), and even evaluation of reproductive parameters (17). Because VOCs are constantly emitted during metabolic processes, the detection of VOC profiles might enable the development of novel non-invasive diagnostic tools (7).

The identification of VOCs produced by pathogens, host-pathogen interactions, and biochemical pathways, either associated with homeostasis or pathophysiological responses, has become the volatilome into an approach of growing interest for the diagnosis of infectious diseases (18). Pathologic processes have the capacity to modify VOCs' patterns either by producing new volatile substances or by the metabolic consumption of VOC substrates that are normally present (19). Consequently, the diagnostic approach of VOC analysis provides two perspectives, the search of new biomarkers and the identification of biomarkers lost along a pathological process (1).

Infection of livestock by slow-growing mycobacteria, such as those grouped under *Mycobacterium tuberculosis* complex (MTBC), especially *Mycobacterium bovis*, as well as *M. avium* subsp. *paratuberculosis* (MAP), might take advantage of the development of faster and sensitive diagnostic techniques. Considering the growth requirements of these mycobacteria, as well as other factors associated with the host immune response after infection, diagnosis of mycobacterial infections becomes a challenge, especially in the livestock sector. The diagnosis of the infection by mycobacteria is currently based on different tedious, expensive, laborious, and time-consuming methodologies (20–22). Thus, the analysis of VOCs could be proposed as an innovative strategy to improve the diagnostic field of these infections (**Table 1**) supported by the fact that, historically, people suffering from tuberculosis had a characteristic breath smell (24). The research carried out in this context has used different biological matrices, such as serum (33, 34), breath (34, 35), feces (13, 28), and microbiological culture (36–39) to identify biomarkers related to diseases produced by mycobacteria.

Although the use of VOCs obtained from different biological samples to diagnose diseases is considered as a big hope with a promising future, now it remains at a developing stage (40). One of the main hurdles against the development of this new strategy is the lack of standardization between studies which often leads to non-comparable results (40, 41). Few detailed *in vivo* studies are available on the analysis of VOCs as a diagnostic tool for mycobacterial infection in animals. In light of these premises, the present review collects the available literature from the volatilome approach to evaluate the recent methodologies and procedures used as an attempt of improvement of the diagnosis of infection by mycobacteria in livestock, focusing on the infection by MTBC (*Mycobacterium bovis*) and MAP, to point out future research lines of interest to be implemented.

MYCOBACTERIA TARGET OF STUDY

Mycobacteria belong to the genus *Mycobacterium* which includes the MTBC, with all the causative species of human and mammal tuberculosis; the *M. avium* complex (MAC), which also comprises species of relevance in human and veterinary medicine, such as MAP; as well as environmental rapid and slow-growing non-tuberculous mycobacteria. These all are aerobic and immobile bacilli with specific growing conditions which include pathogenic, opportunistic, and saprophytic species (42, 43). While there are many species, such as *M. tuberculosis* and *M. bovis*, known for being the etiological agents of important human and animal diseases, rapid- and slow-growing non-tuberculous mycobacteria used to be minority species, which should be considered because of their interference with the currently established diagnostic strategies (44).

Mycobacterium tuberculosis Complex (*Mycobacterium bovis*)

MTBC is composed by a broad group of mycobacteria species characterized for its genetic proximity and its pathogenic ability of affecting humans, such as *M. tuberculosis* and *M. africanum*, and a wide variety of wild and domestic animals, such as *M. bovis* and *M. caprae*. *M. bovis* stands out for being the primary etiological agent responsible for bovine tuberculosis (bTB), also considered as the main cause of animal tuberculosis due to the multi-host character of this bacterium (45). Animal tuberculosis is a zoonotic disease with great impact on public health, agriculture, wildlife, and trade areas (20, 46). In this sense, although most cases reported as human tuberculosis are caused by *M. tuberculosis*, ~30% of these cases are related to *M. bovis* infection (zoonotic tuberculosis) (28), especially in developing countries (47) where prevalence of livestock bTB becomes substantial (48–50). Despite huge efforts that are currently focused on the eradication of bTB, there are many difficulties mainly associated with the performance of the different diagnostic techniques as well as with other geographical and epidemiological conditions, which make it very difficult in endemic countries (51). Therefore, zoonotic tuberculosis is often under-reported, emphasizing the importance of providing appropriate diagnostic tools in livestock to reach the eradication of *M. bovis* and reduce zoonotic tuberculosis cases.

TABLE 1 | *In vivo* studies evaluating VOC analysis as a diagnostic tool for mycobacterial infection in animals.

Mycobacteria species and animal species	Matrix	Analytical technique	Kind of infection	Sensitivity	Specificity	References
Mycobacterium bovis						
Cattle	Serum	EN	Experimental	–	–	(23)
Badger	Serum	EN	Natural and experimental	–	–	(23)
Badger	Serum	SIFT-MS	Natural	88%	62%	(24)
Cattle	Exhaled breath	GC-MS EN	Natural	– 100%	– 79%	(25)
Cattle	Exhaled breath	ATD-GC-MS	Experimental	–	–	(26)
Cattle	Exhaled breath	GC-MS	Experimental	83.8–96.4%	97.4–99.2%	(18)
Cattle	Serum	EN	Natural	–	–	(27)
White-tailed deer	Feces	GC-MS	Experimental	78.6%	91.4%	(13)
Cattle	Feces	GC-MS	Experimental	83–100%	100%	(28)
Wild boar	Exhaled breath	GC-MS	Natural	100%	90%	(29)
Wild boar	Feces	GC-MS	Natural	100%	80%	(29)
Mycobacterium avium subsp. *paratuberculosis*						
Cattle	Serum	EN	Natural	–	–	(30)
Goat	Exhaled breath and feces	DMS	Experimental	–	–	(1)
Goat	Exhaled breath and feces	GC-MS	Experimental	–	–	(31)
Goat	Exhaled breath and feces	GC-MS	Experimental	Exhaled breath: 90.3% Feces: 86.6%	Exhaled breath: 81.8% Feces: 85.0%	(32)

ATD-GC-MS, thermal desorption–gas chromatography–mass spectrometry; DMS, differential mobility spectrometry; EN, electronic nose; GC-MS, gas chromatography–mass spectrometry; GC-GC-MS, two-dimensional gas chromatography–mass spectrometry; SIFT-MS, selected ion flow tube mass spectrometry.

Mycobacterium avium subsp. *paratuberculosis*

MAP is the causative agent of paratuberculosis (PTB) or Johne's disease, a chronic infection that affects the small intestine of ruminants resulting in a marked reduction of animal productivity (31) and sometimes in death (1). MAP is also believed to be related to Crohn's disease, a chronic bowel disease in humans, although this fact is yet to be defined (52–54).

The main importance of PTB comes from the great economic losses in animals due to reduced milk and meat yields as well as slaughter value (32). MAP diagnosis becomes a challenge because of its pathogenesis: while the main clinical signs are only present in the late progression of the disease, when the body condition is severely affected, the animals intermittently spread bacteria during a previous subclinical phase. These features result in a low sensitivity of the current direct (fecal culture and genome detection) and indirect (specific antibodies detection) diagnostic methods (55, 56) (**Table 2**). Hence, reliable and complementary diagnostic methodologies are of key importance to enhance the current diagnostic repertoire of techniques focused on the identification of infected animals so as to improve the sensitivity of the diagnosis.

ROUTINE DIAGNOSTIC TECHNIQUES AGAINST MTBC AND *M. avium* SUBSP. *paratuberculosis*

The diagnosis of mycobacterial infection is currently at the center of attention because, although well-established and reliable, it

has its own limitations. Apart from being a tedious process, special consideration must be given to the lack of an optimal diagnostic sensitivity (**Table 2**) and the different variables which may interfere with the methods and techniques in use (2, 21). Therefore, an accurate and reliable diagnostic methodology of the infection by mycobacteria, or a combination of various strategies, is the cornerstone of their control (23).

Current *Ante-mortem* and *Post-mortem* Diagnostic Techniques Against MTBC

Field and *ante-mortem* surveillance tests against MTBC infection are mainly based on the detection of a delayed-type hypersensitivity response to the intradermal skin test (IST) through the inoculation of purified protein derivative from *M. bovis* (bPPD; tuberculin protein), and on quantifying the concentration of gamma interferon (IFN-γ) after culturing blood samples in the presence of tuberculin, in the case of IFN-γ assay test, a supplemental or confirmatory test (25). IST is the OIE prescribed test for international trade and is currently considered as the official diagnostic screening technique in many countries worldwide; it is the primary *ante-mortem* test to support control and eradication programs in different geographical areas (46), responsible for its effectiveness as it is compulsory in the slaughtering of those animals with a positive result (64). In Europe, the aforementioned information is regulated by the Council Directive 64/432/EEC. Although IST and IFN-γ assay have reasonable sensitivity and good specificity (**Table 2**), both techniques require a minimum of 48–72 h to obtain a result 21, 65) besides presenting other disadvantages and limitations. On the one hand, IST requires visiting the farm and restraint

TABLE 2 | Sensitivity and specificity parameters from conventional diagnostic techniques.

Technique	Sensitivity	Specificity	References
Mycobacterium bovis			
Intradermal skin test			
Caudal fold test	68–96.8%	96–98.8%	(46)
Cervical intradermal test	80–91%	75.5–96.8%	(46)
Comparative cervical test	55.1–93.5%	88.8–100%	(46)
Gamma interferon evaluation	74.00%	≥99%	(57)
	73–100%	80–90%	(46)
Microbiological culture	72.9–82.8%	97.1–100.0%	(58)
Serologic assays—ELISA			
From milk samples (MPB70+MPB83)	50.0%	97.5%	(59)‡
From sera samples (recombinant antigen cocktails)	40.6–93.1%	69.7–99.1%	(60)‡
From sera or plasma samples (recombinant antigen cocktails)	62.7–69.5%	97.2–98%	(IDEXX)†,‡
PCR			
IS6110	82.5–92.3%	94.3–99.0%	(58)
MPB70	94.59%	96.03%	(61)
Mycobacterium avium subsp. *paratuberculosis*			
Microbiological culture	23–70%	100%	(62)
Serologic assays—ELISA	7–94%	40–100%	(62)
PCR			
IS900	79.3–91.0%	88.3–93.9%	(63)

†*Mycobacterium bovis antibody test kit, IDEXX Laboratories Inc.*
‡*ELISA results compared with culture or single intradermal comparative cervical test positive and negative status.*

of the animals twice, and a delicate and difficult administration and interpretation of skin results, which may vary due to differences in tuberculin doses, site of application (**Table 2**), and interpretation schemes (25, 27, 66); on the other hand, IFN-γ assay implies a complex laboratory methodology (18), a considerably more expensive price than a skin test (65, 67), and suffers from cross-reactivity with other related mycobacteria resulting in false-positive results (2). In addition, performance of these tests can be compromised by factors associated with the immune response and health status of the animal leading to a misinterpretation of the results. Development and use of a pre-screening test before field tests would be useful to reduce work efforts and diagnostic time (27).

Although microbiological culture is considered the gold-standard approach for the diagnosis of mycobacterial infection, it is characterized by a long incubation time to confirm the presence of mycobacteria (around 8–12 weeks) (2). Furthermore, the isolation of mycobacteria sometimes requires specific compounds such as mycobactin, a siderophore which determines the viability and growth of some mycobacteria species, as is the case of MAP; and, sometimes, additional steps such as decontamination. For all these reasons, culture becomes a tedious and laborious, although necessary, option in *M. bovis* diagnosis.

Other *in vitro* assays, such as serologic assays (ELISA) or PCR, have limitations associated with accuracy and execution that restrict their use (66). While ELISA sensitivity is affected by the delayed and irregular antibodies response in bTB (68), PCR is considered a postmortem diagnostic option with promising

findings but still under development, focused on the search of markers that ensure diagnostic sensitivity (61) (**Table 2**). Therefore, the reliability of these tests depends on the stage of infection and, in addition, these require transporting of animal samples to the laboratory, which finally increases diagnostic time too (40), highlighting the interest on the availability of portable equipment.

Current *Ante-mortem* and *Post-mortem* Diagnostic Techniques Against *M. avium* subsp. *paratuberculosis*

The intermittent and sometimes low shedding of the mycobacteria as well as the irregular seroconversion in the subclinical phase of PTB (69, 70) gives a limited sensitivity to the *in vivo* diagnosis (32), currently based on serological assays (ELISA) and PCR from feces. Although ELISA has a limited sensitivity (**Table 2**), the irregular spread of bacteria *via* feces has raised serology as the most common technique used for the monitoring of PTB (71) due to its cheap and easy use. In addition, fecal shedding and immune response vary individually to a large extent (72). For example, the sensitivity of PCR methods can be affected by the variable bacterial load in samples and the co-purification of PCR inhibitors during DNA extraction (73). Therefore, and although the current combination between serology, vaccination (when regulation allows this option due to its possible interference on bTB eradication campaigns), and slaughtering constitutes a strategy with remarkable effectiveness, there is a need for diagnostic tests with higher sensitivity and decreased processing time to reduce false-negative results and enable effective disease control strategies, as different authors have highlighted before (31, 32). Volatilome evaluation has been capable of discriminating MAP infection before clinical illness occurs, offering an early diagnosis and significant time savings (1). This could be considered as one of the main advantages against the current techniques in use.

In short, against the current situation, it would be of help to have an *ante-mortem* diagnostic methodology capable of detecting mycobacterial infection with repeatability, a good quality/price ratio, high sensitivity and specificity, and rapid detection and obtaining of results. VOC strategy could be a complementary option because it mostly fulfills these requirements, and it has been successfully used for mycobacterial diagnosis in many animal species (**Table 3**). In this sense, an initial approximation analyzing stable air as matrix has been proposed to evaluate MAP infection in cattle (74); however, due to the low number of infected animals included within each infected group, further studies are required to confirm the suitability of this approach.

IMPACT OF THE EXPERIMENTAL SETTING ON THE VOCs PROFILE

In vitro vs. *in vivo* Studies

Analysis of VOCs as a diagnostic option for mycobacterial disease has been evaluated both *in vivo* and *in vitro*. Compared with *in vivo* assays, the large number of existing *in vitro* studies, which basically consist in mycobacteria culturing, reveals the early stage of development where this research area stands (36–38, 75, 76). The reviewed literature in the present study suggests some drawbacks related to those *in vitro* studies.

First, mycobacteria growth, which as aforementioned requires several weeks or even months, is required to identify changes in the analysis of VOCs from microbiological culture to allow the distinction between negative and positive samples. In other words, although *in vitro* experiments can detect VOC changes related to different stages of the mycobacteria growth (76, 77), it still takes a long time to identify these changes, which is one of the main disadvantages linked to the current diagnostic methodology. Accordingly, researchers point to reduce the diagnostic time by avoiding the limiting step of culturing and suggesting other innovative techniques such as VOC measurement directly *in vivo* (32).

It is also important to highlight the low correlation existing between results obtained from cultured bacteria compared with those VOCs produced from other biological samples studied in *in vivo* experiments (40). For example, (32) detected two compounds only present above MAP cultures which were ranked among the top discriminating VOCs in their statistical analysis. However, in the comparison with their *in vivo* results, these two compounds tended to be in lower concentration in MAP-inoculated animals compared with non-inoculated animals. This situation emphasizes the caution required when adopting *in vitro* findings to *in vivo* conditions since the influence from the host, its microbiome and host–microbiome interactions

(78), as well as the influence from environmental factors, such as diet, age, or drug use (40), needs to be considered. In addition, another hurdle of the *in vitro* settings is related to the different VOC profiles obtained depending on the substrate where the mycobacteria grow resulting in inconclusive findings (79).

The effectiveness of *in vivo* approach is supported by the results of many studies where VOCs from biological samples have been used to distinguish between infected animals with different mycobacteria species and non-infected animals (1, 18, 31, 80). Many different biological matrices such as serum, breath, or feces have been studied as a source of information for VOC analysis in this field, existing great differences between their nature and characteristics. This constitutes another problem in the comparison between *in vitro* vs. *in vivo* experiments, giving inconsistent results. When (31) compared *in vivo* results obtained from feces and breath samples with the *in vitro* VOC profiles obtained from different MAP strains' culture by (77), their conclusions were not very clarifying: from more than 100 substances detected in feces and breath, only 15 and 5 of them, respectively, were found in the bacterial *in vitro* pattern.

Experimental vs. Natural Infection

Another variable to consider when evaluating VOCs as an option for mycobacterial diagnosis in animals is the type of infection: natural or experimental. Although experimental infections are logically the most common and easy option for this kind of approximation, studies in naturally infected animals are of paramount importance. Experimental infections allow controlling different environmental conditions that may impact on the results, being the most studied option in the analysis of VOCs for mycobacterial diagnosis (**Table 1**). However, assays with natural infections are needed to validate the results obtained from any new diagnostic tool, such as volatilome analysis, in experimental settings. Along this review, only a single article has been found to include the analysis of VOCs from both experimentally and naturally infected animals (23). These researchers found that differences between negative and positive animals were more pronounced in the natural infection group than in the experimentally infected one. This fact highlights the importance of performing studies in field conditions in the future to compare with those with experimentally infected animals and to validate the results from the latter ones.

SPECIES UNDER STUDY

The analysis of VOCs has been used in many species for the diagnosis of mycobacterial infection. Livestock species are the most frequent ones, probably because of the importance and repercussion of bTB and PTB for farm animals. As expected, bovine is the most studied animal model with this innovative approach, followed by goats (**Table 1**). Our findings are consistent with the wide variety of diseases that have been tested through this methodology in cattle, such as bovine respiratory disease (11), mastitis (81), brucellosis (30), ketosis (82), or ketoacidosis (83, 84).

TABLE 3 | VOCs related to mycobacterial infection in different animal species (targeted analysis).

Mycobacteria species	Potential discriminatory compounds or type of compounds	Animal species	Matrix	Analytical technique	References
Mycobacterium bovis	2,3-Dimethyl, 1,3- pentadiene 1,3-Dimethylbutyl cyclohexane	Cattle	Exhaled breath	GC-MS	(25)
Mycobacterium bovis	>100 compounds (acetone, dimethyl sulfide, and 2-butanone as the most abundant)	Cattle	Exhaled breath	ATD-GC-MS	(26)
Mycobacterium bovis	4-Hydroxy-4-methyl-2-pentanone Benzaldehyde 1-Ethyl-2-pyrrolidinone α, α-Dimethyl-benzenemethanol **Nonanal**	Cattle (1 year old)	Exhaled breath	GC-MS	(18)
Mycobacterium bovis	Methylbenzene **Hexanal** 2-Methyl pyridine 2,4-Dimethyl pyridine 2-(1,1-Dimethoxy)-ethanol[†] **2-Ethyl-1-hexanol** Benzene acetaldehyde 3,7-Dimethyl-6-octenyl-(2E)-2-butanoate Acetophenone[†] 4-Methyl-phenol 2-Decanone[†] (–)-Beta-fenchol 1-Decanol **Indole** 3-(1,1-Dimethylethyl)-4-methoxy-phenol 1-Octadecanol 2-Dodecanone	White-tailed deer (12–18 months old)	Feces	GC-MS	(13)
Mycobacterium bovis	Thioether Thiophene Aldehyde Organosulfur (sulfone) Imine Pyridine derivative Amino acid Ketone Alcohol **Indole** Diterpenoid alkane Fatty acyl (amino acid derivative) Diterpene alcohol Dicarboxylic acid and derivative	Cattle (120–121 days old)	Feces	GC-MS	(28)

Mycobacterium bovis	Adult animals (>2 years):
	  O-Cymene
	Juvenile animals (<12 months):
	  Acetic acid, methyl ester
	  3-Methylpentane
	  Trichloromethane
	  α-Methylstyrene
	  Decane
	  4,6,8-Trimethyl-1-nonene
	  1,3-Bis(1,1-dimethylethyl)-benzene
	  2,5-Dimethylhexane-2,5-dihydroperoxide
	  2,5-Bis(1,1-dimethylethyl)-phenol
	  Heptacosane
	  5-Butyl-5-ethylheptadecane
	  11-Decyl-tetracosane
	  11-(1-Ethylpropyl)-heneicosane
	  3-Ethyl-5-(2-ethylbutyl)-octadecane
		Wild boar (juveniles, sub-adults, adults)	Exhaled breath	GC-MS	(29)

Mycobacterium bovis	Sub-adult animals (12–24 months): 10,18-Bisnorabieta-8,11,13-triene Juvenile animals (<12 months):	Wild boar (juveniles, sub-adults, adults)	Feces	GC-MS	(29)

TABLE 3 | Continued

Mycobacteria species	Potential discriminatory compounds or type of compounds	Animal species	Matrix	Analytical technique	References
	Acetone Toluene 2,6-Bis(1,1-dimethylethyl)-4-(1-methylpropyl)-phenol				
Mycobacterium avium subsp. *paratuberculosis*	1-Propanol **2-Butanone** **Acetone** Benzene 2-Methyl-butanal Ethylbenzene **Hexanal** **Nonanal** Styrene	Goat (21–55 weeks old)	Exhaled breath	GC-MS	(31)
Mycobacterium avium subsp. *paratuberculosis*	Pentane Hexane Heptane **Acetone** **2-Butanone** 2-Pentanone 2-Hexanone 2-Heptanone 3-Octanone 3-Methyl-2-butanone 3-Methyl-2-pentatone Methyl isobutyl ketone Isoprene **Methyl acetate** Dimethyl sulfide Dimethyl disulfide Furan 2-Ethylfuran 2-Methylfuran **3-Methylfuran** 2-Pentylfuran	Goat (21–55 weeks old)	Feces	GC-MS	(31)
Mycobacterium avium subsp. *paratuberculosis*	45 compounds. Top-3 (random-forest): **3-Methylfuran** 2,3-Butanedione **Methyl acetate**	Goat (2–3 weeks old)	Feces	GC-MS	(32)
Mycobacterium avium subsp. *paratuberculosis*	51 compounds. Top-3 (random-forest): **3-Methylpentane** **2-Ethyl-1-hexanol** 2-Methylpentane	Goat (2–3 weeks old)	Exhaled breath	GC-MS	(32)

ATD-GC-MS, thermal desorption–gas chromatography–mass spectrometry; GC-MS, gas chromatography–mass spectrometry; GC-GC-MS, two-dimensional gas chromatography–mass spectrometry.

[†]*Statistically significant trends identified for vaccinated and infected animals but not in non-vaccinated and infected animals.*

Consistent compounds between different assays are highlighted in bold.

Remarkably, diagnosis through volatilome has been also performed in wildlife, more specifically in deer (13), badger (23, 24), and recently in wild boar (29), with much effort put into the development of a better disease surveillance methodology on these species. Among laboratory animals, although outside the scope of this review, non-human primates have been used to study the mycobacteria species which usually affect humans, *M. tuberculosis* (80, 85), as well as the murine model, which has been also employed to assess the use of breath for mycobacterial infection (41).

The encouraging results obtained in these studies with different animal species highlight the great potential of this methodology in MTBC and MAP diagnosis. However, there is a lack of studies in other species of interest, such as the pig, an animal model with an increasing interest in biomedical research (86). Furthermore, the marked differences that exist among different animal species make feasible that different approaches may be necessary for each species. This review highlights the starting point where this new diagnostic approach stands and the necessity of further studies and research before its setting up as an alternative routine or field technique.

BIOLOGICAL MATRICES

VOCs can be detected directly from different biological samples such as blood, serum, breath, feces, sweat, skin, urine, or vaginal fluids (13, 27, 87–89), opening up huge opportunities for this new diagnostic methodology. Although samples should be initially selected according to the disease and the pathogenesis of the agent, there are multiple options that allow collection of alternative samples. For example, the predominantly respiratory character of bTB would place exhaled breath as the most appropriate sample to study this disease. However, there are studies that show interesting results for the analysis of VOCs from *M. bovis*-infected animals using different biological matrices such as feces (13, 28) or serum (24, 27). A similar situation occurs with PTB. MAP is a mycobacteria characterized by causing digestive disorders, making feasible to find these alterations directly reflected in the fecal volatilome. Despite of this, exhaled breath (1, 31, 32) and serum (30) have given promising findings in different animal species.

The rationale for analyzing exhaled breath in a model of chronic intestinal infection or feces in a primarily respiratory disease is based on the hypothesis that they do not only contain substances originated from the airways or from the digestive system. These also contain metabolites released *via* the lung or the intestine but originated and related to the whole metabolic or health state of the subject (1).

The three most used biological samples for VOC analysis of mycobacterial diseases in animals are exhaled breath, serum, and feces (**Table 1**).

Exhaled Breath

The principle of using exhaled breath lies in its capability for discerning disease-related changes and biomarkers in the organism that are reflected into the breath through exchange *via* the lungs (25), because of its ability to cross the alveolar membranes before being exhaled (26). The use of exhaled breath offers several advantages because it is a non-invasive sample produced in ample supply, having the potential for direct, inexpensive, and eventually real-time monitoring (25, 90). Although in the literature it is considered as a sample that is relatively easy to obtain, its sampling methodology in animals is diverse, revealing a lack of standardization: from modified equine nebulization masks or nostril samplers for cattle, specific ventilators for mice or intubation for macaques, to automated alveolar sampling devices for goats. Furthermore, some factors can affect the sampling methodology, such as eructation in ruminants, which has been shown to significantly affect exhaled VOC profile (91). VOCs from breath are normally concentrated to sorbent materials, such as Tenax or Carbopack Y, Carbopack X, and Carboxen 1000 (18, 80), which simplify its transport and storage, and later these are used to quantify and evaluate the volatile substances with different analytical techniques.

Healthy and diseased animals have been successfully distinguished in mycobacterial infections by identifying volatile molecules in exhaled breath (**Table 3**). (18) performed breath collection and analysis in *M. bovis*-inoculated cattle with two strains obtaining good sensitivity and specificity: 83.8–96.4% and 97.4–99.2%, respectively, using the microbiological culture as reference technique. In addition, (25) reported the measurement of two VOCs from breath linked with *M. bovis* infection and other two VOCs associated with samples from negative individuals, obtaining sensitivity and specificity values of 100 and 79%, respectively.

The studies included in this revision evaluating exhaled breath in the context of mycobacteria infection highlight some important variables to be considered (41). The use of different animal species models, the *Mycobacterium* species and strain used, the infection phase, the breath volume collected, and the sorbent phases used to concentrate VOCs are factors that often differ between the existing assays. Considering all the aforementioned information, a comparison between the existing results is a challenge.

Feces

Feces are regarded as the most accessible sample for research (92). Considering that feces constitute the main media for eliminating metabolic products, these are an important source of information about the internal homeostasis (17). The reason for testing changes in VOCs in feces is based on the common assumption that any abnormality in the activity or composition of the intestinal microbiota and in the whole organism may alter the odor of this matrix (1), which is supported by studies from both human (93–96) and animal medicine (97–100). Consequently, examination of volatile fecal emission could be a very useful non-invasive diagnostic approach (1).

However, as a remarkable fraction of VOCs found in feces is generated by gut commensal microbiota (101), a well-matched control group and knowledge on these bacteria are necessary to identify VOC patterns of pathogenic conditions (31). Despite this shortcoming, using feces as matrix has many advantages; besides an easier sampling, it is not necessary to restrain the animals, eliminating the stressful situation that it implies. Moreover, and in contrast with human medicine, feces offer many different possibilities in terms of sampling protocol: per rectum, after sacrifice, using laboratory animal cages, or just after defecation are some options in veterinary research. The studies using feces reviewed in the present work highlight the existing heterogeneity between the published results (**Tables 1, 2**). However, the obtained results have placed fecal volatilome analysis as an innovative diagnostic approach in the current research context for mycobacterial infections. In this sense, attention has been focused not only on the discrimination between infected and healthy individuals (1, 13, 31, 32) but also in the use of fecal VOC profile for other purposes, such as identification of vaccinated animals in white-tailed deer (13) and cattle (28).

Serum

Serum is the sample of choice in many studies because of its relative ease to obtain and store, and safe distribution (24). Blood or serum is the means of transport of many different substances, compounds, and markers through the organism, existing a complex exchange with the lung or the intestine, among other systems (102). Alterations in VOCs from serum can be detected when a disease, an infection, or a pathologic condition occurs (103).

Serum has been used to distinguish the infection by *M. bovis* or MAP in different animal species through volatilome evaluation (**Table 3**) obtaining very interesting results. For example (30), were able to discriminate MAP and *Brucella* spp. infection in cattle through VOC analysis; and (27) reported an analyzing time of only 20 min to differentiate between bTB-infected and bTB-free bovine sera. However, and although blood and serum could be the most routine samples used in diagnostic field, its collection supposes a stressful situation as it is an invasive method that requires individual immobilization.

In conclusion, three different biological samples have been discussed as source of information in mycobacterial diagnosis in animals through volatilome analysis. Although interesting and useful findings have been shown, there is still a lack of homogeneity among many different study conditions. This often leads to non-comparable and inconsistent results. For example, despite studying the same pathogen (MAP), and using the same biological samples (exhaled breath and feces) and animal species (goats), contradictory conclusions can be found in the literature: while some showed that differences in VOC profiles were less pronounced from breath than those obtained in feces (31, 32), others suggest that volatilome evaluation from exhaled breath might be superior compared with the one from feces (1). In fact, the researchers usually acknowledge that their hypotheses should be verified by future studies, considering their findings as starting points (1, 32). Hence, no reliable comparisons or conclusions can be made with the available information, being advisable to carry out studies where the biological matrices are used simultaneously with the same methodological conditions.

INSTRUMENTAL TECHNIQUES

Some analytical instrumentation techniques allow VOC evaluation. Although gas chromatography with mass spectrometry (GC-MS) is referred very often as the "gold standard" for VOC analysis (104, 105), selected ion flow tube–mass spectrometry (SIFT-MS), proton transfer reaction mass spectrometry (PTR-MS), and secondary electrospray ionization mass spectrometry (SESI-MS) are other mass spectrometry–based options available for bacterial VOC analysis (40). Moreover, various types of ion mobility spectrometers (IMS), such as classical time of flight IMS (IMS-ToF), aspiration IMS (a-IMS), differential mobility spectrometers (DMS), field-asymmetric wave IMS (FAIMS), or multi-capillary column IMS-ToF (MCC-IMS-ToF) have been successfully used in identification of bacterial VOCs as well (22).

In the present review, different analytical techniques have been evaluated to assess VOCs as a diagnostic methodology for mycobacterial infection in animals (**Table 3**): different GC-MS modalities, various electronic nose (EN) models, and DMS, being the first two options by far the most frequent approaches. In this

sense, as other researchers have previously indicated, the diverse methods of VOC collection and analytical systems that have been used are likely to have contributed to the results' variability (18). Supporting this context, each analytical method offers both advantages and limitations.

Gas Chromatography Coupled to Mass Spectrometry

GC-MS has become one of the most preferred options for marker identification of bacterial origin with a very good sensitivity (40). It has a huge potential for both identification and quantification of unknown VOCs from complex matrices (106, 107). Ellis et al. (18) found that 4-hydroxy-4-methyl-2-pentanone, benzaldehyde, 1-ethyl-2-pyrrolidinone, α,α-dimethyl-benzenemethanol, and nonanal were present in significantly greater concentration in *M. bovis*–infected animals than in control ones. Moreover, Bergmann et al. (31) found 16 and 3 VOCs in feces and breath, respectively, which provide detectable differences at any infection time between MAP-inoculated and non-inoculated animals. GC-MS has the capacity of detecting VOCs within a range of parts per billion range, or lower, with good reproducibility and linearity (22, 25). In other words, GC-MS not only seems to be the most suitable for bacterial biomarkers search; in fact, it is the most used technique to diagnose these infections (40). The present review highlights the usefulness of GC-MS as an analytic tool to evaluate VOC changes due to mycobacteria infection employing different biological samples such as exhaled breath or feces (**Table 3**).

In spite of these many advantages, GC-MS has also several drawbacks: most GC-MS equipment are still not implemented as a portable tool; it requires high levels of expertise, qualified personnel, and pre-concentration techniques; and it is currently an expensive instrumentation (40). Therefore, given the aforementioned cons and the significant sampling and analysis time that it implies, GC-MS is not suitable for being used in end-user or point-of-care sites (25, 40).

It is also worth mentioning that comprehensive two-dimensional GC-MS (GCxGC-MS) stands out for the possibility of analyzing VOCs coming from complex matrices (40) and for providing a more complex and unparalleled separation as well as three-dimensional chromatograms' visualization (108).

Electronic Nose

The electronic nose (EN) is an instrument based on chemical sensors combined with a pattern recognition system (109), able to detect different VOCs, such as odors, flavors, and vapors (110, 111). The main advantages of this methodology are the ease of use, its low price, and the rapid analysis time (27). Furthermore, EN methodology avoids sample transport to laboratory, positioning itself as one of the optimal techniques for pen-side use (27). However, it has problems with background separation, it does not identify substances detected, and sometimes its detection limit is high, giving insufficient sensitivity (31, 112).

The huge variety of applications where EN has shown effectiveness could be also considered as another of its strengths: versatility. In this sense, the reviewed information reveals the applicability of many types of EN sensors for different species of mycobacteria diagnosis through VOC identification (**Table 3**). Despite the good and interesting results obtained, the ease of transport of this device has not been exploited in depth because most studies using EN has analyzed VOCs from serum (**Table 3**) and not from other types of samples, such as feces or exhaled breath. The aforementioned information enhances the importance of carrying out future studies using EN focused on non-invasive biological matrices which would permit to develop a portable tool. In this sense (25), used their GC-MS results to tailor an artificial olfactory system to detect bTB in cattle exhaled breath. Although their new system successfully identified all infected animals (100% sensitivity), it wrongly classified 21% of the non-infected individuals (79% specificity).

Other Minor Techniques

DMS is an IMS modality that has been occasionally used for volatilome assessment in mycobacterial infections (**Table 3**). This instrumentation has a lower cost, and it can be used alone or coupled with a GC column which acts as a pre-separation stage (40). Its relatively low price, robustness, reliability, and miniaturization turn IMS technology into one of the potential alternatives for portable VOC analysis in disease diagnosis (40). As with EN, one of its main drawbacks is its lack of capacity to identify specific VOCs (1). This analytical device used by (1) permitted to discriminate healthy from MAP-infected goats, noting a direct correlation among postmortem findings and *in vivo* measurements.

SIFT-MS is a quantitative technique for trace gas analysis based on the ionization of these volatile compounds by positive precursor ions along a flow tube. Although its main advantages are a rapid analysis time and a lower mass range, biological samples usually provide complex data which need computational assistance to be analyzed (24). Spooner et al. (24) applied multivariate analysis for the first time to SIFT-MS data to evaluate serum headspace analysis as a faster screening tool for *M. bovis* infection in badgers, obtaining a much faster diagnosis. However, the insufficient accuracy achieved (88% of true positive and 38% of false positive) makes this approach unsuitable as an alternative for conventional diagnostic techniques.

The existing differences between the reviewed analytical techniques suggest the importance of using methodologies, such as GC-MS, as a first-line analysis, with the objective to identify and define tentative biomarkers. Then, other approaches, such as IMS or EN, could be developed and adapted to a field or point-of-care use.

TARGETED ANALYSIS VS. NON-TARGETED ANALYSIS

The diagnosis of an infection using VOC analysis can be reached by identifying specific substances related to the pathologic process or by detecting significant alterations in the whole VOC profile. Most of the research has attempted to isolate unique VOC biomarkers (targeted analysis) (**Table 3**) that would indicate the presence of mycobacterial infection, with little work done

investigating potential changes within the whole VOC profile (non-targeted analysis).

There are VOCs that can be present in many different situations, hampering to find a specific substance for a particular infection or process. This is the case of methyl-nicotinate, a compound that, although it is proposed as a *M. tuberculosis* biomarker (28), can be found in the breath of non-tuberculous smokers (113); it is used as a flavoring ingredient, and it is present in coffee, various nuts, alcoholic beverages, and fruits (114, 115). In this sense, although tentative biomarkers have been associated with mycobacterial infection in both human (35, 37, 116, 117) and veterinary medicine (**Table 3**), the influence of different factors as well as the dynamic character of volatilome makes the identification of indicative or unique VOCs difficult (28). According to the literature, these factors may be related to host biological variables, environmental conditions, symbiotic and infectious microbe–host interactions, pathophysiological responses, the method of sample collection, and differences in analytical methods used for sample analysis (30, 85, 89). The bias induced by these factors is exemplified by the comparison of two studies which aimed to use exhaled breath VOCs as a source of information to diagnose *M. bovis* infection in cattle (18, 25); using the same animal species, pathogen, and biological sample, only two VOCs were consistent between both studies, highlighting the challenge that this approach supposes. However, along the present review, several VOCs have been pointed out due to its frequency and consistency between the included studies (**Table 3**); while nonanal, hexanal, 2-ethyl-1-hexanol, acetone, and 3-methylpentane were found to be present in both *M. bovis* and MAP infection, there were also compounds indicative of single infection. This is the case of indole, for *M. bovis*, and 2-butanone, methyl acetate, and 3-methylfuran for MAP, molecules that could be postulated as candidates for the discrimination between MTBC and MAP processes. The aforementioned VOCs were found to be consistent between different studies (13, 18, 28, 29, 31, 32), matrices (feces and exhaled breath), and animal species (cattle, goat, deer, and wild boar), which opens up a huge opportunity to use this approach as a diagnostic option for general mycobacterial infections and specific infections as well. Nonetheless, there is still no specific biomarker for mycobacterial infections, being priority to develop analytical methods adapted to volatilome characteristics which allow adequate identification and quantification of these molecules.

On the other hand, there are already studies in the literature which have used the entire VOC profile (non-targeted analysis) to successfully discriminate between diseased and non-infected animals (28). In this way, many research groups have highlighted the importance of considering the entire profile of VOCs released by specific pathogens and how these profiles can help discriminating between infecting pathogens, rather than relying on a limited number of biomarkers (targeted analysis) (118). However, non-targeted analysis does not identify compounds, making not feasible to gather information about the source of these compounds. In addition, other factors, such as feeding, environmental conditions, or metabolic variables, need to be fixed to draw conclusions from the results obtained using this methodology. In this sense, non-targeted analyses by EN or

DMS (1, 23, 27, 30), although showing volatilome potential, make difficult the comparison with other studies, underlining the importance of a proper VOC identification and quantification to obtain consistent results.

CONCLUDING REMARKS AND FUTURE PROSPECTS

In conclusion, although currently there is an important research trend that evidences the potential of VOCs emitted in mycobacterial infections in animals as a diagnostic tool, it is still in an initial phase and presents some difficulties. The number of *in vivo* assays which study the implementation of the analysis of VOCs for mycobacterial diagnosis in animal research is considered scarce. Furthermore, considering the lack of standardization, the dynamic nature of volatilome, the drawbacks and differences in the current methodology, and the use of biological matrices, inconsistent and non-comparable results are usually obtained. Thus, no singular biomarkers indicative of mycobacterial infections have been described to date. The high number of research groups that have studied this new approach worldwide contributes to the lack of standardization because they usually use different protocols, a reason that makes more difficult to reproduce their results.

In the authors' view, volatilome analysis is considered an innovative approach which is likely to become of interest as a complementary tool for current diagnostic methods; this approach is not presented as an alternative, at least to date,

but it is considered a strategy that could offer significant and complementary advances. Although the strategies based on IST and serology have partly succeeded for control and eradication campaigns of MTBC and MAP, respectively, volatilome features could allow the development of an *ante-mortem*, portable, and non-invasive technique, possibly used as a field screening method able to improve sensitivity and specificity parameters as the collected data highlight (**Table 2**). In addition, the possibility of discrimination of highly related mycobacteria infections and the detection of infected subclinical animals stand as major ambitions. Further and thorough studies using several biological matrices with constant *in vivo* conditions are required to obtain robust results as well as reliable comparisons and check the consistency of this methodology between different assays before its implementation at field level. Against the previously described background, the development of analytical tools to obtain useful and robust information about potential VOC marker identification and quantification is considered of paramount importance. This will open new and complementary possibilities in the questioned diagnosis of mycobacterial infection and help to overcome the described drawbacks in the present revision.

AUTHOR CONTRIBUTIONS

JG-L and PR-H conceived and designed the review. PR-H analyzed the data and wrote the manuscript. JG-L, VR-E, and LA revised the manuscript. All authors read and approved the final manuscript.

REFERENCES

1. Purkhart R, Kohler H, Liebler-Tenorio E, Meyer M, Becher G, Kikowatz A, et al. Chronic intestinal Mycobacteria infection: discrimination *via* VOC analysis in exhaled breath and headspace of feces using differential ion mobility spectrometry. *J Breath Res.* (2011) 5:10. doi: 10.1088/1752-7155/5/2/027103
2. Maurer DL, Ellis CK, Thacker TC, Rice S, Koziel JA, Nol P, et al. Screening of microbial volatile organic compounds for detection of disease in cattle: development of lab-scale method. *Sci Rep.* (2019) 9:14. doi: 10.1038/s41598-019-47907-w
3. Ebert BE, Halbfeld C, Blank LM. Exploration and exploitation of the yeast volatilome. *Curr Metabol.* (2017) 5:102–18. doi: 10.2174/2213235X04666160818151119
4. Rioseras AT, Gomez DG, Ebert BE, Blank LM, Ibanez AJ, Sinues PML. Comprehensive real-time analysis of the yeast volatilome. *Sci Rep.* (2017) 7:9. doi: 10.1038/s41598-017-14554-y
5. Singh KD, del Miguel GV, Gaugg MT, Ibanez AJ, Zenobi R, Kohler M, et al. Translating secondary electrospray ionization-high-resolution mass spectrometry to the clinical environment. *J Breath Res.* (2018) 12:10. doi: 10.1088/1752-7163/aa9ee3
6. Sinha R, Khot LR, Schroeder BK, Si YS. Rapid and non-destructive detection of *Pectobacterium carotovorum* causing soft rot in stored potatoes through volatile biomarkers sensing. *Crop Protect.* (2017) 93:122–31. doi: 10.1016/j.cropro.2016.11.028
7. Amann A, Costello B, Miekisch W, Schubert J, Buszewski B, Pleil J, et al. The human volatilome: volatile organic compounds (VOCs) in exhaled breath, skin emanations, urine, feces and saliva. *J Breath Res.* (2014) 8:17. doi: 10.1088/1752-7155/8/3/034001
8. Filipiak W, Mochalski P, Filipiak A, Ager C, Cumeras R,

Davis CE, et al. A compendium of volatile organic compounds (VOCs) released by human cell lines. *Curr Med Chem.* (2016) 23:2112–31. doi: 10.2174/0929867323666160510122913
9. Heddergott C, Calvo AM, Latge JP. The volatome of *Aspergillus fumigatus*. *Eukaryotic Cell.* (2014) 13:1014–25. doi: 10.1128/EC.00074-14
10. Phillips M, Cataneo RN, Chaturvedi A, Kaplan PD, Libardoni M, Mundada M, et al. Detection of an extended human volatome with comprehensive two-dimensional gas chromatography time-of-flight mass spectrometry. *PLoS ONE.* (2013) 8:8. doi: 10.1371/journal.pone.0075274
11. Burciaga-Robles LO, Holland BP, Step DL, Krehbiel CR, McMillen GL, Richards CJ, et al. Evaluation of breath biomarkers and serum haptoglobin concentration for diagnosis of bovine respiratory disease in heifers newly arrived at a feedlot. *Am J Vet Res.* (2009) 70:1291–8. doi: 10.2460/ajvr.70.10.1291
12. Sever A, Abd Elkadir A, Matana Y, Gopas J, Zeiri Y. Biomarkers for detection and monitoring of B16 melanoma in mouse urine and feces. *J Biomarkers.* (2015) 2015:841245. doi: 10.1155/2015/841245
13. Stahl RS, Ellis CK, Nol P, Waters WR, Palmer M, VerCauteren KC. Fecal volatile organic ccompound profiles from white-tailed deer (*Odocoileus virginianus*) as indicators of *Mycobacterium bovis* exposure or *Mycobacterium bovis* Bacille Calmette-Guerin (BCG) vaccination. *PLoS ONE.* (2015) 10:20. doi: 10.1371/journal.pone.0129740
14. Berendsen BJA, Wegh RS, Memelink J, Zuidema T, Stolker LAM. The analysis of animal faeces as a tool to monitor antibiotic usage. *Talanta.* (2015) 132:258–68. doi: 10.1016/j.talanta.2014.09.022
15. Perez-Calvo E, Wicaksono AN, Canet E, Daulton E, Ens W, Hoeller U, et al. The measurement of volatile organic compounds in faeces of piglets as a tool to assess gastrointestinal functionality. *Biosyst Eng.* (2019) 184:122–9. doi: 10.1016/j.biosystemseng.2019.06.005
16. Recharla N, Kim K, Park J, Jeong J, Jeong Y, Lee H, et al. Effects

of amino acid composition in pig diet on odorous compounds and microbial characteristics of swine excreta. *J Anim Sci Technol.* (2017) 59:8. doi: 10.1186/s40781-017-0153-5

17. Karthikeyan K, Muniasamy S, SankarGanesh D, Achiraman S, Saravanakumar VR, Archunan G. Faecal chemical cues in water buffalo that facilitate estrus detection. *Anim Reproduct Sci.* (2013) 138:163–7. doi: 10.1016/j.anireprosci.2013.02.017

18. Ellis CK, Stahl RS, Nol P, Waters WR, Palmer MV, Rhyan JC, et al. A pilot study exploring the use of breath analysis to differentiate healthy cattle from cattle experimentally infected with *Mycobacterium bovis. PLoS ONE.* (2014) 9:12. doi: 10.1371/journal.pone.0089280

19. Probert CSJ, Ahmed I, Khalid T, Johnson E, Smith S, Ratcliffe N. Volatile organic compounds as diagnostic biomarkers in gastrointestinal and liver diseases. *J Gastrointestin Liver Dis.* (2009) 18:337–43.

20. Biet F, Boschiroli ML, Thorel MF, Guilloteau LA. Zoonotic aspects of *Mycobacterium bovis* and *Mycobacterium avium*-intracellulare complex (MAC). *Vet Res.* (2005) 36:411–36. doi: 10.1051/vetres:2005001

21. Nienhaus A, Schablon A, Costa JT, Diel R. Systematic review of cost and cost-effectiveness of different TB-screening strategies. *BMC Health Services Res.* (2011) 11:10. doi: 10.1186/1472-6963-11-247

22. Ratiu IA, Ligor T, Bocos-Bintintan V, Buszewski B. Mass spectrometric techniques for the analysis of volatile organic compounds emitted from bacteria. *Bioanalysis.* (2017) 9:1069–92. doi: 10.4155/bio-2017-0051

23. Fend R, Geddes R, Lesellier S, Vordermeier HM, Corner LAL, Gormley E, et al. Use of an electronic nose to diagnose *Mycobacterium bovis* infection in badgers and cattle. *J Clin Microbiol.* (2005) 43:1745–51. doi: 10.1128/JCM.43.4.1745-1751.2005

24. Spooner AD, Bessant C, Turner C, Knobloch H, Chambers M. Evaluation of a combination of SIFT-MS and multivariate data analysis for the diagnosis of *Mycobacterium bovis* in wild badgers. *Analyst.* (2009) 134:1922–7. doi: 10.1039/b905627k

25. Peled N, Ionescu R, Nol P, Barash O, McCollum M, VerCauteren K, et al. Detection of volatile organic compounds in cattle naturally infected with *Mycobacterium bovis. Sens Actuat B Chemical.* (2012) 171:588–94. doi: 10.1016/j.snb.2012.05.038

26. Turner C, Knobloch H, Richards J, Richards P, Mottram TTF, Marlin D, et al. Development of a device for sampling cattle breath. *Biosyst Eng.* (2012) 112:75–81. doi: 10.1016/j.biosystemseng.2012.03.001

27. Cho YS, Jung SC, Oh S. Diagnosis of bovine tuberculosis using a metal oxide-based electronic nose. *Lett Appl Microbiol.* (2015) 60:513–6. doi: 10.1111/lam.12410

28. Ellis CK, Rice S, Maurer D, Stahl R, Waters WR, Palmer MV, et al. Use of fecal volatile organic compound analysis to discriminate between non-vaccinated and BCG-Vaccinated cattle prior to and after *Mycobacterium bovis* challenge. *PLoS ONE.* (2017) 12:25. doi: 10.1371/journal.pone.0179914

29. Nol P, Ionescu R, Welearegay TG, Barasona JA, Vicente J, Beleno-Saenz KD, et al. Evaluation of volatile organic compounds obtained from breath and feces to detect *Mycobacterium tuberculosis* complex in wild boar (*Sus scrofa*) in Donana National Park, Spain. *Pathogens.* (2020) 9:13. doi: 10.3390/pathogens9050346

30. Knobloch H, Kohler H, Commander N, Reinhold P, Turner C, Chambers M. Volatile organic compound (VOC) analysis for disease detection: proof of principle for field studies detecting paratuberculosis and brucellosis. In: Knobloch H, Kohler H, Commander N, Reinhold P, Turner C, Chambers M, editors, *13th International Symposium on Olfaction and the Electronic Nose.* Brescia: Melville: Amer Inst Physics (2009). p. 195–7. doi: 10.1063/1.3156505

31. Bergmann A, Trefz P, Fischer S, Klepik K, Walter G, Steffens M, et al. *In vivo* volatile organic compound signatures of *Mycobacterium avium* subsp. *paratuberculosis. PLoS ONE.* (2015) 10:20. doi: 10.1371/journal.pone.0123980

32. Kasbohm E, Fischer S, Kuntzel A, Oertel P, Bergmann A, Trefz P, et al. Strategies for the identification of disease-related patterns of volatile organic compounds: prediction of paratuberculosis in an animal model using random forests. *J Breath Res.* (2017) 11:14. doi: 10.1088/1752-7163/aa83bb

33. Fend R, Kolk AHJ, Bessant C, Buijtels P, Klatser PR, Woodman AC. Prospects

for clinical application of electronic-nose technology to early detection of *Mycobacterium tuberculosis* in culture and sputum. *J Clin Microbiol.* (2006) 44:2039–45. doi: 10.1128/JCM.01591-05

34. Weiner J, Parida SK, Maertzdorf J, Black GF, Repsilber D, Telaar A, et al. Biomarkers of inflammation, immunosuppression and stress with active disease are revealed by metabolomic profiling of tuberculosis patients. *PLoS ONE.* (2012) 7:14. doi: 10.1371/annotation/b7f554bc-ad78-4745-9cd6-e14954d6a01d

35. Phillips M, Basa-Dalay V, Bothamley G, Cataneo RN, Lam PK, Natividad MPR, et al. Breath biomarkers of active pulmonary tuberculosis. *Tuberculosis.* (2010) 90:145–51. doi: 10.1016/j.tube.2010.01.003

36. Kuntzel A, Oertel P, Fischer S, Bergmann A, Trefz P, Schubert J, et al. Comparative analysis of volatile organic compounds for the classification and identification of mycobacterial species. *PLoS ONE.* (2018) 13:18. doi: 10.1371/journal.pone.0194348

37. McNerney R, Mallard K, Okolo PI, Turner C. Production of volatile organic compounds by mycobacteria. *Fems Microbiol Lett.* (2012) 328:150–6. doi: 10.1111/j.1574-6968.2011.02493.x

38. Pavlou AK, Magan N, Jones JM, Brown J, Klatser P, Turner APF. Detection of *Mycobacterium tuberculosis* (TB) *in vitro* and *in situ* using an electronic nose in combination with a neural network system. *Biosens Bioelectr.* (2004) 20:538–44. doi: 10.1016/j.bios.2004.03.002

39. Purkhart R, Becher G, Reinhold P, Köhler HU. Detection of mycobacteria by volatile organic compound analysis of *in vitro* cultures using differential ion mobility spectrometry. *J Medical Microbiol.* (2017) 66:276–85. doi: 10.1099/jmm.0.000410

40. Ratiu I-A, Bocos-Bintintan V, Monedeiro F, Milanowski M, Ligor T, Buszewski B. An optimistic vision of future: diagnosis of bacterial infections by sensing their associated volatile organic compounds. *Crit Rev Analyt Chem.* (2019) 2019:1–12. doi: 10.1080/10408347.2019.1663147

41. Franchina FA, Mellors TR, Aliyeva M, Wagner J, Daphtary N, Lundblad LKA, et al. Towards the use of breath for detecting mycobacterial infection: a case study in a murine model. *J Breath Res.* (2018) 12:9. doi: 10.1088/1752-7163/aaa016

42. Pontiroli A, Khera TT, Oakley BB, Mason S, Dowd SE, Travis ER, et al. Prospecting environmental mycobacteria: combined molecular approaches reveal unprecedented diversity. *PLoS ONE.* (2013) 8:13. doi: 10.1371/journal.pone.0068648

43. Rahman SA, Singh Y, Kohli S, Ahmad J, Ehtesham NZ, Tyagi AK, et al. Comparative analyses of nonpathogenic, opportunistic, and totally pathogenic mycobacteria reveal genomic and biochemical variabilities and highlight the survival attributes of *Mycobacterium tuberculosis. Mbio.* (2014) 5:9. doi: 10.1128/mBio.02020-14

44. Biet F, Boschiroli ML. Non-tuberculous mycobacterial infections of veterinary relevance. *Res Vet Sci.* (2014) 97:S69–77. doi: 10.1016/j.rvsc.2014.08.007

45. Michelet L, De Cruz K, Henault S, Tambosco J, Richomme C, Reveillaud E, et al. *Mycobacterium bovis* infection of red fox, France. *Emerg Infect Dis.* (2018) 24:1151–3. doi: 10.3201/eid2406.180094

46. Schiller I, Oesch B, Vordermeier HM, Palmer MV, Harris BN, Orloski KA, et al. Bovine tuberculosis: a review of current and emerging diagnostic techniques in view of their relevance for disease control and eradication. *Transbound Emerg Dis.* (2010) 57:205–20. doi: 10.1111/j.1865-1682.2010.01148.x

47. Muller B, Durr S, Alonso S, Hattendorf J, Laisse CJM, Parsons SDC, et al. Zoonotic *Mycobacterium bovis*-induced tuberculosis in humans. *Emerg Infect Dis.* (2013) 19:899–908. doi: 10.3201/eid1906.120543

48. Cleaveland S, Shaw DJ, Mfinanga SG, Shirima G, Kazwala RR, Eblate E, et al. *Mycobacterium bovis* in rural Tanzania: risk factors for infection in human and cattle populations. *Tuberculosis.* (2007) 87:30–43. doi: 10.1016/j.tube.2006.03.001

49. Cosivi O, Grange JM, Daborn CJ, Raviglione MC, Fujikura T, Cousins D, et al. Zoonotic tuberculosis due to *Mycobacterium bovis* in developing countries. *Emerg Infect Dis.* (1998) 4:59–70. doi: 10.3201/eid0401.980108

50. Grange JM. *Mycobacterium bovis* infection in human beings. *Tuberculosis.* (2001) 81:71–7. doi: 10.1054/tube.2000.0263

51. Skuce RA, Allen AR, McDowell SWJ. Herd-level risk factors

for bovine tuberculosis: a literature review. *Vet Med Int.* (2012) 2012:621210. doi: 10.1155/2012/621210

52. Chiodini RJ, Chamberlin WM, Sarosiek J, McCallum RW. Crohn's disease and the mycobacterioses: a quarter century later. Causation or simple association? *Crit Rev Microbiol.* (2012) 38:52–93. doi: 10.3109/1040841X.2011.638273

53. Mendoza JL, Lana R, Diaz-Rubio M. *Mycobacterium avium* subspecies *paratuberculosis* and its relationship with Crohn's disease. *World J Gastroenterol.* (2009) 15:417–22. doi: 10.3748/wjg.15.417

54. Roda G, Ng SC, Kotze PG, Argollo M, Panaccione R, Spinelli A, et al. Crohn's disease. *Nat Rev Dis Primers.* (2020) 6:1–19. doi: 10.1038/s41572-020-0183-z

55. Köhler H, Gierke F, Möbius P. Paratuberculosis–current concepts and future of the diagnosis. *Magyar Allatorvosok Lapja.* (2008) 130:67–9.

56. McKenna SLB, Keefe GP, Barkema HW, Sockett DC. Evaluation of three ELISAs for *Mycobacterium avium* subsp. *paratuberculosis* using tissue and fecal culture as comparison standards. *Vet Microbiol.* (2005) 110:105–11. doi: 10.1016/j.vetmic.2005.07.010

57. Nunez-Garcia J, Downs SH, Parry JE, Abernethy DA, Broughan JM, Cameron AR, et al. Meta-analyses of the sensitivity and specificity of ante-mortem and post-mortem diagnostic tests for bovine tuberculosis in the UK and Ireland. *Prevent Vet Med.* (2018) 153:94–107. doi: 10.1016/j.prevetmed.2017.02.017

58. Courcoul A, Moyen JL, Brugere L, Faye S, Henault S, Gares H, et al. Estimation of sensitivity and specificity of bacteriology, histopathology and PCR for the confirmatory diagnosis of *Bovine tuberculosis* using latent class analysis. *PLoS ONE.* (2014) 9:8. doi: 10.1371/journal.pone.0090334

59. Buddle BM, Wilson T, Luo DW, Voges H, Linscott R, Martel E, et al. Evaluation of a commercial enzyme-linked immunosorbent assay for the diagnosis of *Bovine tuberculosis* from milk samples from dairy cows. *Clin Vaccine Immunol.* (2013) 20:1812–6. doi: 10.1128/CVI.00538-13

60. Whelan C, Shuralev E, O'Keeffe G, Hyland P, Kwok HF, Snoddy P, et al. Multiplex immunoassay for serological diagnosis of *Mycobacterium bovis* infection in cattle. *Clin Vaccine Immunol.* (2008) 15:1834–8. doi: 10.1128/CVI.00238-08

61. Lorente-Leal V, Liandris E, Castellanos E, Bezos J, Dominguez L, de Juan L, et al. Validation of a real-time PCR for the detection of *Mycobacterium tuberculosis* complex members in bovine tissue samples. *Front Vet Sci.* (2019) 6:9. doi: 10.3389/fvets.2019.00061

62. O.I.E. *Manual of Diagnostic Tests and Vaccines for Terrestrial Animals.* Chapter 3.4.6. World Organization for Animal Health (2018). p. 1058–74. Available online at: https://www.oie.int/es/normas/manual-terrestre/ (accessed January, 2021).

63. Verdugo C, Cardemil C, Steuer P, Salgado M. Bayesian latent class estimation of sensitivity and specificity parameters of the PMS-PCR test for the diagnosis of cattle sub-clinically infected with *Mycobacterium avium* subsp. *paratuberculosis*. *Prevent Vet Med.* (2020) 182:105076. doi: 10.1016/j.prevetmed.2020.105076

64. Bezos J, Casal C, Romero B, Schroeder B, Hardegger R, Raeber AJ, et al. Current ante-mortem techniques for diagnosis of bovine tuberculosis. *Res Vet Sci.* (2014) 97:S44–52. doi: 10.1016/j.rvsc.2014.04.002

65. Schiller I, Vordermeier HM, Waters WR, Whelan AO, Coad M, Gormley E, et al. *Bovine tuberculosis*: effect of the tuberculin skin test on *in vitro* interferon gamma responses. *Vet Immunol Immunopathol.* (2010) 136:1–11. doi: 10.1016/j.vetimm.2010.02.007

66. De la Rua-Domenech R, Goodchild AT, Vordermeier HM, Hewinson RG, Christiansen KH, Clifton-Hadley RS. Ante mortem diagnosis of tuberculosis in cattle: a review of the tuberculin tests, γ-interferon assay and other ancillary diagnostic techniques. *Res Vet Sci.* (2006) 81:190–210. doi: 10.1016/j.rvsc.2005.11.005

67. Katsenos S, Nikolopoulou M, Tsiouri G, Bassukas ID, Constantopoulos SH. The challenging evaluation of patients with severe psoriasis for latent tuberculosis: an important indication for IGRA. *Open Respir Med J.* (2011) 5:59. doi: 10.2174/1874306401105010059

68. Hanna J, Neill SD, Obrien JJ. Elisa tests for antibodies in experimental *Bovine tuberculosis*. *Vet Microbiol.* (1992) 31:243–9. doi: 10.1016/0378-1135(92)90082-5

69. Kruger C, Kohler H, Liebler-Tenorio EM. Sequential development of lesions 3, 6, 9, and 12 months after experimental infection of goat kids with

Mycobacterium avium subsp. *paratuberculosis. Vet Pathol.* (2015) 52:276–90. doi: 10.1177/0300985814533804

70. Miekisch W, Trefz P, Bergmann A, Schubert JK. Microextraction techniques in breath biomarker analysis. *Bioanalysis.* (2014) 6:1275–91. doi: 10.4155/bio.14.86

71. Ezanno P, van Schaik G, Weber MF, Heesterbeek JAP. A modeling study on the sustainability of a certification-and-monitoring program for *paratuberculosis* in cattle. *Vet Res.* (2005) 36:811–26. doi: 10.1051/vetres:2005032

72. Köhler H, Soschinka A, Meyer M, Kather A, Reinhold P, Liebler-Tenorio E. Characterization of a caprine model for the subclinical initial phase of *Mycobacterium avium* subsp. *paratuberculosis* infection. *BMC Vet Res.* (2015) 11:74. doi: 10.1186/s12917-015-0381-1

73. Sevilla IA, Garrido JM, Molina E, Geijo MV, Elguezabal N, Vazquez P, et al. Development and evaluation of a novel multicopy-element-targeting triplex PCR for detection of *Mycobacterium avium* subsp. *paratuberculosis* in feces. *Appl Environ Microbiol.* (2014) 80:3757–68. doi: 10.1128/AEM.01026-14

74. Gierschner P, Küntzel A, Reinhold P, Köhler H, Schubert JK, Miekisch W. Crowd monitoring in dairy cattle—real-time VOC profiling by direct mass spectrometry. *J Breath Res.* (2019) 13:046006. doi: 10.1088/1752-7163/ab269f

75. Chingin K, Liang JC, Liu YL, Chen LF, Wu XP, Hu LH, et al. Rapid detection of *Mycobacterium tuberculosis* cultures by direct ambient corona discharge ionization mass spectrometry of volatile metabolites. *RSC Adv.* (2016) 6:59749–52. doi: 10.1039/C6RA12107A

76. Kuntzel A, Fischer S, Bergmann A, Oertel P, Steffens M, Trefz P, et al. Effects of biological and methodological factors on volatile organic compound patterns during cultural growth of *Mycobacterium avium* subsp. *paratuberculosis. J Breath Res.* (2016) 10:14. doi: 10.1088/1752-7155/10/3/037103

77. Trefz P, Koehler H, Klepik K, Moebius P, Reinhold P, Schubert JK, et al. Volatile emissions from *Mycobacterium avium* subsp. *paratuberculosis* mirror bacterial growth and enable distinction of different strains. *PLoS ONE.* (2013) 8:10. doi: 10.1371/journal.pone.0076868

78. Zhu JJ, Bean HD, Wargo MJ, Leclair LW, Hill JE. Detecting bacterial lung infections: *in vivo* evaluation of *in vitro* volatile fingerprints. *J Breath Res.* (2013) 7:7. doi: 10.1088/1752-7155/7/1/016003

79. Dang NA, Janssen HG, Kolk AHJ. Rapid diagnosis of TB using GC-MS and chemometrics. *Bioanalysis.* (2013) 5:3079–97. doi: 10.4155/bio.13.288

80. Mellors TR, Nasir M, Franchina FA, Smolinska A, Blanchet L, Flynn JL, et al. Identification of Mycobacterium tuberculosis using volatile biomarkers in culture and exhaled breath. *J Breath Res.* (2019) 13:13. doi: 10.1088/1752-7163/aacd18

81. Dervishi E, Zhang G, Dunn SM, Mandal R, Wishart DS, Ametaj BN. GC-MS metabolomics identifies metabolite alterations that precede subclinical mastitis in the blood of transition dairy cows. *J Proteome Res.* (2017) 16:433–46. doi: 10.1021/acs.jproteome.6b00538

82. Zhang HY, Wu L, Xu C, Xia C, Sun LW, Shu S. Plasma metabolomic profiling of dairy cows affected with ketosis using gas chromatography/mass spectrometry. *BMC Vet Res.* (2013) 9:13. doi: 10.1186/1746-6148-9-186

83. ElliottMartin RJ, Mottram TT, Gardner JW, Hobbs PJ, Bartlett PN. Preliminary investigation of breath sampling as a monitor of health in dairy cattle. *J Agri Eng Res.* (1997) 67:267–75. doi: 10.1006/jaer.1997.0168

84. Mottram TT, Dobbelaar P, Schukken YH, Hobbs PJ, Bartlett PN. An experiment to determine the feasibility of automatically detecting hyperketonaemia in dairy cows. *Livestock Product Sci.* (1999) 61:7–11. doi: 10.1016/S0301-6226(99)00045-7

85. Mellors TR, Blanchet L, Flynn JL, Tomko J, O'Malley M, Scanga CA, et al. A new method to evaluate macaque health using exhaled breath: a case study of M-tuberculosis in a BSL-3 setting. *J Appl Physiol.* (2017) 122:695–701. doi: 10.1152/japplphysiol.00888.2016

86. Kaser T, Renois F, Wilson HL, Cnudde T, Gerdts V, Dillon JAR, et al. Contribution of the swine model in the study of human sexually transmitted infections. *Infect Genet Evol.* (2018) 66:346–60. doi: 10.1016/j.meegid.2017.11.022

87. Klemm WR, Hawkins GN, Santos EDL. Identification of compounds in bovine cervico-vaginal mucus extracts that evoke male sexual behavior. *Chemical Senses.* (1987) 12:77–87. doi: 10.1093/chemse/12.1.77

88. Ma WD, Clement BA, Klemm WR. Cyclic changes in volatile

constituents of bovine vaginal secretions. *J Chem Ecol.* (1995) 21:1895–906. doi: 10.1007/BF02033850

89. Shirasu M, Touhara K. The scent of disease: volatile organic compounds of the human body related to disease and disorder. *J Biochem.* (2011) 150:257–66. doi: 10.1093/jb/mvr090

90. Amann A, Miekisch W, Schubert J, Buszewski B, Ligor T, Jezierski T, et al. Analysis of exhaled breath for disease detection. In: Cooks RG, Pemberton JE, editors. *Annual Review of Analytical Chemistry, Vol 7.* Palo Alto, CA: Annual Reviews (2014). p. 455–82. doi: 10.1146/annurev-anchem-071213-020043

91. Oertel P, Küntzel A, Reinhold P, Köhler H, Schubert JK, Kolb J, et al. Continuous real-time breath analysis in ruminants: effect of eructation on exhaled VOC profiles. *J Breath Res.* (2018) 12:036014. doi: 10.1088/1752-7163/aabdaf

92. Deda O, Gika HG, Wilson ID, Theodoridis GA. An overview of fecal sample preparation for global metabolic profiling. *J Pharmaceut Biomed Anal.* (2015) 113:137–50. doi: 10.1016/j.jpba.2015.02.006

93. Aggio RBM, White P, Jayasena H, Costello BD, Ratcliffe NM, Probert CSJ. Irritable bowel syndrome and active inflammatory bowel disease diagnosed by faecal gas analysis. *Aliment Pharmacol Therapeut.* (2017) 45:82–90. doi: 10.1111/apt.13822

94. Garner CE, Smith S, Costello BD, White P, Spencer R, Probert CSJ, et al. Volatile organic compounds from feces and their potential for diagnosis of gastrointestinal disease. *FASEB J.* (2007) 21:1675–88. doi: 10.1096/fj.06-6927com

95. Tait E, Hill KA, Perry JD, Stanforth SP, Dean JR. Development of a novel method for detection of *Clostridium* difficile using HS-SPME-GC-MS. *J Appl Microbiol.* (2014) 116:1010–9. doi: 10.1111/jam.12418

96. Ubeda C, Lepe-Balsalobre E, Ariza-Astolfi C, Ubeda-Ontiveros JM. Identification of volatile biomarkers of *Giardia duodenalis* infection in children with persistent diarrhoea. *Parasitol Res.* (2019) 118:3139–47. doi: 10.1007/s00436-019-06433-4

97. Blake AB, Guard BC, Honneffer JB, Lidbury JA, Steiner JM, Suchodolski JS. Altered microbiota, fecal lactate, and fecal bile acids in dogs with gastrointestinal disease. *PLoS ONE.* (2019) 14:21. doi: 10.1371/journal.pone.0224454

98. Garner CE, Smith S, Elviss NC, Humphrey TJ, White P, Ratcliffe NM, et al. Identification of Campylobacter infection in chickens from volatile faecal emissions. *Biomarkers.* (2008) 13:413–21. doi: 10.1080/13547500801966443

99. Kizil U, Genc L, Genc TT, Rahman S, Khaitsa ML. E-nose identification of *Salmonella enterica* in poultry manure. *Br Poultry Sci.* (2015) 56:149–56. doi: 10.1080/00071668.2015.1014467

100. Summers S, Quimby JM, Phillips RK, Stockman J, Isaiah A, Lidbury JA, et al. Preliminary evaluation of fecal fatty acid concentrations in cats with chronic kidney disease and correlation with indoxyl sulfate and p-cresol sulfate. *J Vet Internal Med.* (2020) 34:206–15. doi: 10.1111/jvim.15634

101. Guarner F, Malagelada JR. Gut flora in health and disease. *Lancet.* (2003) 361:512–9. doi: 10.1016/S0140-6736(03)12489-0

102. Harper RG, Workman SR, Schuetzner S, Timperman AT, Sutton JN. Low-molecular-weight human serum proteome using ultrafiltration, isoelectric focusing, and mass spectrometry. *Electrophoresis.* (2004) 25:1299–306. doi: 10.1002/elps.200405864

103. Kurada S, Mao R, Singh A, Li JN, Lin SN, Wang J, et al. A validated serum headspace metabolome profile discriminates Crohn's disease from non-Crohn's disease. *Gastroenterology.* (2019) 156:S656. doi: 10.1016/S0016-5085(19)38545-2

104. Phillips M, Basa-Dalay V, Blais J, Bothamley G, Chaturvedi A, Modi KD, et al. Point-of-care breath test for biomarkers of active pulmonary tuberculosis. *Tuberculosis.* (2012) 92:314–20. doi: 10.1016/j.tube.2012.04.002

105. Zhang J, Fang AQ, Wang B, Kim SH, Bogdanov B, Zhou ZX, et al. iMatch: a retention index tool for analysis of gas chromatography-mass spectrometry data. *J Chromatogr A.* (2011) 1218:6522–30. doi: 10.1016/j.chroma.2011.07.039

106. Buszewski B, Ratiu IA, Milanowski M, Pomastowski P, Ligor T. The effect of biosilver nanoparticles on different bacterial strains' metabolism reflected in their VOCs profiles. *J Breath Res.* (2018) 12:8. doi: 10.1088/1752-7163/aa820f

107. Ratiu IA, Ligor T, Bocos-Bintintan V, Szeliga J, Machala K, Jackowski M, et al. GC-MS application in determination of volatile profiles emitted by infected and uninfected human tissue. *J Breath Res.* (2019) 13:15. doi: 10.1088/1752-7163/aaf708

108. Ibrahim W, Wilde M, Cordell R, Salman D, Ruszkiewicz D, Bryant L, et al. Assessment of breath volatile organic compounds in acute cardiorespiratory breathlessness: a protocol describing a prospective real-world observational study. *BMJ Open.* (2019) 9:13. doi: 10.1136/bmjopen-2018-025486

109. Gardner JW, Bartlett PN. A brief history of electronic noses. *Sens Actuat B Chemical.* (1994) 18:210–1. doi: 10.1016/0925-4005(94)87085-3

110. Macias MM, Manso AG, Orellana CJG, Velasco HMG, Caballero RG, Chamizo JCP. Acetic acid detection threshold in synthetic wine samples of a portable electronic nose. *Sensors.* (2013) 13:208–20. doi: 10.3390/s130100208

111. Rock F, Barsan N, Weimar U. Electronic nose: current status and future trends. *Chem Rev.* (2008) 108:705–25. doi: 10.1021/cr068121q

112. Majchrzak T, Wojnowski W, Piotrowicz G, Gebicki J, Namiesnik J. Sample preparation and recent trends in volatolomics for diagnosing gastrointestinal diseases. *Trends Anal Chem.* (2018) 108:38–49. doi: 10.1016/j.trac.2018.08.020

113. Scott-Thomas A, Syhre M, Epton M, Murdoch DR, Chambers ST. Assessment of potential causes of falsely positive *Mycobacterium tuberculosis* breath test. *Tuberculosis.* (2013) 93:312–7. doi: 10.1016/j.tube.2013.01.005

114. Wishart DS, Knox C, Guo AC, Eisner R, Young N, Gautam B, et al. HMDB: a knowledge base for the human metabolome. *Nucl Acids Res.* (2009) 37(Suppl.1):D603–10. doi: 10.1093/nar/gkn810

115. Wishart DS, Jewison T, Guo AC, Wilson M, Knox C, Liu Y, et al. HMDB 3.0—the human metabolome database in 2013. *Nucl Acids Res.* (2012) 41:D801–7. doi: 10.1093/nar/gks1065

116. Nawrath T, Mgode GF, Weetjens B, Kaufmann SHE, Schulz S. The volatiles of pathogenic and non-pathogenic mycobacteria and related bacteria. *Beilstein J Organ Chem.* (2012) 8:290–9. doi: 10.3762/bjoc.8.31

117. Phillips M, Cataneo RN, Condos R, Erickson GAR, Greenberg J, La Bombardi V, et al. Volatile biomarkers of pulmonary tuberculosis in the breath. *Tuberculosis.* (2007) 87:44–52. doi: 10.1016/j.tube.2006.03.004

118. Graham JE. Bacterial volatiles and diagnosis of respiratory infections. In: Sariaslani S, Gadd GM, editors. *Advances in Applied Microbiology, Vol 82.* San Diego, CA: Elsevier Academic Press Inc. (2013). p. 29–52. doi: 10.1016/B978-0-12-407679-2.00002-8

15

Evaluation of P22 Antigenic Complex for the Immuno-Diagnosis of Tuberculosis in BCG Vaccinated and Unvaccinated Goats

Claudia Arrieta-Villegas [1]*, José Antonio Infantes-Lorenzo [2], Javier Bezos [3,4],
Miriam Grasa [5], Enric Vidal [1], Irene Mercader [6], Mahavir Singh [7], Mariano Domingo [1,8],
Lucía de Juan [3,4] and Bernat Pérez de Val [1]

[1] IRTA, Centre de Recerca en Sanitat Animal (CReSA, IRTA-UAB), Campus Universitat Autònoma de Barcelona, Barcelona, Spain, [2] Servicio de Inmunología Microbiana, Centro Nacional de Microbiología, Instituto de Investigación Carlos III, Madrid, Spain, [3] VISAVET Health Surveillance Center, Universidad Complutense de Madrid, Madrid, Spain, [4] Departamento de Sanidad Animal, Universidad Complutense de Madrid, Madrid, Spain, [5] Agrupació de Defensa Sanitària de Cabrum i Oví Lleter de Catalunya, Barbens, Spain, [6] Departament d'Agricultura, Ramaderia, Pesca i Alimentació de la Generalitat de Catalunya, Barcelona, Spain, [7] Lionex Diagnostics and Therapeutics GmbH, Braunschweig, Germany, [8] Departament de Sanitat i Anatomia Animals, Universitat Autònoma de Barcelona (UAB), Barcelona, Spain

*Correspondence:
Claudia Arrieta-Villegas
claudia.arrieta@irta.cat

Current eradication strategies of tuberculosis (TB) in goats mainly rely on the single intradermal tuberculin test (SIT) and single intradermal cervical comparative tuberculin tests (SICCTs). TB vaccination has been proposed as a cost-effective option in high-prevalence herds or countries where economic compensation for the slaughter of positive animals is not affordable. However, TB vaccination compromises the efficiency of tuberculin-based diagnostic tests. In this study, the performance of a new diagnostic platform, based on the P22 antigenic complex, was assessed for skin test (ST), interferon-gamma release assay (IGRA), and serology under different TB scenarios. The sensitivity (Se) of diagnostic tests was assessed in TB-infected goats from the same farm (herd A, $N = 77$). The specificity (Sp) was assessed in two TB-negative farms (both vaccinated against paratuberculosis): one TB unvaccinated (herd B, $N = 77$) and another vaccinated with bacille Calmette-Guérin (BCG) (herd C, $N = 68$). The single (s) P22-IGRA showed the highest Se among IGRA tests (91%), and the comparative (c) P22-ST showed the highest Sp (100% in herd B and 98% in herd C). Combined interpretation of techniques enabled the best diagnostic performances. Combining the SICCT + sP22-IGRA improved Se (97%) compared to SICCT + tuberculin-based IGRA (95%), with a reduction of Sp (95 and 100%, respectively). Besides, combination of P22-ELISA with cP22-ST or SICCT elicited a similar performance in the non-vaccination context (Se: 94 and 95%; Sp: 95 and 95%, respectively), but Sp was significantly higher for the combination with cP22-ST compared to SICCT in the TB vaccination context (95 and 79%, respectively). The combination of serological tests based on P22 and MPB83 showed higher complementarity and improved 13 percentage points the Se of P22-ELISA alone. These findings suggest that either cell-mediated or antibody-based diagnostic techniques, using the P22 antigen complex, can contribute to improve the immunodiagnostics of TB in goats under different TB control strategies.

Keywords: tuberculosis, diagnosis, goats, bacille Calmette-Guérin (BCG), skin test, interferon-gamma release assay (IGRA), serology, P22

INTRODUCTION

Tuberculosis (TB) in goats is a chronic infectious disease, mainly caused by *Mycobacterium bovis* and *Mycobacterium caprae*, members of the *Mycobacterium tuberculosis* complex (MTBC). This disease entails important economic costs for livestock industries (1) and could be a source of TB for cattle (2), other domestic animals (3, 4), wildlife (5), and humans (6).

Spain has the second-highest goat census of the EU, with 2.7 million goat heads (data extracted from FAOSTAT on 17/02/2020). Besides, the high TB burden in goats could explain a number of new bovine TB breakdowns, hampering the goal of TB eradication in cattle (7). Therefore, some regions with a high concentration of caprine herds carry out TB eradication campaigns in caprine flocks (8); however, goat herds are still not subjected to a national eradication program, except for those epidemiologically linked with cattle (9).

The cornerstone of an efficient caprine TB eradication program is the diagnosis. The Spanish bovine TB eradication program effectiveness is highly dependent on the routine tuberculin skin testing (10). Current bovine TB testing is based on the single intradermal tuberculin test (SIT) and single intradermal cervical comparative tuberculin tests (SICCTs), and the interferon-gamma release assay (IGRA). However, in goats under certain epidemiological contexts, those diagnostic tests have some drawbacks in terms of sensitivity (Se) and specificity (Sp) (8, 11).

Another concern for TB diagnostics is the vaccination against *Mycobacterium avium* subsp. *paratuberculosis* (MAP), which has been largely implemented in small ruminants, to prevent the development of clinical disease (12). Nevertheless, even though MAP vaccines are authorized (e.g., Gudair® vaccine), it has been demonstrated that paratuberculosis (PTB) vaccination interferes with STs and IGRA used for TB diagnosis (13, 14). In addition, the efficacy of *M. bovis* bacille Calmette-Guérin (BCG) vaccine has also been assessed in goats during the last decade in different vaccination trials (15–19). Even though these trials showed that BCG conferred certain protection to experimentally and naturally infected goats, it was evidenced that vaccination interfered with current TB diagnostic tests (16, 20).

To overcome diagnostic interferences due to BCG vaccination, defined antigens to differentiate infected from vaccinated animals (DIVA) have been developed (14, 21); nevertheless, those antigens have shown lower Se compared to tests based on standard tuberculins (22). Recently, a new multi-protein complex called P22, obtained from purified protein derivative of *M. bovis* (PPD-B) by affinity chromatography, has been developed (23), yielding high Se and variable Sp, depending on the animal species and epidemiological contexts (24). To date, this antigen has been tested to detect humoral response against MTBC in different species (25–30); however, there is a lack of information regarding its performance for cell-mediated immunity (CMI)-based diagnostics.

The aim of this study was to evaluate the performance of different cell-mediated and humoral immunodiagnostic tests, based on the P22 antigenic complex, for the diagnosis of TB in goats under different epidemiological and control scenarios.

MATERIALS AND METHODS

Herds and Experimental Design

A total of 222 goats from three herds were included in the study (**Table 1**): 77 infected goats (infection was confirmed postmortem by gross lesions, histopathology or mycobacterial culture, or both) from a TB-positive herd of murciana-granadina goats (herd A); 77 goats belonging to an officially TB-free herd of alpine goats (herd B) that were vaccinated against PTB with Gudair (CZ Vaccines, Porriño, Spain), around 2 years before sampling; and 68 goats from another TB-free herd (herd C) of Blanca de Rasquera autochthonous breed, that were vaccinated against PTB (Gudair®) and against TB with *M. bovis* BCG Danish 1,331 strain (ATCC, Ref. 35733) as described previously (15). In herd C, 50% of goats were vaccinated with BCG and Gudair® 9–10 months before sampling, and the remaining 50% were vaccinated more than 1 year before. STs, IGRAs, and immunoglobulin G (IgG) enzyme-linked immunosorbent assays (ELISAs) were carried out in the 77 infected goats, as well as in 138, 142, and 142 noninfected goats, respectively (**Table 1**).

Two TB control scenarios were hypothesized in order to study the performance of each diagnostic test: the conventional (TB unvaccinated) scenario, using data from herds A and B, and the BCG-vaccinated (TB-VAC) scenario, using data from herds A and C. Se was calculated using data from herd A, and Sp was calculated using data from herds B and C depending on TB control scenario (**Table 2**).

Antigens

M. tuberculosis var. *bovis* (PPD-B) and *M. avium* (PPD-A) tuberculins (2,500 IU/ml) were obtained from CZ Vaccines

TABLE 1 | Herd and treatment distribution of tested animals.

Herd	TB status	BCG[1]	Gudair®[2]	No. of animals tested		
				ST	IGRA	ELISA
A	Positive	No	No	77	77	77
B	Free	No	Yes	77	74	74
C	Free	Yes	Yes	61	68	68

[1]BCG, bacilli Calmette-Guérin Mycobacterium bovis vaccine. [2]Gudair vaccine, vaccine against paratuberculosis (Mycobacteium avium subspecies paratuberculosis).
TB, tuberculosis; ST, skin test; IGRA, interferon-gamma release assay.

TABLE 2 | TB control scenarios distribution of tested animals.

Control scenario	Herds	BCG[1]	Gudair®[2]	No. of animals tested		
				ST	IGRA	ELISA
Conventional[a]	A+B	No	Yes	154	151	151
TB-VAC[b]	A+C	Yes	Yes	138	145	145

[a]Conventional scenario: composed by TB unvaccinated goats. [b]TB-VAC Scenario: TB negative animals from herd C were vaccinated with BCG and TB-positive animals from herd A were not vaccinated. [1]BCG, bacilli Calmette-Guérin Mycobacterium bovis vaccine. [2]Gudair vaccine, vaccine against paratuberculosis (Mycobacteium avium subspecies paratuberculosis).
TB, tuberculosis; ST, skin test; IGRA, interferon-gamma release assay.

and used at concentrations recommended by the Spanish Ministry (9). The protein complex P22 was produced by immunopurification of PPD-B (CZ Vaccines) as described previously (23) and prepared at a concentration of 500 µg/ml (unpublished data). The DIVA reagent based on a cocktail of recombinant ESAT-6 and CFP-10 proteins (500 µg/ml) (31) and the recombinant MPB83 (MPT83) protein (500 µg/ml) (32) were purchased from Lionex (Braunschweig, Germany).

Skin Tests

SIT was performed by intradermal inoculation of 0.1 ml of PPD-B in the left-hand side of the neck by using a Dermojet® syringe (Akra Dermojet, Pau, France). In the same way, SICCT was performed by intradermal inoculation of 0.1 ml of PPD-B and PPD-A, both in the left-hand side of the neck, at the proximal and distal parts of the neck, respectively. Besides, 0.1 ml of P22 (at 500 µg/ml) was inoculated in the right-hand side of the neck. The increase in skinfold thickness (SFT) was measured just before the inoculation and after 72 h. Severe interpretations of SIT and SICCT were performed, as previously described in the manual of the Spanish bovine TB eradication program (9). Briefly, positive criterion for SIT: SFT PPD-B > 2 mm (severe); and for SICCT: positive to SIT and SFT PPD-B - SFT PPD-A > 1 mm (severe) or presence of clinical signs in the PPD-B inoculation site. P22 single and comparative STs (sP22-ST and cP22-ST) were interpreted using the same criteria as SIT and SICCT, respectively, i.e., considering SFT P22 and SFT P22 - SFT PPD-A measures, respectively.

Whole-Blood Interferon-Gamma Release Assays

Blood samples were collected from the jugular vein prior to ST performance using heparinized tubes and were processed as described previously (16). Shortly, blood samples were stimulated with PPD-B, PPD-A, and P22 at a final concentration of 20 µg/ml, and with DIVA reagent (ESAT-6/CFP-10) at 20 µg/ml, while PBS was added as an unstimulated control. Samples were incubated at $37 \pm 1°C$ with 0.5% CO_2 overnight. Finally, plasma supernatant was collected and analyzed by ELISA (BOVIGAM®, Thermo Fisher Scientific, Waltham, MA, USA) and read at 450 nm using a spectrophotometer (Biotek Power Wave XS). The interpretation of tuberculin-based IGRA (STAND-IGRA) results was performed according to the cutoff point recommended by the manufacturer, i.e., the criterion for positivity: PPD-B OD - PBS OD ≥ 0.05 and PPD-B OD > PPD-A OD. Similarly, cP22-IGRA was considered positive when P22 OD - PBS OD ≥ 0.05 and P22 OD > PPD-A OD, whereas sP22-IGRA and DIVA-IGRA were considered positive when P22 OD - PBS OD ≥ 0.05 and DIVA OD - PBS OD ≥ 0.05, respectively.

Antibody Detection Tests

Plasma samples were analyzed for antibody detection by using two in-house indirect ELISA, one for detecting MPB83 antigen, performed and interpreted as described previously (33), and another one for detecting P22, performed as described previously (24, 25). P22-ELISA was interpreted as follows: ELISA percentage (E%) = [mean sample OD/(2 × mean negative control OD)] ×

100. A sample E% <100% was classified as negative, and a sample E% ≥100% was classified as positive.

Post-mortem Examination

Seventy-seven goats from the positive herd (herd A) were euthanized after ST reading by intravenous injection of a sodium pentobarbital overdose. A complete necropsy procedure was conducted for TB lesion examination. Lesions were collected and immediately fixed in 10% buffered formalin for histopathological confirmation by hematoxylin/eosin staining. Mediastinal and tracheobronchial lymph nodes (LNs) were removed and stored at −20°C for bacterial culture.

Bacteriology

Whole pulmonary LNs of each animal were thawed, pooled, homogenized, and decontaminated as previously described (34) and plated on Middlebrook 7H11 medium (BD diagnostics, Sparks, MD, USA). Then, cultured plates were incubated at 37°C for 28 days. Finally, plates were read, and colonies were confirmed as MTBC by multiplex PCR (35).

Data Analysis

The Sp was calculated in TB-free farms (herds B and C) using the formula Sp = True negatives/(True negatives + False positives). The Se was calculated in the TB-infected farm by the formula Se = True positive/(True positive + False negative). Clooper-Pearson 95% confidence intervals were calculated for Sp and Se. Differences in diagnostic results, between tests, were evaluated by the McNemar test. Moreover, agreement between tests was calculated by Cohen's Kappa coefficient (k) and interpreted as follows: <0.00 poor, 0.00–0.20 slight, 0.21–0.4 fair, 0.41–0.60 moderate, 0.61–0.80 substantial, and 0.81–1.00 almost perfect. The diagnostic performance of each test was calculated using the diagnostic odds ratio (DOR) (36). All statistical tests and 95% confidence intervals were calculated using the Epitools calculator (Sargento, ESG, 2018, Epitools Epidemiological Calculators, Ausvet, Pty., Ltd., Australia; available in www.epitools.ausvet.com.au).

RESULTS

The results of Se of herd A and Sp of herds B and C are summarized in **Table 3**. The TB-positive status of all animals from herd A was confirmed by positive mycobacterial culture and/or positive lesions in histopathological analysis.

Skin Tests

The Se of the cP22-ST was the lowest among tests, but the Sp in herd B was the highest, being identical to the Sp of the SICCT, and a 6 percentage point (p.p.) and 8 p.p. more specific than the SIT and the sP22-ST, respectively. Regarding the herd C, the cP22-ST and the sP22-ST displayed similar Sp, being significantly more specific than the SIT (31 p.p. of increase, p < 0.001, and 30 p.p. of increase, p = 0.005, for cP22-ST and sP22-ST, respectively) and the SICCT (18 p.p. of increase, p = 0.0026, and 17 p.p. of increase, p = 0.0094, for cP22-ST and sP22-ST, respectively).

TABLE 3 | Sensitivity (Se) and specificity (Sp) of diagnostic tests.

Diagnostic test	TB positive (farm A)		Unvaccinated (farm B)		BCG vaccinated (farm C)	
	N[9]	Se (95% CI)[10]	N	Sp (95% CI)[11]	N	Sp (95% CI)[11]
sP22-ST[1]	77	87% (77–94)	77	92% (84–97)	61	97% (89–100)
cP22-ST[2]	77	74% (63–83)	77	100% (95–100)	61	98% (91–100)
SIT[3]	77	94% (85–98)	77	94% (85–98)	61	67% (54–79)
SICCT[4]	77	91% (82–96)	77	100% (95–100)	61	80% (68–89)
sP22-IGRA[5]	77	91% (82–96)	74	95% (87–99)	68	84% (73–92)
cP22-IGRA[6]	77	86% (76–93)	74	96% (89–99)	68	85% (75–93)
STAND-IGRA[7]	77	77% (66–86)	74	100% (95–100)	68	96% (88–99)
DIVA-IGRA[8]	77	71% (60–81)	74	100% (95–100)	68	100% (95–100)
P22-ELISA	77	74% (63–83)	74	93% (85–98)	68	96% (88–99)
MPB83-ELISA	77	75% (64–84)	74	92% (83–97)	68	94% (86–98)

[1]sP22-ST, single P22 skin test; [2]cP22-ST, comparative P22 skin test; [3]SIT, single intradermal tuberculin test; [4]SICCT, single intradermal cervical comparative tuberculin test; [5]sP22-IGRA, single P22 IGRA test; [6]cP22-IGRA, comparative P22 IGRA test; [7]STAND-IGRA, standard tuberculin IGRA test; [8]DIVA-IGRA, differentiating Infected from Vaccinated animals (ESAT-6/CFP-10 peptide cocktail) IGRA test. [9]Number of animals tested. [10]Clopper–Pearson 95% confidence interval for Se. [11]Clopper–Pearson 95% confidence interval for Sp.
TB, tuberculosis; BCG, bacille Calmette-Guérin; IGRA, interferon-gamma release assay.

Interferon-Gamma Release Assays

The sP22-IGRA showed the highest Se among tests, being a 5, 14, and 20 p.p. more sensitive than the cP22-IGRA, the STAND-IGRA, and the DIVA-IGRA, respectively. Indeed, the sP22-IGRA detected 12 positive goats more than the STAND-IGRA, without significant agreement between tests ($k = 0.4$, $p = 0.098$) and diagnostic results significantly different (**Supplementary Data**, $p = 0.005$). The sP22-IGRA and the cP22-IGRA showed similar specificities in both herds B and C, being a 4–5 p.p. less specific than the STAND-IGRA and the DIVA-IGRA. In herd C, both cP22-IGRA and sP22-IGRA were a 10–9 p.p. and a 16–15 p.p. less specific than the STAND-IGRA and the DIVA-IGRA, respectively.

Serological Tests

In terms of Sp and Se, diagnostic results of P22-ELISA were similar to diagnostic results of MPB83-ELISA. In herd A, the MPB83-ELISA detected 10 TB positive animals more than the P22-ELISA, and the P22-ELISA detected nine TB positive animals more than the MPB83-ELISA, and the agreement between tests was considered fair although statistically significant ($k = 0.35$, $p = 0.001$). In herd B, diagnostic results of Sp showed a moderate but significant agreement between ELISA tests ($k = 0.51$, $p < 0.001$), but in herd C, no agreement was observed ($k = -0.05$, $p = 0.33$).

TABLE 4 | Sensitivity (Se) and specificity (Sp) combined results of P22-based diagnostic tests.

Diagnostic tests	TB positive (farm A)		Unvaccinated (farm B)		BCG vaccinated (farm C)	
	N[8]	Se (95% CI)[9]	N	Sp (95% CI)[10]	N	Sp (95% CI)[10]
SIT[1] + sP22-IGRA[2]	77	97% (91–100)	73	89% (80–95)	61	59% (46–71)
SIT + cP22-IGRA[3]	77	97% (91–100)	73	90% (81–96)	61	61% (47–73)
SIT + P22-ELISA	77	96% (89–99)	73	89% (80–95)	61	66% (52–77)
SICCT[4] + sP22-IGRA	77	97% (91–100)	73	95% (87–98)	61	67% (54–79)
SICCT + cP22-IGRA	77	97% (91–100)	73	96% (89–99)	61	67% (54–79)
SICCT + P22-ELISA	77	95% (87–99)	73	95% (87–98)	61	79% (66–88)
sP22-ST[5] + sP22-IGRA	77	95% (87–99)	73	88% (78–94)	61	82% (70–91)
sP22-ST + P22-ELISA	77	94% (85–98)	73	88% (78–94)	61	93% (84–98)
cP22-ST[6] + sP22-IGRA	77	95% (87–99)	73	95% (87–98)	61	84% (72–92)
cP22-ST + P22-ELISA	77	94% (85–98)	73	95% (87–98)	61	95% (86–99)
sP22-IGRA + STAND-IGRA[7]	77	92% (84–97)	74	95% (87–99)	68	84% (73–92)
P22-ELISA + sP22-IGRA	77	95% (87–99)	74	89% (80–95)	68	79% (68–88)
P22 ELISA + cP22-IGRA	77	95% (87–99)	74	91% (81–96)	68	81% (70–89)
P22-ELISA + MPB83-ELISA	77	87% (77–94)	74	92% (83–97)	68	90% (80–96)
P22-ELISA + STAND-IGRA	77	90% (81–95)	74	93% (85–98)	68	91% (82–97)
SIT + STAND-IGRA	77	95% (87–99)	73	93% (85–98)	61	67% (54–79)
SICCT + STAND-IGRA	77	95% (87–99)	73	100% (95–100)	61	80% (68–89)

[1]SIT, single intradermal tuberculin test; [2]sP22-IGRA, single P22 IGRA test; [3]cP22-IGRA, comparative P22 IGRA test; [4]SICCT, single intradermal cervical comparative intradermal tuberculin test; [5]sP22-ST, single P22 skin test; [6]cP22-ST, comparative P22-ST; [7]STAND-IGRA, standard tuberculin IGRA test. [8]Number of animals tested. [9]Clopper–Pearson 95% confidence interval for Se. [10]Clopper–Pearson 95% confidence interval for Sp.
TB, tuberculosis; BCG, bacille Calmette-Guérin; IGRA, interferon-gamma release assay.

Complementarity of Diagnostic Tests

Combined interpretation of P22-based tests was evaluated. Results of Sp and Se of complementarity of diagnostic tests are shown in **Table 4**. In general, complementarity between tests yielded an overall rise of Se with a variable reduction in the Sp.

The combination of cP22-ST + P22 ELISA improved the Se in 20 p.p. and displayed a similar Sp in both herds B and C, being the combined interpretation with the best results in all situations. The combination of SICCT + P22 ELISA showed similar results of Se and Sp in herd B. In herd C, the latter combination detected

10 false-positives more than the cP22-ST + P22-ELISA, reducing its Sp in 16 p.p., and with diagnostic results significantly different between tests ($p = 0.004$). The combination of cP22-ST + cP22-IGRA improved the Se and Sp in herd B at a similar level than the combined interpretations above described, but in herd C, the Sp was reduced in 11 p.p. respect to the cP22-ST + P22-ELISA test.

The combination of current diagnostic tests, e.g., SIT and SICCT, with other diagnostic tests increased the Se but not the Sp, except for the SICCT + STAND-IGRA. The latter combination improved the Se in 4 and 18 p.p. compared to the SICCT and the STAND-IGRA alone, respectively, and maintained the Sp in herd B but not in herd C (reduction of 16 p.p. compared to the STAND-IGRA alone). In herd A, the combined results of MPB83-ELISA + P22-ELISA improved the Se in 12 and 13 p.p. with respect to the MPB83-ELISA and the P22-ELISA alone, respectively, and maintained the Sp in herd B, and in herd C showed a mild reduction of Sp (4 and 6 p.p. of reduction with respect to the MPB83-ELISA and the P22-ELISA alone, respectively). Other combinations of tests did not improve the Se and the Sp, as did the aforementioned combined interpretations.

Performance of Diagnostic Tests

The results of DOR to assess the diagnostic performance for each test are represented in **Figure 1**. In general, a reduced DOR in TB-VAC scenario was observed compared to the conventional one (0.47, 95% CI: 0.28–0.654, of mean reduction in log DOR). In the conventional context, SICCT + STAND-IGRA (3.38, 95% CI: 2.35–4.41), SICCT alone (3.16, 95% CI: 2.36–3.97), SICCT + cP22-IGRA (2.94, 95% CI: 1.12–4.76), and SICCT + sP22-IGRA (2.81, 95% CI: 1.08–4.54) showed the best performances (**Figure 1A**). In TB-VAC context, the best performances were observed in DIVA IGRA (2.53, 95% CI: 1.98–3.8), cP22-ST + P22 ELISA (2.44, 95% CI: 0.97–3.92), and sP22-ST + P22 ELISA (2.31, 95% CI: 0.95–3.67) (**Figure 1B**).

DISCUSSION

Efficient and accurate diagnosis is of paramount importance for the success of eradication programs based on test and slaughter strategy. Here, the performance of new P22 antigenic complex-based cell-mediated and humoral tests for the diagnosis of TB in goats was assessed under different epidemiological and TB control scenarios.

Recently, the P22 antigenic complex has been evaluated for the detection of IgG in ELISA tests in different species: cattle goat, sheep, pigs, and wild boar (24–27), red deer (28), badgers (29), and alpacas and llamas (30). In the present study, the performance of the P22 antigenic complex for diagnostic tests based on CMI, namely, STs and IGRA, was evaluated for the first time in goats. Indeed, the use of P22 for IGRA tests has only been reported in red deer experimentally infected with *M. bovis* (37).

The combined interpretation of tests leads to a substantial improvement of Se at the expense of a variable loss of Sp. As expected, in the conventional context, the SICCT alone or combined with the STAND-IGRA (8, 11, 38) showed the best

performances by DOR analysis. The performances of tuberculin-based tests were followed by the combinations of SICCT with the P22-IGRAs, which increased Se at the cost of a certain loss in Sp. Moreover, the combination of cP22-ST + P22-ELISA clearly increased the Se with the benefit of a minimal decrease of Sp, showing similar results than the combination of SICCT + P22-ELISA. These findings are in concordance with previous studies of P22-ELISA and tuberculin-based skin testing. In cattle, the combination of SIT + P22-ELISA showed an improvement of Se of 30 and 6 p.p. compared to the SIT and the P22-ELISA alone, respectively (25). In another study conducted in goats (39), the same combination improved the Se of the SIT and the P22-ELISA in 19 and 9.5 p.p., respectively. Also, in the same study in goats, the combination of SICCT + P22-ELISA improved the Se of the SICCT in a 24 p.p. These results confirmed the benefits of the strategic use of serological and CMI-based diagnostic tests in parallel to maximize the Se in infected settings.

In the TB-VAC context, the combination of P22-ELISA with the two P22-based STs showed similar performances than the DIVA-IGRA. However, the latter showed considerably lower Se than the combinations of P22-ELISA with P22-based STs (reduction in 23–24 p.p.). Previous studies reported the excellent Sp (16) and the lack of Se (40) of DIVA-IGRA, although the DOR analysis tended to overestimate the Sp in this study. The Se of vaccine-associated diagnostic tests is an essential requirement for the development of an integral vaccination strategy (41), and the combination of cP22-ST + P22-ELISA showed an efficient and innovative diagnostic approach in the TB-VAC context, showing the highest combined Se and Sp values (94 and 95%, respectively).

Concerning the use of the ST in solitary, the P22-based STs showed lower Se compared to both the SIT and the SICCT tests, although previous studies in dairy goat flocks, with larger samples and different epidemiological situations, have shown lower Se for SIT (65%, 95% CI: 63.3–68.2) (8) and SICCT (44.5%, 95% CI: 35–55) (42). However, the Se of the cP22-ST (74%, 95% CI: 63–83) was similar to Se observed in two previous studies using DIVA STs (based on the peptide cocktails ESAT-6, CFP-10, and Rv3616c) developed for the diagnosis of TB in cattle: 76%, 95% CI: 59–93 (43) and 75%, 95% CI: 47.7–97.7 (44). In the latter, the addition of the Rv3020c peptide improved the Se to reach 87.5% (95% CI: 61.7–98.5), being similar to the Se of sP22-ST (87%, 95% CI: 74–94) obtained in the present study. On the other hand, in BCG-vaccinated animals, the Sp of SIT and SICCT decreased dramatically (27 and 20 p.p. of reduction, respectively), whereas the Sp of sP22-ST and cP22-ST remained high (97 and 98%, respectively). These findings again highlight the suitability of P22-based STs as TB vaccine-associated diagnostic candidates, although improvements to increase the Se should be necessary.

Moreover, herd PTB status and MAP vaccination may also affect the interpretation of the results. MAP infection was not reported in farms B and C, and no recent clinical history of PTB was observed by the veterinarians. Despite this, vaccination against MAP is a common practice in small ruminants in Spain (12), and diagnostic interferences due to MAP vaccination

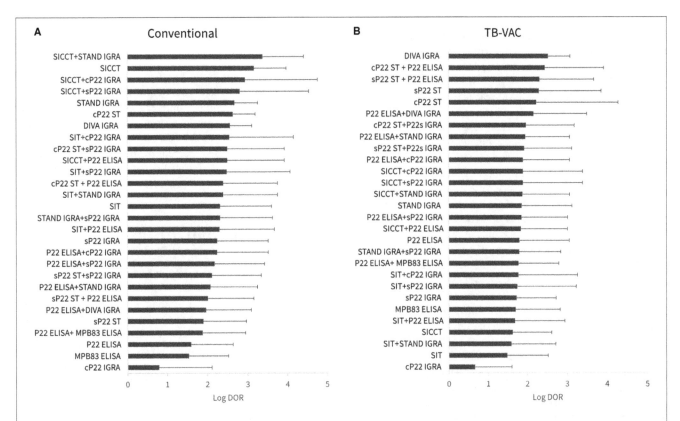

FIGURE 1 | Diagnostic test performance measured by diagnostic odds ratio (DOR). **(A)** Conventional (unvaccinated scenario). **(B)** Tuberculosis (TB)-VAC scenario, animals were vaccinated with *Mycobacterium bovis* bacille Calmette-Guérin (BCG). sP22-ST, single P22 skin test; cP22-ST, comparative P22 intradermal skin test; SIT, single intradermal tuberculin test; SICCT, single intradermal cervical comparative tuberculin test; sP22-IGRA, single P22 interferon-gamma release assay (IGRA) test; cP22-IGRA, comparative P22 IGRA test; STAND-IGRA, standard tuberculin IGRA test; DIVA-IGRA, differentiating infected from vaccinated animals (ESAT-6/CFP-10 peptide cocktail) IGRA test.

on TB diagnosis cannot be ruled out in these two MAP-vaccinated herds. In this sense, strong reactions to PPD-A were observed at skin testing (**Supplementary Data**), but the results of comparative tests (cP22-ST and SICCT) showed higher Sp compared to their respective single STs (i.e., sP22-ST and SIT). These findings indicate that some degree of cross-reactivity due to MAP vaccination was still maintained. Similarly, interferences of MAP vaccination on TB diagnosis, mainly in CMI-based diagnostic tests, were previously observed in MAP-vaccinated goats (14, 45).

Surprisingly, the P22-based IGRAs, particularly the sP22-IGRA, showed higher Se compared to STAND-IGRA and even higher compared to DIVA-IGRA. However, the Se of sP22-IGRA was similar to that previously observed by the STAND-IGRA (92%, 95% CI: 84–96) in other studies conducted in goats (26). The results of Se of the cP22-IGRA in the present study were also similar to those previously observed in experimentally *M. bovis*-infected red deer (37). However, a slight loss of Sp in the P22-IGRAs was detected compared to STAND-IGRA. Even so, the Sp was within ranges (95–100%) described for STAND-IGRA in previous studies (11, 38, 45). This mild reduction in Sp could be explained by the high concentration of P22 used for stimulation of whole blood (20 μg/ml) and by the

fact that P22 complex contains 21 proteins also present in *M. avium* (23), which can cause cross-reactivity with MAP vaccination and/or infection. Indeed, the interference of MAP vaccination on STAND-IGRA has been previously observed in adult MAP-vaccinated goats (13, 14, 45). The Sp of P22-IGRAs considerably decreased in BCG-vaccinated herds compared to that previously described for the STAND-IGRA (16). Overall, the results of sP22-IGRA suggest that this test could be a potentially valuable tool for TB eradication in endemic areas, although further studies to determine the optimal concentration of P22 are required to improve its Sp with a minimal loss of Se.

Serological diagnostics is a cost-effective alternative for TB diagnostics. However, the Se of antibody-based diagnostic tests was generally lower compared to tests based on CMI (46, 47). In the present study, the Se of P22-ELISA was slightly lower than that in previous studies in goats and cattle (25, 39). This loss of Sp might be explained by the fact that animals from herd A were not vaccinated against MAP nor subjected to frequent intradermal testing, factors that could enhance humoral responses against MTBC antigens (48). Interestingly, the Se was significantly enhanced when using P22 and MPB83 ELISAs in parallel. Thus, even though MPB83 is a major component of the P22 complex, specific IgGs of some infected animals were only detectable using the MPB83 purified recombinant protein alone, while others were only detected using the P22 complex, which contains additional serodominant epitopes (23).

Finally, Sp of the P22-ELISA reached considerably higher Sp in MAP-vaccinated (and BCG-unvaccinated, i.e., herd B) goats (93%) compared to that previously found in Spanish (78%) and Norwegian MAP-vaccinated goats (58%) (24). In the latter study, besides MAP vaccination, MAP coinfection and/or contact with environmental mycobacteria was not discarded as a source of diagnostic interference. Interestingly, in the present study, the Sp was also high in BCG- and MAP-vaccinated goats (96%), suggesting that BCG vaccination does not induce antibody responses that cause interference on the diagnosis by the P22-ELISA. The absence of antibody responses was consistent with the fact that the BCG Danish strain used for vaccination expresses low levels of MPB83 and MPB70 (49), which are the most abundant proteins of the P22 antigenic complex (23). Moreover, tuberculin skin testing after 42 days of MAP or BCG vaccination caused a boosting effect on humoral responses against tuberculin antigens, resulting in false-positive cattle for an MPB83-based ELISA (50). Here, minimal or no boosting effects of MAP/BCG vaccination due to skin testing were observed on the P22-ELISA. Indeed, goats from herd B were sampled around 2 years after vaccination against MAP, and ST was performed once or twice after MAP vaccination. Also, 34/68 goats from herd C were vaccinated with BCG and Gudair® at 9–10 months before the sampling, whereas the rest of the animals were vaccinated more than 1 year before, and no ST was performed since. Based on the results herein, the P22-ELISA seemed to be a useful ancillary

diagnostic tool, either in BCG or MAP vaccination context, although it should be confirmed in further studies with larger sized herds.

In conclusion, this study reinforces the applicability of the P22 antigen complex as a complementary instrument for TB diagnostics in goats under different control scenarios. The P22 serological diagnostic is a cost-effective alternative, and combined interpretation with STs, either with PPD-B or P22, showed promising results. Moreover, the use of P22 antigenic complex in CMI-based diagnostic tests showed encouraging results, being suitable for further research on the improvement of TB diagnostics.

AUTHOR CONTRIBUTIONS

BP and JB contributed to conceptualization. CA-V, BP, and MG contributed to data curation. CA-V and BP performed the formal analysis. BP and LJ acquired funding. CA-V, BP, MG, EV, MD, IM, JI-L, and JB contributed to the investigation. CA-V, BP, JI-L, EV, and MD contributed to the methodology. BP and LJ contributed to project administration. JI-L and MS acquired resources. CA-V and BP wrote the original draft. JB, LJ, JI-L, EV, and MD contributed to writing, reviewing, and editing.

ACKNOWLEDGMENTS

We are grateful to Maite Martín, Zoraida Cervera, Carlos Lopez-Figueroa, and the staff of Field Studies Unit of IRTA-CReSA for their technical support.

REFERENCES

1. Daniel R, Evans H, Rolfe S, de la Rua-Domenech R, Crawshaw T, Higgins RJ, et al. Outbreak of tuberculosis caused by *Mycobacterium bovis* in golden Guernsey goats in Great Britain. *Vet Rec.* (2009) 165:335–42. doi: 10.1136/vr.165.12.335

2. Napp S, Allepuz A, Mercader I, Nofrarías M, López-Soria S, Domingo M, et al. Evidence of goats acting as domestic reservoirs of bovine tuberculosis. *Vet Rec.* (2013) 172:663. doi: 10.1136/vr.101347

3. Vidal E, Grasa M, Peralvarez T, Martín M, Mercader I, Pérez de Val B. Transmission of tuberculosis caused by *Mycobacterium caprae* between dairy sheep and goats. *Small Rumin Res.* (2018) 158:22–25. doi: 10.1016/j.smallrumres.2017.11.010

4. Cano-Terriza D, Risalde MA, Rodríguez-Hernández P, Napp S, Fernández-Morente M, Moreno I, et al. Epidemiological surveillance of *Mycobacterium tuberculosis* complex in extensively raised pigs in the south of Spain. *Prev Vet Med.* (2018) 159:87–91. doi: 10.1016/j.prevetmed.2018.08.015

5. Rodríguez S, Bezos J, Romero B, de Juan L, Álvarez J, Castellanos E, Moya N, et al. *Mycobacterium caprae* infection in livestock and wildlife, Spain. *Emerg Infect Dis.* (2011) 17:532–5. doi: 10.3201/eid1703.100618

6. Prodinger WM, Indra A, Koksalan OK, Kilicaslan Z, Richter E. *Mycobacterium caprae* infection in humans. *Expert Rev Anti Infect Ther.* (2014) 12:1501–13. doi: 10.1586/14787210.2014.974560

7. Guta S, Casal J, Napp S, Saez JL, Garcia-Saenz A, Perez De Val B, et al. Epidemiological investigation of bovine tuberculosis herd breakdowns in Spain 2009/2011. *PLoS One.* (2014) 9:e104383. doi: 10.1371/journal.pone.0104383

8. Bezos J, Marqués S, Álvarez J, Casal C, Romero B, Grau A, Mínguez O, et al. Evaluation of single and comparative intradermal tuberculin tests for tuberculosis eradication in caprine flocks in Castilla y León (Spain). *Res Vet Sci.* (2014) 96:39–46. doi: 10.1016/j.rvsc.2013.10.007

9. MAPA. *Ministerio de Agricultura y Pesca, Alimentación y Medio Ambiente.* Programa Nacional de Erradicación de la Tuberculosis Bovina presentado por España para el año (2019). Available online at: https://www.mapa.gob.es/es/ganaderia/temas/sanidad-animal-higiene-ganadera/sanidad-animal/enfermedades/tuberculosis/Tuberculosis_bovina.aspx

10. Napp S, Ciaravino G, Pérez de Val B, Casal J, Saéz JL, Alba A. Evaluation of the effectiveness of the surveillance system for tuberculosis in cattle in Spain. *Prev Vet Med.* (2019) 173:104805. doi: 10.1016/j.prevetmed.2019.104805

11. Bezos J, Álvarez J, Mínguez O, Marqués S, Martín O, Vigo V, Pieltain C, et al. Evaluation of specificity of tuberculosis diagnostic assays in caprine flocks under different epidemiological situations. *Res Vet Sci.* (2012) 93:636–40. doi: 10.1016/j.rvsc.2011.10.009

12. Bastida F, Juste RA. Paratuberculosis control: a review with a focus on vaccination. *J Immune Based Ther Vaccines.* (2011) 9:8. doi: 10.1186/1476-8518-9-8

13. Chartier C, Mercier P, Pellet MP, Vialard J. Effect of an inactivated paratuberculosis vaccine on the intradermal testing of goats for tuberculosis. *Vet J.* (2012) 191:360–3. doi: 10.1016/j.tvjl.2011.03.009

14. Pérez de Val B, Nofrarías M, López-Soria S, Garrido JM, Vordermeier HM, Villarreal-Ramos B, et al. Effects of vaccination against paratuberculosis on tuberculosis in goats: diagnostic interferences and cross-protection. *BMC Vet Res.* (2012) 8:191. doi: 10.1186/1746-6148-8-191

15. Pérez De Val B, Vidal E, Villarreal-Ramos B, Gilbert SC, Andaluz A, Moll X, et al. A multi-antigenic adenoviral-vectored vaccine improves

BCG-induced protection of goats against pulmonary tuberculosis infection and prevents disease progression. *PLoS One.* (2013) 8:e81317. doi: 10.1371/journal.pone.0081317

16. Pérez de Val B, Vidal E, López-Soria S, Marco A, Cervera Z, Martín M, et al. Assessment of safety and interferon gamma responses of *Mycobacterium bovis* BCG vaccine in goat kids and milking goats. *Vaccine.* (2016) 34:881–6. doi: 10.1016/j.vaccine.2016.01.004

17. Roy A, Tomé I, Romero B, Lorente-Leal V, Infantes-Lorenzo JA, Domínguez M, et al. Evaluation of the immunogenicity and efficacy of BCG and MTBVAC vaccines using a natural transmission model of tuberculosis. *Vet Res.* (2019) 50:82. doi: 10.1186/s13567-019-0702-7

18. Vidal E, Arrieta-Villegas C, Grasa M, Mercader I, Domingo M, Pérez de Val B. Field evaluation of the efficacy of *Mycobacterium bovis* BCG vaccine against tuberculosis in goats. *BMC Vet Res.* (2017) 13:252. doi: 10.1186/s12917-017-1182-5

19. Bezos J, Casal C, Álvarez J, Roy A, Romero B, Rodríguez-Bertos A, Bárcena C, et al. Evaluation of the *Mycobacterium tuberculosis* SO$_2$ vaccine using a natural tuberculosis infection model in goats. *Vet J.* (2017) 223:60–7. doi: 10.1016/j.tvjl.2017.04.006

20. Bezos J, Casal C, Puentes E, Díez-Guerrier A, Romero B, Aguiló N, et al. Evaluation of the immunogenicity and diagnostic interference caused by *M. tuberculosis* SO$_2$ vaccination against tuberculosis in goats. *Res Vet Sci.* (2015) 103:73–9. doi: 10.1016/j.rvsc.2015.09.017

21. Vordermeier HM, Jones GJ, Buddle BM, Hewinson RG. Development of immune-diagnostic reagents to diagnose bovine tuberculosis in cattle. *Vet Immunol Immunopathol.* (2016) 181:10–14. doi: 10.1016/j.vetimm.2016.02.003

22. Vordermeier HM, Whelan A, Cockle PJ, Farrant L, Hewinson RG. Use of synthetic peptides derived from the antigens ESAT-6 and CFP-10 for differential diagnosis of bovine tuberculosis in cattle use of synthetic peptides derived from the antigens ESAT-6 and CFP-10 for Differential diagnosis of bovine tuberculosis in Ca. *Cell Host Microbe.* (2001) 8:571–8. doi: 10.1128/CDLI.8.3.571-578.2001

23. Infantes-Lorenzo JA, Moreno I, Risalde MDLA, Roy Á, Villar M, Romero B, et al. Proteomic characterisation of bovine and avian purified protein derivatives and identification of specific antigens for serodiagnosis of bovine tuberculosis. *Clin Proteomics.* (2017) 14:1–10. doi: 10.1186/s12014-017-9171-z

24. Infantes-Lorenzo JA, Moreno I, Roy A, Risalde MA, Balseiro A, De Juan L, et al. Specificity of serological test for detection of tuberculosis in cattle, goats, sheep and pigs under different epidemiological situations. *BMC Vet Res.* (2019) 15:70. doi: 10.1186/s12917-019-1814-z

25. Casal C, Infantes JA, Risalde MA, Díez-Guerrier A, Domínguez M, Moreno I, et al. Antibody detection tests improve the sensitivity of tuberculosis diagnosis in cattle. *Res Vet Sci.* (2017) 112:214–21. doi: 10.1016/j.rvsc.2017.05.012

26. Bezos J, Roy Á, Infantes-Lorenzo JA, González I, Venteo Á, Romero B, et al. The use of serological tests in combination with the intradermal tuberculin test maximizes the detection of tuberculosis infected goats. *Vet Immunol Immunopathol.* (2018) 199:43–52. doi: 10.1016/j.vetimm.2018.03.006

27. Thomas J, Infantes-Lorenzo JA, Moreno I, Cano-Terriza D, de Juan L, García-Bocanegra I, et al. Validation of a new serological assay for the identification of *Mycobacterium tuberculosis* complex-specific antibodies in pigs and wild boar. *Prev Vet Med.* (2019) 162:11–17. doi: 10.1016/j.prevetmed.2018.11.004

28. Thomas J, Infantes-Lorenzo JA, Moreno I, Romero B, Garrido JM, Juste R, et al. A new test to detect antibodies against *Mycobacterium tuberculosis* complex in red deer serum. *Vet J.* (2019) 244:98–103. doi: 10.1016/j.tvjl.2018.12.021

29. Infantes-Lorenzo JA, Dave D, Moreno I, Anderson P, Lesellier S, Gormley E, et al. New serological platform for detecting antibodies against *Mycobacterium tuberculosis* complex in European badgers. *Vet Med Sci.* (2019) 5:61–9. doi: 10.1002/vms3.134

30. Infantes-Lorenzo JA, Whitehead CE, Moreno I, Bezos J, Roy A, Domínguez L, et al. Development and evaluation of a serological assay for the diagnosis of tuberculosis in alpacas and llamas. *Front Vet Sci.* (2018) 5:189. doi: 10.3389/fvets.2018.00189

31. Cockle PJ, Gordon SV, Lalvani A, Buddle BM, Hewinson RG, Vordermeier HM. Identification of novel *Mycobacterium tuberculosis* antigens with potential as diagnostic reagents or subunit vaccine candidates by comparative genomics identification of novel *Mycobacterium tuberculosis* antigens with potential as diagnostic reagents or Su. *Infect Immun.* (2002) 70:6996–7003. doi: 10.1128/IAI.70.12.6996-7003.2002

32. Vordermeier HM, Cockle PC, Whelan A, Rhodes S, Palmer N, Bakker D, et al. Development of diagnostic reagents to differentiate between *Mycobacterium bovis* BCG vaccination and *M. bovis* infection in cattle. *Clin Diagn Lab Immunol.* (1999) 6:675–82. doi: 10.1128/CDLI.6.5.675-682.1999

33. Pérez de Val B, Napp S, Velarde R, Lavín S, Cervera Z, Singh M, et al. Serological follow-up of tuberculosis in a wild boar population in contact with infected cattle. *Transbound Emerg Dis.* (2017) 64:275–83. doi: 10.1111/tbed.12368

34. Pérez De Val B, López-Soria S, Nofrarías M, Martín M, Vordermeier HM, Villarreal-Ramos B, et al. Experimental model of tuberculosis in the domestic goat after endobronchial infection with Mycobacterium caprae. *Clin Vaccine Immunol.* (2011) 18:1872–81. doi: 10.1128/CVI.05323-11

35. Wilton S, Cousins D. Detection and identification of multiple mycobacterial pathogens by DNA amplification in a single tube. *Genome Res.* (1992) 1:269–73. doi: 10.1101/gr.1.4.269

36. Glas AS, Lijmer JG, Prins MH, Bonsel GJ, Bossuyt PMM. The diagnostic odds ratio: a single indicator of test performance. *J Clin Epidemiol.* (2003) 56:1129–35. doi: 10.1016/S0895-4356(03)00177-X

37. Risalde MÁ, Thomas J, Sevilla I, Serrano M, Ortíz JA, Garrido J, et al. Development and evaluation of an interferon gamma assay for the diagnosis of tuberculosis in red deer experimentally infected with *Mycobacterium bovis*. *BMC Vet Res.* (2017) 13:341. doi: 10.1186/s12917-017-1262-6

38. Bezos J, Álvarez J, Romero B, Aranaz A, Juan Ld. Tuberculosis in goats: assessment of current *in vivo* cell-mediated and antibody-based diagnostic assays. *Vet J.* (2012) 191:161–5. doi: 10.1016/j.tvjl.2011.02.010

39. Roy A, Infantes-Lorenzo JA, Domínguez M, Moreno I, Pérez M, García N, et al. Evaluation of a new enzyme-linked immunosorbent assay for the diagnosis of tuberculosis in goat milk. *Res Vet Sci.* (2020) 128:217–23. doi: 10.1016/j.rvsc.2019.12.009

40. Bezos J, Álvarez J, de Juan L, Romero B, Rodríguez S, Fernández-de-Mera IG, Hewinson RG, et al. Assessment of *in vivo* and *in vitro* tuberculosis diagnostic tests in *Mycobacterium caprae* naturally infected caprine flocks. *Prev Vet Med.* (2011) 100:187–92. doi: 10.1016/j.prevetmed.2011.03.012

41. Vordermeier HM, Pérez de Val B, Buddle BM, Villarreal-Ramos B, Jones GJ, Hewinson RG, et al. Vaccination of domestic animals against tuberculosis: review of progress and contributions to the field of the TBSTEP project. *Res Vet Sci.* (2014) 97:S53–S60. doi: 10.1016/j.rvsc.2014.04.015

42. Buendía AJ, Navarro JA, Salinas J, McNair J, de Juan L, Ortega N, et al. Ante-mortem diagnosis of caprine tuberculosis in persistently infected herds: Influence of lesion type on the sensitivity of diagnostic tests. *Res Vet Sci.* (2013) 95:1107–13. doi: 10.1016/j.rvsc.2013.10.003

43. Srinivasan S, Jones G, Veerasami M, Steinbach S, Holder T, Zewude A, et al. A defined antigen skin test for the diagnosis of bovine tuberculosis. *Sci Adv.* (2019) 5:eaax4899. doi: 10.1126/sciadv.aax4899

44. Jones GJ, Whelan A, Clifford D, Coad M, Vordermeier HM. Improved skin test for differential diagnosis of bovine tuberculosis by the addition of Rv3020c-derived peptides. *Clin Vaccine Immunol.* (2012) 19:620–2. doi: 10.1128/CVI.00024-12

45. Roy Á, Infantes-Lorenzo JA, Blázquez JC, Venteo Á, Mayoral FJ, Domínguez M, et al. Temporal analysis of the interference caused by paratuberculosis vaccination on the tuberculosis diagnostic tests in goats. *Prev Vet Med.* (2018) 156:68–75. doi: 10.1016/j.prevetmed.2018.05.010

46. de la Rua-Domenech R, Goodchild AT, Vordermeier HM, Hewinson RG, Christiansen KH, Clifton-Hadley RS. Ante mortem diagnosis of tuberculosis in cattle: a review of the tuberculin tests, γ-interferon assay and other ancillary diagnostic techniques. *Res Vet Sci.* (2006) 81:190–210. doi: 10.1016/j.rvsc.2005.11.005

47. Bezos J, Casal C, Romero B, Schroeder B, Hardegger R, Raeber AJ, et al. Current ante-mortem techniques for diagnosis of bovine tuberculosis. *Res Vet Sci.* (2014) 97(Suppl):S44–S52. doi: 10.1016/j.rvsc.2014.04.002

48. O'Brien A, Whelan C, Clarke JB, Hayton A, Watt NJ, Harkiss GD. Serological analysis of tuberculosis in goats by use of the enferplex caprine TB multiplex test. *Clin Vaccine Immunol.* (2017) 24:e00518-16. doi: 10.1128/CVI.00518-16

49. Charlet D, Mostowy S, Alexander D, Sit L, Wiker HG, Behr MA. Reduced

expression of antigenic proteins MPB70 and MPB83 in *Mycobacterium bovis* BCG strains due to a start codon mutation in sigK. *Mol Microbiol.* (2005) 56:1302–13. doi: 10.1111/j.1365-2958.2005.04618.x

50. Coad M, Clifford DJ, Vordermeier HM, Whelan AO. The consequences of vaccination with the Johne's disease vaccine, Gudair, on diagnosis of bovine tuberculosis. *Vet Rec.* (2013) 172:266. doi: 10.1136/vr.101201

16

Scrapie Control in EU Goat Population: Has the Last Gap been Overcome?

Sergio Migliore*, Roberto Puleio and Guido Ruggero Loria

Istituto Zooprofilattico Sperimentale Della Sicilia "A. Mirri", Palermo, Italy

Keywords: TSEs: transmissible spongiform encephalopathies, scrapie, PRNP: prion gene name, goat, EU regulation, genetic−disease resistance, biodiversity

INTRODUCTION

*Correspondence:
Sergio Migliore
migliore.sergio@gmail.com

Scrapie is a fatal, neurodegenerative disease that affects sheep and goat worldwide, belonging to the group of transmissible spongiform encephalopathies (TSEs).

Since 2002, Member States (MS) of European Union (EU) have implemented active surveillance to control the risk of scrapie. The EU scrapie eradication policy is mainly aimed to eradicate classical scrapie. The choice of population groups and sample sizes have evolved in the years, as well as the eradication measures and control of disease (selective culling, movement restrictions, reinforced surveillance measures, etc.). In this context, over the past two decades, breeding programs to increase the frequency of the resistance-associated ARR allele in sheep populations have been introduced to minimize TSE risk in MS, but there was not a regulatory effort in adoption of analogous measures for goats. However, scientific knowledge related to scrapie resistance associated with goat PRNP gene polymorphisms has considerably expanded in the last 10 years.

Classical scrapie is considered endemic in many MS. Since its publication, the only measures applicable for TSE control in goat contained in Regulation (EC) No 999/2001 obliged farmers to provide a complete culling of whole flock, with great economic loss and serious concerns for the risk of extinction of endangered breeds. However, over the years, additional measures have been introduced such as monitoring of the infected herd without the obligation of total culling and the possibility of reintroducing goats with unknown genotype after biosafety practices. Nevertheless, these measures could allow the goat population to become the main reservoir of scrapie, affecting the disease eradication program in small ruminant population.

Following a request from the European Commission (EC), the European Food Safety Authority (EFSA) was asked to deliver scientific opinions on the scrapie situation in EU to evaluate the introduction of breeding policies in goats. From 2014, EFSA advised to promote selection and introduction of resistant bucks in EU caprine population (1). More recently, in 2017, based on the latest scientific evidence, EFSA concluded that breeding programs for scrapie resistance in goats should be implemented in MS, taking particular attention to potential negative effects of extinction in rare and endangered breeds (2).

With Regulation (EC) No 2020/772 of June 11, 2020, amending Regulation (EC) No 999/2001, EC laid down new approaches as regards eradication measures for TSEs in goats and in endangered breeds. In this context, the authors discuss advantages and critical points related to the different control measures introduced by EU regulations during the last two decades.

STATE OF THE ART

Legislative Basis

Regulation (EC) No 999/2001 establishes rules for the prevention, control, and eradication of certain TSEs, including scrapie in small ruminants. This Regulation dates back to 2001 and, after many subsequent amendments, is still in force today.

In 2003, Regulation (EC) No 260/2003 revised the requirements for eradication measures in case of the detection of TSE in a farm by selective culling of susceptible sheep and by requiring the implementation of measures to increase TSE resistance in the outbreak. Simultaneously, decision 2003/100 (EC) laid down requirements for the establishment of breeding programs for resistance to TSE in sheep, aimed to increase the level of alleles associated with resistance (ARR) and decreasing the frequency of alleles associated with susceptibility (VRQ) in EU sheep population. Commission Regulation (EC) No 1923/20065 and No 727/2007 then integrated the breeding program requirements into Regulation (EC) No 999/2001. In 2006, EFSA confirmed the efficacy of breeding program for TSE resistance in sheep (3).

More recently, on June 11, 2020, Regulation (EC) No 2020/772 amended Annexes I, VII, and VIII to Regulation (EC) No 999/2001 introducing the possibility for the MS to limit slaughtering/culling and destruction to goats which are genetically susceptible to classical scrapie. In addition, the definition of "endangered breed" of Regulation (EU) 2016/1012 replaced the expression of "local breed in danger of being lost to farming" as laid down in Regulation (EU) No 807/2014 (4).

Scrapie in EU Goats

Classical scrapie shows similar epidemiological features in sheep and goats and the involvement of both species in outbreaks is common. Even if the incidence in goats is much lower than in sheep, milk and placenta of infected goats may serve as sources of infection to sheep (5, 6). Scrapie in goat was described for the first time in 1942 (4); since then, clinical cases have been recorded throughout Europe. Animal movements between herds and environmental contamination play relevant roles as risk factors.

In 2019, a total of 325,386 sheep and 138,128 goats were tested in EU. In sheep, 821 cases of classical scrapie were detected in seven MS, whereas 517 cases were reported in goats in seven MS (7). Scrapie in goat is considered endemic in the EU countries with the largest caprine populations with more than 10,500 cases from 2002 to 2017. Between 2002 and 2015, classical scrapie was detected in 10 MS with 2.4 cases out of 10,000 tested heads. In this prevalence study, Cyprus was excluded due to an epidemic over the last 10 years (2).

Genetic Basis

In the last two decades, an extensive review of literature was conducted to identify relevant alleles of goat PRNP to which a breeding program could be based. These studies were conducted within different MS and goat breeds. A considerable dataset has been produced for the following alleles: S127, M142, R143, D145, D146, S146, H154, Q211, and K222. Among them, K222,

D146, and S146 alleles confer higher genetic resistance to classical scrapie strains circulating in the EU goat population (2). In 2017, based on a combination of the "weight of evidence" and the "strength of resistance," EFSA provided a ranking of resistance to classical scrapie, as follows: K222 > D146 = S146 > Q211 = H154 = M142 > S127 = H143 > wild type (2).

Goat Breeding in EU

Goat farming plays an important socioeconomic role in several countries, particularly where there are hills and mountains, and remote, marginal, and even semi-arid areas (8, 9). Europe is the continent with the widest caprine biodiversity with 187 goat breeds, which is 33% of the goat breeds acknowledged worldwide (10). In this context, there are breeds with large population sizes, cosmopolitan and often characterized by a high production, and breeds with small population sizes not yet subjected to conservation programs because of their remoteness or because they are less competitive in terms of production than other selected breeds (9). Such different scenarios obviously have required a different scrapie control strategy.

DISCUSSION

In 2017, EFSA, based on prolonged field experience and experimental studies, concluded that the K222, D146, and S146 variants confer genetic resistance to the classical scrapie strain circulating in the EU goat population (2). EFSA highlighted that the protective effect of K222 is greater than D146 and S146 variants and of ARR allele in sheep, when the 2002 Scientific Steering Committee opinion was published (2). In this regard, a substantial difference between sheep and goats in the new Regulation (EC) No 2020/772 still remains. In sheep, the ARR/ARR homozygous genotype in reproductive males is an essential requirement, whereas in goats, heterozygosity for at least one of K222 and D/S146 alleles is sufficient to avoid the stamping out. It should be remembered that heterozygous variants Q222K and N146S/D in goats do not confer full protection against classical scrapie as reported in natural outbreaks in Greece (11) and in Cyprus (12). In addition, the subsequent restocking of outbreak without genotype consideration after biosafety practices is a considerable risk. These are critical points whose efficacy will be assessed in the future.

The EFSA opinion also highlights that a high selective pressure in some breeds with a low frequency of resistant variants would likely have an adverse effect on genetic diversity and that each MS should be able to design its own genetic selection strategy depending on the breed concerned.

Estimating the frequency of candidate alleles is a preliminary step in understanding the feasibility of a breeding program. Several investigations on goat PRNP were performed in MS in recent years, and some breed-related differences emerged (**Table 1**). Higher frequency (>24.5%) of 146D or S variants was described in cosmopolitan Boer goat in Great Britain and Netherlands (13–15) and in native Damascus and related breeds in Cyprus (16.5%) (17). A lower frequency (3%) was also described in local and crossbred in Greece (16). To date,

TABLE 1 | Breeds with S146/D146 and K222 haplotypes reported in literature and their frequencies reported in EU.

Country	Breed	Geographical classification	Local status*	Frequency (%)	Source
146D or 146S					
UK	Boer	Cosmopolitan	At risk	24.5–35.5	(13, 14)
Netherlands	Boer	Cosmopolitan	Unknown	31	(15)
	Nubian	Cosmopolitan	At risk	7.1	
Greece	Local/crossbred	Local	Unknown	3.0	(16)
Cyprus	Damascus and related breeds	Cosmopolitan	Not at risk	16.5	(17)
222K					
UK	Toggenburg	Cosmopolitan	At risk	1.9	(13)
Netherlands	Saanen	Cosmopolitan	Unknown	1.9	(15)
	Toggenburg	Cosmopolitan	At risk	29.5	
Greece	Local/crossbred	Local	Unknown	5.6	(16)
France	Saanen	Cosmopolitan	Not at risk	4.9	(18)
Spain	Saanen	Cosmopolitan	Unknown	1.2	(19)
	Alpine	Cosmopolitan	Unknown	6.4	
	Local breeds	Local	At risk	0–0.03	
Italy (Northern breeds)	Camosciata	Cosmopolitan	Not at risk	2.4	(20)
	Saanen	Cosmopolitan	Not at risk	3.0	
	Roccaverano	Local	Endangered	4.3	
	Valdostana	Local	Critical	1.3	
Italy (Southern breeds)	Garganica	Local	Endangered	17.2	
	Jonica	Local	Critical	7.3	
	Southern crossbred	Local	Unknown	22.5	
	Girgentana	Local	Endangered	18.7	(21)
	Rossa Mediterranea	Local	Critical	12.7	(22)
	Argentata dell'Etna	Local	Endangered	16.3	
	Aspromontana	Local	No at risk	10.3	(23)
	Cilentana	Local	Critical	18.2	

*DAD-IS database—FAO (22).

this mutation does not seem to be widespread in other MS. In contrast, 222 K variant seems to be more common across the MS. Frequencies between 1.2 and 7.5% were described in cosmopolitan and large population size breeds such as Saanen (1.2–4%) and Alpine (6.4–7.5%) reared in Spain, Netherlands, Italy, France, and Greece (15, 16, 18–20). Very high frequency (29.5%) was described in Dutch Toggenburg in Netherlands (15). Variable frequencies were described in small size of native breeds such as local and crossbred in Greece (0.3–5.6%) (16). In Italy, where a great caprine biodiversity is present, a difference between northern and southern native breeds was described (20), with higher frequencies of 222 K in Southern breed such as Garganica (17.2%), Ionica (7.2%), southern crossbred (22.5%), Girgentana (18.7%), Rossa Mediterranea (12.7%), Argentata dell'Etna (16.3%), Aspromontana (10.3%), and Cilentana (18.2%) (20–23). Many of these breeds are considered in critical or endangered status (24) and for this reason any breeding program should consider the endangered status of each goat population to preserve the genetic variability and the biodiversity together with disease control (21).

Various mutations in the PRNP in different breeds have potentially been positively selected in relation to local circulating scrapie strains originating in specific environmental conditions (25).

A recent study (26) assessed the impact of different breeding strategies in goat using a mathematical model, and it concluded that breeding programs for scrapie resistance could be implemented also in a context of so high biodiversity and also different size of the populations of goats. Nevertheless, the growth rate of resistant goats in some breeds may be slow due to the initial genetic profile not being particularly favorable inside the breed. In cosmopolitan breeds with a large population size, a breeding program in the overall population would be desirable. In contrast, in endangered breeds with a small population, a breeding program should be implemented starting from reproductive nuclei. This scheme is less expansive and protects the endangered breeds even if it takes longer to reach the expected results.

As well as goat breeds, a breeding program for scrapie resistance should consider the particular situation of each MS in terms of the presence of resistant alleles and their relative frequency. For example, in Greece, which has one of the largest goat populations in Europe, a goat-scrapie resistance program targeting the Q211, S146, and K222 alleles was designed (27), whereas in Italy, pilot projects selected positively a singular variant K222.

Although there is a strong interest in disease control among goat farmers in the Northern MS, breeding for resistance is often compromised by the low frequency of resistant alleles. By contrast, in Southern MS where a satisfying frequency of resistant alleles is present, goat farming is mainly related to pastoralism and in several cases there is a lack of interest in starting genetic programs. For this reason, to be successful, new regulations have to consider engaging farmers' cooperation by appropriate risk communication and involving them in the genetic program as well as providing an adequate financial support for goat genotyping.

Regulation (EC) No 2020/772 laid down an alternative tool for scrapie control in EU goat population. It particularly recognized the genetic resistance to classical scrapie in goats carrying at least one of the most recognized alleles (K222, D146, and S146) and preserving them from culling in the case of outbreak. In addition, the new regulation introduces possible derogation measures for endangered breeds according to Regulation (EU) 2016/1012. This new measure will finally strengthen the control of TSEs in small ruminants in the EU and will also have beneficial effects on farming system and for the conservation of goat breed biodiversity.

AUTHOR CONTRIBUTIONS

SM drafting of the article. RP and GL revised the article. All authors contributed to the article and approved the submitted version.

REFERENCES

1. EFSA BIOHAZ Panel. Scientific Opinion on the scrapie situation in the EU after 10 years of monitoring and control in sheep and goats. *EFSA J.* (2014) 12:3781. doi: 10.2903/j.efsa.2014.3781

2. EFSA BIOHAZ Panel. Genetic resistance to transmissible spongiform encephalopathies. (TSE) in goats. *EFSA J.* (2017) 15:4962. doi: 10.2903/j.efsa.2017.4962

3. EFSA BIOHAZ Panel. Opinion of the Scientific Panel on Biological Hazards on "the breeding programme for TSE resistance in sheep". *EFSA J.* (2006) 4:382. doi: 10.2903/j.efsa.2006.382

4. Chelle PL. A case of scrapie in goats. *Bull de l'Academie Vet de France.* (1942) 15:294–5.

5. Schneider DA, Madsen-Bouterse SA, Zhuang D, Truscott TC, Dassanayake RP, O'Rourke KI. The placenta shed from goats with classical scrapie is infectious to goat kids and lambs. *J Gen Virol.* (2015) 96:2464–9. doi: 10.1099/vir.0.000151

6. Konold T, Thorne L, Simmons HA, Hawkins SA, Simmons MM, González L. Evidence of scrapie transmission to sheep via goat milk. *BMC Vet Res.* (2016) 12:208. doi: 10.1186/s12917-016-0807-4

7. EFSA. Annual report of the scientific network on BSE-TSE 2019. *EFSA Supp Pub.* (2019) 16:1771E. doi: 10.2903/sp.efsa.2019.EN-1771

8. Boayzouglu J, Hatziminaoglou I, Morand-Fehr P. The role of the goat in society: past, present and perspectives for the future. *Small Rumin Res.* (2005) 60:13–23. doi: 10.1016/j.smallrumres.2005.06.003

9. Dubeuf JP, Boyazoglu J. An international panorama of goat selection and breeds. *Livest Sci.* (2009) 120:225–31. doi: 10.1016/j.livsci.2008.07.005

10. Gahal S. Biodiversity in goats. *Small Rum Res.* (2005) 60:75–81. doi: 10.1016/j.smallrumres.2005.06.021

11. Fragkiadaki EG, Vaccari G, Ekateriniadou LV, Agrimi U, Giadinis ND, Chiappini B, et al. PRNP genetic variability and molecular typing of natural goat scrapie isolates in a high number of infected flocks. *Vet Res.* (2011) 42:104. doi: 10.1186/1297-9716-42-104

12. Papasavva-Stylianou P, Windl O, Saunders G, Mavrikiou P, Toumazos P, Kakoyiannis C. PrP gene polymorphisms in Cyprus goats and their association with resistance or susceptibility to natural scrapie. *Vet J.* (2011) 187:245–50. doi: 10.1016/j.tvjl.2009.10.015

13. Goldmann W, Ryan K, Stewart P, Parnham D, Xicohtencatl R, Fernandez N, et al. Caprine prion gene polymorphisms are associated with decreased incidence of classical scrapie in goat herds in the United Kingdom. *Vet Res.* (2011) 42:110. doi: 10.1186/1297-9716-42-110

14. Goldmann W, Marier E, Stewart P, Konold T, Street S, Langeveld J, et al. Prion protein genotype survey confirms low frequency of scrapie-resistant K222 allele in British goat herds. *Vet Rec.* (2016) 178:168. doi: 10.1136/vr.103521

15. Windig JJ, Hoving RA, Priem J, Bossers A, Keulen LJ and Langeveld JP. Variation in the prion protein sequence in Dutch goat breeds. *J Anim Breed Gen.* (2016) 133:366–74. doi: 10.1111/jbg.12211

16. Bouzalas IG, Dovas CI, Banos G, Papanastasopoulou M, Kritas S, Oevermann A, et al. Caprine PRNP polymorphisms at codons 171, 211, 222 and 240 in a Greek herd and their association with classical scrapie. *J Gen Vir.* (2010) 91:1629–34. doi: 10.1099/vir.0.017350-0

17. EFSA. Scientific and technical assistance on the provisional results of the study on genetic resistance to Classical scrapie in goats in Cyprus. *EFSA J.* (2012) 10:2972. doi: 10.2903/j.efsa.2012.2972

18. Barillet F, Mariat D, Amigues Y, Faugeras R, Caillat H, Moazami-Goudarzi K, et al. Identification of seven haplotypes of the caprine PrP gene at codons 127, 142, 154, 211, 222 and 240 in French Alpine and Saanen breeds and their association with classical scrapie. *J Gen Vir.* (2009) 90:769–76. doi: 10.1099/vir.0.006114-0

19. Acìn C, Martin-Burriel I, Monleon E, Lyahyai J, Pitarch JL, Serrano C, et al. Prion protein gene variability in Spanish goats. Inference through susceptibility to classical scrapie strains and pathogenic distribution of peripheral PrP(sc.). *PLoS ONE.* (2013) 8:e61118. doi: 10.1371/journal.pone.0061118

20. Acutis PL, Colussi S, Santagada G, Laurenza C, Maniaci MG, Riina MV, et al. Genetic variability of the PRNP gene in goat breeds from Northern and Southern Italy. *J App Microbiol.* (2008) 104:1782–9. doi: 10.1111/j.1365-2672.2007.03703.x

21. Migliore S, Agnello S, Chiappini B, Vaccari G, Mignacca SA, Di Marco Lo Presti V, et al. Biodiversity and selection for scrapie resistance in goats: genetic polymorphism in "Girgentana" breed in Sicily, Italy. *Small Rum Res.* (2015) 125:137–41. doi: 10.1016/j.smallrumres.2015.01.029

22. Vitale M, Migliore S, La Giglia M, Alberti P, Di Marco Lo Presti V, Langeveld JP. Scrapie incidence and PRNP polymorphisms: rare small ruminant breeds of Sicily with TSE protecting genetic reservoirs. *BMC Vet Res.* (2016) 12:141. doi: 10.1186/s12917-016-0766-9

23. Fantazi K,Migliore S, Kdidi S, Racinaro L, Tefiel H, Boukhari R, et al. Analysis of differences in prion protein gene (PRNP) polymorphisms between Algerian and southern Italy's goats. *Ital J Ani Sci.* (2018) 17:578 -85. doi: 10.1016/S1474-4422(18)30205-9

24. FAO. Available online at: http://www.fao.org/dad-is/browse-by-country-and-species/en/ (accessed June 30, 2020).

25. Migliore S, Agnello S, D'Avola S, Goldmann W, Di Marco Lo Presti V, et al. A cross-sectional study of PRNP gene in two native Sicilian goat populations in Italy: a relation between prion gene polymorphisms

and scrapie incidence. *J Genet.* (2017) 96:319–25. doi: 10.1007/s12041-017-0776-9

26. Sacchi P, Rasero R, Ru G, Aiassa E, Colussi S, Ingravalle F, et al. Predicting the impact of selection for scrapie resistance on PRNP genotype frequencies in goats. *Vet Res.* (2018) 49:26. doi: 10.1186/s13567-018-0518-x

27. Kanata E, Humphreys-Panagiotidis C, Giadinis ND, Papaioannou N, Arsenakis M, Sklaviadis T. Perspectives of a scrapie resistance breeding scheme targeting Q211, S146 and K222 caprine PRNP alleles in Greek goats. *Vet Res.* (2014) 45:43. doi: 10.1186/1297-9716-45-43

17

A Retrospective Survey of the Abortion Outbreak Event Caused by Brucellosis at a Blue Fox Breeding Farm in Heilongjiang Province, China

Yulong Zhou[1†], Ye Meng[2†], Yachao Ren[3], Zhiguo Liu[4*] and Zhenjun Li[4*]

[1] College of Animal Science and Veterinary Medicine, Heilongjiang Bayi Agricultural University, Daqing, China, [2] Department of Heilongjiang Key Laboratory for Animal Disease Control and Pharmaceutical Development, College of Veterinary Medicine, Northeast Agricultural University, Harbin, China, [3] Pharmacy Department, Harbin Medical University-Daqing, Daqing, China, [4] Chinese Center for Disease Control and Prevention, National Institute for Communicable Disease Control and Prevention, Beijing, China

*Correspondence:
Zhiguo Liu
wlcblzg@126.com
Zhenjun Li
lizhenjun@icdc.cn

†These authors have contributed equally to this work

Brucellosis is a common zoonosis in China, resulting in abortion in animals. Outbreaks of abortion in blue foxes caused by Brucella infection have rarely been reported. In the present study, 3–5 mL blood samples collected from the femoral veins of 10 abortuses of blue foxes were assessed by RBPT (Rose Bengal plate test) and SAT (serum tube agglutination test) to preliminarily investigate the source of infection for the clustering of abortion events at a blue fox farm in Heilongjiang Province. Screening experiments showed that all 10 blood samples were positive in the RBPT, while only eight blood samples out of the 10 were positive in the SAT. Subsequently, 10 tissue samples (spleen, lungs, stomach contents, and afterbirth) from the same 10 foxes were assessed using AMOS (acronym for B. abortus, melitensis, ovis, and suis)-PCR (polymerase chain reaction), and sequencing analysis was performed on amplification products to verify the results of the serology survey. Results showed a spectral band of ~731 bp in these samples. BLAST showed sequences of AMOS-PCR products in this study to be 100% similar ($E = 0.0$) to sequences in B. melitensis strain from GenBank. These data preliminarily indicated that the blue fox's outbreak of abortion events was caused by brucellosis via the B. melitensis strain. Then 726 serum samples were tested by RBPT and SAT to determine the prevalence of brucellosis on the farm. A comprehensive epidemiological and reproductive status survey of the infected blue fox population was performed. The seropositive rate was found to be 67.90% (493/726) by RBPT and 41.32% (300/726) by SAT. The technicians had stopped feeding the foxes with chicken carcasses and instead fed them raw ground sheep organs (lungs, tracheae, placentae, and dead sheep fetuses) infected by B. meliteneis strains, and that this change in diet caused the outbreak of abortion events. The high abortion rate (55%) and low cub survival rate (65%) were the most distinctive features of the outbreak; these factors led to severe economic losses. Feeding cooked sheep/goat offal and strict breeding management is necessary for disease prevention.

Keywords: Brucella melitensis, abortion, reproductive, blue fox, goats (sheep) offal

INTRODUCTION

Brucellosis is a widespread zoonotic disease that is caused by bacteria and is categorized as a bacterial human disease (1). The World Organization for Animal Health (OIE) lists brucellosis as a multi-animal comorbidity (2), and brucellosis is a second-category animal infectious disease in China (3). The disease mainly affects the reproductive systems of animals (4, 5). Although 12 *Brucella* species have been identified, *B. melitensis*, *B. abortus*, and *B. suis* are the most common pathogens occurring in human and animal infections (6). Among domestic animals, cattle, sheep, and pigs are infected most frequently, and the disease can be transmitted to bison, elk, wild boars, foxes, hares, African buffalo, and reindeer (7). Brucellosis has caused huge economic losses in the animal husbandry and economic animal breeding industries worldwide (8, 9). The highest and lowest prevalence rates of brucellosis among different fox species were found in red fox (*Vulpes vulpes*) (100%) and hoary fox (*Lycalopex vetulus*) (9%), respectively (10). A study showed *Gardnerella vaginalis* to be the main pathogen that causes miscarriage in foxes in China; the seropositivity rate range of fox population in China is 0.9–21.9%, and in some farms it exceeds 75% (11). Canine distemper virus, pseudorabies virus, and *Staphylococcus aureus* are common pathogenic agents in the fox population (12), but there is no report of fox abortion caused by *Brucella* spp. Moreover, the incidence of brucellosis in China has continued to rise in recent years. Heilongjiang Province was designated a Type I brucellosis severe epidemic region due to the ongoing high incidence rate of animal brucellosis (13, 14). The animal husbandry industry is a main economic pillar of this province, and fox and raccoon breeding are the main sources of income for many farmers in this region. In March 2017, an outbreak of abortion of unknown origin occurred at a blue fox breeding farm in Heilongjiang Province, resulting in a high rate of abortion in pregnant blue foxes and causing serious economic losses. At present, serological techniques remains the mainstay for brucellosis diagnosis (15). These include the Rose Bengal Plate Test (RBPT), serum agglutination test (SAT), and complement-fixation test (CFT) (16–18). However, CFT is a technically complex test, and it requires good laboratory facilities and well-trained personnel to perform it accurately and maintain its reagents (19). Moreover, identification of *Brucella* sp. by conventional tests involves considerable time, risk of human infection, and expert interpretation, whereas PCR is fast, safe, and easy to interpret (20, 21). Previous works described a *Brucella* PCR assay that can distinguish *Brucella abortus* (biovars 1, 2, and 4), *Brucella melitensis* (biovars 1, 2, and 3), *Brucella ovis*, and *Brucella suis* (biovar 1) from each other (22). In this study, RBPT, SAT, and AMOS (*B. abortus*, *B. melitensis*, *Brucella ovis*, and *Brucella suis*)—PCR were used to determine the cause of the outbreak of abortions at a blue fox farm. Our investigation will provide important data for technical guidance in the prevention of blue fox brucellosis as well as promote better management of blue foxes in Heilongjiang province, China.

Abbreviations: RBPT, Rose-Bengal plate test; SAT, serum tube agglutination test; AMOS-PCR, *B. abortus-melitensis-ovis-suis* polymerase chain reaction.

METHODS

Serological Testing

Blood samples were collected from the femoral vein, 3–5 mL per blue fox. A total of 10 serum samples (HBF001–010) were collected from 10 female foxes that had miscarried during 15–20 days in April 2017, and 726 serum samples [65 male foxes, 34 male cub foxes (<1 year old), 564 female foxes, and 61 female cub foxes (<1 year old)] from the blue fox farm were collected in October 2017 to implement the epidemiological survey. Both the Rose Bengal plate test (RBPT) and the Serum Agglutination Test (SAT) were performed according to standard serological procedures (23). RBPT and SAT were used to diagnose human brucellosis (23). RBPT antigen (production batch number: 201701) and SAT antigen (production batch number: 201702) were purchased from Qingdao Yibang Bioengineering Co., Ltd.; brucellosis positive control serum (production batch number: 201702) and negative control serum (production batch number: 201701) were purchased from China Veterinary Drug Supervision Institute. Sperm samples collected from male foxes were preliminarily screened for quality by microscopic examination. Some medicines, including oxytetracycline, astragalus polysaccharides, Vitamin E, and other herbs, were used to treat the blue foxes.

AMOS-PCR

The 10 tissue samples (liver, spleen, lungs, stomach contents, and afterbirth) from the same 10 aborted blue fox fetuses were collected following biosafety regulations. DNA of all samples was extracted using a Qiagen genome DNA prepare kit (Qiagen, Germany) according to the manufacturer's instructions. Subsequently, AMOS-PCR was employed to discriminate the species/biovar of *Brucella* strains. Amplification and detection procedures were as previously described (24). Briefly, the concentration of the four primer pairs was 25 μM/L, and primer A 1 μL, primer M 1.5 μL, primer O 1.5 μL, primer S 1 μL, primer IS711 2 μL, Taq DNA polymerase 1.25 U, and DNA template 2 μL. Finally, sterilized double distilled water was added to a final volume of 50 μL. Amplification parameters: 94°C pre-denaturation 5 min; 94°C 1 min, 60°C 1.5 min, 72°C 10 min, for 40 cycles; final extension at 72°C for 10 min. Five microliter products and 1 μL loading buffer were uploaded to agarose gels to determine the sizes of products. The target gene size was 498 bp for *B. abortus* (bv. 1, 2, and 4), 731 bp for *B. melitensis*, 976 bp for *B. ovis*, and 285 bp for *B. suis* (bv. 1). Then, 10 AMOS-PCR products were sequencing using M primer (F) and comparison was performed using the Basic Local Alignment Search Tool (BLAST).

The Evaluation of Reproductive Performance in Female Blue Foxes

The breeding conditions, estrus rate, weak cub rate, abortion rate, disease occurrence, and medication use of the blue fox farm from 2017 to 2019 were investigated to determine the production performance impact of a female blue fox infected with *B. melitensis*.

TABLE 1 | Brucellosis epidemic situation as detected by serological tests in 726 serum samples from blue fox breeding farm.

Methods	Male	Male cub foxes	Female foxes	Female cub foxes	Total (%)
RBPT (%)	61.58 (40/65)	11.76 (4/34)	78.55 (443/564)	8.20 (5/61)	67.90 (493/726)
SAT (%)	38.49 (25/65)	0	48.58 (274/564)	1.63 (1/61)	41.32 (300/726)

RBPT, Rose Bengal plate test; SAT, serum tube agglutination test.

RESULTS

Serological Tests

In order to investigation the cause of the outbeak abortus event. First, ten samples from female foxes were collected and examined by RBPT and SAT. The RBPT results in all 10 serum samples from female foxes were positive. However, eight samples were positive for the SAT (titer 1:50, ++), while the two remaining samples were all suspect cases (titer 1:50, +) (**Supplementary Table 1**). A preliminary serological survey indicated that infection with *Brucella* spp. could be a cause of spontaneous abortion in blue foxes. Subsequently, for further survey the situation the infection in blue fax farming, a total of 726 serum samples were collected and detected by RBPT and SAT. The positive rate of the RBPT was 67.90% (493/726) (**Table 1**), and the positive rate of the SAT was 41.32% (300/726) (**Table 1**). The SAT titer in 125 samples was 1:25 + (**Table 1**). Finally, eight of the human staff of this far were screened for serum antibodies against *Brucella* infection in eight staff in this farming were performed, five staff members of the farm were diagnosed with brucellosis, while there were no brucellosis antibodies detected in the other three staff members. The obvious clinical symptoms (swollen testicles, bedridden, back pain, leg pain) were observed in five brucellosis patients. They frequently ground the raw internal organs of sheep/goat to feed the blue foxes.

AMOS-PCR Amplification

The AMOS-PCR showed that the expected 731 bp size amplified result was observed in three positive controls (*B. melitensis* M5; 6. *B. abortus* A19, and *B. suis* S2), and there were no bands in the negative control *E. coli* strain. Moreover, an expected 731 bp band was detected among four different tissue types in the samples from aborted fetuses, including spleen, lung, stomach contents, and fetal coats, consistent with the target gene fragment of *B. melitensis* strains (**Figure 1**). PCR product sequencing showed that sequences ~700 bp in size were obtained from all 10 samples. Further BLAST showed that these sequences were 100% similar (*E* = 0.0, sort by percent identity as 100%) to sequences of *B. melitensis* strain hosted in GenBank (**Supplementary Figure 1**). This result further verified the results from serological tests as well as confirming that *B. melitensis* was the pathogen involved in the blue fox cluster of abortion events.

The Epidemiology Investigation

The farm began breeding blue foxes in 2014. In 2016, there were 2,000 female foxes and 110 male foxes, and the abortion rate was 5%. Blue foxes started mating in March 2017, and miscarriages occurred 10–40 days after pregnancy [in general, around 53 days (49–56) for the entire pregnancy]. Although

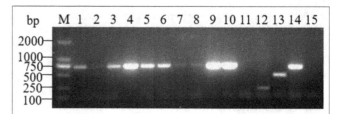

FIGURE 1 | AMOS-PCR typing of the sample from three aborted fetuses of the blue fox. M, marker, DL2000 bp; lane 1–3, spleen, lungs and stomach contents samples from HBF001; lane 4–6, spleen, lungs and stomach contents samples from HBF002; lane 7–8, spleen and lungs samples from HBF003; lane 9–11, Fetal coats samples from three aborted fetus (HBF001-3); lane 12, *B. suis* S2; lane 13, *B. abortus* A19; lane 14, *B. melitensis* M5; lane 15. Negative control, *E. coli*.

the female fox's estrus rate was 85% (1,700/2,000) in that year, the miscarriage rate was 50% (850/1,700); weak cubs accounted for 5% (250/5,000), and the mortality rate of foxes reached 35% (1,750/5,000) (**Table 2**). After the brucellosis was diagnosed, oxytetracycline, astragalus polysaccharides, Vitamin E, and other herbs were used for treatment, but these had no effect. Therefore, only 18 brucellosis-positive female foxes were kept for breeding in 2018, and the remainder were eliminated. The investigation found that from August 2016 to November 2016, previously used chicken carcasses were replaced by raw ground sheep internal organs (lungs, tracheae, placentae, and dead fetuses) to feed breeding foxes, and clustering of female fox abortions occurred a few months later. After being infected, female blue foxes were without any obvious manifestations; however, reduced sperm counts and deformed sperm in male foxes were observed in microscopic examinations (unpublished).

DISCUSSION

Brucellosis is one of the most important infectious causes of reproductive disorders in various species of animals (25). Various *Brucella* species are well-known causes of contagious abortion in cattle, sheep, goats, swine, and other animals (26). In the present study, both serological and AMOS-PCR methods confirmed that a *Brucella* spp. strain was the cause of the outbreak of abortion among blue foxes on this farm. Similarly, a previous study reported that brucellosis was found in a fox farm (27). Molecular tools can support the results from serological tests to avoid cross-reaction with other pathogens (28). AMOS-PCR results showed the presence of this special 731 bp band in many aborted fetuses' samples. Moreover, sequences from PCR products have 100% similarity to *B. melitensis* sequences from GenBank. These data

TABLE 2 | The reproduction profile of the blue fox in this farm during 2016–2018.

Years	Female no.	Estrus rate (%)	Abortion rate (%)	Survival rate (%)
2016	2,000	93.33	5	98
2017	2,000	85.00	50	65
2018	18	77.78	7.14	33.33

2017 is the year the infection occurred.

indicate that the outbreak at the blue fox farm was causing by the *B. melitensis* infected. A similar study showed that *B. melitensis* biovar 3 was the main pathogen responsible for cow and sheep abortion in China, and that this variant posed a human health risk (29). The seroprevalence of brucellosis in sheep and goat flocks was higher in eastern China, with 7.00% positive rate, than in any other region (30). Heilongjiang Province is one of the severe animal brucellosis epidemic regions in northern China (30). Moreover, ~9% (56/621) of the samples from yaks were seropositive for *Brucella* tested via SAT at the Qinghai-Tibet Plateau, China (31). Similarly, the individual yak seroprevalence of brucellosis was 2.8% and herd level seroprevalence was 18.2% (32). Also, *Brucella* strains were isolated from the wildlife in China, such as blue sheep (*Pseudois nayaur*), yaks (*Bos mutus grunniens*), and Tibetan gazelle (*Procapra picticaudata*) (33). *B. melitensis* biovar 3 from the spleen of an Asian badger (*Meles leucurus*) showed a MLVA-16 genotype similar to that of isolates from local aborted sheep fetuses (34).

Our surveys showed that sporadic abortion events occurred in 5% of pregnancies on this farm during 2016. However, a >50% abortion rate was observed in 2017. The blue fox farm did not introduce new foxes during the period 2014–2017, and the breeding environment had not changed. The only changed factor was the feed for the blue foxes, where raw ground offal of sheep from the local slaughterhouse was used to feed the breeding foxes instead of chicken carcasses as used previously. Subsequently, an outbreak abortion event occurred during March and April in 2017. Moreover, serological screening showed that the seropositive rate of brucellosis in the fox breeding farm was 41.32% (300/726), being 38.49% (40/64) in male foxes and 48.58% (274/564) in female foxes. Moreover, five out of eight staff in this farm were diagnosed with brucellosis. This evidence indirectly showed that feeding the raw viscera of sheep infected with *Brucella* spp. were the main cause for the outbreak of abortion events on the blue fox breeding farm. Due to the high abortion rate (55%), low cub survival rate (65%), and human infections, this farm was closed at the beginning of 2019. The study showed that the highest-threat organs of ruminants are the lungs, and the trend analysis also highlighted the cattle intestine as a potentially high-threat organ (35). Moreover, our previous study reported that *B. melitensis* was obtained from dogs that were often fed with sheep offal (36). Moreover, hares have been considered as a possible source of *B. suis* biovar 2 outbreaks in domestic pigs via swill feeding with offal from hunted infected hares (37).

In order to identify the causative pathogen of blue fox abortion, we tried to isolate and cultivate *Gardnerella vaginalis* and other common abortion-related pathogens, but only a few *Staphylococcus* and *Streptococcus* strains were detected in abortion afterbirth. What we particularly regret is that our laboratory (Heilongjiang Bayi Agricultural University) did not meet the expected biosafety requirements necessary for bacteriological experiments, so *Brucella* strains isolation were not performed. Isolated *Brucella* from the (wild) red fox (*Vulpes vulpes*) (38, 39), gray fox (40), and tundra wolf (41) have been reported. Therefore, our conclusion is a reasonable explanation for this outbreak of abortion events. In addition, blue foxes infected by *Brucella* strains were without any obvious symptoms except the abortion after pregnancy at 10–40 days. This observation agrees with a previous report that *B. melitensis* in the adult ewe is generally asymptomatic and self-limiting within about 3 months. However, because the bacteria may enter and cause necrosis of the chorionic villi and fetal organs, abortion or stillbirths may occur (42, 43). Another study showed that brucellosis is essentially a disease of sexually mature animals, the preferred site being the reproductive tracts of males and females. If the animal is not pregnant, the infected animal may be without clinical symptoms and may have a negative serological reaction. However, if such an animal becomes pregnant, the production of the simple carbohydrate erythritol in the fetus and its membranes causes rapid multiplication of bacteria in the uterus, and this is likely to end in abortion (44). In this study, a 77.78% (14/18) estrus rate was recorded in blue foxes after infection by *B. melitensis*. In comparison with 2016, the estrus rate had declined; the abortion rate was 10 times higher than previously, and the survival rate of the pups dropped significantly. *B. melitensis* primarily affects the reproductive tracts of sheep and goats, and the infection is characterized by late abortion, stillbirth, a weakened fetus, and to a lesser extent orchitis and infection of the accessory sex glands and impaired fertility in males (45). The stillbirths and weakened fetuses in this case resulted in economic losses. The infected staff member often participated in the offal grinding, and thus the specific source of infection needs further investigation. *B. melitensis* infects mainly sheep and goats and other animals, resulting in an important zoonosis that has a significant effect on the husbandry economy and the public health of many developing countries.

Our study has several limitations. Due to restrictions by the limited lab facilities, the isolation and culture of *Brucella* from abortus samples were not carried out. Moreover, a tracing-back survey of the source of sheep (goats) offal is lacking. Animal offal samples have been collected from the local slaughterhouse for further bacteriological experiments, and genetic phylogenetic analysis will provide the available information to reveal the complete transmission chain of events.

CONCLUSION

In the present study, we combined RBPT, SAT, and AMOS-PCR to investigate the cause of an abortion outbreak event in a blue fox farm in Heilongjiang province. Our experiments showed that blue foxes ingesting sheep offal infected with *B. melitensis* was the main cause of the outbreak. These data indirectly verified the severe animal brucellosis epidemic trend in this region, where *B. melitensis* infection was a spillover from the main host to the blue fox. These events pose a public health risk to people in the fur and catering industries and to workers in other breeding industries that provide animal feed. It is thus time to launch an animal brucellosis prevention program against the spread of *Brucella*.

AUTHOR CONTRIBUTIONS

YZ, YM, and YR collected the samples and performed the serology and AMOS-PCR amplifications. ZLiu performed data analysis and drafted the manuscript. YZ and ZLiu conducted epidemiological investigations. YZ and ZLi participated in the design of the study, critically reviewed the manuscript, and

managed the project. All authors have read and approved the final version of the manuscript.

FUNDING

This study was supported by Heilongjiang Bayi Agricultural University Funds (No. XDB201820) and Natural Science Talent Support Program (No. ZRCPY201807), the Natural Science Foundation Project of Heilongjiang Province (LH2020C083), the National Natural Science Foundation of China (No. 81703426), and the China Postdoctoral Science Foundation (No. 2019M651312), and National Key R&D Program of China, Grant Numbers 2019YFC1200700, 2019YFC1200601-6; and the National Natural Science Foundation of China (No. 82073624). The funding agencies had no role in the study design, data collection, analysis, decision to publish, or manuscript preparation.

ACKNOWLEDGMENTS

We are grateful to the staff of the blue fox breeding farm for assistance with the sample collection and for their cooperation with the epidemiological investigation.

REFERENCES

1. Ackelsberg J, Liddicoat A, Burke T, Szymczak WA, Levi MH, Ostrowsky B, et al. *Brucella* exposure risk events in 10 clinical laboratories, New York City, USA, 2015 to 2017. *J Clin Microbiol.* (2020) 58:e01096-19. doi: 10.1128/JCM.01096-19

2. Zhou K, Wu B, Pan H, Paudyal N, Jiang J, Zhang L, et al. ONE Health approach to address zoonotic brucellosis: a spatiotemporal associations study between animals and humans. *Front Vet Sci.* (2020) 7:521. doi: 10.3389/fvets.2020.00521

3. Shang D, Xiao D, Yin J. Epidemiology and control of brucellosis in China. *Vet Microbiol.* (2002) 90:165-82. doi: 10.1016/S0378-1135(02)00252-3

4. Silbereisen A, Tamborrini M, Wittwer M, Schürch N, Pluschke G. Development of a bead-based luminex assay using lipopolysaccharide specific monoclonal antibodies to detect biological threats from *Brucella* species. *BMC Microbiol.* (2015) 15:198. doi: 10.1186/s12866-015-0534-1

5. Tadesse G. Brucellosis seropositivity in animals and humans in ethiopia: a meta-analysis. *PLoS Negl Trop Dis.* (2016) 10:e0005006. doi: 10.1371/journal.pntd.0005006

6. Hull NC, Schumaker BA. Comparisons of brucellosis between human and veterinary medicine. *Infect Ecol Epidemiol.* (2018) 8:1500846. doi: 10.1080/20008686.2018.1500846

7. Godfroid J, Nielsen K, Saegerman C. Diagnosis of brucellosis in livestock and wildlife. *Croat Med J.* (2010) 51:296. doi: 10.3325/cmj.2010.51.296

8. Charypkhan D, Sultanov AA, Ivanov NP, Baramova SA, Taitubayev MK, Torgerson PR. Economic and health burden of brucellosis in Kazakhstan. *Zoo Public Health.* (2019) 66:487-94. doi: 10.1111/zph.12582

9. Dadar M, Alamian S, Behrozikhah AM, Yazdani F, Kalantari A, Etemadi A, et al. Molecular identification of *Brucella* species and biovars associated with animal and human infection in Iran. *Vet Res Forum.* (2019) 10:315-21. doi: 10.30466/vrf.2018.89680.2171

10. Dadar M, Shahali Y, Fakhri Y, Godfroid J. The global epidemiology of *Brucella* infections in terrestrial wildlife: a meta-analysis. *Transbound Emerg Dis.* (2020) 1-15. doi: 10.1111/tbed.13735

11. Li ZY, Chen ZG. Research progress of *Gardnerella vaginalis* in fox. *Agric Sci Res.* (2006) 27:65-7. doi: 10.3969/j.issn.1673-0747.2006.04.019

12. Wei ZF. Major diseases affecting fox reproduction. *Sci Cultivat.* (2007) 10:49-50.

13. Jiang W, Chen J, Li Q, Jiang L, Huang Y, Lan Y, et al. Epidemiological characteristics, clinical manifestations and laboratory findings in 850 patients with brucellosis in Heilongjiang Province, China. *BMC Infect Dis.* (2019) 19:439. doi: 10.1186/s12879-019-4081-5

14. Liang PF, Zhao Y, Zhao JH, Pan DF, Guo ZQ. Human distribution and spatial-temporal clustering analysis of human brucellosis in China from 2012 to 2016. *Infect Dis Poverty.* (2020) 9:142. doi: 10.1186/s40249-020-00754-8

15. Sathyanarayan MS, Suresh DR, Sonth SB, Krishna S, Surekha YA. A comparative study of agglutination tests, blood culture & Elisa in the laboratory diagnosis of human brucellosis. *Int J Biol Med Res.* (2011) 2:569-72.

16. Mcgiven JA, Tucker JD, Perrett LL, Stack JA, Brew SD, Macmillan AP. Validation of FPA and cELISA for the detection of antibodies to *Brucella* abortus in cattle sera and comparison to SAT. CFT, and iELISA. *J Immunol Methods.* (2003) 278:171-8. doi: 10.1016/S0022-1759(03)00201-1

17. Salisu US, Kudi CA, Bale JOO, Babashani M, Kaltungo BY, Saidu SNA, et al. Seroprevalence of *Brucella* antibodies in camels in Katsina State, Nigeria. *Trop Anim Health Prod.* (2017) 49:1041-6. doi: 10.1007/s11250-017-1297-5

18. Shome R, Kalleshamurthy T, Natesan K, Jayaprakash KR, Byrareddy K, Mohandoss N, et al. Serological and molecular analysis for brucellosis in selected swine herds from Southern India. *J Infect Public Health.* (2019) 12:247-51. doi: 10.1016/j.jiph.2018.10.013

19. Erdenlig Gürbilek S, Tel OY, Keskin O. Comparative evaluation of three serological tests for the detection of *Brucella* antibodies from infected cattle herds. *J Appl Anim Res.* (2017) 45:557-9. doi: 10.1080/09712119.2016.1222942

20. Vaid RK, Thakur SD, Barua S. Brucella diagnosis by PCR. *J Immunol Immunopathol.* (2004) 6:1-8.

21. Al-Garadi MA, Khairani-Bejo S, Zunita Z, Omar AR. Isolation and identification of *Brucella* melitensis in goats. *J Animal Vet Adv.* (2011) 10:972-9. doi: 10.3923/javaa.2011.972.979

22. Bricker BJ, Halling SM. Enhancement of the *Brucella* AMOS PCR assay for differentiation of *Brucella* abortus vaccine strains S19 and RB51. *J Clin Microbiol.* (1995) 33:1640-2. doi: 10.1128/JCM.33.6.1640-1642.1995

23. Yagupsky P, Morata P, Colmenero JD. Laboratory diagnosis of human brucellosis. *Clin Microbiol Rev.* (2019) 33:e00073-19. doi: 10.1128/CMR.00073-19

24. Du SN, Wang ZJ, Yu GW, Cui YL, Chen JJ, Hu N, et al. Epidemiological characteristics of human brucellosis in Tongliao city of Inner Mongolia Autonomous Region, 2004-2018. *Zhonghua Liu Xing Bing Xue Za Zhi.* (2020) 41:1063–7. doi: 10.3760/cma.j.cn112338-20190901-00642

25. Woldemeskel M. Zoonosis due to *Bruella suis* with special reference to infection in dogs (Carnivores): a brief review. *Open J Vet Med.* (2013) 3:213–21. doi: 10.4236/ojvm.2013.33034

26. Puri M, Patel N, Gaikwad V, Despande H, Pandey P. A study of prevalence of brucellosis in cases of spontaneous abortions. *Res J Pharm Biol Chem Sci.* (2015) 6:312–20.

27. Tworek R, Serokowa D, Machnicka B. Brucellosis on a fox farm. *Przegl Epidemiol.* (1957) 11:307–8.

28. Ntirandekura JB, Matemba LE, Kimera SI, Muma JB, Karimuribo ED. Association of brucellosis to abortions in humans and domestic ruminants in Kagera ecosystem, Tanzania. *Transbound Emerg Dis.* (2020) 67:1879–87. doi: 10.1111/tbed.13516

29. Zhang H, Deng X, Cui B, Shao Z, Zhao X, Yang Q, et al. Abortion and various associated risk factors in dairy cow and sheep in Ili, China. *PLoS ONE.* (2020) 15:e0232568. doi: 10.1371/journal.pone.0232568

30. Ran X, Chen X, Wang M, Cheng J, Ni H, Zhang XX, et al. Brucellosis seroprevalence in ovine and caprine flocks in China during 2000-2018: a systematic review and meta-analysis. *BMC Vet Res.* (2018) 14:393. doi: 10.1186/s12917-018-1715-6

31. Xulong L, Hailong Q, Zhaoyang B, Yanling Y, Chunhui S, Xiaoyan L, et al. Seroprevalence of *Brucella* infection in yaks (Bos grunniens) on the Qinghai-Tibet plateau of China. *Trop Anim Health Prod.* (2011) 43:305–6. doi: 10.1007/s11250-010-9726-8

32. Zeng J. *Epidemiology of Brucellosis in Yaks in the Tibet Autonomous Region of China.* Perth, WA: Murdoch University (2017).

33. Ma JY, Wang H, Zhang XF, Xu LQ, Hu GY, Jiang H, et al. MLVA and MLST typing of *Brucella* from Qinghai, China. *Infect Dis Poverty.* (2016) 5:26. doi: 10.1186/s40249-016-0123-z

34. Liu X, Yang M, Song S, Liu G, Zhao S, Liu G, et al. *Brucella* melitensis in Asian badgers, Northwestern China. *Emerging Infect Dis.* (2020) 26:804–6. doi: 10.3201/eid2604.190833

35. Večerek V, Kozak A, Malena M, Chloupek P, Pištěková V. Viscera of slaughtered ruminants and potential threats to human health. *Acta Vet Brno.* (2003) 72:631–8. doi: 10.2754/avb200372040631

36. Wang H, Xu WM, Zhu KJ, Zhu SJ, Zhang HF, Wang J, et al. Molecular investigation of infection sources and transmission chains of brucellosis in Zhejiang, China. *Emerg Microbes Infect.* (2020) 9:889–99. doi: 10.1080/22221751.2020.1754137

37. Godfroid J, Garin-Bastuji B, Saegerman C, Blasco JM. Brucellosis in terrestrial wildlife. *Rev Sci Tech.* (2013) 32:27–42. doi: 10.20506/rst.32.1.2180

38. Scholz HC, Hofer E, Vergnaud G, Le Fleche P, Whatmore AM, Al Dahouk S, et al. Isolation of *Brucella* microti from mandibular lymph nodes of red foxes, Vulpes vulpes, in lower Austria. *Vect Borne Zoo Dis.* (2009) 9:153–6. doi: 10.1089/vbz.2008.0036

39. Hofer E, Revilla-Fernández S, Al Dahouk S, Riehm JM, Nöckler K, Zygmunt MS, et al. A potential novel *Brucella* species isolated from mandibular lymph nodes of red foxes in Austria. *Vet Microbiol.* (2012) 155:93–9. doi: 10.1016/j.vetmic.2011.08.009

40. Szyfres B, Tomé JG. Natural *Brucella* infection in Argentine wild foxes. *Bull World Health Organ.* (1965) 34:919–23.

41. Tessaro SV, Forbes LB. Experimental *Brucella* abortus infection in wolves. *J Wildl Dis.* (2004) 40:60–5. doi: 10.7589/0090-3558-40.1.60

42. Olsen SC, Palmer MV. Advancement of knowledge of *Brucella* over the past 50 years. *Vet Pathol.* (2014) 51:1076. doi: 10.1177/0300985814540545

43. Djangwani J, Ooko Abong G, Gicuku Njue L, Kaindi DWM. Brucellosis: prevalence with reference to East African community countries - a rapid review. *Vet Med Sci.* (2021) 1–17. doi: 10.1002/vms3.425

44. Tesfaye G, Wondimu A, Asebe G, Regasa F, Mamo G. Sero-prevalence of bovine brucellosis in and Around Kombolcha, Amhara Regional State, Ethiopia. *Mycobact Dis.* (2017) 7:2. doi: 10.4172/2161-1068.1000242

45. Ren J, Peng Q. A brief review of diagnosis of small ruminants brucellosis. *Curr Med Chem.* (2020) 1–8. doi: 10.2174/0929867328666620123121226

18

Evaluation of the Control Options of Bovine Tuberculosis in Ethiopia using a Multi-Criteria Decision Analysis

Fanta D. Gutema[1]*, Getahun E. Agga[2], Kohei Makita[3], Rebecca L. Smith[4], Monique Mourits[5], Takele B. Tufa[1], Samson Leta[1], Tariku J. Beyene[6], Zerihun Asefa[1], Beksissa Urge[7] and Gobena Ameni[8,9]

[1] College of Veterinary Medicine and Agriculture, Addis Ababa University, Bishoftu, Ethiopia, [2] U. S. Department of Agriculture, Agricultural Research Service, Food Animal Environmental Systems Research Unit, Bowling Green, KY, United States, [3] Department of Veterinary Medicine, School of Veterinary Medicine, Rakukno Gakuen University, Ebetsu, Japan, [4] Department of Pathobiology, College of Veterinary Medicine, University of Illinois Urbana-Champaign, Urbana, IL, United States, [5] Business Economics Group, Wageningen University, Wageningen, Netherlands, [6] Department of Preventive Veterinary Medicine, Ohio State University, Columbus, OH, United States, [7] Ethiopian Institute of Agricultural Research, Addis Ababa, Ethiopia, [8] Aklilu Lemma Institute of Pathobiology, Addis Ababa University, Addis Ababa, Ethiopia, [9] Department of Veterinary Medicine, College of Agriculture, United Arab Emirates University, Al Ain, United Arab Emirates

*Correspondence:
Fanta D. Gutema
fantadesissa@gmail.com

Bovine tuberculosis (BTB) is a zoonotic bacterial infection caused by *Mycobacterium bovis* and is characterized by the development of granulomatous lesions in the lymph nodes, lungs and other tissues. It poses serious public health impacts and food security challenges to the agricultural sector in terms of dairy and meat productions. In Ethiopia, BTB has been considered as a priority disease because of its high prevalence in urban and peri-urban dairy farms. However, there has not been any national control program in the country. Thus, in order to initiate BTB control program in the country, information on control options is needed to tailor the best option for the Ethiopian situation. The objective of this study was to identify, evaluate and rank various BTB control options in Ethiopia using a multi-criteria decision analysis based on preference ranking organization method for enrichment evaluations (PROMETHEE) approach while accounting for the stakeholders' preferences. Control options were evaluated under two scenarios: with (scenario 1) and without (scenario 2) bacillus Calmette–Guérin (BCG) vaccination. Nine potential control options were identified that include combinations of three control options (1) test and slaughter with or without government support, (2) test and segregation, and (3) BCG vaccination. Under scenario 1, BCG vaccination, BCG vaccination and test and slaughter with partial compensation by government, and BCG vaccination and test and slaughter with full compensation by government were the top three ranked control options. Under scenario 2, test and slaughter with full compensation by government was the preferred control option, followed by test and segregation supported by test and slaughter with full government compensation, and test and slaughter with half compensation by government. Irrespective of the variability in the weighting by the stakeholders, the sensitivity analysis showed the robustness of the ranking method.

In conclusion, the study demonstrated that BCG vaccination, and test and slaughter with full compensation by government were the two most preferred control options under scenarios 1 and 2, respectively. National level discussions were strongly recommended for further concretization and implementation of these control measures.

Keywords: bovine tuberculosis, multi-criteria decision analysis, stakeholders, control, Ethiopia

INTRODUCTION

BTB is a zoonotic bacterial infection caused by *M. bovis,* a member of the *Mycobacterium tuberculosis* complex (1). It causes a serious public health impact and food security and safety challenges (2). Contaminated dairy products are the main sources of BTB infections in humans, mainly resulting in extra-pulmonary infections such as lymphadenitis (3). According to the World Health Organization, there were 147,000 new cases of zoonotic TB and 12,500 human TB related deaths in 2016 with higher incidence and death rates in Africa than other parts of the world (4). Even though there are no comprehensive studies to estimate the global socio-economic costs of BTB, it causes significant economic losses due to production losses such as reduced milk yield, cost of surveillance and control programs and trade barriers with a major impact on the livelihoods of poor and marginalized communities (5).

In high income countries, public health risk and economic loss associated with *M. bovis* were considerably reduced or eliminated through the implementation of strict test-and-slaughter and meat inspection protocols for cattle, milk pasteurization, financial compensation to farmers and public education (6, 7). However, in most low and middle income countries where BTB is endemic, like in Ethiopia, such measures are hampered by financial constraints particularly for farmer compensation, and by inadequate veterinary services (8). Currently, there are several ongoing efforts to address zoonotic BTB to end the global TB epidemic by 2030 globally (4). However, there are no policies and implementation activities aligning to this global endeavor in the control of BTB in Ethiopia.

The conventional disease prevention and control interventions can have important environmental, social and economic impacts (9). For instance, test and slaughter policy is effective for control of BTB (10). However, it has several impacts such as killing large numbers of test positive animals, raising welfare concerns, and incurring costs for testing and compensation to cattle owners, making it economically difficult to apply particularly in resource limited countries. As a result, decision-making requires systems approach to integrate these multiple aspects of interventions. Multi-criteria decision analysis (MCDA) is an important and effective emerging system approach that can increase the understanding, acceptability and robustness of a decision problem of controlling zoonotic TB considering an integration of epidemiologic, economic and social-ethics value judgments (9, 11).

BTB was reported from 55% of herds and 32.3% of cattle in urban and peri-urban dairy farms in central Ethiopia (12). The national BTB prevalence estimate was 5.8% in individual cattle,

with higher prevalence of 21.6% in exotic breeds and their crosses and 16.6% in herds kept under intensive and semi-intensive production systems in urban and peri-urban areas (13). Thus, it is particularly a problem for intensive dairy systems that raise dairy cattle with improved breed. For example, in the years 2005–2011, the maximum production loss due to BTB was estimated at \$4.9 million in the urban livestock production systems in Ethiopia (14). Currently, there are no national policies and strategies for the control of BTB although the disease is considered among the top three diseases in dairy producing urban and peri-urban areas of the country in terms of prevalence and household impact (15). Researchers have recommended implementation of control in intensive and semi-intensive dairy farms due to the public health importance of BTB and concerns about spreading the disease through dairy cattle trade from the high prevalence urban system to low prevalence sedentary rural production systems (13, 15). To that end, information for decision making is needed to select and implement control options that are optimally tailored to the country's situations by considering the interests of the dairy farmers and the government. The objective of this study was to identify, evaluate and rank various BTB control options using a multi-criteria decision analysis tool. The outcome of the study would ultimately inform decision makers toward policy formulation and national level discussion to implement BTB control under semi-intensive and intensive dairy farming systems in Ethiopia.

MATERIALS AND METHODS

Assembling Team

The study was conducted between July 2018 and June 2019. A multidisciplinary research team composed of researchers in the fields of veterinary public health, public health, veterinary epidemiology, infectious disease modeling, veterinary animal health economics, biostatistics and multi criteria decision analysis was assembled and involved in the study.

Multi-Criteria Decision Analysis (MCDA)

The comprehensive and stepwise consecutive approaches of MCDA tool for managing zoonotic diseases as developed by Aenishaenslin et al. (9) was used to identify, evaluate and rank various BTB prevention and control options according to stakeholders' preferences to indicate the potential BTB control option under Ethiopian conditions. The approach consists of ten steps that were categorized into seven problem structuring and three decision analysis steps. In the context of the present study, stakeholders refer to key players in the control of BTB include representatives of governmental organizations, animal health professionals, public health professionals and experts (11).

Problem Structuring

The problem structuring step consisted of the following steps: define the problem, identify the stakeholders, identify key decision issues, define criteria and indicators, identify intervention options, evaluate performance of each intervention option and weight criteria. Before conducting the MCDA, literature review was conducted on the available success stories on BTB controls in other countries to identify different control options. A non-systematic literature review approach was followed to search for focused available information on BTB control options using search engines such as Google scholars and PubMed with key phrases like "control of BTB," "control of TB in cattle" and "control of zoonotic TB." The generated articles were read in-depth for the targeted information and the citations in the articles were further referred when deemed necessary. Moreover, experts working on BTB in the academia and veterinary and medical government offices were consulted through face to face discussions and Skype meeting using check list of the important elements of the problem structuring steps of MCDA. Accordingly, they were consulted to contextualize the key decision issues related to BTB control in Ethiopia in terms of the prevalence of BTB in intensive and semi-intensive dairy farms, the need for BTB control, potential control options and measurements for the evaluation of the control options.

The actual MCDA analysis was performed through an interactive group discussion for which key stakeholders ($n = 15$) from various pertinent organizations in Ethiopia were invited. Out of the 15 stakeholders invited, 10 of them agreed to participate in the MCDA process (**Table 1**). The participating stakeholders conducted thorough interactive discussions to lay out problem structuring phase of the analysis, such as defining the problem and identifying key decision issues, defining the measurement scale on criteria, listing potential BTB control options, and evaluating the control options. The stakeholders identified 10 specific criteria (C1–C10) categorized into six clusters, namely epidemiology (1 criterion), practical applicability (1), economics (3), social ethics (3), public health (1) and animal welfare (1). All criteria were categorical ordinal variables (**Table 2**). Each stakeholder independently weighted each of the identified clusters and criteria and evaluated the performance of each of the control options based on three-point qualitative scale as low, medium or high (9).

Decision Analysis

The decision analysis step included: constructing a matrix based on multi-criteria analysis, sensitivity analysis and interpretation of the results. Since two differing opinions were made during the discussion by the stakeholders regarding inclusion and exclusion of BCG vaccination of calves as a control option under Ethiopian conditions, the comparison and option ranking were performed under two scenarios. Scenario 1 was modeled with the inclusion of BCG vaccination while scenario 2 was modeled by excluding it. The academic version of preference ranking organization method for enrichment evaluations (PROMETHEE) software 1.4

was used to perform pair-wise comparisons of the performance of control options using the preferences of the stakeholders to compute the overall outranking scores (16).

Based on the scores, the identified control options were listed from the most to the least preferred option. For ranking of the control options and visual display of the analysis results, the Geometrical analysis for interactive aid (GAIA) with two dimension (U-V) views and PROMETHEE table were used. The action profiles of the control options were performed for the top ranked control options to evaluate their relative performance on each criterion. The GAIA and sensitivity analysis were performed for scenario 1. GAIA walking weights were run to conduct sensitivity analysis to see the effect of weighing the evaluation criteria by stakeholders on the group ranking when the weights of the criterion were changed and to assess the robustness of the results.

RESULTS

From the 10 stakeholders participate in the MCDA process (S1–S10), nine were from the government organization and one stakeholder represented an association of privately owned dairy farmers (**Table 1**). The stakeholders agreed that BTB is a major problem and that the prevalence is particularly high in dairy herds with exotic cattle breeds and their crosses kept under semi intensive or intensive production system in urban and peri-urban dairy farming. They also emphasized the need for pooling collective efforts toward the control of BTB in the country targeting intensive and semi-intensive dairy farms in urban and peri-urban areas, noting the lack of national BTB control or eradication program in Ethiopia. The research team and stakeholders indicated the occurrence of high prevalence of BTB in semi-intensive and intensive dairy farms and the need for designing and implementing potential control option. The stakeholders identified nine possible control options including combinations of three specific options: test and slaughter with or without financial compensation, test and segregation, and BCG vaccination, with the assumption

---

TABLE 1 | Composition of the stakeholders participated in the multi-criteria decision analysis for the evaluation of bovine tuberculosis control options in Ethiopia.

Organizations	Number of participants
Ministry of Agriculture	1
Ethiopian Commercial Dairy Producers Association	1
Ethiopian Public Health Institute	1
Adama General Hospital and Medical College	1
Ethiopian Meat and Dairy Industry Development Institute	1
Addis Ababa University, Pathobiology Institute	1
Addis Ababa University, College of Veterinary Medicine and Agriculture	2
Debre Berhan University	1
Ethiopian Institute of Agricultural Research Center	1

that each option can be implemented independently (**Table 3**). For effective implementation of BTB control option in the country, the stakeholders emphasized also the need for stringent prerequisites such as legal framework for implementation, preliminary BTB status testing of each animal and herd, animal identification and animal movement control, biosecurity measures at dairy farms, public education and BTB herd certification as supplementary/complementary measures to the implementation of potential intervention option(s).

All stakeholders generated a specific weighting scheme based on their perceived relative importance of each criterion as defined for the intended decision-making process. For this, each stakeholder was provided 100 points, and was asked to distribute the points to all specified criteria. The weighting of the stakeholders varied among the clusters and within the cluster criteria. Three stakeholders (S2, S3, and S10) gave the highest weight for the economic criteria, while the other seven stakeholders gave the highest weight to the epidemiologic cluster: reduction of BTB prevalence. The social ethics cluster and criteria generally received the least weight by all stakeholders (**Table 4**). Under scenario 1, the ranking of the control options showed that BCG vaccination (OP1), BCG vaccination combined with test and slaughter with cost sharing (OP6), and BCG vaccination combined with test and slaughter with full compensation of the cost by the government (OP7) as the top three potential control options. **Figure 1** shows the relative performance of the top three control options on each criterion. The first ranked option, BCG vaccination, performs well on C2, C6, and C10 while poorly performing on C1 i.e., reduction in the prevalence/incidence of BTB. Conversely, the second and the third control options relatively perform well on C1 while poorly performed significantly on C8 and C10, respectively.

TABLE 2 | Criteria used in the evaluation of bovine tuberculosis control options in Ethiopia.

Criteria cluster	Brief description of criterion
Epidemiology (EPI)	Reduction in BTB incidence or prevalence (C1)
Practical applicability (PA)	Level of difficulty in implementing the control option under Ethiopian condition (C2)
Economics (ECO)	Cost to the farmers -cost of test, loss of milk, replacement cost and other related costs (C3)
	Cost to the government- compensation of slaughtered animals, cost of laboratory test, veterinary costs (cost of farm visit, administrative cost to implement the control option (C4)
	Cost to the industry- inadequate milk supply to processing industries (C5)
Social ethics (SOE)	Acceptability by the Government (C6)
	Acceptability by dairy farmers (C7)
	Social impact - social crisis as a result of the intervention in terms of loss of high performing cow or loss of employment for labor workers (C8)
Public health (PH)	Public health impact - exposure to bovine tuberculosis during implementation of the intervention (C9)
Animal welfare (AW)	Impact on animal - welfare problems as a result of the intervention like slaughtering positive cattle, stress during vaccination and segregation (C10)

TABLE 3 | Descriptions of single and combined control options identified by stakeholders for control of bovine tuberculosis (BTB) in Ethiopia.

BTB control option	Description
BCG vaccination (OP1)	Calf vaccination with BCG vaccine at 6 weeks of age.
Test and segregation (OP2)	Testing and segregating infected animals at early stage of the disease and calf at birth, and switching to test-and-slaughter method in the final stage.
Test and slaughter with cost sharing (OP3)	Testing and slaughtering positive animals with the government and the owner equally sharing the cost of compensation for the slaughtered animals.
Test and slaughter with government support (OP4)	Testing and slaughtering positive animals with the government compensating full cost of the slaughtered animals to the owner.
BCG vaccination and test and segregation (OP5)	Calf vaccination to reduce the prevalence of the disease in the herd, and switch to test and segregation.
BCG vaccination and test and slaughter with cost sharing (OP6)	Calf vaccination and switching to testing and slaughtering of positive animals with the government and the owner equally sharing the cost of compensation for the slaughtered cattle.
BCG vaccination and test and slaughter with government support (OP7)	Calf vaccination, and switch to testing and slaughtering of positive animal with the government compensating full cost of the slaughtered animals to the owner.
Test and segregation and test and slaughter with cost sharing (OP8)	Testing and segregating infected animals, and switch to testing and slaughtering positive animals with the government and the owner equally sharing the cost of compensation for the slaughtered animals.
Test and segregation and test and slaughter with government support (OP9)	Testing and segregating infected animals, and switch to testing and slaughtering positive animals with the government compensating full cost of the slaughtered animals to the owner.

*BTB test refers to application of tuberculin skin test that consists of injecting bovine tuberculin, a purified protein extract derived from M. bovis, intradermally and measuring the skin thickness at the site of injection after 72 h to detect any subsequent swelling at the injection site-sign of delayed hypersensitivity reaction associated with infection.

TABLE 4 | The relative weight given by stakeholders based on their preference for each cluster and specific criteria for the control of bovine tuberculosis (BTB) in Ethiopia.

Cluster	Criteria	Weights									
		S1	S2	S3	S4	S5	S6	S7	S8	S9	S10
Epidemiology	Reduction in BTB incidence (C1)	**25**	**20**	**20**	**30**	**25**	**25**	**25**	**25**	**30**	**20**
Practical applicability	Practical applicability (C2)	**15**	**10**	**10**	**15**	**15**	**15**	**15**	**15**	**20**	**10**
Economics	Cost to the farm owner (C3)	10	15	20	10	15	15	15	15	10	20
	Cost to the government (C4)	10	10	15	9	10	10	10	10	10	20
	Cost to the industry (C5)	10	15	15	6	10	10	10	10	10	10
	Sub total	**30**	**40**	**50**	**25**	**35**	**35**	**35**	**35**	**30**	**50**
Social ethics	Acceptance by government (C6)	6	10	5	5	5	5	5	5	5	5
	Acceptance by owner (C7)	4	5	5	5	5	5	5	5	5	5
	Social impact (C8)	4	5	5	4	5	5	5	5	5	2
	Sub total	**14**	**20**	**25**	**14**	**15**	**15**	**5**	**15**	**15**	**12**
Public health	Public health impact (C9)	**10**	**6**	**5**	**10**	**5**	**5**	**7**	**5**	**3**	**3**
Animal welfare	Impact on animal welfare (C10)	**6**	**4**	**5**	**6**	**5**	**5**	**3**	**5**	**2**	**5**
	Total	**100**	**100**	**100**	**100**	**100**	**100**	**100**	**100**	**100**	**100**

The bold numbers indicate the weight given for each cluster out of 100 points by each stakeholder.

Under scenario 2, test and slaughter with full government compensation (OP4) was the preferred control option followed by test and segregation combined with test and slaughter with full government compensation (OP9), and test and slaughter with half compensation by government (OP3) (**Table 5**).

Figure 2 is the GAIA-scenarios plane visually displaying the positions of the control options and the stakeholders' preferences for scenario 1. As indicated in the GAIA plane, the options OP1, OP7, and OP6 are located on the right positions close to the decision axis representing the preferred control options while OP2 and OP8 are positioned in the left away from the decision axis representing the less preferred options that agreed with the results generated by the PROMETHEE table (**Table 5**). In the plane, most of the stakeholders (8/10) preferences were pointed toward the positive direction of the x-axis, having less variation in their preferences of the control options, while stakeholders 5 and 10 had major deviation from the group. BCG vaccination was not among the top three ranked control options for these two stakeholders. The sensitivity analysis showed that when equal weight was given to each criterion, the ranking of the three top control options remained stable except shifting in the order between the second (OP7) and third option (OP6), indicating the robustness of the study.

DISCUSSION

To the best of our knowledge this is the first study to identify, evaluate and rank different BTB control options using MCDA tool based on the stakeholders' opinions and preferences in Ethiopia. Despite high prevalence of the disease in dairy cattle in the country, currently there is no BTB control and /or eradication program. The participation of stakeholders to achieve the purpose and use of participatory approaches such as MCDA are helpful to identify and evaluate BTB control options. In the present study, we generated the desired data from stakeholders

who represented organizations with direct responsibilities or had specific interests in BTB prevention and control in Ethiopia.

In addition to identifying, evaluating and ranking of BTB control options, the stakeholders also identified various pre-requisite measures such as legal framework for the implementation and allied issues as an integral part of a control program prior to its application. Similarly, these measures were identified and their implications on the future prevention and control of BTB in Ethiopia were mentioned as daunting tasks by Dibaba et al. (17). In agreement to these requirements, several BTB eradication programs in many countries succeeded in reducing or eliminating the disease in cattle, by employing such multi-faceted approaches in place (10). Thus, creating enabling conditions, particularly formulation of BTB control policy and implementation guidelines, should be the primary steps in order to implement prevention and control of BTB effectively in the country. This will serve as a springboard toward initiation and implementation of the identified BTB control options in Ethiopia. The role of pertinent stakeholders and researchers would be indispensable in this regard in advising policy and decision makers by creating platforms for national level sensitization and discussion.

In the present study, nine potential BTB control options consisting of three single and six combined options were identified based on the stakeholders' preferences. Under scenario 1, the stakeholders ranked BCG vaccination as the number one control option and complementary measure to the second and third control options in cattle under Ethiopian conditions. BCG vaccination refers to vaccination of calves at 6 weeks of age. Calves are immune-competent at birth and are naturally sensitized to antigens of environmental mycobacteria at a young age. By 6 weeks of age, calves usually show a strong immunological response to such antigens. BCG vaccination of calf at birth induced a high level of immunity. However, it is recommendable to vaccinate calf at 6 weeks of age (18).

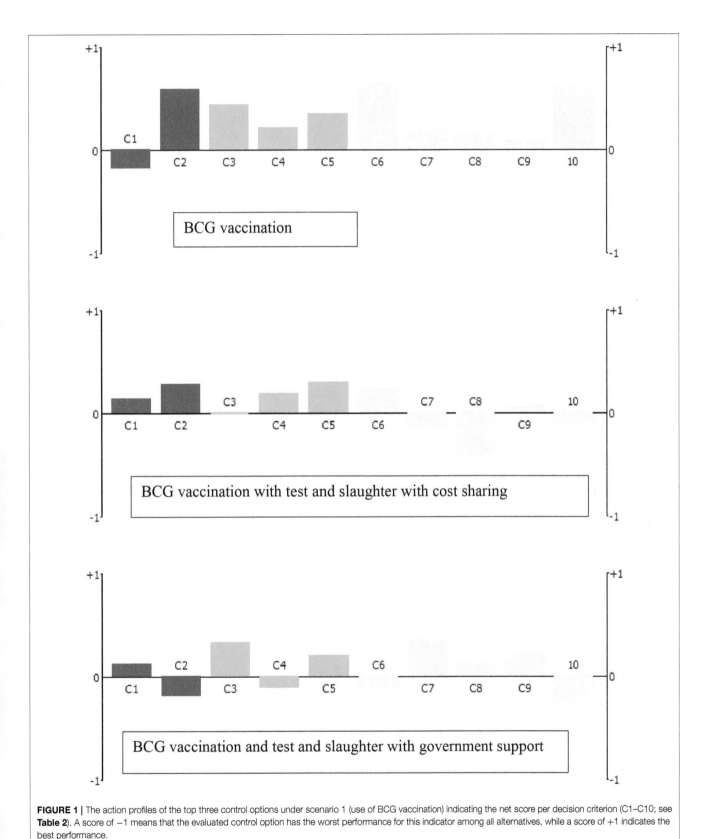

FIGURE 1 | The action profiles of the top three control options under scenario 1 (use of BCG vaccination) indicating the net score per decision criterion (C1–C10; see **Table 2**). A score of −1 means that the evaluated control option has the worst performance for this indicator among all alternatives, while a score of +1 indicates the best performance.

Despite significant knowledge gaps regarding the real impact of BCG vaccination on the incidence of BTB and the inability to distinguish between infected and vaccinated cattle using purified protein derivative (PPD) skin test (19, 20), recent experimental studies have indicated the significance of vaccinating cattle with BCG vaccine in reducing the prevalence, progression and severity

TABLE 5 | Group ranking for bovine tuberculosis control options in Ethiopia.

Alternative control option	Scenario 1		Scenario 2	
	Score	Rank	Score	Rank
BCG vaccination (OP1)	0.250	1	NA	NA
BCG vaccination, and test and slaughter with government support (OP7)	0.111	2	NA	NA
BCG vaccination, and test and slaughter with cost sharing (OP6)	0.071	3	NA	NA
Test and slaughter with government support (OP4)	0.006	4	0.100	1
BCG vaccination, and test and segregation (OP5)	−0.015	5	NA	NA
Test and segregation, and test and slaughter with government support (OP9)	−0.068	6	0.019	2
Test and slaughter with cost sharing (OP3)	−0.074	7	0.018	3
Test and segregation (OP2)	−0.141	8	−0.070	5
Test and segregation, and test and slaughter with cost sharing (OP8)	−0.140	9	−0.067	4

NA, not applicable.

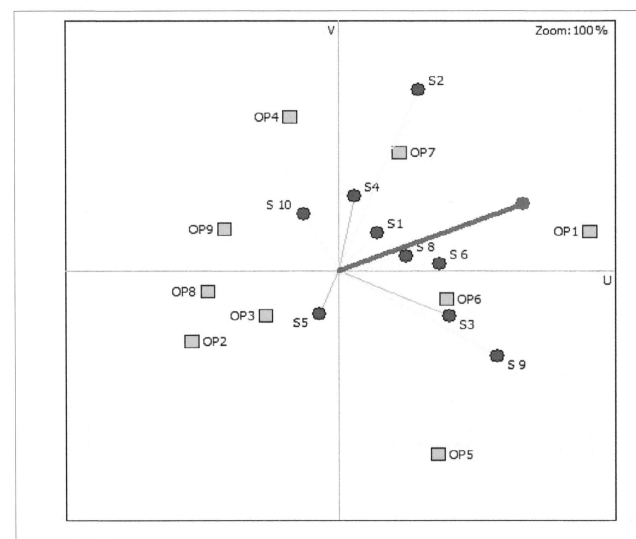

FIGURE 2 | Geometrical analysis for interactive aid decision map for the intervention options under scenario 1 involving BCG vaccination (Delta = 71%, meaning that 71% of the information is conserved in the two-dimensional plane).

of BTB and recommended BCG vaccine as a valuable tool in the control of BTB (21, 22). The use of BCG vaccination has been encouraged because of the development of a new skin test which could differentiate *M. bovis* infected animals from BCG-vaccinated animals (i.e., DIVA role) (23). The experiment conducted in Ethiopia on the evaluation of the efficacy BCG under natural challenge model demonstrated good performance of BCG particularly in reducing the severity and dissemination of the lesion (22). However, approved commercial BCG vaccines for use in cattle are not yet present on the market.

According to the stakeholders, BCG vaccination poorly reduces the prevalence of BTB in cattle. This is likely influenced by the role of BCG in sensitizing cattle to respond to the conventional BTB diagnostic test, combined with the low level of protection of BCG vaccine in cattle compared to its relative effectiveness in humans (22). To overcome the diagnostic limitations of PPD skin test, an alternative skin test that can differentiate infected from vaccinated animals (DIVA) was developed (24). Thus, in the presence of the alternative test with DIVA role BCG vaccination would be the preferred control option for control of BTB, particularly in low and middle income countries like Ethiopia (24).

The second and the third control options involve prior application of BCG vaccination to reduce the number of positive cattle followed by test and slaughter with half and full compensation by the government, respectively. In high income countries, test and slaughter is the most preferred and a widely applied approach to control and eventually eradicate BTB, since the prevalence is low (6, 7, 10). For instance, Australia is among the few countries that eradicated BTB successfully (25) while USA is on the verge of controlling BTB through tracing of infected herds identified through meat inspection, followed by test and slaughter program (26). Many European Union countries also were successful to be recognized as officially TB free countries (27). However, BTB control is not practically feasible in low and middle income countries like Ethiopia through test and slaughter method alone due to lack of resources for rigorous testing, tracing, slaughtering of large number of positive cattle, and compensations to farmers (28).

Alternatively, as revealed by the present study, applying BCG vaccination to reduce the prevalence and progression of BTB and subsequent integration with other control options such as test and slaughter, could be a novel approach for Ethiopia which can also be adopted by other low and middle income countries where BTB is endemic and implementation of test and slaughter policy is practically challenging. To that end, the availability and accessibility of commercial BCG vaccine is critically needed. In addition, mutual understanding, acceptability and cooperation between dairy cattle owners and the government are profoundly needed particularly regarding cost recovery scheme for the implementation of the approach.

Under scenario 2 (which did not consider BCG vaccination as a feasible option), test and slaughter with full compensation by the government ranked the number one preferred control option. Indeed, this could be the most preferred and acceptable option for the cattle owner from the perespective of relatively practical applicability and lower socio-economic impacts. However, this might not be acceptable to the government, as it would be too costly vis-a-vis to other priorities of the government (29). Besides the cost implication, implementation of the test and slaughter approach involves slaughtering and culling of large number of test positive cattle, especially at the beginning of the program, raising concerns of animal welfare and loss of cattle with good milk yield. This might affect the social acceptability of the control option.

Preferably, the second (test and segregation combined with test and slaughter with government support) and third (test and slaughter with cost sharing) options, would be the preferred options in developing countries. There are compelling evidences that test and segregation method significantly reduced the incidence of BTB (30, 31). The method involves segregating test negative animals at early stage of the disease from positive reactors based on whole herd testing. This is particularly important in countries where BTB control is lacking such as in Ethiopia and when BTB control is planned for the first time. For long term surveillance and application of BTB control with this method, testing the herd of all animals >6 weeks of age annually (depending on the incidence rate) and segregating between the positive and negative reactor. For positive reactor pregnant cow and segregating calf at birth is recommended (32). In case of milk from positive reactor cows, pasteurization of milk is effective treatment to avoid public risk and economic loss associated with discarding of milk. *M. bovis* is killed at pasteurization temperature and holding time (33). Use of small scale milk pasteurization and boiling of milk would be an alternative option for smallholder dairy farmers. More specifically, the authors suggested the third control option of scenario 2- test and slaughter with cost sharing as a reliable, feasible and acceptable option from economic point of view in Ethiopia. However, this requires as well advocacy and promotion to create awareness and to convince all stakeholders, particlularly the cattle owners to actively enagage in the implementation of the control options and share the associated costs. However, the social acceptance of slaughtering animals for disease control in this era would be very unlikely since BTB is not a public health emergency and due to the presence of effective public health measures such as meat inspection and milk pasteurization. These measures are not strictly followed in developing countries like Ethiopia and control of BTB in cattle contributed to breaking the cycle of trasmission of zoonotic BTB through meat and milk consumption. Given the high prevalence of BTB in the Ethiopian dairy herds, raising awareness of the public and communities at risk such as dairy farmers about the economic and public health of the diseases by the government would support the initiation of BTB control program.

In this study, the majority (70%, $n = 10$) of the stakeholders gave the highest weight to the epidemiologic criterion (reduction in the prevalence/incidence of BTB) in evaluating the identified control options, while the social ethics criteria generally received the least weight. The epidemiologic criterion is practically important for the control and eradication of BTB. For instance, the application of test and slaughter policy is challenged mainly due to economic and animal welfare reasons, and this impact is lower when the prevalence of BTB is low (6).

The study has some limitations. The MCDA was based on the stakeholder's opinion and preferences which might result in the difference of the weighing clusters and criteria due to personal bias. In addition, some of the invited stakeholders did not participate. Future nationwide large-scale surveys involving all stakeholders from dairy farmers, academia, veterinary associations, research institutions, NGOs, commodity associations, federal and state agencies would remedy the limitation of small size of stakeholder participation. The other limitation is the absence of commercially licensed BCG vaccine for use in calves at the moment. In this study, BCG vaccine is identified by the stakeholders as a potential control option given its importance in lowering the prevalence and progression of BTB and the development of new skin test, DIVA, which could differentiate *M. bovis* infected animals from BCG-vaccinated animals.

Based on the insights obtained from this MCDA, the following important long-term stepwise approaches were suggested to initiate national level discussions and to create awareness regarding the need for BTB control and eventually work toward controlling/eradicating the disease. First, establishing a national multidisciplinary BTB organizing body/council is needed that is composed of representatives from all stakeholders that would support the government in the formulation of a national level BTB control/eradication program and implementation guidelines. Second, the economic feasibility of the top ranked control options should be assessed, and resources should be mobilized to validate the best control option in a sentinel population (i.e., applying it in selected urban and peri-urban intensive dairy farms where the prevalence of BTB is presumably high). Third, it is necessary to critically evaluate the outcomes of the control program in the selected areas and then extend the best practices to scale up the program to other regions of the country. Finally, conducting persistent surveillance and monitoring of the status of BTB across the country will be needed to develop a national database that would help in periodic evaluation of the effectiveness of the control measures put in place and taking timely corrective actions as needed. An effective and safe BCG vaccine for use in cattle is critical for this approach.

In conclusion, the study used an MCDA tool in identifying and evaluating BTB control options in Ethiopia. According to the stakeholders' preferences, calf vaccination and test and slaughter with full cost compensation by government are the best control options under a scenario that included BCG vaccination and a scenario with no BCG vaccination, respectively. Moreover, the study showed that integrating calf BCG vaccination with other potential control options, in minimizing the number of test positive cattle thereby decreasing the cost of compensation for culled/slaughtered cattle and maintain animal welfare as the most suitable BTB control option in Ethiopia that can also be used by other countries, especially low income countries.

AUTHOR CONTRIBUTIONS

FG, GEA, KM, TB, MM, and GA designed the study. FG, SL, TT, ZA, BU, and GA collected and summarized the data during multi-criteria decision process. FG analyzed the data. FG wrote the manuscript. FG, GEA, KM, TB, TT, MM, RS, SL, ZA, BU, and GA critically revised and edited the manuscript and approved its submission.

ACKNOWLEDGMENTS

We thank the stakeholders for participating in the study and Tsedale Teshome for technical support. We are also grateful to Cécile Aenishaenslin for providing practical guide on the use of PROMETHEE software.

REFERENCES

1. Langer AJ, LoBue PA. *Public Health Significance of Zoonotic Tuberculosis Caused by the Mycobacterium tuberculosis Complex. Zoonotic Tuberculosis: Mycobacterium bovis and Other Pathogenic Mycobacteria.* 3rd ed. Wiley-Blackwell (2014). p. 21–33.

2. OIE. *Manual of Diagnostic Tests and Vaccines for Terrestrial Animals.* Paris: Office Internationale des Epizooties (OIE) (2016).

3. Oloya J, Opuda-Asibo J, Kazwala R, Demelash AB, Skjerve E, Lund A, et al. Mycobacteria causing human cervical lymphadenitis in pastoral communities in the Karamoja region of Uganda. *Epidemiol Infect.* (2008) 136:636–43. doi: 10.1017/S09502688070 09004

4. WHO/FAO/OIE, World Health Organization (WHO), Food and Agriculture Organization of the United Nations (FAO) and World Organisation for Animal Health (OIE). *Road Map for Zoonotic Tuberculosis.* (2017). Available online at: https://www.visavet.es/bovinetuberculosis/data/Roadmap_zoonotic_TB_OIE.pdf (accessed July 3, 2020).

5. OIE. *The Socio-Economic Costs of Bovine Tuberculosis - OIE Bulletin.* (2019). Available online at: https://oiebulletin.com/?panorama=3-05-tb-costs-en (accessed July 3, 2020).

6. Schiller I, RayWaters W, Vordermeier HM, Jemmi T, Welsh M, Keck N, et al. Bovine tuberculosis in Europe from the perspective of an officially tuberculosis free country: trade, surveillance and diagnostics. *Vet Microbiol.* (2011) 151:153–9. doi: 10.1016/j.vetmic.2011.02.039

7. Olmstead AL, Rhode PW. The eradication of bovine tuberculosis in the united states in a comparative perspective. In: Zilberman D, Otte J, Roland-Holst D, and Pfeiffer D, editors. *Health and Animal Agriculture in Developing Countries.* New York, NY: Springer (2012). p. 7–30.

8. Zinsstag J, Schelling E, Roth F, Bonfoh B, De Savigny D, Tanner M. Human benefits of animal interventions for zoonosis control. *Emerg Infect Dis.* (2007) 13:527. doi: 10.3201/eid1304.060381

9. Aenishaenslin C, Hongoh V, Cissé HD, Hoen AG, Samoura K, Michel P, et al. Multi-criteria decision analysis as an innovative approach to managing zoonoses: results from a study on Lyme disease in Canada. *BMC Public Health.* (2013) 13:897. doi: 10.1186/1471-2458-13-897

10. OIE, World Organization for Animal Health. *Bovine Tuberculosis.* (2020). Available online at: https://www.oie.int/en/animal-health-in-the-world/animal-diseases/Bovine-tuberculosis/ (accessed May 3, 2020).

11. Mourits MC, Van Asseldonk MA, Huirne RB. Multi criteria decision making to evaluate control strategies of contagious animal diseases. *Prev Vet Med.* (2010) 96:201–10. doi: 10.1016/j.prevetmed.2010.06.010

12. Firdessa R, Tschopp R, Wubete A, Sombo M, Hailu E, Erenso G, et al. High prevalence of bovine tuberculosis in dairy cattle in central Ethiopia: implications for the dairy industry and public health. *PLoS ONE.* (2012) 7:e52851. doi: 10.1371/journal.pone.0052851

13. Sibhat B, Asmare K, Demissie K, Ayelet G, Mamo G, Ameni G. Bovine tuberculosis in Ethiopia: a systematic review and meta-analysis. *Prev Vet Med.* (2017) 147:149–57. doi: 10.1016/j.prevetmed.2017.09.006

14. Tschopp R, Hattendorf J, Roth F, Choudhoury A, Shaw A, Aseffa A, et al. Cost estimate of bovine tuberculosis to Ethiopia. *Curr Top Microbiol Immunol.* (2012) 365:249–68. doi: 10.1007/978-3-662-45792-4_245

15. LMP. *Livestock Health Priorities in the Ethiopian Livestock Master Plan. Ethiopia LMP Brief 3.* Nairobi: LMP (2015).

16. Visual PROMETHEE. *The Academic Version of PROMETHEE (Preference Ranking Organization Method for Enrichment Evaluations) Software 1.4.* Available online at: http://www.promethee-gaia.net/software.html (accessed June 11, 2020).

17. Dibaba AB, Kriek NP, Thoen CO. *Tuberculosis in Animals: An African Perspective.* Switzerland: Springer (2019). p. 15–30.

18. Buddle BM, Wedlock DN, Parlane NA, Corner LAL, De Lisle GW, Skinner MA. Revaccination of neonatal calves with *Mycobacterium bovis* BCG reduces the level of protection against bovine tuberculosis induced by a single vaccination. *Infect Immun.* (2003) 71:6411–9. doi: 10.1128/IAI.71.11.6411-6419.2003

19. Chambers MA, Carter SP, Wilson GJ, Jones G, Brown E, Hewinson RG, et al. Vaccination against tuberculosis in badgers and cattle: an overview of the challenges, developments and current research priorities in Great Britain. *Vet Rec.* (2014) 175:90–6. doi: 10.1136/vr.102581

20. Buddle BM. Tuberculosis vaccines for cattle: the way forward. *Expert Rev Vaccines.* (2010) 9:1121–4. doi: 10.1586/erv.10.112

21. Nugent G, Yockney IJ, Whitford J, Aldwell FE, Buddle BM. Efficacy of oral BCG vaccination in protecting free-ranging cattle from natural infection by *Mycobacterium bovis. Vet Microbiol.* (2017) 208:181–9. doi: 10.1016/j.vetmic.2017.07.029

22. Buddle BM, Vordermeier HM, Chambers MA, de Klerk-Lorist LM. Efficacy and safety of BCG vaccine for control of tuberculosis in domestic livestock and wildlife. *Front Vet Sci.* (2018) 5:259. doi: 10.3389/fvets.2018.00259

23. Srinivasan S, Jones G, Veerasami M, Steinbach S, Holder T, Zewude A, et al. A defined antigen skin test for the diagnosis of bovine tuberculosis. *Sci Adv.* (2019) 5:1–8. doi: 10.1126/sciadv.aax4899

24. Chandran A, Williams K, Mendum T, Stewart G, Clark S, Zadi S, et al. Development of a diagnostic compatible BCG vaccine against Bovine tuberculosis. *Sci Rep.* (2019) 9:17791. doi: 10.1038/s41598-019-54108-y

25. More SJ, Radunz B, Glanville RJ. Lessons learned during the successful eradication of bovine tuberculosis from Australia. *Vet Rec.* (2015) 177:224. doi: 10.1136/vr.103163

26. USDA. *USDA National Tuberculosis Eradication Program.* (2018). Available online at: https://www.aphis.usda.gov/aphis/ourfocus/animalhealth/animal-disease-information/cattle-disease-information/national-tuberculosis-eradication-program (accessed June 22, 2020).

27. EFSA, ECDC, European Food Safety Authority and European Centre for Disease Prevention and Control. The European Union one health 2018 zoonoses report. *EFSA J.* (2019) 17:05926. doi: 10.2903/j.efsa.2019.5926

28. Meiring C, van Helden PD, Goosen WJ. TB control in humans and animals in South Africa: a perspective on problems and successes. *Front Vet Sci.* (2018) 5:298. doi: 10.3389/fvets.2018.00298

29. Ameni G, Tafess K, Zewde A, Eguale T, Tilahun M, Hailu T, et al. Vaccination of calves with *Mycobacterium bovis* Bacillus Calmette–Guerin reduces the frequency and severity of lesions of bovine tuberculosis under a natural transmission setting in Ethiopia. *Transboundary Emerg Dis.* (2018) 65:96–104. doi: 10.1111/tbed.12618

30. AdeaneCRW, Gaskell, JF. A segregation method for eliminating tuberculosis from cattle. *Epidemiol Infect.* (1928) 27:248–56. doi: 10.1017/S0022172400031983

31. Ameni G, Aseffa A, Sirak A, Engers H, Young DB, Hewinson GR, et al. Effect of skin testing and segregation on the incidence of bovine tuberculosis, and molecular typing of *Mycobacterium bovis* in Ethiopia. *Vet Rec.* (2007) 161:782–6.

32. Brooks-Pollock E, Conlan AJ, Mitchell AP, Blackwell R, McKinley TJ, Wood JL. Age-dependent patterns of bovine tuberculosis in cattle. *Vet Res.* (2013) 44:97. doi: 10.1186/1297-9716-44-97

33. Bolaños CAD, Paula, CLD, Guerra ST, Franco MMJ, Ribeiro MG. Diagnosis of mycobacteria in bovine milk: an overview. *Rev Inst Med Trop S Paulo.* (2017) 59:1–13. doi: 10.1590/s1678-9946201759040

19

Field-Adapted Full Genome Sequencing of Peste-Des-Petits-Ruminants Virus using Nanopore Sequencing

Emeli Torsson[1]*, Tebogo Kgotlele[2], Gerald Misinzo[2], Jonas Johansson Wensman[3], Mikael Berg[1] and Oskar Karlsson Lindsjö[4]

[1] Department of Biomedical Sciences & Veterinary Public Health, Swedish University of Agricultural Sciences, Uppsala, Sweden, [2] Department of Veterinary Microbiology and Parasitology, Sokoine University of Agriculture, Morogoro, Tanzania, [3] Department of Clinical Sciences, Swedish University of Agricultural Sciences, Uppsala, Sweden, [4] Department of Animal Breeding and Genetics, Swedish University of Agricultural Sciences, Uppsala, Sweden

*Correspondence:
Emeli Torsson
e.torsson@gmail.com

Peste-des-petits-ruminants virus (PPRV) is currently the focus of a control and eradication program. Full genome sequencing has the opportunity to become a powerful tool in the eradication program by improving molecular epidemiology and the study of viral evolution. PPRV is prevalent in many resource-constrained areas, with long distances to laboratory facilities, which can lack the correct equipment for high-throughput sequencing. Here we present a protocol for near full or full genome sequencing of PPRV. The use of a portable miniPCR and MinION brings the laboratory to the field and in addition makes the production of a full genome possible within 24 h of sampling. The protocol has been successfully used on virus isolates from cell cultures and field isolates from tissue samples of naturally infected goats.

Keywords: peste-des-petits-ruminants virus, eradication, molecular epidemiology, full genome sequencing, MinION, miniPCR

INTRODUCTION

With the development of new and portable sequencing equipment, it is now possible to perform—in very basic laboratories—sequencing that was previously limited to well-equipped laboratories (1–4). With a small thermocycler such as the miniPCR (Amplyus, Cambridge, United States), the hand-held MinION sequencer (Oxford Nanopore Technologies, Oxford, United Kingdom), and portable computational resources, full genome sequencing and advanced molecular epidemiology can be performed in almost any setting (1–4). This is highly advantageous for the diagnosis and control of viral diseases. This approach enables rapid sequencing-based technologies in resource constrained environments, in addition to bringing the laboratory analysis closer to the disease outbreak and reducing the time from diagnosis to full genome and epidemiological investigations.

Peste des petits ruminants (PPR) is a highly contagious and deadly disease in small ruminants (5). The cause is the peste-des-petits-ruminants virus (PPRV), a single-stranded negative-sense RNA virus belonging to the genus *Morbillivirus* (6). Other morbilliviruses include canine distemper virus, measles virus, feline morbillivirus, marine morbilliviruses, and the now eradicated rinderpest virus (RPV) (7).

PPR has a large socioeconomic impact, as small ruminants are mainly kept by poor and rural populations that depend on their animals for income and livelihood. Due to this, the Food and Agriculture Organization of the United Nations (FAO) and the World Animal Health Organization (OIE) have launched a control and eradication program for PPRV to eliminate the disease by 2030 (8). To reach this goal, accurate and well-functioning diagnostic and epidemiological tools need to be in place (9). The Global Strategy for Control and Eradication of PPR (8) highlights that countries in stage 2 in the eradication program (out of four stages), have to strengthen laboratory capacity with molecular methods able to better characterize the collected virus isolates (8). Use of the full genome to characterize isolates, rather than only a partial sequence or genetic marker, ensures detection of important changes within the genome (10).

PPRV is widely distributed in Africa and Asia. In many of these areas, efficient transport of samples, with an unbroken cold chain to a laboratory with the correct equipment, is hard to achieve (9, 11). A broken cold chain during sample transport risks degradation of the sensitive nucleic acid of single-stranded RNA viruses such as PPRV. Analyses performed as close to possible to the sample collection site avoids these long transports (12). More accessible, less expensive, and more timely full genome sequencing will lead to better comprehensive surveillance and detection in the control of a disease such as PPR. The implementation of these mobile methodologies for molecular epidemiology will also increase the chances for successful eradication.

Here we have developed a protocol for a quick, on-site, field-adapted full genome sequencing of veterinary significant virus diseases, with PPRV as an important example. The protocol uses the highly portable miniPCR thermocycler and the MinION sequencer.

MATERIALS AND METHODS

The full wet lab protocol is available at DOI:dx.doi.org/10.17504/protocols.io.pnxdmfn.

Samples

A selection of samples of different origins was used to verify the protocol. These included: (i) viral RNA collected from a cell-culture grown virus (Vero-SLAM cell line), isolate Nigeria 75/1, kindly provided by Dr. Siamak Zohari, National Veterinary Institute (SVA), Uppsala, Sweden; (ii) RNA from field samples representing all currently known lineages of PPRV (cultured on the CV-1-SLAM cell line), kindly provided by Dr. William G. Dundon, International Atomic Energy Agency (IAEA), Vienna, Austria, [KP789375 (13), KR781450, KR781449 (14) and KM463083 (15)]; and, (iii) two field isolates (tissue) collected by Tebogo Kgotlele and Prof. Gerald Misinzo from an outbreak in goats in Dakawa, Morogoro region, Tanzania, in 2013 (16).

Primer Design

Two sets of multiplex full-genome primers were designed using Primal Scheme (http://primal.zibraproject.org) (17). One primer set had an amplicon length of 800 base pairs (bp) and an overlap

TABLE 1 | Complete genomes used to generate the multiplex primers with the primal scheme.

Accession no.	Lineage	Country	Year
EU267273.1	I	Cote d'Ivoire	1989
KR781451.1	II	Cote d'Ivoire	2009
KR828814.1	II	Nigeria	2012
X74443.2	II	Nigeria	1975
KJ867540.1	III	Ethiopia	1994
KJ867543.1*	III	Uganda	2012
KJ867541.1	IV	Ethiopia	2010
KR828813.1	IV	Nigeria	2013

*First genome in file.

of 100; the other primer set had an amplicon length of 600 bp and an overlap of 40. Primers were designed using eight full genome sequences representing all known lineages available at the NCBI GenBank (**Table 1**). Primers, for the 600-bp and 800-bp amplicons, are available in the Supplementary Material (**Tables S1, S2**).

RNA Extraction, cDNA Synthesis, and PCR Amplification

QIAamp Viral RNA Mini kit (Qiagen) was used according to the manufacturer's instructions to extract RNA from tissue samples from Tanzania (sample type iii). The other samples were shared with us as extracted RNA. cDNA synthesis was performed using Superscript IV First-Strand Synthesis System (Invitrogen) with 11 µl of RNA, according to the manufacturer's instructions. PCR amplification was performed using the Q5 Hot Start High Fidelity Polymerase (New England BioLabs) according to the protocol in (17). The protocol divided the multiplex primers into two pools with an even amount of primer pairs, and was run on the miniPCR thermocycler. The amplicons were then purified using AMPure XP magnetic beads (Beckman Coulter) or HighPrep PCR Clean-up System (MagBio Genomics Inc.) with a 1.8× bead ratio and quantified using Qubit 1.0 Fluorometer dsDNA HS assay (Thermo Fisher Scientific). To verify the amplification, a 1% agarose gel electrophoresis (6–7 V/cm, 50–60 min) was performed, this is however optional in the final protocol.

Nanopore Library Preparation and Sequencing

Sequencing libraries were prepared using the SQK-LSK109 Ligation Sequencing Kit and EXP-NBD104 Native Barcode expansion (Oxford Nanopore Technologies) according to manual and previously suggested modifications (17, 18). The purified PCR amplicons were repaired and A-tailed using the NEBNext Ultra II End Repair/dA-Tailing module (New England BioLabs). Native barcodes and adaptors were ligated to amplicons using Blunt/TA Ligase Master Mix (New England BioLabs). The library was then sequenced on a MinION Flowcell R9.4. for 10 h.

Data Analysis

The docker, as well as guidance for replication of the study is available at (www.github.com/Ackia/Field_Seq). In addition to this, a suggested user protocol is included in the protocol at protocols.io (DOI: dx.doi.org/10.17504/protocols.io.pnxdmfn). The process in short; raw reads were basecalled using GUPPY (version 3.1.5. used for the publication. FASTQ files are available in repository PRJEB35549). Read-set composition

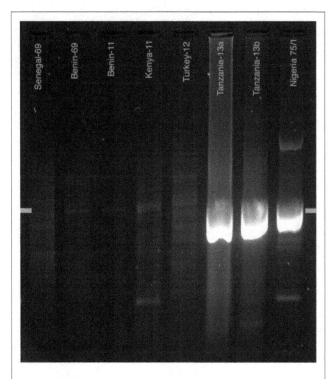

FIGURE 1 | Gel electrophoresis of purified 800-bp PCR amplicons. The blue marker indicates the 800-bp size marker. Full gel image available in **Supplementary Material**.

and quality were assessed using plots produced by PycoQC (19). Demultiplexed read-sets were checked for purity using Kraken 2, and results were visualized in Pavian (20, 21). The read-sets were aligned to the reference genome (RefSeq assembly accession: GCF_000866445.1) using minimap2 (22). The resulting alignment file was sorted and converted into an index bam-file for further processing with samtools (23). BED files were created, representing the coverage of the sequence reads against the reference genome. BED files were further visualized using R and ggplot (24, 25). Consensus sequence were extracted using samtools and bcftools (23). Whole-genome comparison of sequence identity was performed using sourmash with the sequences of good quality (coverage x50 > 80%) reported from MinION sequencing (26). Based on the sourmash results, representative sequences were selected and whole genome comparison was performed between the consensus sequences produced with the FieldSeq protocol and the reference sequences using Mashtree (27). The tree from Mashtree was visualized using R and ggtree.

RESULTS

Gel electrophoresis following PCR amplification of Nigeria 75/1 virus cultured on Vero-SLAM cells showed two bands—one very clear at 800 bp, and a second, weaker band at approximately 2400 bp (**Figure 1**). These longer amplicons are not seen on the gel electrophoresis image for the Tanzanian field samples. However, a strong band is seen at 800 bp. For the samples cultured on CV-1 cells, the gel electrophoresis image shows a narrow band at 800 bp, together with a wide selection of bands of all sizes.

Sequencing of the Nigeria 75/1 isolate produced 741,787 raw reads for the 800-bp primer set and 629,875 raw reads for the 600-bp primer set. The 800-bp primers gave a genome coverage (>50×) of 98.6% and an average coverage of 4,602 reads, whereas the 600-bp primers produced a genome coverage of 99.5%, with an average coverage of 4,586 reads (**Table 2**). Following this first evaluation of the primer sets, we found that the 800-bp primer set

TABLE 2 | Results from sequencing using the Oxford Nanopore MinION sequencer.

Sample (lineage)	Raw reads	Total bp	N50 length (bp)	Reads mapped to PPRV	Average coverage	Genome coverage >50× (%)	Genome coverage >25× (%)	Source
Nigeria 75/1*, 800 bp (II)	741,787	660,217,802	870	672,805	4601	98.6	99.4	Cultured on Vero-SLAM
Nigeria 75/1, 600 bp (II)	629,875	500,972,391	630	597,110	4586	99.5	99.5	Cultured on Vero-SLAM
Senegal-69 (I)	721,283	483,015,988	753	10,196	416	49.6	71.8	Cultured on CV-1**
Benin-69 (II)	945,266	619,883,689	826	35,716	554	78.9	87.5	Cultured on CV-1**
Benin-11 (II)	354,531	221,621,251	779	47,828	460	66.4	79.2	Cultured on CV-1**
Kenya-11 (III)	1,123,782	662,242,080	736	178,526	2311	85.0	88.8	Cultured on CV-1**
Turkey-12 (IV)	776,693	500,690,835	748	11,554	493	67	79.8	Cultured on CV-1**
Tanzania-13a (III)	947,742	707,688,820	782	771,053	4340	91.2	93.0	Field isolate
Tanzania-13b (III)	1,418,713	1,089,046,940	780	1,197,778	4506	93.5	93.5	Field isolate

*Mean from duplicate runs.
**Stably transfected with a plasmid expressing the goat SLAM receptor.

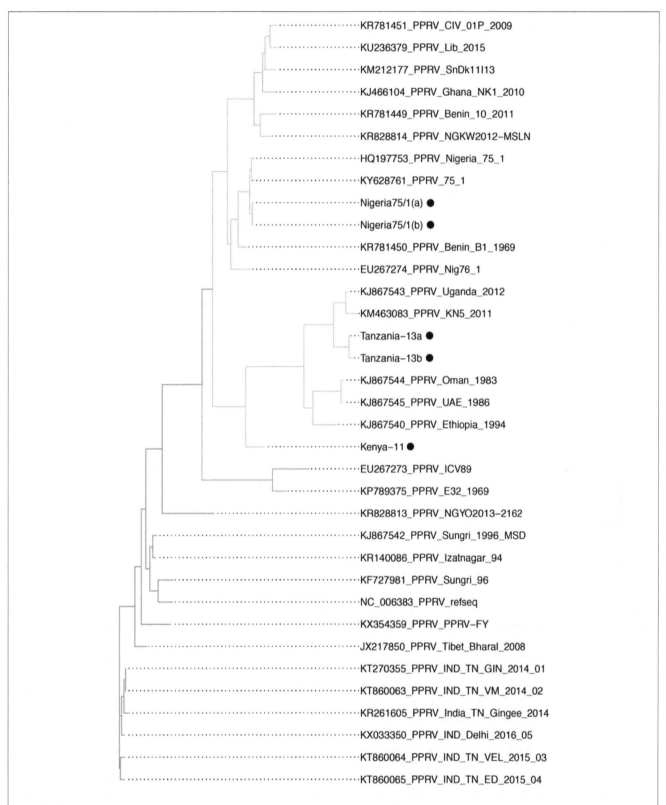

FIGURE 2 | Genomic comparison of whole genome sequences of PPRV from the NCBI GenBank and the isolates with consensus sequences from the minION sequencing that produced quality sequences (>80% of the full genome). All isolates placed in the comparison according to their previously known lineage. Included consensus sequences are indicated by black dots. Isolates with purple branches indicated lineage I, isolates with green branches indicate lineage II, isolates with blue branches indicate lineage III, and isolates with red indicate lineage IV.

gave more even coverage of the PPRV genome, including a higher coverage of the ends of the genome. A possible explanation of this could be the increase overlap of the amplicons for the 800 bp primer set, around 100 bp instead of around 40 bp. On the basis of this result, we decided to continue working with only the 800-bp amplicon primer set for further samples (coverage comparison of both primer sets is available in **Supplementary Material, Figure 1**).

The Nigeria 75/1 isolate, the first trial sample, was run in duplicate to evaluate the reproducibility within a single run. The duplicates produced 709,440 and 636,171 reads that mapped against PPRV, with an average coverage of 4,454 and 4,749 reads. This was considered as an equal performance of the duplicates, which were henceforth presented as a mean of the two (**Table 2**). A total of 672,805 reads was mapped to the PPRV genome to give a coverage (above 50×) of 98.4% of the full genome (**Table 2**). For the isolates cultured on CV-1 cells, the protocol was run using the 800-bp multiplex primers. The total number of raw reads varied between 354,531 and 1,123,782; however, most reads did not map against the PPRV reference genome (**Table 2**). Despite this, an average of 69.4% of the genome was covered above 50×. For the two field isolates from Tanzania, the sequencing results were 947,742 and 1,418,713 raw reads, respectively, out of which 771,053 and 1,197,778 reads mapped to the PPRV reference genome (**Table 2**). For these isolates, 91.9% and 93.5% of the genome had coverage above x50. The whole genome sequences with good quality were compared based on nucleic acid similarity and grouped based on distance using mashtree (**Figure 2**). The sequences produced on MinION showed good conformity with previously sequenced genomes based on lineage and previous sequencing.

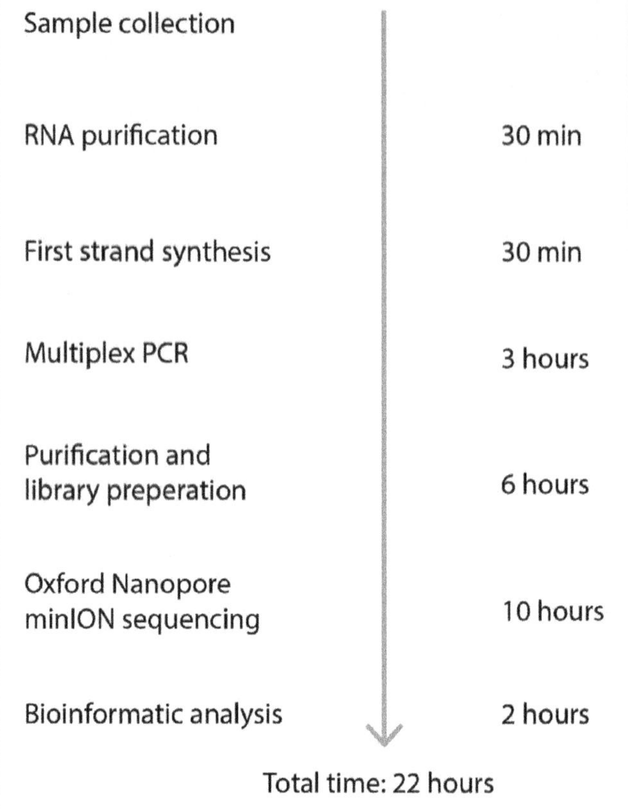

DISCUSSION

Here we have presented a protocol for full genome sequencing of the peste-des-petits-ruminants virus (PPRV) using the miniPCR thermocycler and Oxford Nanopore MinION. Both are suitable for use in a minimally equipped laboratory facility or even directly in the field. PPRV is currently the target of a control and eradication program, launched by the FAO and OIE in 2015, with a goal of eradication by 2030 (8). The success of this program depends on vaccination campaigns and the ability to quickly diagnose and trace the source of an outbreak (8). PPRV most often occurs in areas that lack infrastructure and laboratory facilities (11), making it difficult to reach a quick diagnosis or do adequate epidemiological investigations. Moreover, long transports of samples increase the risk of degrading the sensitive viral nucleic acid in the sample, leading to false negative results (5). By bringing the laboratory closer to the outbreak, these risks are minimized and the time from recognizing clinical signs to a molecular epidemiological investigation is significantly reduced.

The proposed protocol does not require an expert laboratory- or sequencing technician, but it does need a basic understanding of contamination avoidance and handling of laboratory equipment. We estimate that, assuming previous training in basic pipetting skills, this protocol can easily be performed

FIGURE 3 | Workflow and estimated time required for each step of the protocol.

following one full run-through auscultation. The loading of reagents to the MinION flow cell requires the most practice, which can be done on used flow cells, or this single step can be performed by more experienced personnel. The time needed to run the full protocol, from the purification of RNA to analyzed sequences, is around 22–24 h (**Figure 3**). The protocol does not include instructions for RNA purification. In a field setting, either a spin column protocol using a small battery-driven centrifuge would be a good option or a magnetic bead-based system (as the latter is also needed in other steps of the protocol). **Table 3** gives a full list of reagents and cost calculation. With our protocol, a full genome is possible to produce for under USD 100 per sample. Washing and reusing the flow cells reduces the cost even further, to around USD 80 per sample.

With good quality virus isolates, this protocol performed well and yielded a full genome with a mean coverage of around 4,500 reads. To standardize the quality assessment of the many new high-throughput sequences being produced, Ladner et al. suggest five standard sequenced viral genomes could be placed in (10). For molecular epidemiology, they suggest the standard "Coding complete," which means 90–99% of the genome is sequenced with no gaps, all open reading frames (ORFs) are complete, and the average coverage is 100×. The sequences produced using our method meet these requirements when the virus isolates are of good quality.

TABLE 3 | Reagents used within the protocol, with cost calculations based on prices stated on suppliers' homepages in September 2019.

Reagent	Product number	Source	Cost/unit	Cost/sample (USD)
RNA extraction			variable	
SuperScript IV first-strand synthesis system	18091050	ThermoFisher Scientific	USD 2978 (200 reactions)	14.89
Multiplex primers		SigmaAldrich	variable, our 800-bp primers cost USD 158 for 100 μM/primer	0.02
Q5 hot start high-fidelity DNA polymerase	M0493L	New England Biolabs	USD 532 (500 reactions)	1.10
dNTPs (10 μM each)	R0192	ThermoFisher Scientific	USD 88 (1 ml)	0.13
HighPrep™ PCR clean-up system	AC-60050	MagBio Genomics	USD 526 (50 ml)	1.40
Qubit dsDNA HS assay kit	Q32854	ThermoFisher Scientific	USD 289 (500 reactions)	1.73
NEBNext Ultra II End Repair/dA-tailing module	E7546L	New England Biolabs	USD 795 (96 reactions)	4.10
Native barcoding expansion 1-12	EXP-PBC001	Oxford Nanopore	USD 288*	4
Blunt/TA ligase master mix	M0367L	New England Biolabs	USD 520 (250 reactions)	20.80
Ligation sequencing kit (incl. FlowCell priming Kit)	SQK-LSK109	Oxford Nanopore	USD 599 (6 reactions)	8.30
MinION flow cell	R9.4.1	Oxford Nanopore	USD 500–900/flow cell, depending on the quantity ordered**	42
Total				USD 98.5

*Contains 12 unique barcodes and enough of each to use in 12 different sequencing libraries.
**Possible to wash up to 5 times, then USD 8.4/sample and total USD 81/sample (including the cost of Flow Cell Wash kit).

For the first run using the cell culture grown Nigeria 75/1 isolate the coverage is over 100× for the entire genome, missing only a piece of the virus poly-A tail (**Figure 4**). There is a slight decrease in coverage in the intergenic region between the matrix (M) and the fusion (F) protein gene (nucleotide position 4,445–5,526), as well as a short region close to the end of the genome. The M and F intergenic region is the longest intergenic region in the PPRV genome and is rich in GC content and secondary structures (28). These properties makes the region difficult for both primer design and amplification. This region have the lowest coverage in all the sequenced isolates, and was problematic for both studied primer sets. In the isolate from Tanzania it is the only region with low coverage (**Figure 5**), however the coverage is above zero and for molecular epidemiology the ORF are of most importance (10).

In the isolates cultured on CV-1 cells, we did not get equally good coverage over the full genome as we did for the Nigeria 75/1 and Tanzanian isolates (**Figure 6**, **Table 2**). The majority of the reads from the CV-1 samples instead mapped against the human genome. We suspect this is due to the low concentration of viral RNA, degradation of the viral genomes in the samples, and that the human sequences were mistakenly interpreted as such but in fact, had originated from the CV-1 cells (African Green monkey kidney cells). Even though this is not a perfect result, it shows how this protocol works with degraded and damaged samples. Despite the reduced coverage of the genome, we were able to extract 49.6–85.0% (with >50× coverage) of the full genomes in these five samples with an average coverage well above 100× for them (**Table 2**). The regions with lowest coverage for these isolates were the same for these as for the isolates of better quality, the M-F intergenic region and a region toward the end of the genome within the large protein, exemplified by the Kenya-11

isolate in **Figure 6**. Coverage plots for all sequenced isolates are available as **Supplementary Material**.

The four samples that produced above 80% of the full genome (Nigeria 75/1, Tanzania-13a/b, and Kenya-11) were used in a genomic comparison together with other available whole genomes (**Figure 2**). The Nigeria 75/1 isolate that performed excellent in the protocol placed together with the Nigeria 75/1 sequence collected from the database. The isolate from Kenya (Kenya-11) was previously sequenced with the accession number KM463083 (15) which is also included in the comparison. These two whole genome sequences is slightly seperated. This is probably due to the sequences produced using the protocol suggested here is not covering 100% of the genome, wheras the published sequence is full and produced by Sanger sequencing. They do, however, place within the same branch, together with other islolates from lineage III of PPRV. Within the same branch, the two samples from Tanzania (-13a and -13b) are also placed closed together, as expected due to the samples being collected from the same outbreak. By comparing, the consensus sequences produced by the described protocol with previously published sequences produced using the other sequencing techniques; we were able to evaluate the performance of the protocol. Other comparisons of the minION sequencing technique to other more traditional, and labor and equipment intensive have equally found that the method produces high quality sequences (29).

A common practice is to use only the genetic marker, the partial nucleoprotein sequence, to study the phylogeny of a PPRV isolate, as these 255 nts is what the lineage is based on. This increases the risk of missing important changes in the genome outside of the marker, but these changes could be important in the transmission routes and the virus evolution (10). Using the full genome also enables the use of advanced phylogenies such as

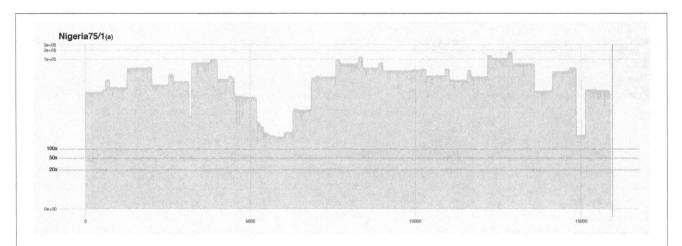

FIGURE 4 | Coverage plot of Nigeria 75/1(a) duplicate. The x-axis represents the length of the genome (15.948 nucleotides). The y-axis represents the sequencing depth on a logarithmic scale. BED files, representing the coverage of the sequence reads against the reference genome, were visualized using R and ggplot.

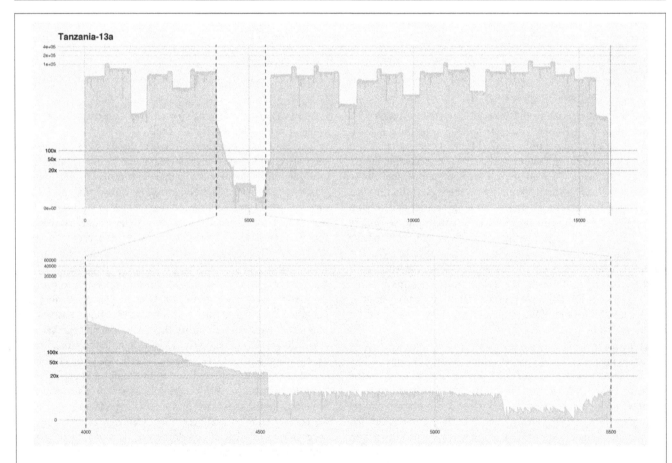

FIGURE 5 | Coverage plot of the Tanzania-13a isolate. The x-axis represents the length of the genome (15.948 nucleotides). The y-axis represents the sequencing depth on a logarithmic scale. BED files, representing the coverage of the sequence reads against the reference genome, were visualized using R and ggplot. A majority of the genome was covered with over 100× sequencing depth, however in the intergenic region between the matrix and the fusion protein genes the sequencing depth falls below ×20 (framed by red dotted lines and showed in detailed in lower half of figure).

those produced by alignments with VIRULIGN (30). The isolates used to verify our protocol are from very different timepoints and geographic regions. If the sequences had belonged to an ongoing outbreak within the same area, this improved resolution of the comparison could help determine the start and transmission route of the outbreak. It would also have made it possible to

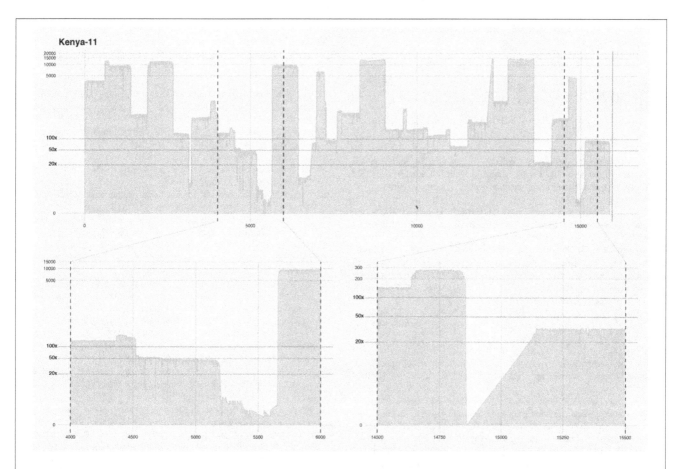

FIGURE 6 | Coverage plot of the Kenya-11 isolate cultured on CV-1 cells. The x-axis represents the length of the genome (15.948 nucleotides). The y-axis represents the sequencing depth on a logarithmic scale. BED files, representing the coverage of the sequence reads against the reference genome, were visualized using R and ggplot. The coverage of this isolate was more uneven, however 85% was covered with ×50 sequencing depth. The lower part of the figure shows a detailed view of two regions with lower coverage, the intergenic region between the matrix and the fusion protein genes (framed by red dotted lines) and a region close to the end of the genome within the large protein gene (framed by blue dotted lines).

track the outbreak in real-time using tools such as Nextstrain (12, 31). For such analyses during outbreaks, the viruses need to be thoroughly sequenced. With our protocol, the production of complete genomes from PPRV field isolates are simplified and will hopefully lead to more full genomes being produced and published.

The use of full genome sequencing for epidemiology and disease surveillance is dependent on the sharing of data and the uploading of the sequences to freely available databases. A genome sequence viewed in isolation can only give limited information (1). Currently, there are 74 complete PPRV genomes available in the NCBI GenBank. Only two are isolated from a wild ruminant: a Dorcas gazelle from a zoological collection in the United Arab Emirates in 1986 (32, 33), and a Capra Ibex in China in 2015 (34). One of the questions in PPR epidemiology is the role of wild ruminants in the spread of the disease. Identified cases in African wildlife are so far considered to be spill-overs from domestic animals, but outbreaks of PPR have occurred

several times in Asian wildlife (35). With additional full genome sequences available, this question could possibly be solved.

In conclusion, we have presented a field-adapted, easy to follow, protocol for full genome sequencing of PPRV using the miniPCR thermocycler and the MinION sequencer. With high-quality isolates, the protocol produces a near-complete genome for <USD 100 per sample. We hereby hope to increase the number of complete genomes available for PPRV. More genomes would allow evaluation of the virus evolution and more precise molecular epidemiological investigations. In addition, they would provide a basis for vaccine and drug development (3).

AUTHOR CONTRIBUTIONS

Conceptualization: ET and OK. Formal analysis: ET, TK, and OK. Writing—original draft preparation: ET. Writing—review and editing: OK, JJ, MB, and ET. Visualization: OK.

Supervision: MB, GM, and JJ. Funding acquisition: ET, JJ, and OK. All authors contributed to the article and approved the submitted version.

REFERENCES

1. Gardy J, Loman NJ, Rambaut A. Real-time digital pathogen surveillance—the time is now. *Genome Biol.* (2015) 16:155. doi: 10.1186/s13059-015-0726-x

2. Rambo-Martin BL, Keller MW, Wilson MM, Nolting JM, Anderson TK, Vincent AL, et al. Mitigating pandemic risk with influenza A virus field surveillance at a swine-human interface. *bioRxiv [Preprint].* (2019) 585588. doi: 10.1101/585588

3. Faria NR, Sabino EC, Nunes MR, Alcantara LCJ, Loman NJ, Pybus OG. Mobile real-time surveillance of Zika virus in Brazil. *Genome Med.* (2016) 8:97. doi: 10.1186/s13073-016-0356-2

4. Krehenwinkel H, Pomerantz A, Henderson JB, Kennedy SR, Lim JY, Swamy V, et al. Nanopore sequencing of long ribosomal DNA amplicons enables portable and simple biodiversity assessments with high phylogenetic resolution across broad taxonomic scale. *GigaScience.* (2019) 8:giz006. doi: 10.1093/gigascience/giz006

5. Parida S, Muniraju M, Mahapatra M, Muthuchelvan D, Buczkowski H, Banyard AC. Peste des petits ruminants. *Vet. Microbiol.* (2015) 181:90–106. doi: 10.1016/j.vetmic.2015.08.009

6. Gibbs E, Taylor W, Lawman M, Bryant J. Classification of peste des petits ruminants virus as the fourth member of the genus Morbillivirus. *Intervirology.* (1979) 11:268–74. doi: 10.1159/000149044

7. Woo PC, Lau SK, Wong BH, Fan RY, Wong AY, Zhang AJ, et al. Feline morbillivirus, a previously undescribed paramyxovirus associated with tubulointerstitial nephritis in domestic cats. *Proc. Natl. Acad. Sci. U.S.A.* (2012) 109:5435–40. doi: 10.1073/pnas.1119972109

8. FAO, OIE. Global strategy for the control and eradication of PPR2015. In: *FAO and OIE International Conference for the Control and Eradication of peste des petits ruminants.* Abidjan (2015).

9. FAO. Supporting livelihoods and building resilience through Peste des petits ruminants (PPR) and small ruminant disease control. In: Animal Production and Health Position Paper. Rome (2013).

10. Ladner JT, Beitzel B, Chain PS, Davenport MG, Donaldson E, Frieman M, et al. Standards for sequencing viral genomes in the era of high-throughput sequencing. *mBio.* (2014) 5:e01360–14. doi: 10.1128/mBio.01360-14

11. OIE. (2019). Available online at: http://www.oie.int/wahis_2/public/wahid.php/Wahidhome/Home (accessed February 2, 2020).

12. Wohl S, Schaffner SF, Sabeti PC. Genomic analysis of viral outbreaks. *Annu. Rev. Virol.* (2016) 3:173–95. doi: 10.1146/annurev-virology-110615-035747

13. Dundon WG, Yu D, Lô MM, Loitsch A, Diop M, Diallo A. Complete genome sequence of a lineage I peste des petits ruminants virus isolated in 1969 in West Africa. *Genome Announc.* (2015) 3:e00381–15. doi: 10.1128/genomeA.00381-15

14. Adombi C, Waqas A, Dundon W, Li S, Daojin Y, Kakpo L, et al. Peste des petits ruminants in Benin: persistence of a single virus genotype in the country for over 42 years. *Transbound. Emerg. Dis.* (2017) 64:1037–44. doi: 10.1111/tbed.12471

15. Dundon W, Kihu S, Gitao G, Bebora L, John N, Oyugi J, et al. Detection and genome analysis of a lineage III peste des petits ruminants virus in Kenya in 2011. *Transbound. Emerg. Dis.* (2017) 64:644–50. doi: 10.1111/tbed.12374

16. Kgotlele T, Kasanga CJ, Kusiluka LJ, Misinzo G. Preliminary investigation on presence of peste des petits ruminants in Dakawa, Mvomero district, Morogoro region, Tanzania. *Onderstepoort J. Vet. Res.* (2014) 81:a732. doi: 10.4102/ojvr.v81i2.732

17. Quick J, Grubaugh ND, Pullan ST, Claro IM, Smith AD, Gangavarapu K, et al. Multiplex PCR method for MinION and illumina sequencing of Zika and other virus genomes directly from clinical samples. *Nat. Protoc.* (2017) 12:1261. doi: 10.1038/nprot.2017.066

18. Hu Y, Schwessinger B. Amplicon sequencing using MinION optimized from 1D native barcoding genomic DNA. *protocols.io.* (2018). doi: 10.17504/protocols.io.mhkc34w

19. Leger A, Leonardi T. pycoQC, interactive quality control for Oxford nanopore sequencing. *J. Open Source Softw.* (2019) 4:1236. doi: 10.21105/joss.01236

20. Breitwieser FP, Salzberg SL. Pavian: interactive analysis of metagenomics data for microbiomics and pathogen identification. *biorxiv [Preprint].* (2016):084715. doi: 10.1101/084715

21. Wood DE, Lu J, Langmead B. Improved metagenomic analysis with Kraken 2. *biorxiv [Preprint].* (2019):762302. doi: 10.1101/762302

22. Li H. Minimap2: pairwise alignment for nucleotide sequences. *Bioinformatics.* (2018) 34:3094–100. doi: 10.1093/bioinformatics/bty191

23. Li H, Handsaker B, Wysoker A, Fennell T, Ruan J, Homer N, et al. The sequence alignment/map format and SAMtools. *Bioinformatics.* (2009) 25:2078–9. doi: 10.1093/bioinformatics/btp352

24. R Core Team. *R: A Language and Environment for Statistical Computing.* R Foundation for Statistical Computing. Vienna, Austria (2020). Available online at: https://www.R-project.org/ (accessed April 16, 2020).

25. Wickham H. *ggplot2: Elegant Graphics for Data Analysis.* New York, NY: Springer-Verlag (2016). doi: 10.1007/978-3-319-24277-4_9

26. Brown C, Irber L. sourmash: a library for MinHash sketching of DNA. *J. Open Source Softw.* (2016) 1:27. doi: 10.21105/joss.00027

27. Katz L, Griswold T, Morrison S, Caravas J, Zhang S, Bakker H, et al. Mashtree: a rapid comparison of whole genome sequence files. *J. Open Source Softw.* (2019) 4:1762. doi: 10.21105/joss.01762

28. Munir M, Zohari S, Berg M. Genome organization of peste des petits ruminants virus. In: Munir M, Zohari S, Berg M, editors. *Molecular Biology and Pathogenesis of Peste des Petits Ruminants Virus.* Berlin; Heidelberg: Springer-Verlag (2013). p. 1–22. doi: 10.1007/978-3-642-31451-3_1

29. Lewandowski K, Xu Y, Pullan ST, Lumley SF, Foster D, Sanderson N, et al. Metagenomic nanopore sequencing of influenza virus direct from clinical respiratory samples. *J. Clin. Microbiol.* (2019) 58:e00963–19. doi: 10.1128/JCM.00963-19

30. Libin PJ, Deforche K, Abecasis AB, Theys K. VIRULIGN: fast codon-correct alignment and annotation of viral genomes. *Bioinformatics.* (2018) 35:1763–5. doi: 10.1093/bioinformatics/bty851

31. Hadfield J, Megill C, Bell SM, Huddleston J, Potter B, Callender C, et al. Nextstrain: real-time tracking of pathogen evolution. *Bioinformatics.* (2018) 34:4121–3. doi: 10.1093/bioinformatics/bty407

32. Furley C, Taylor W, Obi T. An outbreak of peste des petits ruminants in a zoological collection. *Vet. Rec.* (1987) 121:443–7. doi: 10.1136/vr.121.19.443

33. Muniraju M, Munir M, Banyard AC, Ayebazibwe C, Wensman J, Zohari S, et al. Complete genome sequences of lineage III peste des petits ruminants viruses from the Middle East and East Africa. *Genome Announc.* (2014) 2:e01023–14. doi: 10.1128/genomeA.01023-14

34. Zhu Z, Zhang X, Adili G, Huang J, Du X, Zhang X, et al. Genetic characterization of a novel mutant of peste des petits ruminants virus isolated from Capra ibex in China during 2015. *BioMed. Res. Int.* (2016) 2016:7632769. doi: 10.1155/2016/7632769

35. Aguilar XF, Fine AE, Pruvot M, Njeumi F, Walzer C, Kock R, et al. PPR virus threatens wildlife conservation. *Science.* (2018) 362:165–6. doi: 10.1126/science.aav4096

ACKNOWLEDGMENTS

We would like to acknowledge the kind assistance given by Tomas Bergström and Anna Van Der Heiden during this study.

20

Early Life Inoculation with Adult-Derived Microbiota Accelerates Maturation of Intestinal Microbiota and Enhances NK Cell Activation in Broiler Chickens

Nathalie Meijerink[1†], Jannigje G. Kers[2,3†], Francisca C. Velkers[2], Daphne A. van Haarlem[1], David M. Lamot[4], Jean E. de Oliveira[5], Hauke Smidt[3], J. Arjan Stegeman[2], Victor P. M. G. Rutten[1,6] and Christine A. Jansen[1*]

[1] Division Infectious Diseases and Immunology, Department Biomolecular Health Sciences, Faculty of Veterinary Medicine, Utrecht University, Utrecht, Netherlands, [2] Division Farm Animal Health, Department Population Health Sciences, Faculty of Veterinary Medicine, Utrecht University, Utrecht, Netherlands, [3] Laboratory of Microbiology, Wageningen University & Research, Wageningen, Netherlands, [4] Cargill Animal Nutrition and Health Innovation Center, Velddriel, Netherlands, [5] Cargill R&D Center, Vilvoorde, Belgium, [6] Department of Veterinary Tropical Diseases, Faculty of Veterinary Science, University of Pretoria, Pretoria, South Africa

*Correspondence:
Christine A. Jansen
c.a.jansen@uu.nl

† These authors have contributed
equally to this work

Studies in mammals, including chickens, have shown that the development of the immune system is affected by interactions with intestinal microbiota. Early life microbial colonization may affect the development of innate and adaptive immunity and may contribute to lasting effects on health and resilience of broiler chickens. We inoculated broiler chickens with adult-derived-microbiota (AM) to investigate their effects on intestinal microbiota composition and natural killer (NK) cells, amongst other immune cells. We hypothesized that AM inoculation directly upon hatch (day 0) would induce an alteration in microbiota composition shortly after hatch, and subsequently affect (subsets of) intestinal NK cells and their activation. Microbiota composition of caecal and ileal content of chickens of 1, 3, 7, 14, 21, and 35 days of age was assessed by sequencing of 16S ribosomal RNA gene amplicons. In parallel, subsets and activation of intestinal NK cells were analyzed by flow cytometry. In caecal content of 1- and 3-day-old AM chickens, a higher alpha-diversity (Faith's phylogenetic diversity) was observed compared to control chickens, whereas ileal microbiota were unaffected. Regarding beta-diversity, caecal microbiota profiles could be clustered into three distinct community types. Cluster A represented caecal microbiota of 1-day-old AM chickens and 1- and 3-day-old control chickens. Cluster B included microbiota of seven of eight 3- and 7-day-old AM and 7-day-old control chickens, and cluster C comprised microbiota of all chickens of 14-days and older, independent of inoculation. In 3-day-old AM chickens an increase in the percentages of intestinal IL-2Rα[+]NK cells and activated NK cells was observed compared to control chickens of the same age. In addition, an increase in relative numbers of intestinal cytotoxic CD8αα[+]T cells was observed in 14- and 21-day-old AM chickens. Taken together, these results indicate that early exposure to AM shapes and accelerates the maturation of caecal microbiota, which is paralleled by an increase in IL-2Rα+NK cells and enhanced NK cell activation. The observed association between early life development of intestinal microbiota and immune system indicates possibilities to apply microbiota-targeted strategies that can accelerate maturation of intestinal microbiota and strengthen the immune system, thereby improving the health and resilience of broiler chickens.

Keywords: poultry, avian immunology, intestinal microbiota, intraepithelial lymphocytes, innate immunity, NK cells

INTRODUCTION

Health and production efficiency of broiler chickens are of major importance, as chicken meat is a key sustainable source of animal protein for the growing human population (1, 2). In poultry production, restrictions of the use of antimicrobials have made other strategies to maintain or improve poultry health, such as enhanced immune responsiveness, increasingly important.

A crucial role in chicken health and production performance is played in many physiological processes by intestinal microbiota, including nutrient digestion and absorption, metabolism, intestinal barrier function, and development of intestinal immunity (3, 4). The maturation of the intestinal microbiota of chickens entails rapid successional changes, developing from a simple, to a more complex and diverse composition due to gradual colonization with microbiota (5–7). Early life exposure to microbiota is an important driver of this development, which can also affect health later in life. This has been shown in human infants (8–10), and other mammals and hatchlings treated with antibiotics early in life or raised under extreme hygienic conditions, e.g., germ-free or SPF environments (11–15). Also, in commercial chickens under normal circumstances, early transiently colonizing bacteria have been shown to have a large effect on intestinal microbiota composition later in life (16–18). However, due to hatching in a hatchery environment, colonization in commercial chickens starts with microbiota from environmental, rather than parental sources. As these environmental microorganisms may include pathogenic bacteria, competitive exclusion products derived from intestinal microbiota of healthy adult chickens have been developed to compete with colonization by pathogenic bacteria and are widely used in poulty production systems to induce a healthy microbiota (19). When supplied *in ovo* or to hatchlings, adult-derived microbiota has been shown to accelerate bacterial colonization (20–22) and to decrease the occurrence of undesirable bacteria such as *Salmonella* and *Escherichia coli* (19, 23, 24).

The intestinal immune system plays an important role in the defense against pathogens that enter a host via the gut. Underneath the mucus layer [the first protective barrier in the intestinal tract (25)], a layer of epithelial cells including immune cells such as the intraepithelial lymphocytes (IEL) is observed. The population of IEL consists of high numbers of γδ T cells, adaptive CD8+ T cells and innate natural killer (NK) cells (26). During embryonic development and early life, when resistance against pathogens relies on innate immune responses since the adaptive immune system is not yet fully developed, NK cells are important players (27, 28). Chicken NK cells have also been reported in multiple organs including the intestine, lung, spleen, and blood (26, 29, 30). Previously, we and others showed that a high percentage of intestinal NK cells in chickens are recognized by the marker 28-4 (26), which was identified as CD25 or IL-2Rα (26). In mammals, the IL-2Rα chain is expressed on NK cells early upon activation (31), and this is followed by enhanced NK cell mediated killing and IFNγ production (31). Another marker found to be expressed on intestinal NK cells was 20E5 (32). It is also expressed on cells that show NK cell activation (29). Furthermore, elsewhere in the body, increased surface expression of CD107 indicative of NK cell activation was observed on primary chicken NK cells in lung, spleen and blood upon infections with avian viruses (30, 33, 34).

In the intestinal tract many interactions occur between the microbiota and immune cells (35, 36). These interactions are important for the development of the immune system, as was shown in mammals (21, 37, 38) and chickens (14, 39). For example, early life transplantation of adult microbiota has resulted in increased natural antibody titers in laying chickens (40) paralleled by long lasting effects on mRNA levels of pro-inflammatory cytokines (41). Disturbing the early life microbiota in 1-day-old broiler chickens by antibiotics resulted in reduced numbers of macrophage-like cells in the jejunum (14), whereas differences in rearing environment, e.g., a reduction in environmental microbial exposure resulted, in two phylogenetically distinct lines of broiler chickens, in lower expression levels of β-defensins (42).

Studies in rodents and humans have shown that specific probiotic microorganisms enhance intestinal NK cell activity and cytokine production (43) either directly via their interaction with receptors expressed on NK cells (44, 45), or indirectly via cytokine production of resident myeloid or epithelial cells (46). Also the adaptive immune system can be modulated via interactions with the microbiota (47–50), or indirectly through innate immune cell activities. As other studies in rodents and humans have shown, the microbiota affects activation of γδ T cells (51, 52) and CD8+ T cells (53). Taken together, this indicates that the composition and activity of the microbiota and its effects on the immune system in early life may have long term consequences on the health of individuals.

In chickens, previous studies addressed the effect of microbiota on innate immune responses in the intestine, spleen and blood by studying mRNA levels of immune related genes (41, 42) by immunohistochemistry (14) and by analysis of natural antibody titers (40). In this study, we used tools that we developed previously for the analysis of the phenotype and the function of chicken innate immune cells (29, 54) to assess whether and to what extent differences in early life microbial colonization would affect the development of NK cells locally (in the intestine) and systemically (in spleen and blood).

We hypothesized that inoculation with adult-derived microbiota(AM) upon hatch would induce an alteration in microbiota development and affect the presence and activation of intestinal NK cells. To induce early colonization with a rich, complex microbiota to stimulate immune development, we used Aviguard® (MSD Animal Health, the Netherlands), as this product derived from microbiota of healthy adult chickens has been shown to be able to colonize the intestinal tract and induce early maturation of the intestinal microbiota in previous studies with hatchlings (22, 55). In this study, AM inoculation resulted in an accelerated maturation of the intestinal microbiota, an increase of IL-2Rα^+ NK cells and enhanced activation of NK cells. The observed association between early life development of intestinal microbiota and the immune system indicates possibilities to apply microbiota-targeted strategies that can accelerate maturation of intestinal microbiota and strengthen the immune system to improve the health and resilience of broiler chickens.

MATERIALS AND METHODS

Birds and Husbandry

Ross 308 broiler 17- and 18-day old embryonated eggs were obtained from the same parent flock of a commercial hatchery (Lagerwey, the Netherlands). ED17 (hatch group A, $n = 52$) and ED18 eggs (hatch group B, $n = 52$) were disinfected with 3% hydrogen peroxide and placed in disinfected egg hatchers. All eggs hatched at ED21. Directly upon hatch, chickens (day 0 in age) were randomly divided into two treatment groups, weighed, labeled and inoculated. Next, the chickens of the two treatment groups were placed in separate floor pens of 2×1.5 m (pens 1 and 2), with a solid wall separating the pens. Each pen was divided in two equal parts of 1×1.5 m for chickens from hatch group A and B. The pens were lined with wood shavings (2 kg/m^2, sterilized by autoclavation). Non-sterilized standard commercial starter and grower feeds (Research Diet Services, the Netherlands) and water was provided *ad libitum*. No antibiotics, coccidiostatic drugs or commercial vaccines were applied during the experiment. A standard lighting, temperature scheme for Ross broiler chickens was used, and conditions were kept the same for all compartments. The chickens were observed daily for clinical signs, abnormal behavior or mortality and were also evaluated for presence of abnormalities during post-mortem. No signs of disease or impaired health were observed in both groups throughout the experiment. Feed intake and body weight were assessed in both groups at each sampling moment and followed the expectations based on the Ross 308 broiler performance standards in both groups.

The experimental room was equipped with a mechanical negative pressure ventilation system.

The animal experiment was approved by the Dutch Central Authority for Scientific Procedures on Animals and the Animal Experiments Committee (registration number AVD1080020174425) of Utrecht University (the Netherlands) and all procedures were done in full compliance with all relevant legislation.

Experimental Design

Chickens were inoculated once immediately after hatch to reduce opportunities for prior exposure to microbiota. First, the control group received an oral inoculation with 0.5 ml PBS (Lonza, Basel, Switzerland). The other group, henceforth referred to as the AM group, was inoculated with 0.5 ml of PBS containing 0.05 g/ml of competitive exclusion product Aviguard® (MSD Animal Health, the Netherlands). This is a freeze-dried powder, soluble in water, consisting of fermented, undefined cultures from intestinal microbiota of healthy specific-pathogen-free birds and was used according to manufacturer's instructions. To determine the microbial composition of the AM inoculum and compare this to the microbiota in the chickens, four aliquots of 2 ml were stored at −80°C for DNA extraction. The experimental design of the study is shown in **Supplementary Figure 1**.

Sample Collection

At day 0 (upon hatch), four non-inoculated chickens per hatch group were randomly selected and sacrificed, to collect caecal and ileal content for microbiota analyses, as has been described in (56). Ileal content was collected distal and close to the Meckel's diverticulum. The intestinal content was gently squeezed into a 2 ml sterile cryotube, snap frozen on dry ice and stored at −80°C for DNA extraction. The time between sacrificing and placing the intestinal samples on dry ice was between 3–5 min. To avoid cross contamination, all management and biotechnical procedures were completed first with the control group and for each compartment at the same time. At days 1 (24 h after inoculation), 3, 7, 14, 21, and 35, eight chickens (four from the control and four from the AM group) were randomly selected per hatch group (A/B) and sacrificed to collect caecal and ileal content as described above. At day 0 and day 1, the chickens were too small to collect sufficient cells for immunological analyses. Therefore, ileum tissue, spleen and blood were collected from day 3 onwards from six of these eight chickens ($n = 3$ per hatch group). All chickens were weighed prior to post-mortem analyses.

DNA Extraction

In total, 104 caecal and 104 ileal content samples, consisting of 52 samples per treatment group, and four samples of the AM inoculum were analyzed for microbiota composition. DNA was extracted from 0.25 g content, using 700 µl of Stool Transport and Recovery (STAR) buffer (Roche Diagnostics Nederland BV, the Netherlands). All samples were transferred to sterile screw-capped 2 ml tubes (BIOplastics BV, the Netherlands) containing 0.5 g of zirconium beads (0.1 mm; BioSpec Products, Inc., USA), and 5 glass beads (2.5 mm; BioSpec Products). All samples were treated in a bead beater (Precellys 24, Bertin technologies, France) at a speed of 5.5 m/s for 3×1 min, followed by incubation at 95°C with agitation (15 min and 300 rpm). The lysis tube was centrifuged (13,000 g for 5 min at 4°C), and the supernatant was transferred to a 2 ml microcentrifuge tube. Thereafter, the above-described process was repeated with 300 μl STAR buffer. An aliquot (250 μl) of the combined supernatants from the sample lysis was then transferred into the custom Maxwell® 16 Tissue LEV Total RNA Purification Kit cartridge. The remainder of the extraction protocol was then carried out in the Maxwell® 16 Instrument (Promega, the Netherlands) according to the manufacturer's instructions. DNA concentrations were measured with a NanoDrop ND-1000 spectrophotometer (NanoDrop® Technologies, DE, USA), and the DNA samples were stored at −20°C until further use.

qPCR, 16S rRNA Gene Amplification, Sequencing, and Data Processing

Extracted DNA was diluted to 20 ng μl^{-1} in nuclease free H$_2$O. All PCR plastics were UV irradiated for 15 min before use. To validate the AM inoculation, absolute quantification of the bacterial 16S rRNA genes by real-time PCR amplification was performed for the caecal content samples of day-old chickens. For ileal content samples the amount of DNA was too low to reliably determine gene copy numbers. All qPCR assays (CFX384™ real-time PCR detection system, Bio-Rad, Hercules, CA, USA) were performed in triplicate with 25 μl reactions and was described previously (57). For 16S ribosomal RNA (rRNA) gene-based microbial composition profiling, barcoded amplicons covering the variable regions V5–V6 of the bacterial 16S rRNA gene were generated by PCR using the 784F and 1064R primers as described before (58). Each sample was amplified in duplicate using Phusion hot start II high fidelity polymerase (Finnzymes, Finland), checked for correct size and concentration on a 1% agarose gel and subsequently combined and purified using CleanNA magnetic beads (CleanNA, the Netherlands). A detailed description of the PCR conditions is given elsewhere (56). Positive and negative controls were added to the data set to ensure high quality sequencing data. As positive controls we used synthetic mock communities of known composition (58), and as negative controls we used nuclease free water. The resulting libraries were sent to Eurofins Genomics GmbH (Germany) for sequencing on an Illumina Hiseq2500 instrument. The 16S rRNA data was analyzed using NG-tax 2.0 (59). In short, paired-end libraries were filtered to contain only read pairs with a perfect match to the primers and perfectly matching barcodes, to demultiplex reads by sample. Amplicon sequence variants (ASVs) were defined as unique sequences. The ASV picking strategy was based on a *de novo* reference approach. Taxonomy was assigned using the SILVA 128 16S rRNA gene reference database (60). Caecal content samples of day 0 and ileal content samples of day 0 and 1 were excluded from the analysis, because these contained a large number of families associated with the negative control samples, and therefore did not pass our quality control standards. Raw sequence data were deposited into the Sequence Read Archive (SRA) at NCBI under accession number PRJNA670739.

Isolation of Tissues and Cells

Ileum segments (±10 cm distal from Meckel's diverticulum), spleens and blood (5 ml) were collected. Ileum segments were washed with PBS to remove contents and cut in sections of 1 cm^2 and washed again. Subsequently, IELs were collected by incubating three times in EDTA-medium [HBSS 1x (Gibco BRL) supplemented with 10% heat-inactivated FCS (Lonza); 1% 0.5M EDTA (Sigma-Aldrich)] at 200 rpm for 15 min at 37°C. Supernatants were collected and centrifuged 5 min at 1,200 rpm at 20°C. Cells were then resuspended in PBS, lymphocytes were isolated using Ficoll-Paque Plus (GE Healthcare, the Netherlands) density gradient centrifugation for 12 min at 1,700 rpm, washed in PBS using centrifugation for 5 min at 1,300 rpm and resuspended at 4.0 × 10^6 cells/ml in NK medium [IMDM supplemented with 8% heat-inactivated FCS (Lonza); 2% heat-inactivated chicken serum, 100 U/ml penicillin/ streptomycin, and 2 mM glutamax I; Gibco BRL, United Kingdom]. Spleens were homogenized using a 70 μm cell strainer [Beckton Dickinson (BD) Biosciences, NJ, USA] to obtain a single cell suspension. Next, lymphocytes in spleen and blood were isolated by Ficoll-Paque density gradient centrifugation (20 min at 2,200 rpm), washed in PBS and resuspended at 4.0 × 10^6 cells/ml in NK medium as described for ileum.

Flow Cytometry

Presence and activation of NK and T cell subsets were determined in IEL, spleen, and blood. Unless described otherwise, all antibodies were obtained from Southern Biotech (AL, USA). Markers known to be expressed on chicken NK cells (hybridomas provided by Göbel), such as mouse-anti-chicken-28-4 (IL-2Rα; IgG3) and—20E5-BIOT (IgG1) were co-stained with mouse-anti-chicken-CD45-FITC (IgM) and -CD3-APC (CT3; IgG1) mAb to exclude T cells. The T cell panel included the following markers: mouse-anti-chicken-CD3-PE (CT3; IgG1), -CD4-APC (CT4; IgG1), -TCRγδ-FITC (TCR-1, IgG1), -CD8α (EP72, IgG2b), and -CD8β-BIOT (EP42, IgG2a). Secondary antibody staining was performed using goat-anti-mouse-IgG3-PE and streptavidin-PercP (BD Biosciences) in the NK cell panel, and goat-anti-mouse-IgG2b-APC/Cy7 and streptavidin-PercP in the T cell panel. To asses CD107 expression on NK cells, lymphocytes were washed in PBA and stained with mouse-anti-chicken-CD3-PE, -TCRγδ-BIOT (TCR-1, IgG1),-28-4, and -CD41/61-FITC (11C3, IgG1, Serotec) to exclude thrombocytes from analysis. Secondary antibody staining was performed using streptavidin-PercP and goat-anti-mouse-IgG3-APC/Cy7. All staining procedures were incubated for 20 min at 4°C in the dark, washed in PBA and subsequently stained with a live/dead marker (Zombie Aqua™ Fixable Viability Kit, Biolegend) for 15 min at RT in the dark to exclude dead cells. Finally, lymphocytes were fixed using 2% paraformaldehyde (Merck, Germany) for 10 min at RT, washed and resuspended in 200 μl PBA. Fluorescence of cells was assessed in 150 μl or 50,000 lymphocytes in the live gate using a FACSCANTO II Flowcytometer (BD Biosciences), and data was analyzed with software program FlowJo (Tree star Inc, OR, USA).

NK Cell Activation Assay

NK cell activation was determined using the CD107-assay, which measures increased surface expression of CD107 as a result of degranulation of perforin and granzymes (29).

Briefly, lymphocytes isolated from IEL, spleen, and blood were resuspended in NK medium, and 1×10^6 lymphocytes per sample were used. Lymphocytes were cultured in presence of 1 µl/ml Golgistop (BD Biosciences) and mouse-anti-chicken-CD107-APC mAb (5G10, IgG1, hybridomas provided by Göbel, T.W., Ludwig Maximilians University, Germany) during 4 h at 37°C, 5% CO_2. Next, cells were washed, stained with monoclonal antibodies and analyzed by flow cytometry.

Data Analysis

Statistical analyses for microbiota and the relation between microbiota and the immune system were performed in R version 3 (R Foundation for Statistical Computing, Austria), using the packages Phyloseq, Microbiome, Vegan, and DirichletMultinomial (61–64). A Kruskal-Wallis test was used to test for difference in 16S rRNA gene counts in caecal content of day-old chickens between treatment groups.

Alpha and beta diversity metrics and multivariate statistical analyses were applied to determine differences in the measured intestinal microbiota between the two treatment groups and with age. The alpha diversity (within sample) data was determined using Faith's phylogenetic diversity. Faith's phylogenetic diversity not only takes the number of different taxa (ASVs) into account, but also the phylogenetic relatedness of these taxa (65). To test for differences in relative abundance of genera between treatment groups, we used a Wilcoxon rank-sum test and corrected for multiple comparisons using the Benjamini-Hochberg (BH) procedure. The beta diversity (between samples) was determined using weighted and unweighted UniFrac metrics (66). Multivariate microbiota data were visualized using principal coordinates analysis (PCoA, multidimensional scaling method), and non-parametric permutational analysis of variance (PERMANOVA) tests were used to analyze group differences within multivariate community data (67).

To assess whether the development of the microbiota proceeded through different stages of maturation in the two treatment groups, Dirichlet Multinomial Mixtures (DMM) modeling was applied, using a probabilistic model, to identify possible clusters (types) of microbial composition 16S rRNA gene sequence data (68) based on the relative abundance of the microbial groups at genus level. Two separate DMM models were used to study clustering of the microbiota data of the caecal content and ileal content separately. Next, to test whether the observed differences in the microbial development between treatments were associated with differences in immune development, Wilcoxon rank-sum test, corrected for multiple comparisons using BH, was used to test for associations between the identified DMM clusters of microbial composition and immunological parameters. As ileal microbiota clustering did not indicate differences in microbial development between treatments, only the clusters identified for the caecal microbiota profiles were used. Associations were tested for a subset of immunological parameters that showed differences between AM and control chickens of the same age. Furthermore, parameters with fewer than four observations per treatment group and day of age were omitted. The final selection of parameters included

percentages and absolute numbers of intestinal IL-2Rα$^+$, 20E5$^+$ and CD107$^+$ NK cells, and CD8αα$^+$ T cells.

Statistical analyses for the immunological parameters were done with GraphPad Prism 7.0 software (GraphPad Software Inc., USA), using the Mann-Whitney U-test to test differences between treatment groups at a specific day of age. A p-value of <0.05 was considered statistically significant.

RESULTS

AM Treatment Influences the Composition and Development of the Intestinal Microbiota in Newly Hatched Chickens

The total bacterial 16S rRNA gene copy numbers 24 h after inoculation were significantly higher in caecal content samples at day 1 in AM inoculated compared to control chickens, indicating the presence of a higher quantity of bacteria after inoculation with AM (**Supplementary Figure 2**).

To investigate the effect of AM inoculation on the microbiota composition at different ages in the broiler chickens, alpha and beta diversities, as well as differences in relative abundance of individual microbial taxa, were assessed. The phylogenetic diversity metric, providing information on the number as well as phylogenetic relatedness of observed microbial taxa at the ASV level, was used as an alpha diversity measure to determine differences between AM and control chickens. The phylogenetic diversity of the caecal content was higher in 1- and 3-day-old AM chickens compared to controls, but not for any of the other ages (**Figure 1A**). In contrast, the phylogenetic diversity of ileal content microbiota did not differ between treatment groups at any age (**Figure 1B**).

Beta diversity, i.e., the similarity in composition between samples, was determined using the weighted and unweighted UniFrac distance metrics to determine the influence of age and treatment on the composition. Two dimensional visualization of the caecal content microbiota profiles in PCoA plots placed 3- and 7-day-old AM inoculated chickens closely together, indicating high similarity in microbiota composition between these age groups (**Figure 2**). PERMANOVA of caecal content microbiota showed that treatment explained 6–9% of the variation in caecal microbiota composition between samples ($p < 5e-04$; unweighted UniFrac, $p < 2e-04$, weighted UniFrac), whereas age explained 49–41% of the variation between samples ($p < 5e-04$; unweighted UniFrac, $p < 2e-04$, weighted UniFrac). PERMANOVA of ileal content samples showed that treatment explained 4% of the variation in ileal microbiota composition based on unweighted UniFrac, whereas treatment did not significantly contribute to explaining the observed variation using the weighted UniFrac distance metrics ($p = 0.038$; unweighted UniFrac, $p = 0.355$, weighted UniFrac, **Figure 2B**), indicating that differences in microbial profiles of ileal samples between treatment groups concerned mostly the presence/absence of taxa occurring at low relative abundance. Age explained 29–24% of the variation between the ileal content samples ($p < 1e-04$; unweighted UniFrac, $p < 1e-04$, weighted UniFrac).

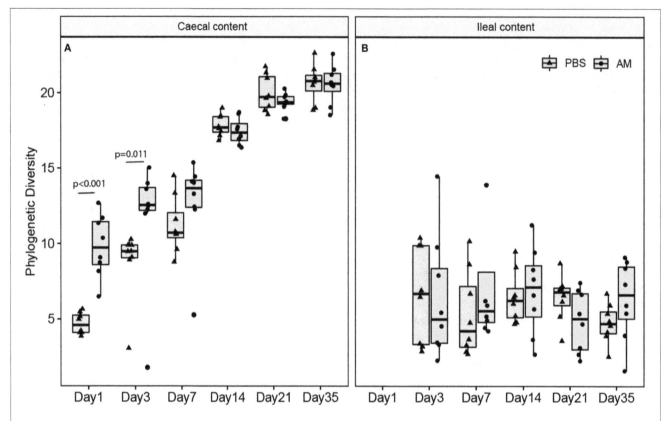

FIGURE 1 | Phylogenetic diversity of the ileal and caecal content microbiota at different ages. **(A)** The phylogenetic diversity (alpha diversity, at ASV level) was only significantly higher in the caecal content of AM chickens compared to controls on day 1 and day 3 (*p* < 0.05). **(B)** In the ileal content microbiota no differences were observed at any of the ages. *n* = 8 chickens per treatment per day of age, whiskers show 95% interval, box 50% interval.

In the AM inoculum 24 different genera were detected, for which the relative abundances in caecal and ileal samples were compared between AM and control chickens. A higher relative abundance in caecal content of AM chickens compared to controls was found for 10 of these 24 genera at day 1, five on day 3, four at day 7, and two at day 14 and 21. At day 35 none of these genera differed in relative abundance between AM and control chickens (**Table 1**). This indicates that AM inoculation had an impact on the relative abundance of genera at an early age, but did not permanently influence the relative abundance of these genera in the caecal content samples. For ileal content, no differences in the relative abundances of the 24 genera of the inoculum were observed at any of the different ages (data not shown).

To assess if AM inoculation affected the development of the microbial composition from hatch toward a mature microbiota, microbial profiles were subjected to DMM clustering of 16S rRNA gene sequencing data based on the relative abundance of microbial taxa at genus level. The DDM method showed the best model fit, based on lowest Laplace approximation, for three clusters in the caecal content profiles (**Figure 3A**). Cluster A contained 26 samples, with all 1-day-old AM and control chickens and all 3-day-old controls. Cluster B consisted of 21 samples, containing seven of the eight 3-day-old AM chickens and 7-day-old AM and control chickens. The remaining 48 samples were in cluster C, which contained all AM and control

chickens of 14, 21, and 35 days old. This difference in distribution of AM and control chickens over cluster A and B in the 1st week of life indicates an accelerated maturation of caecal microbiota profiles for AM chickens. In contrast, clustering for the ileal content profiles only showed an effect of age, with cluster D dominated by 3- and 7-day-old chickens of both treatments, and cluster E by chickens of 14, 21, and 35 days old of both treatments (**Figure 3B**). The relative microbial abundance of the clusters observed in the caecal content was analyzed and although PBS and AM chickens varied in their relative abundance of microbial families, PBS and AM chickens can be part of the same cluster based on relative abundance of genera (**Figure 3C**).

AM Treatment Affects Presence of NK Cell Subsets and Their Activation

Possible differences in subsets and activation of intestinal NK cells from AM and control chickens were determined. Local effects of AM inoculation on intestinal NK cells were compared to systemic effects measured in spleen and blood. Within the live lymphocytes, the CD3 negative IL-2Rα+ or 20E5+ NK cells were quantified (**Figure 4A**). In parallel, NK cell activation was determined by analysis of enhanced CD107 surface expression on CD3 negative and CD41/61 negative cells. At day 3, the percentage of intestinal IL-2Rα+ NK cells tended to be higher

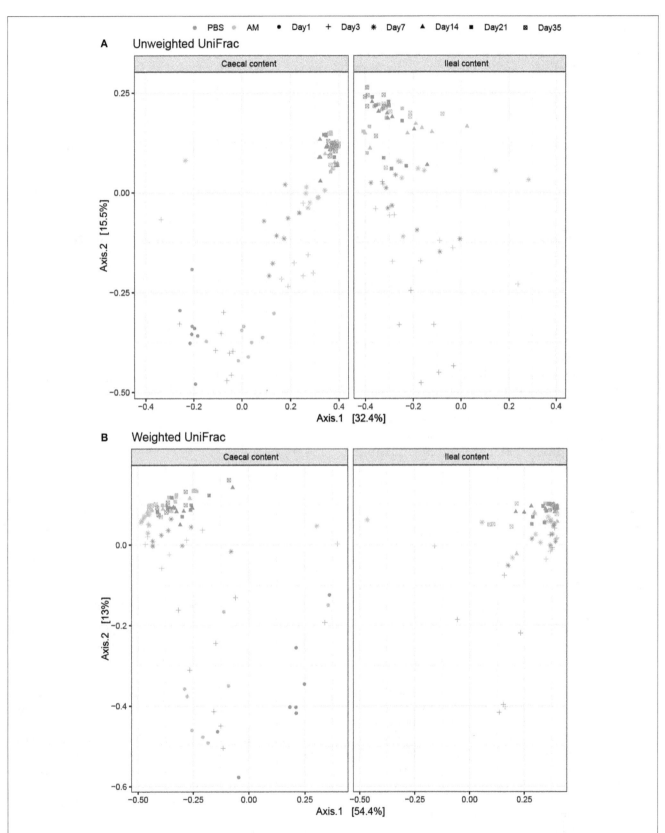

FIGURE 2 | PCoA plot visualizing caecal and ileal content microbial profiles. Unweighted **(A)** and weighted **(B)** UniFrac distance based PCoA on caecal (left) and ileal (right) content samples. **(A)** PERMANOVA of caecal content microbiota showed that treatment explained 6–9% of the variation in caecal microbiota composition

(Continued)

FIGURE 2 | between samples (p < 5e-04; unweighted UniFrac, p < 2e-04, weighted UniFrac), whereas age explained 49–41% of the variation between samples (p < 5e-04; unweighted UniFrac, p < 2e-04, weighted UniFrac). **(B)** PERMANOVA of ileal content samples showed that treatment explained 4% of the variation in ileal microbiota composition based on unweighted UniFrac, whereas treatment did not significantly contribute to explaining the observed variation using the weighted UniFrac distance metrics (p = 0.038; unweighted UniFrac, p = 0.355, weighted UniFrac). n = 8 chickens per treatment per day of age.

in AM chickens (5.61 ± 0.95%) compared to controls (3.25 ± 0.93%, p = 0.09, **Figure 4B**). No differences between treatment groups were observed in intestinal 20E5$^+$ NK cells (**Figure 4C**). Increased CD107 expression on intestinal NK cells was observed at day 3 in AM chickens (10.52 ± 0.70%), when compared to controls (8.07 ± 0.47%, p = 0.06, **Figure 4D**). At day 35, an increase in activation of intestinal NK cells was observed in AM chickens (14.86 ± 1.27%) compared to the controls (11.71 ± 0.75%, p = 0.04, **Figure 4D**). No differences between treatment groups were observed in CD107 expression of intestinal NK cells at other ages (**Figure 4D**).

Relative numbers of IL-2Rα$^+$ and 20E5$^+$ NK cells in spleen and blood were similar in both treatment groups (**Figures 4E,F, Supplementary Figures 3A,B**). However, NK cell activation was significantly increased in splenic NK cells in 3-day-old AM chickens (20.74 ± 1.10%) compared to controls (15.35 ± 0.40%, p = 0.004, **Figure 4G**). No difference in CD107 surface expression on blood-derived NK cells was found between treatment groups (**Supplementary Figure 3C**). Furthermore, AM inoculation did not affect total lymphocyte numbers in the intestine, spleen and blood (**Supplementary Figures 4A,E,I**). In addition to the percentages of the different NK subsets, absolute numbers were determined. Similar trends were observed in absolute number of IL-2Rα$^+$, 20E5$^+$, and CD107$^+$ NK cells although the differences between treatments were less pronounced (**Supplementary Figure 4**).

AM Treatment Affects Intestinal Cytotoxic CD8αα T Cells in 14- and 21-Day-Old Chickens

In addition to NK cell subsets and NK cell activation, effects of AM inoculation on presence and function of γδ T cells and presence of cytotoxic CD8$^+$ T cells were studied. Within the CD3$^+$ and CD4$^-$ lymphocytes, both TCRγδ$^+$ and TCRγδ$^-$ cell populations were analyzed for CD8αα and CD8αβ expression (**Figure 5A**). In parallel, activation of γδ T cells was determined at day 7, 14, and 21 by analyzing increased surface expression of CD107 on CD3$^+$CD41/61$^-$ TCRγδ$^+$ cells (**Figure 5A**). No differences between AM and control chickens were observed in the percentage of intestinal γδ T cells (**Figure 5B**), CD8$^-$, CD8αα$^+$, and CD8αβ$^+$ gamma delta subsets (data not shown) and activation of γδ T cells (**Figure 5C**). The percentage of intestinal CD8αα$^+$ T cells tended to be higher in 14- (25.3 ± 1.5%) and 21-day-old AM chickens (33.2 ± 4.2%) compared to controls (19.5 ± 1.7%, p = 0.08 and 24.0 ± 1.3%, p = 0.07, respectively, **Figure 5D**). No differences between groups were found at any age in the percentages of intestinal CD8αβ$^+$ T cells (**Figure 5E**). Furthermore, no differences between AM and control chickens were observed in the percentage of γδ T cells (**Figure 5F, Supplementary Figure 3D**),

subsets (data not shown), γδ T cell activation (**Figure 5G, Supplementary Figure 3E**) and cytotoxic T cells in spleen and blood (**Figures 5H,I, Supplementary Figures 3F,G**). Absolute numbers of these parameters were investigated and did not show any differences between AM and control chickens, although an increase in numbers of both treatments was observed with age (**Supplementary Figure 5**).

Association Between Caecal Microbiota Clusters and Immune Cells

Clustering of the caecal content profiles suggests that AM chickens showed an earlier maturation of caecal microbiota profiles compared to controls. Also, differences in IL-2Rα$^+$ NK cells, NK cell activation and CD8αα T cells were observed between AM chickens compared to the controls. To assess a possible relationship between the observed differences in the microbial development between treatments and the detected differences in immune parameters, we used the previously identified DMM clusters to test for correlations between the caecal microbiota profiles (i.e., stages of successive microbiota maturation) and immune parameters.

Clusters A, B, and C were based on relative abundance of genera present in the caecal microbiota of chickens and represent different stages during the early life development of caecal microbiota. Correlations to relative and absolute numbers of IL-2Rα$^+$, 20E5$^+$, CD107$^+$ NK cells, and cytotoxic CD8aa$^+$ T cells in the ileum were investigated. The percentage of intestinal IL-2Rα$^+$ NK cells was higher in cluster B compared to cluster A (p = 0.026, **Table 2**), and compared to cluster C (p = 0.044, **Table 2**) regardless of treatment (**Figure 6A**). The percentage of IL-2Rα$^+$ NK cells in cluster C tended to be higher compared to cluster A, but this was not significant (p = 0.068, **Table 2**, **Figure 6A**). Relative numbers of intestinal 20E5$^+$ NK cells were similar between clusters A and B and highest in cluster C (**Figure 6B, Table 2**). Relative numbers of intestinal CD107$^+$ NK cells were highest in cluster C and lowest in cluster A (**Table 2, Figure 6C**). Within cluster C, the percentage of CD107$^+$ NK cells tended to be higher in AM chickens (**Figure 6C**). Relative numbers for intestinal cytotoxic CD8αα$^+$ T cells were higher in cluster B and C compared to cluster A and did not differ between cluster B and C (**Figure 6D, Table 2**). Similar correlations were observed between clusters and absolute numbers of intestinal 20E5$^+$, CD107$^+$ NK cells and cytotoxic CD8αα$^+$ T cells (**Table 2**).

These results indicate significant associations between caecal microbiota clusters and subsets of intestinal immune cells.

DISCUSSION

In this study, we aimed to induce an alteration in the intestinal microbiota shortly after hatch by administration of adult-derived

TABLE 1 | Relative abundance of genera present in the AM inoculum and differences in relative abundance in caecal content for AM compared to control chickens.

| Genera | Relative abundance AM inoculum | | Differences in relative abundance AM vs. control chickens | | | | | | | | | | | | | | | |
| | | | Day 1 | | | Day 3 | | | Day 7 | | | Day 14 | | | Day 21 | | |
	RA%	SD%	AM%	PBS%	P	AM%	PBS%	P	AM%	PBS%	P	AM%	PBS%	P	AM%	PBS%	P
Eubacterium coprostanoligenes group	0.65	0.22	-	-		0.06	-		-	-		0.84	1.12		0.71	0.65	
Bacteroides	0.47	0.06	-	-		3.91	-	**0.045**	2.57	-	**0.018**	2.01	1.12		3.01	3.57	
Blautia	0.30	0.09	9.17	-	**0.006**	5.86	3.92		4.67	16.63		4.35	13.14		6.10	10.68	
Candidatus_Soleaferrea	0.39	0.06	0.56	-	**0.006**	-	-		-	-		-	-		-	-	
Clostridium sensu stricto 1	2.77	0.45	24.32	53.93	**0.033**	1.96	22.30		-	0.19		-	-		0.03	-	
Clostridium sensu stricto 2	0.72	0.12	0.77	-	**0.006**	-	-		-	-		-	-		-	-	
Collinsella	0.53	0.07	0.68	-	**0.034**	4.65	-	**0.018**	3.64	1.04		1.54	4.30		3.60	2.02	
Enterococcus	10.80	1.07	10.12	17.64		16.19	18.55		0.86	0.87		0.32	0.36		0.43	0.48	
Erysipelatoclostridium	2.53	0.09	0.26	0.00		2.56	-	**0.027**	0.05	2.07	**0.018**	0.81	2.01		0.44	1.06	**0.043**
Escherichia-Shigella	0.57	0.02	32.73	3.36	**0.006**	0.72	11.07	**0.044**	0.16	0.73		-	0.03		-	-	
Eubacterium	0.66	0.04	0.30	-	**0.016**	0.46	0.11		0.92	0.28		0.15	0.19		0.07	0.12	
Flavonifractor	1.02	0.14	1.23	-	**0.006**	0.90	0.66		0.13	0.44		0.05	0.43	**0.010**	0.41	-	
Lachnoclostridium	9.78	0.93	2.30	-	**0.006**	3.28	-	**0.018**	0.77	0.85		0.66	0.72		0.41	0.16	
Lactobacillus	14.96	1.33	8.46	-		6.83	1.12		8.05	3.44		5.34	12.34		13.85	10.14	
Megamonas	1.55	0.56	0.02	-		4.05	-		30.21	-	**0.018**	27.46	-	**0.009**	7.46	-	**0.022**
Megasphaera	3.30	0.74	-	-		-	-		-	-		-	-		-	-	
Negativicoccus	3.62	0.66	-	-		-	-		-	-		-	-		-	-	
Oscillibacter	1.94	0.18	-	-		-	-		-	-		-	-		-	-	
Peptostreptococcus	30.97	4.04	0.19	-	**0.034**	-	-		-	-		▪	-		-	-	
Sellimonas	1.31	0.38	-	-		-	-		0.31	0.75		0.60	0.84		0.50	0.88	
Slackia	0.34	0.09	0.02	-		0.03	-		0.43	-	**0.037**	0.01	0.05		0.08	0.10	
Sutterella	1.76	0.21	-	-		-	-		-	-		-	-		-	-	
Uncultured	4.45	3.56	0.00	0.00		1.40	0.27		1.07	2.15		1.37	1.96		1.11	1.48	
unknown	0.08	0.09	-	-		-	-		-	-		-	-		-	-	

The AM inoculum contained 24 different genera and the genera for which significant differences in relative abundance of AM inoculated chickens (AM) vs. controls (PBS) were found for day 1, 3, 7, 14, and 21 are indicated in bold (n = 8). No differences were observed between treatments on day 35. Results are based on differences of relative abundance tested with Wilcoxon rank-sum test. P = adjusted p-values (<0.05) were corrected for multiple testing with Benjamini-Hochberg (BH). - = not detected. RA = Relative abundance (%) in the AM inoculum. AM/PBS = Relative abundance (%) in AM/control treatment.

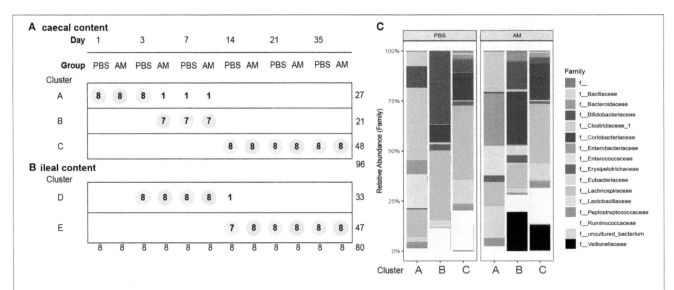

FIGURE 3 | Dirichlet multinomial mixtures (DMM) clustering of 16S rRNA gene sequencing data for caecal and ileal microbial profiles. **(A)** DMM clustering showed the best model fit for three clusters in the caecal content profiles (lowest Laplace approximation, n = 96). Cluster A contains 27 samples, Cluster B 21 samples, and the remaining 48 samples are in cluster C. Cluster B contains 3-day old AM chickens, and seven of eight AM and all control chickens of day 7, indicating acceleration of microbiota maturation in the caecal content. Nodes are colored according to intervention (AM or PBS) and ordered according to age. **(B)** In the ileal content samples two distinct clusters were observed, but no evidence for acceleration of the development of the microbiota (n = 80). **(C)** Relative microbial abundance of the clusters observed in the caecal content stratified by the intervention at family level.

microbiota, and compared presence and function of NK cells, as representatives of developing innate immunity, to those of non-inoculated controls. We hypothesized that early exposure to adult-derived microbiota would accelerate intestinal microbiota colonization and affect subsets and activation of intestinal NK cells. Our results indicate that the inoculation with the adult-derived microbes mostly affected the early development of the caecal microbiota, and induced an earlier maturation of caecal microbiota compared to control broiler chickens. This development was paralleled by an increase in intestinal IL-2Rα⁺ NK cells and enhanced activation of NK cells early in life and CD8αα⁺ T cells later in life.

The AM inoculation delivered immediately after hatch successfully altered intestinal microbiota composition, especially in the 1st week of life, but did not permanently influence the diversity of caecal microbiota. In addition, with respect to the genera found in the AM product, a higher relative abundance was only found shortly after inoculation. More specifically, a higher relative abundance in AM chickens was found for 10 of the 24 genera in the inoculum on day 1, but this quickly declined to two genera by the end of the 1st week. These findings are in line with previous studies with the same product: inoculation with Aviguard *in ovo* enhanced development of intestinal microbiota of broiler chickens and increased diversity and reduced the abundance of *Enterobacteriaceae* (22). Similar to our study, not all genera present in the inoculum permanently colonized the intestine; they were assumed to have been transient colonizers facilitating the development of a complex microbiota by temporarily altering the microenvironment (22). Similar observations have been reported for 1-day-old laying hens

inoculated with Aviguard. Not all bacteria of the product, nor of the mother hen, were effectively transferred to the chickens' gut, but compared to controls, caecal microbiota enriched for the phyla *Bacteroidetes* and *Actinobacteria* was observed within a week in both Aviguard treated chickens and in chickens naturally exposed to a mother hen (55).

Like chickens hatched in commercial hatcheries, the control chickens in our study were gradually exposed to microbiota in the hours and days after hatch from different sources, such as the housing environment, litter, feed, and water. This colonization was delayed compared to the chickens inoculated with AM directly after hatch, as indicated by the clustering of caecal content profiles of 3-day-old controls with 1-day-old AM inoculated chickens, and of 7-day-old controls with 3-day-old AM chickens. This accelerated maturation of caecal microbiota composition has not only been observed in Aviguard studies (22, 55), but also in a study in which topical spray treatment of eggs with adult caecal content significantly altered broiler chicken microbiota immediately after hatch, and accelerated the normal microbiota development (69). As in our study, the effect on the caecal microbiota was highest at 3 days of age, and diminished over time (69). In contrast, swabbing of the egg surface once during incubation with diluted adult caecal content did not lead to significant differences in alpha diversity nor in the pattern of bacterial colonization between treated and control broiler chickens (70). This difference may be a result of the egg inoculation technique, suggesting that perhaps a lower number of spores and vegetative cells was applied to the eggshell in the latter study.

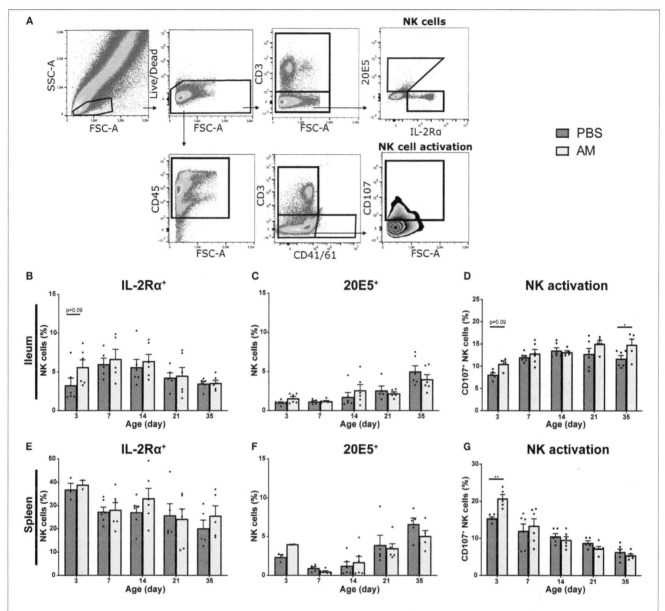

FIGURE 4 | Effect of adult microbiota (AM) on NK cells in broiler chickens. **(A)** Gating strategy after isolation of lymphocytes from IEL to analyze NK cell subsets and activation. **(B,E)** Percentages of NK cell subsets by characterization of surface markers IL-2Rα, **(C,F)** 20E5 during aging in **(B–D)** IEL and **(E–G)** spleen. **(D,G)** Percentages of NK cell activation during aging as assessed by measuring the surface marker CD107. Mean + SEM of chickens is shown ($n = 6$), however, chickens were excluded from analysis when numbers of events acquired in the gate of interest were < 100. Statistical significance is indicated as *$p < 0.05$ and **$p < 0.01$.

Although many of the available poultry microbiota studies have focused on broiler chickens, its relation with the innate immune system has not previously been elaborately investigated. We observed an increase in IL-2Rα+ NK cells and activation of NK cells within the 1st days of life, together with an increase in relative numbers of cytotoxic CD8αα+ T cells from day 14 onwards in chickens that were inoculated with AM.

The increased NK cell activation observed in AM chickens may suggest a mildly increased cytotoxic capacity against potential pathogens, as the CD107 expression can increase up to 30% upon viral infections (33), which is more than 2-fold higher than the NK cell activation observed in this study. This result is in line with the observed increase in IL-2Rα+ NK cells in this study. Studies in humans have shown that increased IL-2Rα expression is associated with an early stage of NK cell activation (31), and this was also observed in chickens (32, 71, 72). In addition to the local effect on NK cell activation, our observation of increased splenic NK cell activation in 3-day-old AM chickens also indicates there is a systemic effect. No

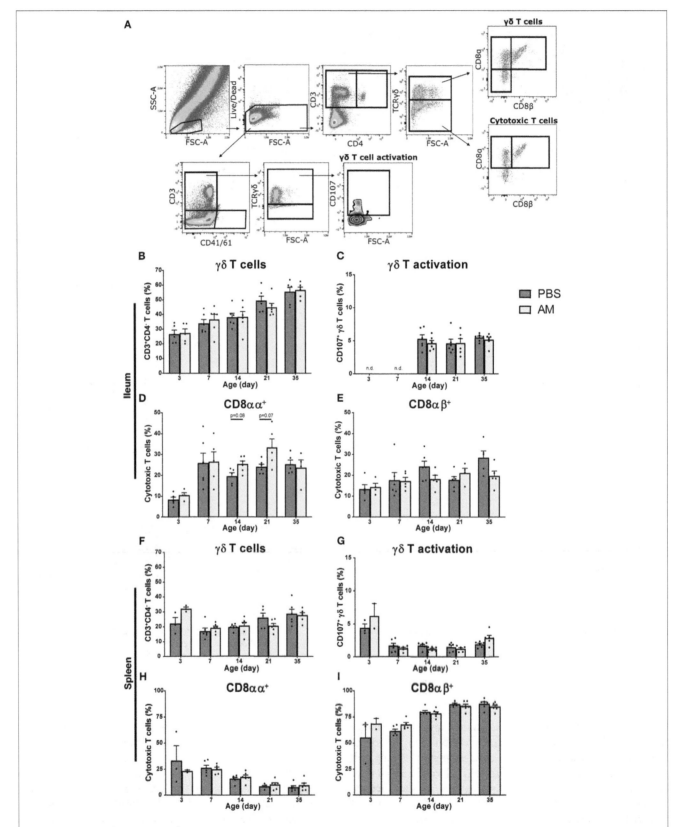

FIGURE 5 | Effect of adult microbiota (AM) on T cells in broiler chickens. **(A)** Gating strategy after isolation of lymphocytes from IEL to analyze T cell subsets and γδ T cell activation. **(B,F)** Percentages of total γδ T cells, subsets (data not shown) and **(C,G)** γδ T cell activation by characterization of surface markers TCRγδ and CD107

(Continued)

FIGURE 5 | during aging in **(B–E)** IEL and **(F–I)** spleen. **(D,H)** Percentages of cytotoxic T cell subsets using the surface markers CD8αα and **(E,I)** CD8αβ during aging. Mean + SEM of chickens is shown ($n = 6$), however, chickens were excluded from analysis when numbers of events acquired in the gate of interest were <100.

TABLE 2 | Statistical differences in relative (%) and absolute (cells/mg) numbers of intestinal immune cells between caecal microbiota clusters.

Immune cells	Cluster A vs. B	Cluster B vs. C	Cluster A vs. C
IL-2Rα$^+$ NK (%)	**0.026**	**0.044**	0.068
20E5$^+$ NK (%)	0.124	**3.0e^{-4}**	**0.001**
CD107$^+$ NK (%)	**0.003**	**0.020**	**0.001**
CD8αα$^+$ T (%)	**0.001**	0.254	**4.1e^{-4}**
IL-2Rα$^+$ NK (cells/mg)	**0.011**	0.051	**2.7e^{-4}**
20E5$^+$ NK (cells/mg)	**0.039**	**5.3e^{-7}**	**2.1e^{-6}**
CD107$^+$ NK (cells/mg)	0.398	**4.0e^{-6}**	**1.1e^{-4}**
CD8αα$^+$ T (cells/mg)	**0.008**	**9.5e^{-6}**	**6.4e^{-4}**

Significant differences are indicated in bold.

effects of AM inoculation on immune cells in the blood were observed.

The observed differences between AM and control chickens with respect to immune parameters suggest an interaction between microbial and immune development. This was further substantiated by the significant associations between IL-2Rα$^+$ NK cells, CD107$^+$ NK, and CD8αα$^+$ T cells and caecal microbiota clusters: cluster A includes chickens with a starting microbiota, cluster B chickens in the middle of the maturation process and cluster C chickens with a more matured successive microbiota composition from day 14 onwards. These clusters follow the successional patterns of microbiota development as previously described for broiler chickens, with bacterial community richness increasing rapidly over time and stabilizing from day 14 onwards (5–7). Our analyses showed that cluster B was associated with an increase in IL-2Rα$^+$ NK cells and an enhanced NK cell activation regardless of treatment. This suggests that the accelerated microbiota colonization due to AM inoculation affected the development of NK cells locally and systemically. Interestingly, the IL-2Rα$^+$ NK cell subset was higher in relative numbers in cluster B compared to the starting microbiota cluster A, but subsequently decreased in relative numbers in the more mature microbiota cluster C. The 20E5$^+$ NK cell subset and NK cells that express CD107 further increased in relative numbers between cluster B and cluster C. This fits with the observation in mammals that an increase in IL-2Rα expression is associated with an early stage of NK cell activation, which is followed by enhanced NK cell mediated killing. Cluster C was associated with an increased relative number of intestinal cytotoxic CD8αα$^+$ T cells. As the caecal microbiota in this cluster shows a matured composition similar in AM and control chickens of the same age, this suggests that early life inoculation with AM also affected the adaptive immune development in the intestine.

Although these results indicate associations between early life microbiota colonization and immune system development, the data from this study cannot elucidate exactly how these processes are related. As has been shown in humans and mice, microbiota can signal to immune cells in various ways either locally or systemically (46, 73). Locally, microorganisms interact directly with NK cells via TLRs and NCRs resulting in cytokine production by NK cells, and indirectly via cytokine production of resident myeloid or epithelial cells that consequently affect NK cell responses (46, 74). Systemically, microbiota can induce instructive signals to non-mucosal antigen-presenting cells and by producing among others IL-15, TNFα and IFN, subsequently prime optimal splenic NK cell responses (73). Since chicken NK cells have been shown to express TLRs (75) and NCRs (76, 77), the interactions between microbiota and NK cells probably follow similar routes to those in humans and mice.

In mammals, specific commensal bacterial strains have been linked to modulation of NK cells. Several reports established that bacteria within the *Lactobacillus* genus can induce IFNγ and cytotoxicity responses in intestinal NK cells as a result of IL-12 production by dendritic cells after TLR engagement with bacteria (43, 78, 79). Furthermore, *Bacteroides fragilis* can stimulate innate and adaptive immune pathways directly through TLR signaling and indirectly by inducing cytokine production (80). Although we did observe significant differences in the relative abundance of genera between AM and control chickens at day 1 and 3, we cannot pinpoint a specific genus responsible for the observed effect on NK cells. Interestingly, the genus *Bacteroides* showed a significantly higher prevalence and relative abundance in 3- and 7-day-old AM chickens and the genus was absent in control chickens of similar age. This could suggest that the observed effects on NK cells in 3-day-old AM chickens may be linked to a higher presence of *Bacteroides* bacteria as shown previously (80). We did not find differences in the prevalence of *Lactobacillus* bacteria due to AM inoculation. Other genera that showed significant differences in their prevalence and/or relative abundance between AM and control chickens at 1 and 3 days of age have not been described as specifically interacting with NK cells.

In addition, microbiota has been shown in mice and humans to interact directly with γδ T cells, and increased frequencies of CD8$^+$ γδ T cells and γδ T cell activation were observed during intestinal inflammation (51, 81). Under non-inflammatory conditions similar to those of our study, application of adult caecal content on eggs altered and accelerated the microbiota of 3-day-old chickens but did not affect γδ T cells in caecal tonsils (69). Furthermore, AM inoculated chickens in our study showed an increased presence of intestinal CD8αα$^+$ T cells at 2 and 3 weeks of age. Although in previous studies with mice no CD8αα and CD8αβ subsets were investigated, microbiota was shown to have direct (53) and indirect (82) effects on cytotoxic T cells, as IFNγ production was induced.

Further research including challenge models is needed to answer the question if chickens with an accelerated maturation of intestinal microbiota and enhanced NK cell responses early in life are indeed more resilient against infections.

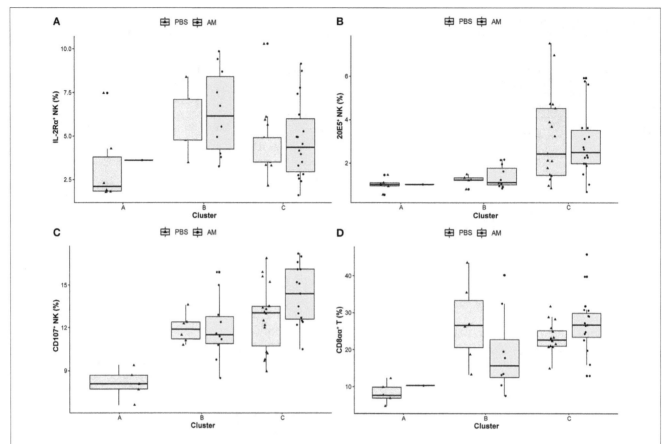

FIGURE 6 | Associations between caecal microbiota clusters and immune cells. Associations between the identified DMM clusters of caecal microbiota composition and relative numbers of intestinal NK cell subsets **(A)** IL-2Rα+, **(B)** 20E5+, **(C)** CD107+, and **(D)** cytotoxic CD8αα+ T cells were analyzed using Wilcoxon rank-sum test. Adjusted p-values (<0.05) were corrected for multiple testing with BH.

Interestingly we observed a relation between changes in caecal microbiota and intestinal NK cell responses. It would have been highly interesting to investigate the interaction between immune system and microbiota at caecum level, but unfortunatelythis was not possible since only few NK cells can be obtained from the caecum in young chickens (83, 84).

Although we set out to analyze the relation between NK cells and microbiota composition in the ileum, we did not observe differences between treatment groups at any age in the phylogenetic diversity of ileal microbiota nor in the relative abundances of genera. Not being able to show a difference at ileal level, especially considering the relatively small number of chickens at each time point, was not surprising, and exactly the reason why we also collected caecal content. Nevertheless, the shift in microbiota composition as measured in the caeca showed that the AM treatment has successfully affected microbiota development in parts of the intestinal tract. For the AM treatment to be able to alter caecal microbiota composition, the microbiota of the AM product at least must have passed, and to some extent may have colonized upstream parts of the intestinal tract as well, albeit not inducing a measurable shift in microbiota composition in ileum. Therefore,

we expect that the observed effects on ileal NK cells are associated with the AM treatment.

In conclusion, our study showed a relation between an accelerated maturation of intestinal microbiota and the enhanced NK cell response early in life.

This interaction between microbiota and the developing innate immune system indicates possibilities in developing strategies to improve health and resilience of broiler chickens. One such possibility is through feed interventions or the use of products with adult-derived microbiota directly after hatch, both of which can affect microbiota composition and may accelerate microbiota maturation. Consequently, this can strengthen the innate immune system, conferring direct protective effects early in life as well as influencing adaptive immunity later in life.

The combination of a well-developed microbiota and immune system may result in more robust broiler chickens with higher resilience against health challenges, such as disturbances in gut health and invading pathogens. Future research including challenge studies are warranted to test this hypothesis.

AUTHOR CONTRIBUTIONS

NM, JK, FV, DL, JO, HS, JS, VR, and CJ contributed to the conception, design of the study, drafting, and critically revising it for important intellectual content. NM, JK, FV, DH, and CJ contributed to acquisition of data. NM and JK performed the analysis of data. FV and CJ supervised the work. All authors approved the final version to be submitted.

ACKNOWLEDGMENTS

We thanked the animal caretakers of the department Population Health Sciences, division Farm Animal Health, Faculty of Veterinary Medicine, Utrecht University, for their help during the animal experiments. We acknowledged R. H. G. A. van den Biggelaar and I. S. Ludwig for their help during the isolation of immune cells. We acknowledged G. J. A. Arkesteijn for maintaining optimal working conditions of the Flow Cytometry and Cell Sorting Facility, Faculty of Veterinary Medicine, Utrecht University. We thanked M. van Gaal and I. Heikamp-de Jong (Laboratory of Microbiology, Wageningen University & Research) for their help with molecular analyses of microbial composition.

REFERENCES

1. OECD/FAO. *OECD-FAO Agricultural Outlook 2019-2028*. Rome: OECD Publishing; Paris/Food and Agriculture Organization of the United Nations (2019). doi: 10.1787/agr_outlook-2019-en

2. Skunca D, Tomasevic I, Nastasijevic I, Tomovic V, Djekic I. Life cycle assessment of the chicken meat chain. *J Clean Prod*. (2018) 184:440–50. doi: 10.1016/j.jclepro.2018.02.274

3. Kogut MH. The effect of microbiome modulation on the intestinal health of poultry. *Anim Feed Sci Technol*. (2019) 250:32–40. doi: 10.1016/j.anifeedsci.2018.10.008

4. Pedroso AA, Lee MD. The composition and role of the microbiota in chickens. In: Niewold T, editor. *Intestinal Health*. Wageningen: Wageningen Academic Publishers (2015). p. 21–50. doi: 10.3920/978-90-8686-792-9_2

5. Cressman MD, Yu Z, Nelson MC, Moeller SJ, Lilburn MS, Zerby HN. Interrelations between the microbiotas in the litter and in the intestines of commercial broiler chickens. *Appl Environ Microbiol*. (2010) 76:6572–82. doi: 10.1128/AEM.00180-10

6. Oakley BB, Kogut MH. Spatial and temporal changes in the broiler chicken cecal and fecal microbiomes and correlations of bacterial taxa with cytokine gene expression. *Front Vet Sci*. (2016) 3:11. doi: 10.3389/fvets.2016.00011

7. Jurburg SD, Brouwer MSM, Ceccarelli D, van der Goot J, Jansman AJM, Bossers A. Patterns of community assembly in the developing chicken microbiome reveal rapid primary succession. *MicrobiologyOpen*. (2019) 8:e00821. doi: 10.1002/mbo3.821

8. Dominguez-Bello M, Costello EK, Contreras M, Magris M, Hidalgo G, Fierer N, et al. Delivery mode shapes the acquisition and structure of the initial microbiota across multiple body habitats in newborns. *Proc Natl Acad Sci USA*. (2010) 107:11971–5. doi: 10.1073/pnas.1002601107

9. Borewicz K, Suarez-Diez M, Hechler C, Beijers R, de Weerth C, Arts I, et al. The effect of prebiotic fortified infant formulas on microbiota composition and dynamics in early life. *Sci Rep*. (2019) 9:2434. doi: 10.1038/s41598-018-38268-x

10. Borewicz K, Gu F, Saccenti E, Hechler C, Beijers R, de Weerth C, et al. The association between breastmilk oligosaccharides and faecal microbiota in healthy breastfed infants at two, six, and twelve weeks of age. *Sci Rep*. (2020) 10:4270. doi: 10.1038/s41598-020-61024-z

11. Coloe PJ, Bagust TJ, Ireland L. Development of the normal gastrointestinal microflora of specific pathogen-free chickens. *J Hyg*. (1984) 92:79–87. doi: 10.1017/S0022172400064056

12. Inman CF, Haverson K, Konstantinov SR, Jones PH, Harris C, Smidt H, et al. Rearing environment affects development of the immune system in neonates. *Clin Exp Immunol*. (2010) 160:431–9. doi: 10.1111/j.1365-2249.2010.04090.x

13. Mulder IE, Schmidt B, Lewis M, Delday M, Stokes CR, Bailey M, et al. Restricting microbial exposure in early life negates the immune benefits associated with gut colonization in environments of high microbial diversity. *PLoS ONE*. (2011) 6:e28279. doi: 10.1371/journal.pone.0028279

14. Schokker D, Jansman AJM, Veninga G, de Bruin N, Vastenhouw SA, de Bree FM, et al. Perturbation of microbiota in one-day old broiler chickens with antibiotic for 24 hours negatively affects intestinal immune development. *BMC Genomics*. (2017) 18:241. doi: 10.1186/s12864-017-3625-6

15. Xi Y, Shuling N, Kunyuan T, Qiuyang Z, Hewen D, ChenCheng G, et al. Characteristics of the intestinal flora of specific pathogen free chickens with age. *Microb Pathog*. (2019) 132:325–34. doi: 10.1016/j.micpath.2019.05.014

16. Ballou AL, Ali RA, Mendoza MA, Ellis JC, Hassan HM, Croom WJ, et al. Development of the chick microbiome: how early exposure influences future microbial diversity. *Front Vet Sci*. (2016) 3:2. doi: 10.3389/fvets.2016.00002

17. Polansky O, Sekelova Z, Faldynova M, Sebkova A, Sisak F, Rychlik I. Important metabolic pathways and biological processes expressed by chicken cecal microbiota. *Appl Environ Microbiol*. (2016) 82:1569–76. doi: 10.1128/AEM.03473-15

18. Volf J, Polansky O, Varmuzova K, Gerzova L, Sekelova Z, Faldynova M, et al. Transient and prolonged response of chicken cecum mucosa to colonization with different gut microbiota. *PLoS ONE*. (2016) 11:e0163932. doi: 10.1371/journal.pone.0163932

19. Mead GC. Prospects for 'Competitive exclusion' treatment to control salmonellas and other foodborne pathogens in poultry. *Vet J*. (2000) 159:111–23. doi: 10.1053/tvjl.1999.0423

20. Crhanova M, Hradecka H, Faldynova M, Matulova M, Havlickova H, Sisak F, et al. Immune response of chicken gut to natural colonization by gut microflora and to Salmonella enterica serovar enteritidis infection. *Infect Immun*. (2011) 79:2755–63. doi: 10.1128/IAI.01375-10

21. Yin Y, Lei F, Zhu L, Li S, Wu Z, Zhang R, et al. Exposure of different bacterial inocula to newborn chicken affects gut microbiota development and ileum gene expression. *ISME J*. (2010) 4:367–76. doi: 10.1038/ismej.2009.128

22. Pedroso AA, Batal AB, Lee MD. Effect of in ovo administration of an adult-derived microbiota on establishment of the intestinal microbiome in chickens. *Am J Vet Res*. (2016) 77:514–26. doi: 10.2460/ajvr.77.5.514

23. Kerr AK, Farrar AM, Waddell LA, Wilkins W, Wilhelm BJ, Bucher O, et al. A systematic review-meta-analysis and meta-regression on the effect of selected competitive exclusion products on *Salmonella* spp. prevalence and concentration in broiler chickens. *Prev Vet Med*. (2013) 111:112–25. doi: 10.1016/j.prevetmed.2013.04.005

24. Ceccarelli D, van Essen-Zandbergen A, Smid B, Veldman KT, Boender GJ, Fischer EAJ, et al. Competitive exclusion reduces transmission and excretion of extended-spectrum-β-lactamase-producing *Escherichia coli* in broilers. *Appl Environ Microbiol*. (2017) 83:e03439-16. doi: 10.1128/AEM.03439-16

25. Uni Z, Smirnov A, Sklan D. Pre- and posthatch development of goblet cells in the broiler small intestine: effect of delayed access to feed. *Poult Sci*. (2003) 82:320–7. doi: 10.1093/ps/82.2.320

26. Göbel TWF, Kaspers B, Stangassinger M. NK and T cells constitute two major, functionally distinct intestinal epithelial lymphocyte subsets in the chicken. *Int Immunol*. (2001) 13:757–62. doi: 10.1093/intimm/13.6.757

27. Klasing KC, Leshchinsky TV. Functions, costs, and benefits of the immune system during development and growth. In: Adams NJ, Slotow RH, editors. *Proceedings of the 22nd International Ornithological Congress*. Durban (1999). p. 2817–35. Johannesburg: BirdLife South Africa.

28. Sharma JM, Tizard I. Avian cellular immune effector mechanisms - a review. *Avian Pathol.* (1984) 13:357–76. doi: 10.1080/03079458408418541

29. Jansen CA, van de Haar PM, van Haarlem D, van Kooten P, de Wit S, van Eden W, et al. Identification of new populations of chicken natural killer (NK) cells. *Dev Comp Immunol.* (2010) 34:759–67. doi: 10.1016/j.dci.2010.02.009

30. Jansen CA, De Geus ED, Van Haarlem DA, Van De Haar PM, Löndt BZ, Graham SP, et al. Differential lung NK cell responses in avian influenza virus infected chickens correlate with pathogenicity. *Sci Rep.* (2013) 3:2478. doi: 10.1038/srep02478

31. Leong JW, Chase JM, Romee R, Schneider SE, Sullivan RP, Cooper MA, et al. Preactivation with IL-12, IL-15, and IL-18 induces cd25 and a functional high-affinity il-2 receptor on human cytokine-induced memory-like natural killer cells. *Biol Blood Marrow Transplant.* (2014) 20:463–73. doi: 10.1016/j.bbmt.2014.01.006

32. Meijerink N, van Haarlem DA, Velkers FC, Stegeman AJ, Rutten VPMG, Jansen CA. Analysis of chicken intestinal natural killer cells, a major IEL subset during embryonic and early life. *Dev Comp Immunol.* (2020) 114:103857. doi: 10.1016/j.dci.2020.103857

33. Vervelde L, Matthijs MGR, van Haarlem DA, de Wit JJ, Jansen CA. Rapid NK-cell activation in chicken after infection with infectious bronchitis virus M41. *Vet Immunol Immunopathol.* (2013) 151:337–41. doi: 10.1016/j.vetimm.2012.11.012

34. Bertzbach LD, van Haarlem DA, Härtle S, Kaufer BB, Jansen CA. Marek's disease virus infection of natural killer cells. *Microorg.* (2019) 7:588. doi: 10.3390/microorganisms7120588

35. Round JL, Mazmanian SK. The gut microbiota shapes intestinal immune responses during health and disease. *Nat Rev Immunol.* (2009) 9:313–23. doi: 10.1038/nri2515

36. Hooper LV, Littman DR, Macpherson AJ. Interactions between the microbiota and the immune system. *Science.* (2012) 336:1268–73. doi: 10.1126/science.1223490

37. Macpherson AJ, Harris NL. Interactions between commensal intestinal bacteria and the immune system. *Nat Rev Immunol.* (2004) 4:478–85. doi: 10.1038/nri1373

38. Rooks MG, Garrett WS. Gut microbiota, metabolites and host immunity. *Nat Rev Immunol.* (2016) 16:341–52. doi: 10.1038/nri.2016.42

39. Broom LJ, Kogut MH. The role of the gut microbiome in shaping the immune system of chickens. *Vet Immunol Immunopathol.* (2018) 204:44–51. doi: 10.1016/j.vetimm.2018.10.002

40. van der Eijk JAJ, Rodenburg TB, de Vries H, Kjaer JB, Smidt H, Naguib M, et al. Early-life microbiota transplantation affects behavioural responses, serotonin and immune characteristics in chicken lines divergently selected on feather pecking. *Sci Rep.* (2020) 10:2750. doi: 10.1038/s41598-020-59125-w

41. Metzler-Zebeli BU, Siegerstetter S, Magowan E, Lawlor PG, O'Connell NE, Zebeli Q. Fecal microbiota transplant from highly feed efficient donors affects cecal physiology and microbiota in low- And high-feed efficient chickens. *Front Microbiol.* (2019) 10:1576. doi: 10.3389/fmicb.2019.01576

42. Butler VL, Mowbray CA, Cadwell K, Niranji SS, Bailey R, Watson KA, et al. Effects of rearing environment on the gut antimicrobial responses of two broiler chicken lines. *Vet Immunol Immunopathol.* (2016) 178:29–36. doi: 10.1016/j.vetimm.2016.06.004

43. Aziz N, Bonavida B. Activation of natural killer cells by probiotics. *Forum Immunopathol Dis Ther.* (2016) 7:41–55. doi: 10.1615/ForumImmunDisTher.2016017095

44. Carrillo-Bustamante P, Kesmir C, de Boer RJ. The evolution of natural killer cell receptors. *Immunogenetics.* (2016) 68:3–18. doi: 10.1007/s00251-015-0869-7

45. Temperley ND, Berlin S, Paton IR, Griffin DK, Burt DW. Evolution of the chicken Toll-like receptor gene family: a story of gene gain and gene loss. *BMC Genomics.* (2008) 9:62. doi: 10.1186/1471-2164-9-62

46. Sonnenberg G, Artis D. Innate lymphoid cell interactions with microbiota: implications for intestinal health and disease. *Immunity.* (2012) 37:601–10. doi: 10.1016/j.immuni.2012.10.003

47. Yitbarek A, Astill J, Hodgins DC, Parkinson J, Nagy É, Sharif S. Commensal gut microbiota can modulate adaptive immune responses in chickens vaccinated with whole inactivated avian influenza virus subtype H9N2. *Vaccine.* (2019) 37:6640–7. doi: 10.1016/j.vaccine.2019.09.046

48. Siwek M, Slawinska A, Stadnicka K, Bogucka J, Dunislawska A, Bednarczyk M. Prebiotics and synbiotics - *In ovo* delivery for improved lifespan condition in chicken. *BMC Vet Res.* (2018) 14:402. doi: 10.1186/s12917-018-1738-z

49. Gao P, Ma C, Sun Z, Wang L, Huang S, Su X, et al. Feed-additive probiotics accelerate yet antibiotics delay intestinal microbiota maturation in broiler chicken. *Microbiome.* (2017) 5:91. doi: 10.1186/s40168-017-0315-1

50. Brisbin JT, Parvizi P, Sharif S. Differential cytokine expression in T-cell subsets of chicken caecal tonsils co-cultured with three species of *Lactobacillus*. *Benefic Microbes.* (2012) 3:205–10. doi: 10.3920/BM2012.0014

51. Nielsen MM, Witherden DA, Havran WL. γδ T cells in homeostasis and host defence of epithelial barrier tissues. *Nat Rev Immunol.* (2017) 17:733–45. doi: 10.1038/nri.2017.101

52. Yang Y, Xu C, Wu D, Wang Z, Wu P, Li L, et al. γδ T cells: crosstalk between microbiota, chronic inflammation, and colorectal cancer. *Front Immunol.* (2018) 9:1483. doi: 10.3389/fimmu.2018.01483

53. Tanoue T, Morita S, Plichta DR, Skelly AN, Suda W, Sugiura Y, et al. A defined commensal consortium elicits CD8 T cells and anti-cancer immunity. *Nature.* (2019) 565:600–5. doi: 10.1038/s41586-019-0878-z

54. De Geus ED, Jansen CA, Vervelde L. Uptake of particulate antigens in a nonmammalian lung: phenotypic and functional characterization of avian respiratory phagocytes using bacterial or viral antigens. *J Immunol.* (2012) 188:4516–26. doi: 10.4049/jimmunol.1200092

55. Kubasova T, Kollarcikova M, Crhanova M, Karasova D, Cejkova D, Sebkova A, et al. Contact with adult hen affects development of caecal microbiota in newly hatched chicks. *PLoS ONE.* (2019) 14:e0212446. doi: 10.1371/journal.pone.0212446

56. Kers JG, Velkers FC, Fischer EAJ, Hermes GDA, Lamot DM, Stegeman JA, et al. Take care of the environment: housing conditions affect the interplay of nutritional interventions and intestinal microbiota in broiler chickens. *Animal Microbiome.* (2019) 1:10. doi: 10.1186/s42523-019-0009-z

57. Verlaet A, van der Bolt N, Meijer B, Breynaert A, Naessens T, Konstanti P, et al. Toll-like receptor-dependent immunomodulatory activity of pycnogenol®. *Nutrients.* (2019) 11:214. doi: 10.3390/nu11020214

58. Ramiro-Garcia J, Hermes GDA, Giatsis C, Sipkema D, Zoetendal EG, Schaap PJ, et al. NG-Tax, a highly accurate and validated pipeline for analysis of 16S rRNA amplicons from complex biomes. *F1000 Res.* (2016) 5:1791. doi: 10.12688/f1000research.9227.1

59. Poncheewin W, Hermes GDA, van Dam JCJ, Koehorst JJ, Smidt H, Schaap PJ. NG-Tax 2.0: a semantic framework for high-throughput amplicon analysis. *Front Genet.* (2020) 10:1366. doi: 10.3389/fgene.2019.01366

60. Quast C, Pruesse E, Yilmaz P, Gerken J, Schweer T, Yarza P, et al. The SILVA ribosomal RNA gene database project: improved data processing and web-based tools. *Nucleic Acids Res.* (2013) 41:590. doi: 10.1093/nar/gks1219

61. McMurdie PJ, Holmes S. phyloseq: an R package for reproducible interactive analysis and graphics of microbiome census data. *PLoS ONE.* (2013) 8:e61217. doi: 10.1371/journal.pone.0061217

62. Lahti L, Shetty S, Blake T, Salojarvi J. *Tools for Microbiome Analysis in R. Version 1.5.28* (2017). Available online at: http://microbiome.github.com/microbiome

63. Oksanen J, Blanchet FG, Kindt R, Legendre P, O'hara R, Simpson GL, et al. *Vegan: community ecology package. R package version 1.17-4* (2010). Available online at: http://cran.r-project.org

64. Morgan M. *DirichletMultinomial: Dirichlet-Multinomial Mixture Model Machine Learning for Microbiome Data. R Package Version 1.28.0* (2019). Available online at: https://bioconductor.org/packages/DirichletMultinomial/

65. Faith DP. The role of the phylogenetic diversity measure, PD, in bio-informatics: getting the definition right. *Evol Bioinform Online.* (2006) 2:277–83. doi: 10.1177/117693430600200008

66. Lozupone CA, Hamady M, Kelley ST, Knight R. Quantitative and qualitative beta diversity measures lead to different insights into factors that structure microbial communities. *Appl Environ Microbiol.* (2007) 73:1576–85. doi: 10.1128/AEM.01996-06

67. Anderson MJ. A new method for non-parametric multivariate analysis of variance. *Austral Ecol.* (2001) 26:32–46. doi: 10.1046/j.1442-9993.2001.01070.x

68. Holmes I, Harris K, Quince C. Dirichlet multinomial mixtures: generative

models for microbial metagenomics. *PLoS ONE.* (2012) 7:e0030126. doi: 10.1371/journal.pone.0030126

69. Richards-Rios P, Leeming G, Fothergill J, Bernardeau M, Wigley P. Topical application of adult cecal contents to eggs transplants spore-forming microbiota but not other members of the microbiota to chicks. *Appl Environ Microbiol.* (2020) 86:e02387-19. doi: 10.1128/AEM.02387-19

70. Donaldson EE, Stanley D, Hughes RJ, Moore RJ. The time-course of broiler intestinal microbiota development after administration of cecal contents to incubating eggs. *PeerJ.* (2017) 5:e3587. doi: 10.7717/peerj.3587

71. Jahromi MZ, Bello MB, Abdolmaleki M, Yeap SK, Hair-Bejo M, Omar AR. Differential activation of intraepithelial lymphocyte-natural killer cells in chickens infected with very virulent and vaccine strains of infectious bursal disease virus. *Dev Comp Immunol.* (2018) 87:116–23. doi: 10.1016/j.dci.2018.06.004

72. Abdolmaleki M, Yeap SK, Tan SW, Satharasinghe DA, Bello MB, Jahromi MZ, et al. Effects of newcastle disease virus infection on chicken intestinal intraepithelial natural killer cells. *Front Immunol.* (2018) 9:1386. doi: 10.3389/fimmu.2018.01386

73. Ganal SC, Sanos SL, Kallfass C, Oberle K, Johner C, Kirschning C, et al. Priming of natural killer cells by nonmucosal mononuclear phagocytes requires instructive signals from commensal microbiota. *Immunity.* (2012) 37:171–86. doi: 10.1016/j.immuni.2012.05.020

74. Poggi A, Benelli R, Venè R, Costa D, Ferrari N, Tosetti F, et al. Human gut-associated natural killer cells in health and disease. *Front Immunol.* (2019) 10:961. doi: 10.3389/fimmu.2019.00961

75. Kannaki TR, Reddy MR, Shanmugam M, Verma PC, Sharma RP. Chicken toll-like receptors and their role in immunity. *World's Poult Sci J.* (2010) 66:727–38. doi: 10.1017/S0043933910000693

76. Straub C, Neulen M, Sperling B, Windau K, Zechmann M, Jansen CA, et al. Chicken NK cell receptors. *Dev Comp Immunol.* (2013) 41:324–33. doi: 10.1016/j.dci.2013.03.013

77. Jansen CA, Van Haarlem DA, Sperling B, Van Kooten PJ, De Vries E, Viertlboeck BC, et al. Identification of an activating chicken Ig-like receptor recognizing avian influenza viruses. *J Immunol.* (2016) 197:4696–703. doi: 10.4049/jimmunol.1600401

78. Fink LN, Zeuthen LH, Christensen HR, Morandi B, Frøkiær H, Ferlazzo G. Distinct gut-derived lactic acid bacteria elicit divergent dendritic cell-mediated NK cell responses. *Int Immunol.* (2007) 19:1319–27. doi: 10.1093/intimm/dxm103

79. Koizumi S, Wakita D, Sato T, Mitamura R, Izumo T, Shibata H, et al. Essential role of Toll-like receptors for dendritic cell and NK1.1+ cell-dependent activation of type 1 immunity by Lactobacillus pentosus strain S-PT84. *Immunol Lett.* (2008) 120:14–9. doi: 10.1016/j.imlet.2008.06.003

80. Troy EB, Kasper DL. Beneficial effects of Bacteroides fragilis polysaccharides on the immune system. *Front Biosci.* (2010) 15:25–34. doi: 10.2741/3603

81. Bhagat G, Naiyer AJ, Shah JG, Harper J, Jabri B, Wang TC, et al. Small intestinal CD8+TCRγδ+NKG2A + intraepithelial lymphocytes have attributes of regulatory cells in patients with celiac disease. *J Clin Invest.* (2008) 118:281–93. doi: 10.1172/JCI30989

82. Luu M, Weigand K, Wedi F, Breidenbend C, Leister H, Pautz S, et al. Regulation of the effector function of CD8+ T cells by gut microbiota-derived metabolite butyrate. *Sci Rep.* (2018) 8:14430. doi: 10.1038/s41598-018-32860-x

83. Chai J, Lillehoj HS. Isolation and functional characterization of chicken intestinal intra-epithelial lymphocytes showing natural killer cell activity against tumour target cells. *Immunology.* (1988) 63:111–7.

84. Gómez Del Moral M, Fonfría J, Varas A, Jiménez E, Moreno J, Zapata AG. Appearance and development of lymphoid cells in the chicken (Gallus gallus) caecal tonsil. *Anat Rec.* (1998) 250:182–9. doi: 10.1002/(SICI)1097-0185(199802)250:2<182::AID-AR8>3.0.CO;2-5

21

Epidemiology of Classical Swine Fever in Japan—A Descriptive Analysis of the Outbreaks in 2018–2019

Yumiko Shimizu, Yoko Hayama, Yoshinori Murato, Kotaro Sawai, Emi Yamaguchi and Takehisa Yamamoto*

Viral Disease and Epidemiology Research Division, National Institute of Animal Health, National Agriculture and Food Research Organization, Tsukuba, Japan

*Correspondence:
Takehisa Yamamoto
mtbook@affrc.go.jp

This study describes the epidemiological characteristics of classical swine fever (CSF) outbreaks in Japan. The first case was confirmed in September 2018, 26 years after the last known case. Outbreaks occurred on 39 farms, 34 commercial farms, and 5 non-commercial farms, between September 2018 and August 2019. In this study, a descriptive analysis was conducted of the epidemiological data on the characteristics of the affected farms, clinical manifestations, intra-farm transmission, association with infected wild boars, and control measures implemented on the farms. Twenty-eight of the 34 affected commercial farms were farrow-to-finish farms. It was assumed that the major risk factors were frequent human-pig interactions and the movement of pigs between farms. Fever and leukopenia were commonly observed in infected pigs. In 12 out of 18 farms where clinical manifestations among fattening pigs was the reason for notification, death was the most frequent clinical manifestation, but the proportion of dead animals did not exceed 0.5% of the total number of animals at most of the affected farms. Therefore, the clinical form of CSF in Japan was considered to be sub-acute. Twenty-three of the 29 farms (79%) with pigs at multiple stages (i.e., piglets, fattening pigs, and sows), had infection across the multiple stages. Many of these farms were within 5 km of the site where the first infected wild boars had been discovered, suggesting that infected wild boars were the source of infection. Infections still occurred at farms that had implemented measures at their farm boundaries to prevent the introduction of the virus into their farms, such as disinfection of vehicles and people, changing boots of the workers, and installation of perimeter fences. It is necessary to continue to strengthen biosecurity measures for farms located in areas with infected wild boars and to continue monitoring the distribution of infected wild boars so that any abnormalities can be reported and inspected at an early stage.

Keywords: classical swine fever (CSF), domestic pig (Sus scrofa), epidemiology, outbreak investigation, Japan

INTRODUCTION

Classical swine fever (CSF) is among the most devastating contagious diseases in pigs. Due to its impact on pig production, the prevention and control of the disease has been a major priority in pig producing countries. In Japan, 9.2 million heads of pigs are reared at about 4,300 farms as of 2019 and pork is produced mainly for domestic consumption (about 900,000 ton/year) and partially for export (about 2,000 ton/year). Although the export of pork is not a major industry in Japan, since the domestic demand for pork in Japan is increasing in recent years to more than 1.8 million ton/year, the protection of domestic pig industry from CSF and the maintenance of productivity is also a major issue.

The disease is caused by the CSF virus (CSFV), a single-stranded RNA virus of the *Pestivirus* genus of the *Flaviviridae* family. Pigs and wild boars are the virus hosts. Infected animals experience non-specific clinical symptoms due to immunosuppression (1, 2). Clinical forms of the disease vary depending on the virulence of the virus, age of host animals, hygiene management at the farm, and the presence of secondary infections; the clinical forms that have been seen in wild boars are similar to those in pigs (2). CSF can be divided into the following forms: acute, chronic, and persistent. The acute form is characterized by atypical clinical signs such as high fever, anorexia, gastrointestinal symptoms, general weakness, and conjunctivitis. This is followed by neurological signs and skin hemorrhages or cyanosis in different locations of the body 2 to 4 weeks after infection, known as the "typical" CSF signs. Animals with this form usually die 10 to 30 days after CSFV infection. In the chronic form, animals show various non-specific symptoms including fever, listlessness, loss of appetite, decreased growth, and death after 1 month from infection. The persistent form is observed in piglets infected as fetuses through vertical transmission (2). These piglets can become immunotolerant to the virus and can be a constant source of infection. They are able to constantly excrete the virus, even without any clinical symptoms, and are a dangerous virus reservoir until the late onset (2).

CSF outbreaks in pigs have been reported in Central and South America, Europe, Asia, and Africa. In the 1990s, large outbreaks occurred in the Netherlands, Germany, Belgium, and Italy but the disease has now been contained in these Western European countries. These countries are now officially recognized as CSF free, according to the World Organization for Animal Health (OIE) Terrestrial Code (3). Japan suffered from CSF since from the 1880s until the development of a live vaccine using the GPE-strain in the 1960s. The live vaccine was used since 1969, resulting in a sharp decline in the number of outbreaks to zero. The last reported case was recorded in 1992 (4). In 2000, the use of the live vaccine began being restricted before totally ceasing in 2006. Japan was officially recognized as CSF free in 2015, when the OIE began officially recognizing CSF disease status (5). This status was subsequently suspended in September 2018 due to the re-occurrence of CSF in central Japan.

On August 24, 2018, a fallow-to-finish pig farm in Gifu Prefecture, located in the central part of Japan, reported an increase in the number of dying animals to their local veterinary service. At the farm, clinical signs such as fever, loss of appetite, and abortion were more frequently observed prior to the deaths. The farm manager consulted the farm veterinarian, who considered the signs to be caused by heatstroke. On September 9, 2018, CSF viral infection was confirmed by laboratory tests conducted at the National Institute of Animal Health, National Agriculture and Food Research Organization (NIAH-NARO), after an absence of 26 years.

By January 2019, six more outbreaks had been reported near the first infected farm, in the southern area of Gifu Prefecture. In February 2019, the first outbreak in Aichi Prefecture was confirmed in Toyota City, located in the northern area of Aichi. The second outbreak in Aichi Prefecture was reported within the same month, in Tahara City, located in the southern peninsula, almost 47 km away from the infected farm in Toyota City. From March to June 2019, a total of 18 outbreaks had been reported in Gifu and Aichi. In July 2019, the first outbreak in Mie Prefecture and the first outbreak in Fukui Prefecture were reported. By August 2019, 39 outbreaks had been confirmed in Gifu, Aichi, Mie, and Fukui Prefectures (**Figures 1, 2**).

The virus strain causing the outbreaks in Japan from 2018 to 2020 was found to be the subgenotype 2.1d (6, 7). Subgenotype 2.1d was firstly isolated from the outbreaks in China in 2014 to 2015 (8) and is reported to cause a chronic or moderate form of infection (9–11). It has also been detected in South Korea (12, 13). A phylogenetic study showed that the CSF virus isolated from the 2018 Japan outbreak index case was different from the strains that had caused previous CSF-outbreaks in Japan (6). It has, therefore, been considered that the virus causing the 2018–2020 CSF outbreaks in Japan was newly introduced from the surrounding Asian countries, though the route of introduction or origin of the virus is unclear.

Control measures implemented to contain the CSF outbreaks were based on the Guideline to Control Classical Swine Fever (hereinafter referred to as "the Guideline." A specific national guideline and the last revised version was published on February 5, 2020 under the Act on Domestic Animal Infectious Disease Control of Japan.) (14). These measures included: stamping-out of all animals in the affected farms, control of movement of animals to a radius of 3 km of the affected farms, control of animal shipment in the area of 3 to 10 km from the affected farms, and disinfection of vehicles at control-points set-up at roads inside the movement control areas. All farms identified as having a relationship with the affected farms were investigated, and all animals confirmed to be infected with CSF virus at these farms were also stamped-out. Killed animals were buried at the affected farms or at burial sites near the affected farms, except for one epidemiologically related farm, whose animals were rendered for incineration due to unavailability of burial sites.

Active surveillance was implemented at farms and in wild boars. Surveillance at farms was implemented within the movement-control areas, within a 3 km radius of the affected farms. Clinical investigation, polymerase chain reaction (PCR), and enzyme-linked immunosorbent assay (ELISA) tests were conducted on blood samples of randomly-selected pigs from the affected farms within 24 h of confirmation of an infection. At

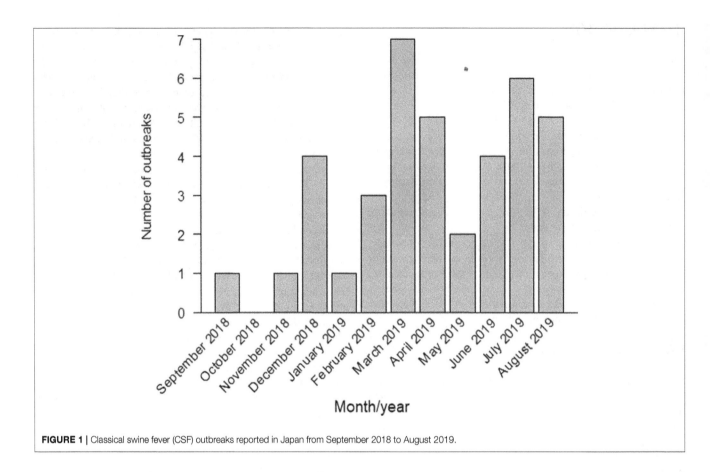

FIGURE 1 | Classical swine fever (CSF) outbreaks reported in Japan from September 2018 to August 2019.

least 30 animals were tested per farm to detect a prevalence of 10% with 95% confidence. When a farm had more than two pig houses, at least five animals per pig house were tested even when the total sample size exceeds 30. In these samplings, pigs with clinical symptoms were sampled with priority. The same set of tests was conducted to all farms present within the movement-control area from 17 days after the completion of all control measures at the affected farm. Shipment restrictions in the area of 3 to 10 km from the affected farms were lifted when all the farms within the movement-control area were confirmed to be CSF free by the second round of tests, while movement controls were lifted 28 days after the completion of all control measures on the affected farms.

A nationwide surveillance in wild boars had been implemented since 2006, after the cessation of the use of vaccine in pigs, and after the official recognition of CSF freedom in 2015, 273, and 389 wild boars were tested in 2016 and 2017, respectively with negative results. After the first pig case was confirmed at a pig farm in Gifu Prefecture in September 2018, intensive CSF surveillance in wild boars targeting the area within 10 km of the affected farm started according to the Guideline. As a result of the intensive surveillance, the first positive case of wild boar was found dead within 10 km of the farm with the first pig case. After the first case of wild boar, hunters captured wild boars within a 10 km radius of the sites where infected wild boars were found, in addition to the area around affected farms. The dead or captured wild boars in the surveillance areas were then tested

for CSF by local veterinary services. Additionally, all prefectures were requested to test dead wild boars found in their jurisdiction.

The vaccination of wild boars, using bait vaccine, started in March 2019 in Gifu Prefecture and in the adjacent prefectures with CSF-positive wild boars. By October 2019, given that the spread of the disease had not been controlled by improving biosecurity measures at farms, preventive vaccination at pig farms using the live CSF-vaccine began in Gifu and in the eight adjacent prefectures. By the end of December 2019, vaccination expanded to the additional 11 surrounding prefectures.

Descriptive epidemiological analyses provide an overview of the epidemic and shed light on the characteristics of the outbreaks, including the possible factors related to the occurrence of the disease. There are descriptive epidemiological studies on CSF outbreaks that have occurred in the Netherlands, Germany, and Belgium (15–18). These are all good references for countries needing to control the disease.

Regarding the epidemic of CSF caused by subgenotype 2.1d virus strain, the isolation of the virus has been reported (9–13), but the features of outbreaks caused by the specific subgenotype virus strain have not been fully described. As for the re-occurrence of CSF in Japan since 2018, there were studies describing genetic characteristic of the virus (6, 7), pathogenicity in experimental infection (19), and estimating the risk of infection from wild boars (20). However, an overall description of the outbreaks and analyses of clinical manifestations observed during outbreaks have not been reported.

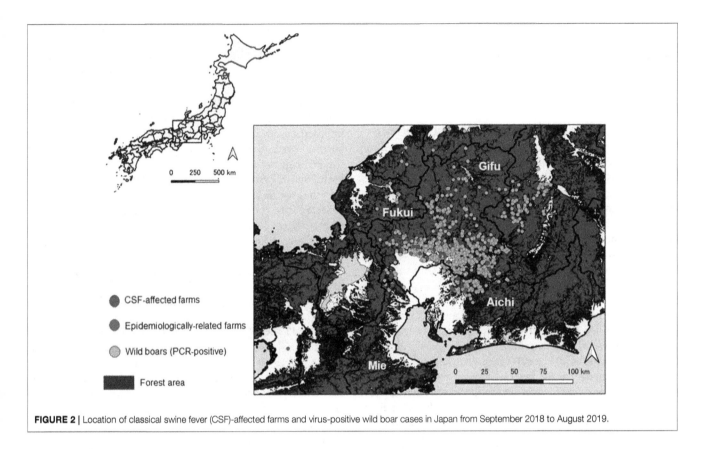

FIGURE 2 | Location of classical swine fever (CSF)-affected farms and virus-positive wild boar cases in Japan from September 2018 to August 2019.

This study is the first report that gives an epidemiological overview of the CSF outbreaks in pig farms by the virus strain of subgenotype 2.1d, which occurred in Japan, for the period from September 2018 to August 2019. The characteristics of the symptoms observed from infected animals and the measures taken at the affected farms described in this study will be a good reference for the countries affected by the epidemic of CSF caused by subgenotype 2.1d, which causes a chronic or moderate form of infection.

MATERIALS AND METHODS

Data Collection

Epidemiological data from the 39 farms where CSF outbreaks occurred in the period from September 2018 to August 2019 were collected using the epidemiological investigation reports. These reports also included information on the preventive measures implemented at the farms. Each epidemiological investigation on an affected farm was conducted by epidemiological investigation team (EIT) from the Ministry of Agriculture, Forestry and Fisheries (MAFF) of Japan. The EIT consisted of veterinary officials of MAFF and veterinary epidemiologists of NIAH-NARO. Most of the investigation activities were implemented on the date or the next date of confirmation of CSF infection and before starting of the stamping-out at the farm. During the epidemiological investigation, managers of affected farms were interviewed and asked about the biosecurity measures implemented at their farms, and about flows of workers and pigs

inside and outside of pig houses. Information on structures of affected pig houses and feedstuff was also collected at the on-site investigation. When fences and/or bird-proof nets were installed at affected farms, the way they were installed was checked by the EIT and the EIT confirmed if there were any possibilities of intrusion of wild animals. Brief list of questions used in the EIT investigations are shown in **Supplementary Table 1**.

Farm locations were extracted from the Domestic Animal Disease Control Map Database of Japan. All farms which did not rear pigs or boars for marketing purposes were classified as non-commercial farms. These included farms being managed by municipalities for breeding or education. Information regarding the number of animals being reared at the affected farms and the duration from infection confirmation to completion of stamping-out was collected from publicly available data from MAFF and prefectural governments.

Data on CSF-positive wild boars, including their location and laboratory test results, were also provided by MAFF.

Data Analysis

All statistical analyses were conducted using R (R Core Team, 2020). The Fisher's exact test was applied for univariate analyses. CSF-cumulative incidence rates by types of farms and clinical symptoms by types of pigs were compared by applying the test to 2×2 contingency tables. The association between the infection in sows and the status of transmission between pig houses was analyzed in the similar method. For the multiple comparisons of CSF-occurrence among farrow-to-finish farms, fattening farms and breeding farms, a 2 × 3 contingency table was prepared and the Fisher's exact test was applied by the "fisher.multcomp" function of the RVAideMemoire package. For the comparison of the number of animals at farms and the number of leucocytes by categories of farms and pigs, the Wilcoxon rank sum test ("wilcox.test" function) was applied.

Clinical Manifestations at Affected Farms

Information on the clinical manifestation, as observed at disease notification, and the type of pigs showing symptoms (piglets, sows, or fattening pigs) was collected from the following sources: (i) the epidemiological investigation reports completed by EIT (provided by MAFF), (ii) the CSF-EIT meeting reports (published on the MAFF web-site), (iii) the emergency notification reports submitted to the MAFF by the prefectural governments (provided by MAFF), and (iv) the verification reports prepared by Gifu Prefecture on their response to the CSF outbreaks (available on the Gifu prefectural government web-site).

The type of pigs affected, that is, piglets, sows, and fattening pigs, were classified as stated in the above sources. However, some farms only provided data on the age of the affected pigs. In such cases, pigs <3 months (or 90 days) of age were classified as piglets; pigs aged 3 months (or 90 days) and above were classified as fattening pigs, and pigs for breeding purposes were classified as sows. Observed clinical manifestations were classified into eight symptoms; loss of appetite, listlessness, respiratory disorders, fever, cyanosis, diarrhea, death, and neurological symptoms.

The association between the type of pigs (fattening/sows/piglets) and the development of any of the major four symptoms, that is, loss of appetite, listlessness, respiratory disorders, and death, was analyzed for each combination.

Results of Laboratory Tests of Pigs at Affected Farms

Farms with confirmed CSF infections, following tests conducted after receiving notification, had five or more pigs from each pig house randomly sampled before being stamped-out. The basic sample size was at least 30 animals per farm, to detect a prevalence of 10% with 95% confidence, and as additional conditions to detect the infection more efficiently, at least five animals per pig house, from all the pig houses, with priority in sampling from pigs with clinical symptoms were sampled in accordance with the Guideline. Investigations were conducted to measure the number of leucocytes, and PCR and ELISA tests performed to determine the infection status and spread of the virus at the farm. Blood sampling was conducted by the prefecture's local veterinary service, based on the Guideline, and antigens and antibodies against CSF were tested using PCR and ELISA, respectively. Following infection by CSF virus, the viral antigen is detected in the blood and/or organs of pigs where it grows, before any antibodies can be detected. Accordingly, the status is indicated as PCR(+)/ELISA(−). As the course of infection proceeds, antibodies against the CSF virus can be detected and the status becomes PCR(+)/ELISA(+). After the virus is eliminated from the pigs, the pigs become immune to CSF virus infection and the status is indicated as PCR(−)/ELISA(+).

Experimental infections using the virus strain isolated from the cases in Gifu Prefecture indicated that antibodies against the virus are developed on or after 14 days from infection, and that antigen detection lasts for more than 28 days after infection (19).

Proportion of Dead Animals at Farms

Obligatory daily reporting of the number of dead animals was imposed on farms located within a 3 km radius of an affected farm, a 10 km radius of an infected wild boar, and that had shipped pigs to the common slaughterhouses shared by affected farms, starting from February 2019, following the detection of the 8th case (the first outbreak in Aichi Prefecture). Reports were collected from the affected farms by the local veterinary service who reported the number to the MAFF. The daily proportion of dead animals was calculated by dividing the number of dead animals per day by the total number of animals at the farm on that day. When the total number of animals at the farm on each day was not available, the number of animals at the farm on the date of stamping-out was used as the denominator.

Data on Geographical Information

Geographical data on administrative divisions (as of 2018) and forested areas (as of 2015) was downloaded from the National Land Numerical Information download service, provided by the Ministry of Land, Infrastructure, Transport and Tourism of Japan, and was used to draw maps. The maps were drawn, and distance measured, by quantum geographic information system (QGIS) version 3.10.

We recorded the distance between the affected farms and the nearest site where a PCR-positive wild boar was found before the farm notified the outbreak. In addition, the shortest distance between affected farms was measured as the distance between an affected farm and the nearest affected farm with a confirmed infection, in which the infection was confirmed before that of the farm in question. This was measured using the distance matrix of the geoprocessing tools of QGIS.

RESULTS

Details of the Affected Farms
Classification and Comparison by Types of Farms
Pig/boar

Out of 39 outbreaks confirmed between September 2018 until August 2019, 38 outbreaks occurred at pig farms and one outbreak at a boar farm. Boars are not common livestock in Japan but there are boar farms where several or a few dozen boars are reared for training hunting dogs or for meat, or often without any particular purpose, as in the affected boar farm. In Gifu Prefecture, 21 out of 44 pig farms and one out of five boar farms were affected. The cumulative incidence rate was 48% (=21/44) for pig farms and 20% (=1/5) for boar farms, and there was no significant difference between the cumulative incidence rate of pig farms and boar farms (*p* > 0.1, Fisher's exact test).

Commercial/non-commercial

Five outbreaks occurred at non-commercial farms; four in Gifu Prefecture from November to December 2018, and one in

TABLE 1 | Number of classical swine fever (CSF) outbreaks at commercial pig farms in Gifu Prefecture from September 2018 to August 2019, by production type.

Production type	Number of farms		
	Affected	Not affected	Total
Farrow-to-finish	13	1	14
Fattening	4	10	14
Multiplier	1	11	12
Total	18	22	40

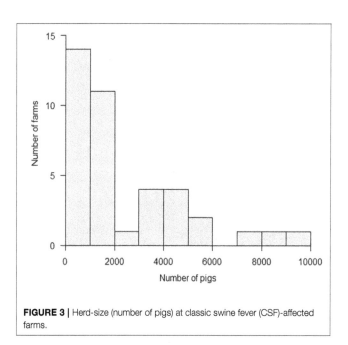

FIGURE 3 | Herd-size (number of pigs) at classic swine fever (CSF)-affected farms.

Aichi Prefecture in August 2019. Affected non-commercial farms included: the livestock research institutes of Gifu and Aichi Prefectures, the Gifu Prefectural College of Agriculture, the Gifu Prefectural Park of Livestock, and a boar farm. Thirty-four outbreaks occurred at commercial pig farms. In Gifu Prefecture, 18 out of 41 commercial pig/boar farms were affected and four out of eight non-commercial pig/boar farms were affected. The cumulative incidence rates were, therefore, 44% (=18/41) in commercial farms and 50% (=4/8) in non-commercial farms, with no significant difference between them ($p > 0.1$, Fisher's exact test).

Farrow-to-finish/fattening/breeding

The affected 34 commercial pig farms consisted of 28 farrow-to-finish farms, 5 fattening farms, and 1 breeding farm. Two out of five fattening farms were group farms comprising a farrow-to-finish and a breeding farm. In Gifu Prefecture, at commercial pig farms, the cumulative incidence rate of the farrow-to-finish farms was 93% (=13/14 farms), fattening farms was 29% (=4/14 farms), and breeding farms was 8.3% (=1/12 farms) (**Table 1**). Comparing the rates among the types of farms, the cumulative incidence rate of the farrow-to-finish farms was significantly higher than that of the fattening and breeding farms ($p < 0.05$, multiple comparison).

Number of Animals

More than half of the affected farms reared <2,000 animals, with a median number of 1,271 (25–75th percentile: 625–3,622) animals (**Figure 3**). The median size of these farms was not significantly different from that of all farms in Japan ($p > 0.1$, Wilcoxon rank sum test) (21). For non-commercial farms, the livestock research institutes of Gifu and Aichi Prefectures reared about 500 and 700 animals each, respectively. The other non-commercial farms reared 10 to 20 animals per farm. For commercial farms, the median number of animals reared per farm was 1,556 (25–75th percentile: 976–4,007) animals, ranging between 250 and 10,000 animals.

In Gifu Prefecture, 22 out of 49 pig/boar farms were affected and 27 farms were not affected. The median number of animals reared at the 22 affected farms was 1,277 (25–75th percentile: 594–2,916) animals, while the median number of animals reared at the 27 non-affected farms was 519 (25–75th percentile: 127–1,584) animals. Therefore, the number of animals reared at

affected farms was significantly higher ($p < 0.05$, Wilcoxon rank sum test).

Number of Days From Diagnosis to Completion of Stamping-Out

The time between definitive diagnosis and the completion of stamping-out ranged between 1 and 5 days, with a median of 2 days (25–75th percentile: 1–3 days) (**Figure 4**). There were 11/39 farms that required 3 days or more to complete stamping-out, of which 10 of these had either more than 4,000 animals or constituted a pig farm complex, resulting in multiple farms needing to be slaughtered simultaneously. The median number of animals at these 11 farms was 4,189 (25–75th percentile: 3,520–5,215) animals and was significantly larger than that of the other 28 farms ($p < 0.01$, Wilcoxon rank sum test).

Clinical Manifestations and Transmission of Virus Within Farms
Common Clinical Manifestations
Fever

Eleven of the 38 pig farms suspected CSF by fever and made notification. After including results from the on-site inspections following notification, pigs with a fever over 40°C were observed at 30/38 pig farms.

Decrease in the number of leucocytes

Pigs from all affected farms were noted to have a decreased leucocyte count to <10,000 cells/μl. Leucocyte counts were not measured at the wild boar farm because of their aggressiveness. The leucocyte level was measured on 939 CSF-positive pigs [PCR(+) and/or ELISA(+)] and 3,005 CSF-negative pigs [PCR(−) and ELISA(−)]. The median leucocyte level within CSF-positive pigs was 8,490 (25–75th percentile: 5,900–13,000)

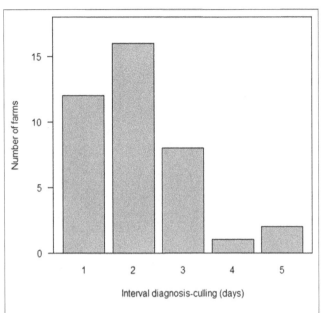

FIGURE 4 | Distribution of the interval between laboratory confirmed diagnosis and the completion of culling at 39 farms affected by classical swine fever (CSF) in Japan, 2018–2019.

cells/µl, which was significantly lower than that of CSF-negative pigs ($p < 0.01$, Wilcoxon rank sum test).

Clinical Manifestations Leading to the Notification and the Results of Laboratory Tests

Clinical manifestations of fattening pigs were the reason for notification at 18 out of 34 commercial farms. Among these 18 farms, death was the common reason for notification in 12 farms.

In 9 out of 34 commercial farms, clinical manifestations of sows led to notification. At all nine farms, the reason for notification was loss of appetite, with death also cited as a reason in one of these nine farms.

In 6 out of 34 commercial farms, clinical manifestations in piglets led to notification. The death of weaning pigs was the reason for notification in four out of six farms while loss of appetite in sows was also cited as a reason in one of the four farms. As for the other two farms, fever and listlessness of weaning pigs were the reasons for notification at one farm, and listlessness of piglets as well as loss of appetite and listlessness of sows were the reasons in the other.

Table 2 shows the observed clinical manifestations and the results of laboratory tests according to farm level.

Other than the farms that notified CSF by clinical manifestations, in 4 out of 34 commercial farms, the clinical manifestations were not observed by farm managers, where the infection was detected by PCR and ELISA tests applied as a part of the movement/shipment-control areas. After the detection by the laboratory tests, pigs with fever were confirmed at two farms, but pigs at the other two farms remained asymptomatic. Pigs tested ELISA(+) at two out of four farms, PCR(+)/ELISA(+) at one farm without fever, and PCR(−)/ELISA(+) at one farm with

fever. In the other two farms, pigs only tested PCR(+)/ELISA(−) but one of the farms had pigs with fever.

As a result of analyses on the association between the type of pigs and the development of symptoms, it was indicated that respiratory disorders and loss of appetite significantly led to notification more frequently in fattening pigs and in sows, respectively ($p < 0.05$ and $p < 0.01$, Fisher's exact test). Death was significantly less frequently cited as a reason for notification in sows ($p < 0.05$, Fisher's exact test).

Abnormal Birth

Abnormal births, including abortion and stillbirth, were reported only by three farms during the epidemiological investigation interviews, while stillbirths were recorded in the daily reports from 10 other farms traced up to 60 days before confirmation of infection. In 9 out of these 13 farms, the pig houses with recorded stillbirths were confirmed to be affected with CSF afterwards. However, none of these farms suspected that the abnormal births were a clinical manifestation of CSF infection.

Death and Proportion of Dead Animals

Based on the records of the daily number of dead animals at the farms traced up to a maximum of 60 days before infection was confirmed, 30 out of 39 affected farms had observed their animals dying before notification. In 12 out of 30 farms, the cause of the death was considered to be due to weakness or being crushed (in suckling pigs), diarrhea (in weaning pigs), streptococcus's infection, pneumonia, gastroenteritis, and stress or growth insufficiency (in weaning and fattening pigs). CSF was not suspected as the cause according to both the local veterinary service and the supervising veterinarian since the other pigs being reared in the same pens or pig houses as the dead pigs did not have any abnormal symptoms. In the other 18 farms, CSF was suspected, and the death led to notification.

Data on the daily number of dead animals before notification were available on 31 of the affected farms. In 6 out of the 31 farms, the proportion of dead animals on the date of notification was more than 0.5% (Case no. 9, 17, 27, 28, 30, 31). Three of these six farms notified due to the increase in the number of dead weaning pigs, and the other three farms due to the death of their fattening pigs. Other than those six farms, there was no observed increased number of dead animals from the other farms on the date of notification (**Figure 5**). For the other 25 farms, temporary increases in the proportion of dead animals to more than 0.5% were observed before the dates of notification in six farms (Case no. 21, 24, 29, 33, 35, 37), but the cause of the increase was crushing death in suckling pigs or abortion.

Transmission Between Pig Houses by Pig Flow (Intra Farm Pig Movement)

In the 34 commercial farms, including the two farms without any clinical manifestations, infection was limited to one pig house in eight farms and confirmed in all the pig houses in the other eight farms. In the other 18 farms, infection was confirmed in more than two, but not all, pig houses. Transmission of the infection between pig houses by pig flow was assumed to have occurred when there was a record of the infected pigs having moved

TABLE 2 | Reported clinical signs by types of pigs and the results of serological tests on CSF at the 34 affected commercial farms.

Type of pigs	Reported clinical manifestation	No. of farms with clinical signs	Results of serological tests on CSF at farm level[a]		
			PCR-positive/ELISA-negative	PCR-positive/ELISA-positive	PCR-negative/ELISA-positive
Fattening pig		18	1	6	11
	Death	12	1	3	8
	Fever	7	0	3	4
	Listlessness	8	0	4	4
	Loss of appetite	7	0	3	4
	Respiratory disorders	5	0	0	5
	Diarrhea	2	0	1	1
	Cyanosis	2	0	0	2
	Decreased growth	1	0	0	1
Sow		9	2	3	4
	Loss of appetite	9	2	3	4
	Fever	4	2	1	1
	Listlessness	2	0	1	1
	Death	1	1	0	0
Piglet		6	1	3	2
	Death	4	1	2	1
	Listlessness	3	0	2	1
	Cyanosis	2	1	0	1
	Fever	2	0	2	0
	Loss of appetite	1	0	1	0
	Neurological symptom	1	0	1	0
	Diarrhea	1	0	0	1

[a]Classification of farms by the results of serological tests. PCR-positive/ELISA-negative, all animals tested at the reporting and before culling were PCR-positive but without CSF-virus-specific antibodies; PCR-positive/ELISA-positive, at least one animal tested at the reporting or before culling was PCR-positive and with CSF-virus-specific antibodies; PCR-negative/ELISA-positive, at least one animal tested at the time of reporting or before culling was with CSF-virus-specific antibodies but PCR-negative.
PCR, polymerase chain reaction; ELISA, enzyme-linked immunosorbent assay.

between pig houses, and when both pig houses were confirmed to be affected. Based on the epidemiological investigations and movement records of the infected pigs, transmission by pig flow was strongly suspected in 7 of the 26 farms, with infection confirmed in multiple pig houses. In five of the farms, the viral spread by pig flow was refuted since the farms were fattening farms and/or the pigs had not moved between pig houses. In the other 14 farms, the transmission routes between pig houses remained unclear because either there were no records of the movement of pigs between pig houses or because almost all of the pig houses in the farm had been found to be infected with no trace as to the source of the infection within the farm.

Transmission Between Stages of Pigs

The infection was not limited to a single stage in 23 out of 29 commercial farms rearing multiple stages of pigs (28 farrow-to-finish farms and one breeding farm). In one the other six farms, infection was confirmed only in fattening pigs (five of the six farms) and in sows (one of the six farms).

The association between the infection in sows and the status of transmission between pig houses is shown in

Table 3. Infection in multiple pig houses was observed more frequently when there was infection of sows ($p < 0.01$, Fisher's exact test).

Surrounding Environment of the Affected Farms

Distribution of Infected Wild Boars

In Gifu Prefecture, wild boars confirmed as PCR-positive were frequently detected near the affected farms. On the other hand, PCR-positive wild boars were not found near the affected farms located at the southern peninsula of the Aichi Prefecture (**Figure 2**).

Twenty-eight out of 38 affected farms, excluding the first affected farm, were located within 5 km from PCR-positive wild boars detected before the notification of an outbreak at each farm. Out of the 28 farms, 23 farms were located in the southern area of Gifu Prefecture or in the adjacent northern area of Aichi Prefecture, two farms were located in the central part of Aichi Prefecture, and the other three farms were located in Mie and Fukui Prefectures.

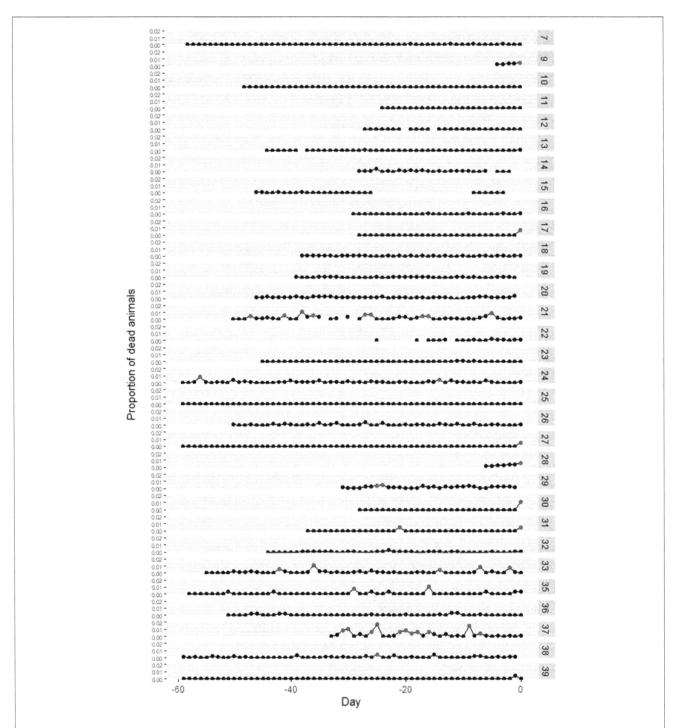

FIGURE 5 | Changes in the proportion of dead animals at classical swine fever (CSF)-affected farms. Numbers at the right side indicate case numbers. The proportion over 0.5% is marked as red point. Day 0 = report date. Data were not available for Case no. 1–6, 8, and 34.

Distance Between Affected Farms

The median distance between affected farms and the nearest other affected farm was 6.95 km (25–75th percentile: 2.35–11.38 km). Four farms were located within a distance of 1 km, with one of these four farms was located in a pig farm complex in the southern peninsula of Aichi Prefecture. The other three farms were located in the northern area of Aichi Prefecture, with two of the three farms adjoining each other and the nearest affected farm being the one in common. One of these farms was an affiliated farm of one of the other two farms.

TABLE 3 | CSF-infection among sows and the spread of classical swine fever (CSF) viruses between pig houses.

Infection in sows	Number of CSF-affected farms rearing multiple stages of pigs		Total
	Spread of CSF viruses in each farm		
	Limited to a single pig house	Observed in multiple pig houses	
Yes	2	19	21
No	5	3	8
Total	7	22	29

TABLE 4 | General characteristics of the 39 farms affected by classical swine fever.

	Number of farms
Structure of affected pig houses	
Windowless	0
Semi-windowless[a]	18
With open windows[b]	21
Feedstuff	
Commercial feed only	33
Other than commercial feed	6

[a] One of the 18 semi-windowless pig-houses had open-air paddocks.
[b] Two of the 21 pig-houses with open windows had open-air paddocks.

Livestock Health Management at Affected Farms

Feed

In 33 out of 39 farms, only commercial feed was used. The other six farms used feed other than commercial feed (**Table 4**), with one of these six farms being the boar farm which used rice bran, wasted rice, breadcrumbs discarded from food factories, and vegetable scraps discarded by neighboring farmers. The other five farms using non-commercial feed were commercial pig farms using confectionery residues such as biscuit crumbs (two farms), breadcrumbs (one farm), weeds around the farm (one farm), and liquid feed made with food wastes including table leftovers and cooking residues (one farm) as feed.

Measures to Prevent Intrusion of Wild Boars

Fences around farms were installed at 26 of the 39 farms, but only 14 farms had complete fences protecting them against intrusion by wild boars. In addition, 15 of the 39 farms had installed electric fences, but the fences were complete at only 12 farms (**Table 5**).

Biosecurity Measures at Farm Boundaries

Disinfection of vehicles, such as feed transporters, at farm boundaries was implemented at 28 of the 39 farms. At 5 of the remaining 11 farms, the ground surface at the entrance of the farms was covered with lime. To prevent farm workers from bringing in the virus, changing of boots and clothes at the farm entrances were implemented in more than half of the affected farms (**Table 5**).

Biosecurity Measures at the Border of Pig Houses

As for the structure of the pig houses, there were no windows or filters installed on the openings of the pig houses at 21 of the 39 farms. Openings were covered with curtains at the other 18 farms. There were three farms with open-air paddocks, one of which was a commercial farm (**Table 4**). To prevent entry of the virus into the pig houses, more than half of the affected farms installed bird-proof netting on the openings of the pig houses, but some of them had gaps or breakages and complete netting was installed at only 15 farms. Changing of boots at each entrance of the pig houses was implemented at more than half of the affected farms (**Table 5**).

DISCUSSION

Details of the Affected Farms

Regarding the type of management, 80% of the affected commercial farms were farrow-to-finish farms. In Gifu Prefecture, the incidence at farrow-to-finish farms was significantly higher than in other farms. This may be due to the fact that in a farrow-to-finish farm, the management of both piglet production and shipment of fattening pigs requires frequent movements of pigs within the farm, with frequent handling, which increases the risk of introducing the virus into the farm. In a case-control study of the outbreaks of foot-and-mouth disease (FMD) in Japan, it was indicated that the risk of infection was higher in farrow-to-finish farms than in fattening farms (22). The reason is considered that sows and piglets in farrow-to-finish farms require more frequent care than pigs in fattening farms and that the disease transmission via direct contact with animals and contaminated fomites tends to occur more frequently in farrow-to-finish farms. Other studies on African swine fever (ASF) outbreaks in Estonia (23) and CSF in the Netherlands (24) have also indicated that the incidence tended to be higher in farms rearing sows with piglets and fattening pigs.

The number of animals at affected farms was significantly larger when comparing affected and non-affected farms in Gifu Prefecture. At large farms, the infection risk may be higher when the number of sows is larger, leading to a larger number of employees engaged in the management of breeding and feeding, as well as the larger number of people entering and leaving the farm for purposes such as transporting feed and shipping fattening pigs. These conditions have not been investigated at non-affected farms, therefore, case-control studies would be necessary for further analysis. On the CSF outbreaks in the Netherlands, a case-control study (25) and a survival analysis (24) reported that the risk of CSF infection was higher on farms with more than 500 animals.

In the CSF outbreak reported in this paper, the median number of days from diagnosis to complete stamping-out was 2 days, including farms with ~10,000 animals. Minimizing the period between infection and stamping-out is important in order to prevent the spread of diseases. In 2010, the spread of FMD in Japan was worsened by delays in stamping-out (22), and due to this fact, the guidelines for specific animal diseases including CSF was revised to include the time limit for the containment

TABLE 5 | Preventive measures implemented at the 39 farms affected by classical swine fever.

	No. of farms	Proportion (N = 39)
1. Measures at the boundaries of the farms		
Installation of fences without electricity[a]	26	67%
- part of fences were left open and/or gaps or damages present	12	31%
- without any defects	14	36%
Installation of electric fences[a]	15	38%
- parts of fences were left open and/or gaps or damages present	3	8%
- without any defects	12	31%
Covering ground with hydrated lime at entry points	15	38%
Disinfection of vehicles at entry points	28	72%
- by power sprayer [b]	25	64%
- by disinfection baths [b]	6	15%
- by portable sprayer [b]	2	5%
- by disinfection mats [b]	2	5%
Changing footwear of persons entering the farms	29	74%
Changing clothes of persons entering the farms	23	59%
2. Measures to prevent intrusion into pig houses		
Covering windows of pig houses with bird-proof nets	25	64%
- gaps or damage present	10	26%
- without any defects	15	38%
Changing boots at the entrances of each pig house	22	56%
Changing gloves and clothes at the entrances of each pig house	6	15%

[a]Fourteen farms had some electric fences and some fences without electricity; 12 farms had fences without electricity only; one farm had electric fences only; and 12 farms did not have any fences.
[b]Farms were applying one or more of the ways to disinfect vehicles at entry points.

measures. The Guideline stipulates that stamping-out should be completed within 24 h, for farms with 1,000 to 2,000 heads of fattening pigs, and that carcasses should be buried or burned within 72 h after confirmation of infection. On the CSF outbreaks in the Netherlands between 1997 and 1998, the median size of the affected farms was 1296.5 animals (25–75th percentile: 800–1,800 animals), and it was reported that 70% of the affected animals were killed within 1 day (26, 27). The relatively longer days required in the affected farms in Japan would reflect relatively large number of animals (median size was 1,271 and 25 and 75th percentile: 625–3,622) reared at infected farms and caused shortage in the available human resources. To complement the shortage of human resources, MAFF coordinated mobilization of official veterinarians of MAFF and surrounding prefectural governments to the affected farms and for several large farms, and the Self-Defense Forces were also deployed to assist activities related to the containment measures. For example, in Gifu Prefecture, a median number of 1,670 (25–75th percentile: 1,108–4,321) people engaged in control activities at an affected farm and the Self-Defense Forces were deployed at 6 out of 20 outbreaks, in which 1,662 to 9,858 animals were subject to stamping-out.

Clinical Manifestations and Transmission of Virus Within Farms

In the recent outbreaks of CSF in Japan, fever and leukopenia were observed in many cases. In the infection experiment of Japanese isolates, fever over 40°C and leukopenia (<10,000 cells/μl) were observed before the fever had started (19). Fever

and leukopenia have been reported as common symptoms of CSF infection in the experiments of other strains (1, 2, 26, 28). Non-specific symptoms such as fever and loss of appetite are common for many diseases and frequently observed at farms, hence they are unlikely to lead to notification. Previous reports have also pointed out that there are cases where notification is delayed due to these symptoms being misdiagnosed as other diseases with clinical symptoms not detected until secondary infection occurs (1, 2, 15, 26).

The results of laboratory tests on the affected farms indicate that the infection in fattening pigs tended to take time to develop clinical manifestations, leading to late notification. Fattening pigs are kept in groups with continuous feeding, therefore, it might be difficult to recognize abnormalities when their appetite is low in the early stages of infection. Notifications may only be made after the appearance of dead pigs, after the number of infected pigs has increased. In addition, there were significantly more cases of respiratory symptoms leading to notifications among fattening pigs than among sows and piglets. It is also possible that CSF infections worsen the clinical symptoms of fattening pigs which have already been infected with other respiratory diseases.

The piglet deaths at the time of notifications were observed in the weaning pigs of each farm. In CSF, piglets suffering from vertical infection are known to be persistently infected and it is possible that these piglets only developed clinical symptoms after weaning. For the piglets showing PCR(+)/ELISA(+), it is thought that viruses are not eliminated despite antibody production. The same condition has been reported in infection experiments with low to moderately pathogenic strains of CSF (29, 30).

In most cases, increases in the number of dead animals to more than 0.5% of the total number was not observed. This result was concordant with the result of the study of experimental infection using the virus strain isolated from the 2018 Japan outbreak. In that study, no infected animals died during the study period up to 28 days post-infection (19). These data suggest that detection of CSF infections by death is difficult in sub-acute CSF infections because the proportion of animals dying does not change significantly.

About 80% of the farms (23/29 farms) had infection in pigs at multiple stages. Infections confined to a single stage were observed mainly in the farms housing only fattening pigs. In addition, this study showed the association between the infection in sows and the occurrence of infection in multiple pig houses. It is also suggested by a previous study using a simulation model that the on-farm infection started in sows could only be noticed clinically when transmitted to weaning or fattening pig groups (31). These studies suggest that infection in sows would cause infection in piglets. These piglets move to other pig houses and become a source of infection to other pig houses and finally detected when they show clinical signs. It is important to note that transmission through the movement of infected pigs cannot be prevented by strengthening biosecurity measures such as disinfection.

Source of Infection to the Farms

The geographical distribution of outbreaks and infected wild boars in Gifu Prefecture suggested that infected wild boars around the farm might have been the source of infection. The fact that many of the outbreak farms were within 5 km of the proximate infected wild boar detection sites suggested that infected wild boars were the source of infection to the farms. A study on the geographic analysis of the risk of infection from infected boars for the recent Japanese CSF outbreak indicated that the risk was dependent on the distance to the infected boar and that the risk of infection extended to farms within 5 km (20). However, among the farms located within 5 km of the proximate infected wild boar, the intrusion of wild boars into farms was not confirmed by witnessing any signs or footprints of food exploring on livestock, except for one outbreak at the Gifu Prefectural Park. This could indicate that the virus carried by wild boars in the area surrounding the farms might have been secondarily carried into the farms by other wild animals or persons. It is also possible that small wild animals, such as rats and wild birds including crows, could also carry the virus into the farms, although it has not been proven that these animals can transmit the virus to date, and further verification is needed (25, 32, 33).

To enhance the biosecurity measures conducted at pig farms, MAFF has provided several rounds of guidance since the first outbreak in September 2018 on how to comply with the biosecurity standards at farms, including countermeasures against the entry of wild animals. Although vaccination for pigs began in prefectures with infected wild boars in October 2019, biosecurity measures at farms will continue to be important.

As for the outbreaks at the southern peninsula of Aichi Prefecture, infected wild boars were not found near the affected farms. Therefore, the involvement of infected wild boars on those outbreaks is unclear. Genetic analysis has shown that the there is a relationship between strains isolated from infected farms in an area with infected wild boars in Gifu Prefecture and strains isolated from some of the outbreak farms in the southern peninsula area of Aichi Prefecture. Since there was no epidemiological relationship found between those farms, it is considered that the long-distance transmission may have occurred indirectly through vehicles or other fomites traveling between these areas (34).

Considering the role of wild boars in the spread of the disease, the surveillance in wild boars is an important issue. At present in Japan, there are difficulties in conducting and continuing the surveillance of wild boars to monitor CSF infection mainly because of the lack of specific legal and organizational system for disease surveillance in wild animals. Future control plans on CSF in Japan should be discussed with more detailed investigation on the interaction between the infection in pigs and that in wild boars.

If the distance between farms is <1 km, there is a possibility of occurrence of local transmission (35). As for the affected farms, the farms possibly affected by local transmission were located in two areas in Aichi Prefecture, that is, one in the southern peninsula area and one in the northern area adjacent to Gifu Prefecture. Full genome analysis showed that the virus strains isolated from two of the three farms in the northern area were closely related to each other, but the remaining one was different. The virus from this one farm and the virus isolated from five farms in the southern peninsula area were closely related (34). This suggests that in some cases, transmission of the virus was considered to be occurring between neighboring farms. In contrast, more farms were located more than 1 km apart from each other, suggesting that in many farms, outbreaks were caused by factors other than local transmission such as transmission through people, fomites, or wildlife that had some contact with infected wild boars.

For the previous CSF outbreaks, feedstuffs such as kitchen residues were considered to be one of the major sources of infection on farms (15). It is unlikely that swill feeding was the cause of the outbreaks during the 2018 Japan outbreak as only one of the six farms using non-commercial feeds was feeding kitchen waste residues. The other four farms using non-commercial feeds mainly used food plant residues which did not include meat. Therefore, there was no possibility of contamination by the meat. For the two farms that also fed vegetable scraps and weeds, the possibility that these feeds were the source of infection cannot be ruled out, as infected wild boars have been found in the areas surrounding the vegetable scrap and weed collections.

This study mainly focuses on the features of the affected farms and the comparison between affected farms and non-affected farms have not been conducted. To elucidate the factors influencing the risk of CSF infection, comparison between infected and non-infected farms will be necessary. Whether there is a difference in the risk of occurrence due to the structure of pig houses or other status of biosecurity measures will need to be verified through case-control studies and other studies in the future.

CONCLUSION

It appears that the current CSF outbreaks in Japan were caused by a virus originating from neighboring countries that spread to pig farms, but the specific route of entry into Japan is unknown. Since most of the infections have occurred in the areas where infected wild boars have been detected and the areas with infected farms are expanding with the expansion of the range of infected wild boars, it is likely that infected wild boars are the main source of infection. Clinical symptoms are non-specific and are difficult to detect during the early stages of the infection. In areas at high risk of infection, daily clinical observation and early testing for pigs showing loss of appetite and listlessness are required. Areas with infected wild boars are still expanding more than a year after the first outbreak. It is necessary to continue to

strengthen biosecurity measures at farms located in areas with infected wild boars and to monitor the distribution of infected wild boars.

AUTHOR CONTRIBUTIONS

YH conceived the study. YS and TY analyzed the data and wrote the main manuscript text. YH, YM, KS, and EY contributed to the interpretation of the results and helped draft the manuscript. All authors reviewed the manuscript.

ACKNOWLEDGMENTS

We appreciate the kind cooperation of the Ministry of Agriculture, Forestry and Fisheries, Government of Japan and the local governments for providing epidemiological information on the CSF outbreaks in Japan.

REFERENCES

1. Moennig V, Floegel-Niesmann G, Greiser-Wilke I. Clinical signs and epidemiology of classical swine fever: a review of new knowledge. *Vet J.* (2003) 165:11–20. doi: 10.1016/S1090-0233(02)00112-0

2. Blome S, Staubach C, Henke J, Carlson J, Beer M. Classical swine fever—an updated review. *Viruses.* (2017) 9:1–24. doi: 10.3390/v9040086

3. OIE. *Recognition of the Classical Swine Fever Status.* (2019). Available online at: https://www.oie.int/fileadmin/Home/eng/Animal_Health_in_the_World/docs/pdf/Resolutions/2019/A_R22_CSF_status.pdf (accessed May 7, 2020).

4. MAFF. *Annual Statistics of Domestic Animal Infectious Diseases.* (1937–2019) (2019). Available online at: https://www.maff.go.jp/j/syouan/douei/kansi_densen/attach/pdf/kansi_densen-162.pdf (accessed May 7, 2020).

5. OIE. *Resolutions adopted by the World Assembly of the OIE Delegates during their 83rd General Session.* (2015). Available online at: https://www.oie.int/fileadmin/Home/eng/About_us/docs/pdf/Session/A_RESO_2015_public.pdf (accessed May 7, 2020).

6. Postel A, Nishi T, Kameyama KI, Meyer D, Suckstorff O, Fukai K, Becher P. Reemergence of classical swine fever, Japan, 2018. *Emerg Infect Dis.* (2019) 25:1228–31. doi: 10.3201/eid2506.181578

7. Nishi T, Kameyama K, Kato T, Fukai K. Genome sequence of a classical swine fever virus of subgenotype 2.1, isolated from a pig in Japan in 2018. *Am Soc Microbiol.* (2019) 8:e01362–18. doi: 10.1128/MRA.01362-18

8. Leng C, Zhang H, Kan Y, Yao L, Li M, Zhai H, et al. Characterisation of newly emerged isolates of classical swine fever virus in China, 2014–2015. *J Vet Res.* (2017) 61:1–9. doi: 10.1515/jvetres-2017-0001

9. Luo Y, Ji S, Liu Y, Lei JL, Xia SL, Wang Y, et al. Isolation and characterization of a moderately virulent classical swine fever virus emerging in china. *Transbound Emerg Dis.* (2017) 64:1848–57. doi: 10.1111/tbed.12581

10. Zhang H, Leng C, Tian Z, Liu C, Chen J, Bai Y, et al. Complete genomic characteristics and pathogenic analysis of the newly emerged classical swine fever virus in China. *BMC Vet Res.* (2018) 14:204. doi: 10.1186/s12917-018-1504-2

11. Zhou B. Classical swine fever in China—an update minireview. *Front Vet Sci.* (2019) 6:187. doi: 10.3389/fvets.2019.00187

12. An DJ, Lim SI, Choe SE, Kim KS, Cha RM, Cho IS et al. Evolutionary dynamics of classical swine fever virus in South Korea: 1987–2017. *Vet Microbiol.* (2018) 225:79–88. doi: 10.1016/j.vetmic.2018.09.020

13. Choe S, Cha RM, Yu D-S, Kim K-S, Song S, Choi S-H, et al. Rapid spread of classical swine fever virus among South Korean wild boars in areas near the border with North Korea. *Pathogens.* (2020) 9:244. doi: 10.3390/pathogens9040244

14. MAFF. *Guideline to Control Classical Swine Fever.* (2020). Available online at: https://www.maff.go.jp/j/syouan/douei/katiku_yobo/k_bousi/attach/pdf/index-25.pdf (accessed May 20, 2020).

15. Fritzemeier J, Teuffert J, Greiser-Wilke I, Staubach C, Schlüter H, Moennig V. Epidemiology of classical swine fever in Germany in the 1990s. *Vet Microbiol.* (2000) 77:29–41. doi: 10.1016/S0378-1135(00)00254-6

16. Mintiens K, Deluyker H, Laevens H, Koenen F, Dewulf J, De Kruif A. Descriptive epidemiology of a classical swine fever outbreak in the Limburg Province of Belgium in 1997. *J Vet Med Ser B.* (2001) 48:143–9. doi: 10.1046/j.1439-0450.2001.00429.x

17. Stegeman A, Elbers A, De Smit H, Moser H, Smak J, Pluimers F. The 1997–1998 epidemic of classical swine fever in the Netherlands. *Vet Microbiol.* (2000) 73:183–96. doi: 10.1016/S0378-1135(00)00144-9

18. Pluimers FH, De Leeuw PW, Smak JA, Elbers ARW, Stegeman JA. Classical swine fever in The Netherlands 1997–1998: a description of organisation and measures to eradicate the disease. *Prev Vet Med.* (1999) 42:139–55. doi: 10.1016/S0167-5877(99)00085-9

19. Kameyama KI, Nishi T, Yamada M, Masujin K, Morioka K, Kokuho T, Fukai K. Experimental infection of pigs with a classical swine fever virus isolated in Japan for the first time in 26 years. *J Vet Med Sci.* (2019) 81:1277–84. doi: 10.1292/jvms.19-0133

20. Hayama Y, Shimizu Y, Murato Y, Sawai K, Yamamoto T. Estimation of infection risk on pig farms in infected wild boar areas—epidemiological analysis for the reemergence of classical swine fever in Japan in 2018. *Prev Vet Med.* (2020) 175:104873. doi: 10.1016/j.prevetmed.2019.104873

21. MAFF. *Census of Livestock Industry 2019.* (2019). Available online at: https://www.e-stat.go.jp/stat-search/files?page=1&layout=datalist&toukei=00500222&tstat=000001015614&cycle=7&year=20190&month=0&tclass1=000001020206&tclass2=000001134566&stat_infid=000031878373 (accessed May 20, 2020).

22. Muroga N, Kobayashi S, Nishida T, Hayama Y, Kawano T, Yamamoto T, et al. Risk factors for the transmission of foot-and-mouth disease during the 2010 outbreak in Japan: a case-control study. *BMC Vet Res.* (2013) 9:150. doi: 10.1186/1746-6148-9-150

23. Nurmoja I, Mõtus K, Kristian M, Niine T, Schulz K, Depner K, Viltrop A. Epidemiological analysis of the 2015–2017 African swine fever outbreaks in Estonia. *Prev Vet Med.* (2018) 181:104556. doi: 10.1016/j.prevetmed.2018.10.001

24. Benard HJ, Stärk KDC, Morris RS, Pfeiffer DU, Moser H. The 1997–1998 classical swine fever epidemic in The Netherlands—a survival analysis. *Prev Vet Med.* (1999) 42:235–48. doi: 10.1016/S0167-5877(99)00078-1

25. Elbers ARW, Stegeman JA, De Jong MCM. Factors associated with the introduction of classical swine fever virus into pig herds in the central area of the 1997/98 epidemic in the Netherlands. *Vet Rec.* (2001) 149:377–82. doi: 10.1136/vr.149.13.377

26. Elbers ARW, Stegeman A, Moser H, Ekker HM, Smak JA, Pluimers FH. The classical swine fever epidemic 1997–1998 in the Netherlands: descriptive epidemiology. *Prev Vet Med.* (1999) 42:157–84. doi: 10.1016/S0167-5877(99)00074-4

27. Boender GJ, Van Den Hengel R, Van Roermund HJW, Hagenaars TJ. The influence of between-farm distance and farm size on the spread of classical swine fever during the 1997–1998 epidemic in the Netherlands. *PLoS One.* (2014) 9:e95278. doi: 10.1371/journal.pone.0095278

28. Postel A, Becher P. Epidemiology, diagnosis and control of classical swine fever : recent developments and future challenges. *Transbound Emerg Dis.* (2018) 65:248–61. doi: 10.1111/tbed.12676

29. Donahue BC, Petrowski HM, Melkonian K, Ward GB, Mayr GA, Metwally S. Analysis of clinical samples for early detectionof classical swine fever during infection with low, moderate, and highly virulent strains in relation to the onset of clinical signs. *J Virol Methods.* (2012) 179:108–15. doi: 10.1016/j.jviromet.2011.10.008

30. Petrov A, Blohm U, Beer M, Pietschmann J, Blome S. Comparative analyses of host responses upon infection with moderately virulent classical swine fever virus in domestic pigs and wild boar. *Virol J.* (2014) 11:1–6. doi: 10.1186/1743-422X-11-134

31. Stegeman A, Elbers ARW, Bouma A, De Smit H, De Jong MCM. Transmission of classical swine fever virus within herds during the 1997–1998 epidemic in The Netherlands. *Prev Vet Med.* (1999) 42:201–18. doi: 10.1016/S0167-5877(99)00076-8

32. Kaden V, Lange E, Steyer H, Bruer W, Langner C. Role of birds in transmission of classical swine fever virus. *J Vet Med Ser B Infect Dis Vet Public Heal.* (2003) 50:357–59. doi: 10.1046/j.1439-0450.2003.00670.x

33. Truong QL, Seo TW, Yoon B Il, Kim HC, Han JH, Hahn TW. Prevalence of swine viral and bacterial pathogens in rodents and stray cats captured around pig farms in Korea. *J Vet Med Sci.* (2013) 75:1647–50. doi: 10.1292/jvms.12-0568

34. MAFF. *Interim Report on the Epidemiological Investigation for Classical Swine Fever Outbreaks in Japan.* (2019). Available online at: https://www.maff.go.jp/j/syouan/douei/csf/pdf/index-281.pdf (accessed April 7, 2020).

35. Stegeman JA, Elbers ARW, Bouma A, De Jong MCM. Rate of inter-herd transmission of classical swine fever virus by different types of contact during the 1997-8 epidemic in The Netherlands. *Epidemiol Infect.* (2002) 128:285–91. doi: 10.1017/S0950268801006483

22

TRIM62 from Chicken as a Negative Regulator of Reticuloendotheliosis Virus Replication

Ling Li[1†], Dongyan Niu[2†], Jie Yang[1], Jianmin Bi[3], Lingjuan Zhang[4], Ziqiang Cheng[1] and Guihua Wang[1*]

[1] College of Veterinary Medicine, Shandong Agricultural University, Tai'an, China, [2] Veterinary Medicine, University of Calgary, Calgary, AB, Canada, [3] China Animal Husbandry Industry Co., Ltd., Beijing, China, [4] Penglai City Animal Epidemic Prevention and Control Center, Penglai, China

*Correspondence:
Guihua Wang
wguihua1126@163.com

[†]These authors have contributed
equally to this work

Emerging evidence suggests that the tripartite motif containing 62 (TRIM62), a member of the TRIM family, plays an important role in antiviral processes. The objective of the study was to explore the role of TRIM62 in reticuloendotheliosis virus (REV) infection and its potential molecular mechanism. We first demonstrated that the REV infection affected the TRIM62 expression first upregulated and then downregulated in CEF cells. Next, we evaluated the effect of TRIM62 on viral replication. Overexpression of TRIM62 decreased REV replication. On the contrary, silencing of endogenously expressed TRIM62 increased viral replication. Then, to explore the necessity of domains in TRIM62's negative regulation on viral replication, we transfected CEF cells with TRIM62 domain deletion mutants. Deletion domain partially abolished TRIM62's antiviral activity. The effect of SPRY domain deletion was the highest and that of coiled-coil was the lowest. Further, we identified 18 proteins that coimmunoprecipitated and interacted with TRIM62 by immunocoprecipitation and mass spectrometry analysis. Strikingly, among which, both Ras-related protein Rab-5b (RAB5B) and Arp2/3 complex 34-kDa subunit (ARPC2) were involved in actin cytoskeletal pathway. Altogether, these results strongly suggest that chicken TRIM62 provides host defense against viral infection, and all domains are required for its action. RAB5B and ARPC2 may play important roles in its negative regulation processes.

Keywords: TRIM62, negative regulation, reticuloendotheliosis virus, domain deletion, RAB5B and ARPC2

INTRODUCTION

TRIM62 (tripartite motif containing 62) is a member of the TRIM family proteins and is also known as DEAR1 (ductal epithelium-associated RING chromosome) (1). TRIM family proteins, also known as RBCC proteins, contain conserved RING finger, B-box, coiled-coil domains, and a variable C terminus (2). Despite their common domain structure, TRIM proteins play critical roles in distinct cellular processes such as intercellular signaling, innate immunity, transcription, autophagy, and carcinogenesis (3, 4). Members of the TRIM family of E3 ligases exhibit antiviral activities (5, 6). More than 20 TRIM proteins, which affected the entry or release of retrovirus such as human immunodeficiency virus 1 (HIV), murine leukemia virus (MIV), or avian leucosis virus (ALV), were screened (6). Expression of low amounts of TRIM62 enhanced HIV gene expression and release, and the E3 mutant of TRIM62 inhibited HIV release more potently than the wild-type protein (6). However, TRIM62 from orange-spotted grouper (EcTRIM62) negatively regulated the innate antiviral immune response against fish RNA viruses (7).

Reticuloendotheliosis virus (REV) is an avian retrovirus that can induce immunosuppression, runting syndrome, lymphomas, and acute reticulum cell neoplasia (8, 9). The occurrence of reticuloendotheliosis (RE) has an immunosuppressive effect and REV as the contaminant within vaccines against Marek's Disease (MD) (10), fowlpox (11, 12), and Gallid herpesvirus 2 (GaHV-2) (13), which may lead to vaccination failures and co-incidence

of RE with other secondary infectious agents. Since breeder and layer flocks are commonly vaccinated against MD, the possible congenital transmission of REV between chickens was also be taking into account. The occurrence of RE has major economic importance. So far, no effective vaccines have been developed against RE; thus, the only protection remains flock renewal with elimination of affected birds or application of experimental antiviral treatment. In a previous study, we have confirmed that TRIM62 possesses restriction of avian leukosis virus subgroup J (ALV-J) replication (14). ALV-J is another avian retrovirus. At present, no data are available regarding the role of TRIM62 from chicken in REV infection.

To explore the role of TRIM62 in REV infection, in the present study, we detected and analyzed the association of TRIM62 expression with viral replication. Then, we evaluated the effects of TRIM62 on viral replication by overexpression, silencing, and domain deletion of TRIM62 in CEF cells with REV infection. Further, with TRIM62 overexpression, we screened key proteins that interacted with TRIM62. Our study provided evidence that chicken TRIM62 negative regulated the REV replication.

TABLE 1 | Primers used for quantitative reverse transcription-PCR.

Gene target	Primer sequence	Fragment size (bp)
TRIM62	Forward: TACTGGGAGGTGGTGGTGTC	246
	Reverse: CGTCGGCGTTGTAGAAGATG	
REV (env)	Forward: TTGTTGAAGGCAAGCATCAG	330
	Reverse: GAGGATAGCATCTGCCCTTT	
RAB5B	Forward: CCCCAGCATCGTCATTG	101
	Reverse: GGCTGTTGTCATCTGCGTAA	
ARPC2	Forward: CGGAAAGGTGTTTATGC	223
	Reverse: CAGGTAGTCTCGGAATGTG	
GADPH	Forward: GAACATCATCCCAGCGTCCA	132
	Reverse: CGGCAGGTCAGGTCAACAAC	

MATERIALS AND METHODS

Cell Culture and Viral Infection

The CEF cells' cultural protocol was conducted as described in a previous study (14). CEF cells were incubated with a diluted stock

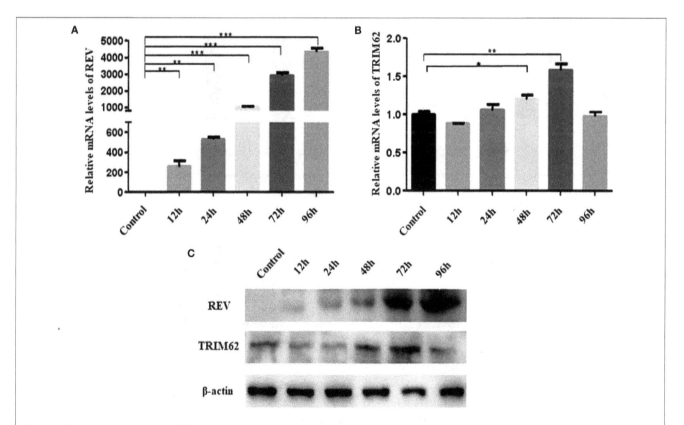

FIGURE 1 | Effect of REV infection on TRIM62 expression. CEF cells were infected with REV. The RNA expression levels of REV **(A)** and of TRIM62 **(B)** at 12, 24, 48, 72, and 96 h post-infection in CEF cells were assessed by qRT-PCR. **(C)** The protein expression levels of REV and TRIM62 were detected by WB. Uninfected CEF cells were used as the control. *$p < 0.05$, **$p < 0.01$, and ***$p < 0.001$.

of SNV strain of REV (China strain: JX0927, maintained in our laboratory) at a multiplicity of infection (MOI) of 0.1. The mRNA expression of TRIM62 and REV in CEF cells were detected at different times (12, 24, 48, 72, and 96 h post-infection). The mRNA expression of TRIM62 in the supernatant was also detected in parallel at the same sampling times.

Plasmid of Chicken TRIM62 and Short Hairpin RNA (shRNA) Transfection

To identify the antiviral function of TRIM62, CEF cells were seeded on six-well-plates for 12 h and transfected with plasmids using a lentiviral vector for TRIM62 overexpression and silence. The transfected plasmids containing chicken TRIM62 (pTRIM62)/domain deletion mutants were for TRIM62 overexpression, and those containing short hairpin RNA targeting TRIM62 (shTRIM62) were for TRIM62 silence. The gene sequence of chicken TRIM62 was obtained from GenBank (XM_015297235.2) (14). These plasmids fused to a Flag tag. The transfected empty vector CEF cells were used as control. The pTRIM62/shTRIM62/pTRIM62-ΔR/B/C/S and empty vector were purchased from Jikai Gene Technology, Inc. (Shanghai, China). After stably expressing TRIM62/shTRIM62 for 12 h/24 h, the transfected CEF cells were incubated with REV. After

72 h, the TRIM62 and viral mRNA/protein levels were detected by qRT-PCR/WB.

Quantitative Real-Time PCR (qRT-PCR)

Total RNA from CEF cells was isolated using the Tiangen RNeasy mini kit according to the manufacturer's instructions. RNA was reverse transcribed to cDNA using the TaqMan Gold Reverse Transcription kit (Applied Biosystems). qRT-PCR was performed according to a previously described protocol (15, 16). Glyceraldehyde 3-phosphate dehydrogenase (GAPDH) was used as a control for basal RNA levels. Primer sequences are listed in **Table 1**.

Western Blotting

The CEF cells were lysed in RIPA lysis buffer [25 mM Tris (pH 7.4), 150 mM NaCl, 1 mM EDTA, 1% NP-40, 5% glycerol] containing protease and phosphatase inhibitor cocktails (Novasygen, Beijing, China). The lysis was separated by SDS-PAGE and transferred to PVDF membranes (Millipore, Bedford, USA) as reported previously (17, 18). The target proteins were detected with specific primary antibodies against TRIM62 (19) and REV env (primary antibodies were prepared by our laboratory, anti-REV gp90) at a 1:200, 1:500, and 1:3,000

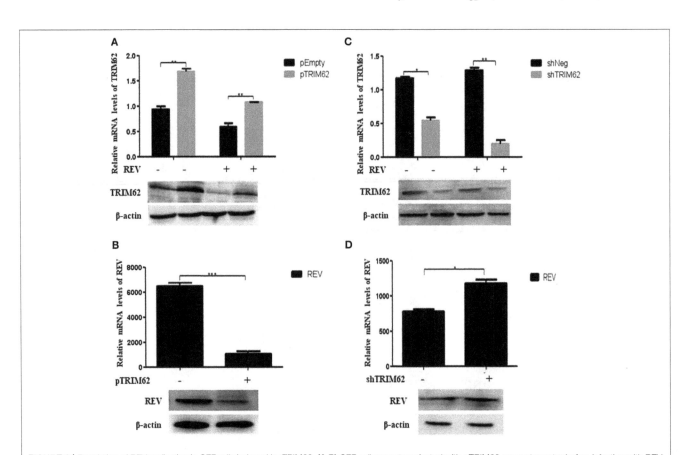

FIGURE 2 | Restriction of REV replication in CEF cells induced by TRIM62. **(A,B)** CEF cells were transfected with pTRIM62 or empty vector before infection with REV. The expression levels of TRIM62 **(A)** and REV **(B)** were assessed by qRT-PCR and Western blotting. **(C,D)** CEF cells were transfected with shTRIM62 or a negative-control shRNA before infection with REV. The expression levels of TRIM62 **(C)** and REV **(D)** were determined by qPCR and Western blotting. *$p < 0.05$, **$p < 0.01$, and ***$p < 0.001$.

dilution, respectively. The secondary antibodies were horseradish peroxidase (HRP)-conjugated enhanced chemiluminescence (ECL) goat. The blots were visualized by the ECL-enhanced chemiluminescence kit (Roche, Basel, Switzerland).

Immunocoprecipitation

According to the instructions of Pierce Co-Immunoprecipitation (Co-IP) Kit (Thermo, Thermo Fisher Scientific, Massachusetts, USA), the 12-h pTRIM62 transfected CEF cells were subjected to REV infection for 72 h. The REV-infected CEF cells were then harvested and lysed. The anti-Flag label antibody was incubated with AminoLink coupling resin for 2 h at room temperature for antibody immobilization. After centrifugation of cell lysates, supernatants were immunoprecipitated with coupling antibody. After another centrifugation of immunoprecipitated

supernatants, the protein complex was washed three times with RIPA lysis buffer. Immunoprecipitates were incubated with elution buffer for 5 min at room temperature and centrifuged. The prey complex was collected and stored at −80°C. CEF cells were transfected with empty vector infected with REV as control.

Liquid Chromatography-Mass Spectrometry Analysis

Ten micrograms of the above prey complex was incubated in SDS-PAGE sample buffer (Solarbio, Beijing, China) for 5 min at 95°C. Proteins of cell lysates were separated by SDS-PAGE gels for 10 min and formed into a line. Each of the SDS-PAGE gel lanes was cut and subjected to trypsin digestion. Mass spectrometry (MS) analysis was performed according to a previously reported protocol (20) for detecting polypeptide

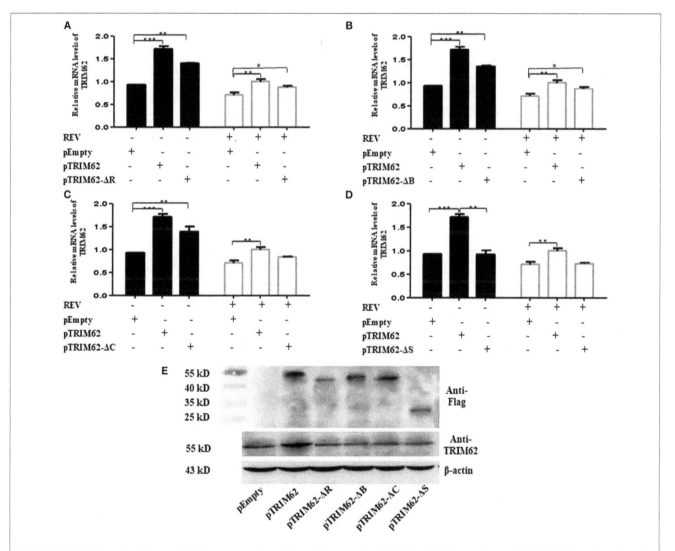

FIGURE 3 | Effect of domain deletion on TRIM62 expression. The relative mRNA expression of TRIM62 in CEF cells transfected with RING (A), B-box (B), coiled-coil (C), or SPRY (D) domain deletion mutant with or without REV infection were measured by qRT-PCR using pEmpty and pTRIM62 as controls. (E) TRIM62 protein expression levels were detected with specific primary antibodies against Flag label and TRIM62 by Western blotting, respectively. pEmpty represent empty vector, pTRIM62 represent TRIM62 full length, pTRIM62-ΔR represent RING domain deletion, pTRIM62-ΔB represent B-box domain deletion, pTRIM62-ΔC represent coiled-coil domain deletion, and pTRIM62-ΔS represent SPRY domain deletion. $^*p < 0.05$, $^{**}p < 0.01$, and $^{***}p < 0.001$.

sequence of proteins. Independent triplicate samples were analyzed. Polypeptide sequence was identified against using the Gallus (chicken) database and viral database (uniport-Gallusgalluschicken_REV_Combined.fasta) using Proteome Discoverer 1.4 (Thermo Fisher Scientific, Massachusetts, USA) software.

Statistical Analysis

Results are presented as the means ± standard deviations (SD) of at least three sample replicates. Statistical analysis was performed using SPSS 19.0 statistical software, and $p < 0.05$ was considered statistically significant.

RESULTS

REV Infection Affected TRIM62 Expression in CEF Cells

To assess association between the expression of TRIM62 and REV, we measured the TRIM62 expression and REV replication in REV-infected CEF cells at the transcriptional and translational level. Time course infection of REV in CEF cells showed that the REV mRNA levels were significantly increased ($p < 0.001$) from 48 to 96 h post-infection (**Figure 1A**), and the TRIM62 mRNA levels were also significantly upregulated at 48 h ($p < 0.1$) and 72 h ($p < 0.1$) as compared to that in uninfected CEF cells. However, compared with control, there were no changes of TRIM62 mRNA levels at another time point (**Figure 1B**). The REV mRNA expression was upregulated and reached the plateau at 96 h post-infection in CEF cells (17).

The protein levels of REV and TRIM62 were detected by WB, which were consistent with the dynamic changes of mRNA levels. Compared with control, the viral protein levels were significantly increased ($p < 0.001$) from 48 to 96 h post-infection, and TRIM62 protein levels were also significantly upregulated at 48 and 72 h ($p < 0.01$). However, there were no changes of TRIM62 protein levels at another time point observed (**Figure 1C**).

TRIM62 Restricted REV Replication in CEF Cells

We overexpressed or silenced TRIM62 to detect the role of TRIM62 in REV replication in infected CEF cells. Compared with non-transfected cells, despite REV infection, the TRIM62 mRNA level was significantly greater ($p < 0.01$) in pTRIM62-transfected CEF cells (**Figure 2A**) and lower ($p < 0.01$) in shTRIM62-transfected CEF cells (**Figure 2C**). The TRIM62 overexpression decreased the REV mRNA expression in transfected cells (**Figure 2B**), whereas silence of TRIM62 increased the mRNA expression of REV (**Figure 2D**). These results were confirmed in protein levels by Western blotting (**Figures 2A–D**). Our results strongly suggest the role of TRIM62 in restricting REV infection.

Domain Deletion-Induced TRIM62's Antiviral Activity Abolished Partially

To further investigate the effect of domain on negative regulation of TRIM62, we explored the effect of TRIM62 domain deletion mutants on TRIM62 expression and REV

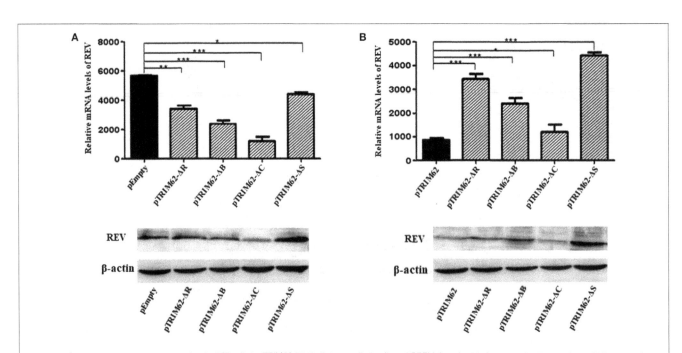

FIGURE 4 | Inhibition of REV RNA expression in CEF cells by TRIM62 RING, B-box, coiled-coil, and SPRY domain deletion mutants. The relative mRNA expression levels of REV in CEF cells transfected with RING, B-box, coiled-coil, or SPRY domain deletion mutants were measured by qRT-PCR and Western blotting. pEmpty **(A)** and pTRIM62 **(B)** were used as controls. pEmpty represent empty vector, pTRIM62 represent TRIM62 full-length, pTRIM62-ΔR represent RING domain deletion, pTRIM62-ΔB represent B-box domain deletion, pTRIM62-ΔC represent coiled-coil domain deletion, and pTRIM62-ΔS represent SPRY domain deletion. $^*p < 0.05$, $^{**}p < 0.01$, and $^{***}p < 0.001$.

replication. The mutants were prepared as previously described (14). Regardless of REV infection, the expression of TRIM62 was significantly higher in cells transfected with deletion of RING (**Figure 3A**) and B-box (**Figure 3B**) than empty vector ($p > 0.1$). When transfected with coiled-coil domain deletion mutant, viral infection decreased the expression of TRIM62 in cells (**Figure 3C**). These results indicated that the effect of REV infection on TRIM62 may associate with the coiled-coil domain. Compared with empty vector, there was no difference

TABLE 2 | Identified proteins interacting with TRIM62.

No.	Accession	Gene	Protein	Coverage
1	A0A1L1RRL2	ACTB	Actin, cytoplasmic 1	30.12
2	A0A1L1RSN4	ACTC1	Actin, alpha cardiac muscle 1	25.61
3	F1NJ08	VIM	Vimentin	17.39
4	E1C2H4	LEMD2	LEM domain containing 2	4.79
5	A0A1L1RWD5	RPL15	Ribosomal protein L15	17.16
6	F1NSP8	HNRNPU	Heterogeneous nuclear ribonucleoprotein U	1.78
7	A0A1D5PW24	RPL19	Ribosomal protein L19	14.05
8	P01994	HBAA	Hemoglobin subunit alpha-A	10.56
9	A0A1L1RLB1	PKM	Pyruvate kinase PKM	5.81
10	**A0A1D5PKU6**	**RAB5**	**Ras-related protein Rab-5**	**5.14**
11	Q05744	CTSD	Cathepsin D	4.52
12	**A0A1L1RPQ9**	**Arp2/3**	**Arp2/3 complex 34 kD subunit**	**3.90**
13	A0A1L1RM78	PPIA	Peptidyl-prolyl cis-trans isomerase	12.00
14	A0A1D5NYW5	N/A	Peptidylprolyl isomerase	7.35
15	A0A1D5PZE3	APOA1	Apolipoprotein A-I	5.70
16	F1NK96	PDIA6	Protein disulfide isomerase family A member 6	6.04
17	A0A1D5PJM6	NUP214	Nucleoporin 214	0.59
18	F1NWX0	LOC425049	Tubulin alpha chain	6.46

The bold means the two proteins are involved in the skeleton pathway.

obtained of TRIM62 expression in cells transfected with deletion of SPRY domain mutant (**Figure 3D**). The qRT-PCR primers located in the SPRY domain may explain this result that deletion of SPRY domain did not result in difference of TRIM62 mRNA expression. To further confirm the results, we measured the TRIM62 protein expression with specific primary antibodies against TRIM62 (**Figure 3E**). The expression of TRIM62 in mutant-transfected cells is lower than that in complete TRIM62-transfected cells.

As compared with pEmpty vector-transfected cells, the level of REV mRNA expression was significant lower ($p < 0.1$) in CEF cells transfected by any of the TRIM62 domain deletion mutants (**Figure 4A**). The effect of coiled-coil domain deletion was the highest (77.9 ± 2.3%), and that of SPRY domain deletion was the lowest (22.8 ± 2.5%). Compared with complete TRIM62, the mRNA expression of REV was significantly higher in cells transfected with domain deletion mutants (**Figure 4B**). The viral expression in SPRY domain deletion-transfected cells was the highest (435.5 ± 6.2%), and that in coiled-coil domain deletion-transfected cells was the lowest (53.2% ± 6.4%). These results suggested that the deletion of domains partially abolished the antiviral activity of TRIM62.

Identification of Cell Proteins That Interact With TRIM62

The REV infection affected the TRIM62 expression first upregulated and then downregulated in CEF cells. We hypothesized that other important interacting proteins besides the domains were involved in TRIM62's negative regulation of REV replication. To identify host cell proteins that interact with TRIM62, we used a tandem affinity purification approach coupled with mass spectrometry-based proteomics technology. These experiments identified 18 cell proteins that coimmunoprecipitated with transiently expressed Flag-tagged TRIM62 (**Table 2**). Decades of HIV research have testified to the integral role of the actin cytoskeleton in both establishing and spreading the infection (21). Of the TRIM62-interacting cell proteins identified, we focused on cytoskeletal proteins RAB5B and ARPC2. To verify the interaction between TRIM62 and RAB5B/ARPC2, CEF cells were transfected with a plasmid expression Flag-tagged RAB5B/APRC2 before REV infection, immunoprecipitated with anti-Flag antibody, and immunoblotted with anti-TRIM62 antibody. CEF cells were

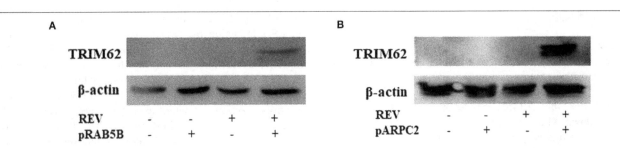

FIGURE 5 | Validation of the interaction of TRIM62 with ARB5B and ARPC2. CEF cells were transfected with a plasmid expression Flag-tagged RAB5B **(A)** and APRC2 **(B)** before REV infection/uninfection and immunoprecipitated with anti-Flag antibody. The TRIM62 in immunoprecipitates was detected by Western blotting with anti-TRIM62 antibody.

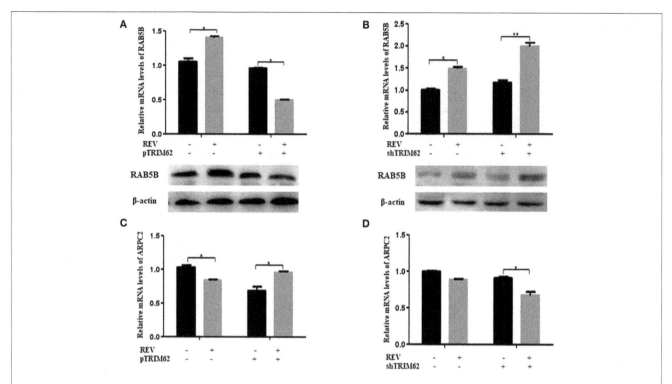

FIGURE 6 | Effect of TRIM62 on the expression of RAB5B and ARPC2. **(A,B)** The relative mRNA and protein expression of RAB5B and in CEF cells were transfected with pTRIM62 **(A)** or shTRIM62 **(B)**. **(C,D)** The relative mRNA expression of ARPC2 in CEF cells were transfected with pTRIM62 **(C)** or shTRIM62 **(D)**. *$p < 0.05$, **$p < 0.01$.

transfected with plasmid or empty vector uninfected with REV and transfected with empty vector infected with REV as control, respectively. Upon REV infection, anti-TRIM62 coprecipitated Flag-tag RAB5B (**Figure 5A**) and Flag-tag ARPC2 (**Figure 5B**).

Further, we found that TRIM62 affected the expression of RAB5B and ARPC2. As shown in **Figures 6A,B**, in CEF cells infected with REV, overexpression of TRIM62 exhibited a decrease of RAB5B expression, and silencing of TRIM62 enhanced the expression of RAB5B. On the contrary, in CEF cells infected with REV, the overexpression of TRIM62 resulted in an increase of ARPC2 expression, and silencing of TRM62 reduced the expression of ARPC2 (**Figures 6C,D**). These results indicated that RAB5B and ARPC2 play important roles in the negative regulation of TRIM62 on REV replication.

DISCUSSION

The host innate immune system senses antigen and elicits local antiviral defense to control infection. However, the REV can evade surveillance by the immune system after infection. TRIM62 is an innate immune regulator (6). In this study, we found that the TRIM62 expression levels were first up and then down with the increase of REV replication in CEF cells. These results suggest that as an innate immune factor, TRIM62 was activated and induced a short periodic significant upregulation at the fast replication period of REV ($p <$ 0.001), and REV may circumvent TRIM62's restrictive effects by reducing its expression levels. However, we did not obtain

valid data of TRIM62 expression in supernatant because the RNA concentration was too low. The reason that TRIM62 expression was first increased and then decreased needed further confirmation.

In the current study, TRIM62 has been identified as a protein that negatively regulates REV replication. Gene silencing of TRIM62 enhanced REV infection, which indicated that TRIM62 contributes to the endogenous restriction of REV in CEF cells. The further characterization of mechanisms by which REV reduces TRIM62 expression is warranted.

Owing to the presence of similar domains, the TRIM proteins were involved in similar antiviral biological processes. However, the domains of TRIM proteins played complicated roles in the inhibition of different viruses. Deletion of the PRY-SPRY domain of TRIM62 from human did not compromise its signal transduction properties. Rather, in addition to the RING domain, both B-box and coiled-coil domains were required for NF-κB and AP-1 induction by TRIM62 (5). Thus, the B-box and/or coiled-coil domains that confer oligomerization/dimerization properties (22) are indispensable for TRIM62-mediated signaling (5). The SPRY domain mediated the affinity for the viral capsid and the function of RING domain to TRIM5α restriction of retrovirus infection was determined by the target virus (23). The antiviral activity of fish TRIM36 required both RING and SPRY domains (24). The RING and C-terminal tail were essential for TRIM56's antiviral activity against flaviviruses (25). Interestingly, the inhibitory effect of fish TRIM62 on interferon immune and inflammation response to negatively regulate virus replication was also dependent on RING and SPRY domains (7). In our study, this varied expression level of mutants (**Figure 3**) could be due to variation in transfection and expression efficiency of different plasmids in primary cells. Even though our results demonstrated that RING, B-box, coiled-coil, and SPRY domains contribute to the antiviral activity of chicken TRIM62, the effect of RING and SPRY was more significant than that of B-box and coiled-coil (**Figures 4A,B**). These results indicated that RING and SPRY domains are related to the antiviral activity of TRIM proteins.

Retroviruses are considered to use vesicular trafficking in infected cells (18, 26, 27). RAB5B is an isoform of RAB5, which is a member of the RAB family, a small GTPase family. RAB5B regulates fusion and motility of early endosomes, and is a marker of the early endosome compartment (28). RAB5B is a major regulator of hepatitis B virus (HBV) production (29). APRC2 is a component of Arp2/3 complex. The T cell-specific deletion of ARPC2 results in compromised peripheral T cell homeostasis (30). T cell survival and proliferation are mediated by complex homeostatic signals. Peripheral T cells are maintained at a constant cell number so that they can efficiently recognize foreign antigens and protect the host from pathogen invasion (31). Thus, of the TRIM62-interacting cell proteins identified, we focused on RAB5B and ARPC2. The interaction between RAB5B/ARPC2 and TRIM62 indicated that they played important roles in TRIM62 negative regulation on REV replication. A detailed understanding of host restriction may lead to antiviral therapies aimed at strengthening the innate immunity to retroviruses at the cellular and molecular level.

In addition, TRIM62 is a putative tumor suppressor and the TRIM62 levels represent an important prognostic marker in lung tumor (32) acute myeloid leukemia (AML) (33) and cervical

cancer (34). ARPC2 promotes proliferation and metastasis (35, 36). REV is an oncogenic retrovirus. Further study is warranted to investigate the potential function of chicken TRIM62 and ARPC2 on REV infection inducing tumor formation.

CONCLUSION

We demonstrated that TRIM62 is a new suppressor that negatively regulates REV replication. The deletion of RING, B-box, coiled-coil, and SPRY domains partially affected TRIM62's antiviral activity, and the effects of RING and SPRY deletion were more significant than that of B-box and coiled-coil. The results suggested that all domains, RING, B-box, coiled-coil, and SPRY domains, are required for chicken TRIM62 to provide host defense against viral replication. Furthermore, both RAB5B and ARPC2 interacted with TRIM62, and maybe played important roles in TRIM62 negative regulation on REV replication. Our study provided a potential antiviral strategy targeting this novel regulator.

AUTHOR CONTRIBUTIONS

GW designed the experiments. LL, DN, and JY performed the experiments. GW, LL, and DN prepared the manuscript. JB, LZ, and ZC analyzed the data. All authors have read and approved the final version of the manuscript.

REFERENCES

1. Lott ST, Chen N, Chandler DS, Yang Q, Wang L, Rodriguez M, et al. DEAR1 is a dominant regulator of acinar morphogenesis and an independent predictor of local recurrence-free survival in early-onset breast cancer. *PLoS Med.* (2009) 6:e1000068. doi: 10.1371/journal.pmed.1000068
2. Reymond A, Meroni G, Fantozzi A, Merla G, Cairo S, Luzi L, et al. The tripartite motif family identifies cell compartments. *EMBO J.* (2001) 20:2140–51. doi: 10.1093/emboj/20.9.2140
3. McNab FW, Rajsbaum R, Stoye JP, O'Garra A. Tripartite-motif proteins and innate immune regulation. *Curr Opin Immunol.* (2011) 23:46–56. doi: 10.1016/j.coi.2010.10.021
4. Napolitano LM, Meroni G. TRIM family: pleiotropy and diversification through homomultimer and heteromultimer formation. *IUBMB Life.* (2012) 64:64–71. doi: 10.1002/iub.580
5. Uchil PD, Hinz A, Siegel S, Coenen-Stass A, Pertel T, Luban J, et al. TRIM protein-mediated regulation of inflammatory and innate immune signaling and its association with antiretroviral activity. *J Virol.* (2013) 87:257–72. doi: 10.1128/JVI.01804-12
6. Uchil PD, Quinlan BD, Chan WT, Luna JM, Mothes W. TRIM E3 ligases interfere with early and late stages of the retroviral life cycle. *PLoS Pathog.* (2008) 4:e16. doi: 10.1371/journal.ppat.0040016
7. Yang Y, Huang Y, Yu Y, Zhou S, Wang S, Yang M, et al. Negative regulation of the innate antiviral immune response by TRIM62 from orange spotted grouper. *Fish Shellfish Immunol.* (2016) 57:68–78. doi: 10.1016/j.fsi.2016.08.035
8. Zavala G, Cheng S, Barbosa T, Haefele H. Enzootic reticuloendotheliosis in the endangered attwater's and greater prairie chickens. *Avian Dis.* (2006) 50:520–25. doi: 10.1637/7655-052806R.1

9. Barth CF, Ewert DL, Olson WC, Humphries EH. Reticuloendotheliosis virus REV-T(REV-A)-induced neoplasia: development of tumors within the T-lymphoid and myeloid lineages. *J Virol.* (1990) 64:6054–62. doi: 10.1128/JVI.64.12.6054-6062.1990
10. Mays JK, Silva RF, Kim T, Fadly A. Insertion of reticuloendotheliosis virus long terminal repeat into a bacterial artificial chromosome clone of a very virulent Marek's disease virus alters its pathogenicity. *Avian Pathol.* (2012) 41:259–65. doi: 10.1080/03079457.2012.675428
11. Awad AM, Abd El-Hamid HS, Abou Rawash AA, Ibrahim HH. Detection of reticuloendotheliosis virus as a contaminant of fowl pox vaccines. *Poult Sci.* (2010) 89:2389–95. doi: 10.3382/ps.2010-00899
12. Koo BS, Lee HR, Jeon EO, Jang HS, Han MS, Min KC, et al. An outbreak of lymphomas in a layer chicken flock previously infected with fowlpox virus containing integrated reticuloendotheliosis virus. *Avian Dis.* (2013) 57:812–17. doi: 10.1637/10551-041113-Case.R1
13. Wozniakowski G, Mamczur A, Samorek-Salamonowicz E. Common occurrence of Gallid herpesvirus-2 with reticuloendotheliosis virus in chickens caused by possible contamination of vaccine stocks. *J Appl Microbiol.* (2015) 118:803–8. doi: 10.1111/jam.12734
14. Li L, Feng W, Cheng Z, Yang J, Bi J, Wang XM, et al. TRIM62-mediated restriction of avian leukosis virus subgroup J replication is dependent on the SPRY domain. *Poult Sci.* (2019) 98:6019–25. doi: 10.3382/ps/pez408
15. Dai M, Feng M, Liu D, Cao W, Liao M. Development and application of SYBR Green I real-time PCR assay for the separate detection of subgroup J Avian leukosis virus and multiplex detection of avian leukosis virus subgroups A and B. *Virol J.* (2015) 12:52–62. doi: 10.1186/s12985-015-0291-7
16. Luan H, Wang Y, Li Y, Cui Z, Chang S, Zhao P. Development of a real-time quantitative RT-PCR to detect REV contamination in live vaccine. *Poult Sci.* (2016) 95:2023–9. doi: 10.3382/ps/pew147

17. Zhou D, Xue J, He S, Du X, Zhou J, Li C, et al. Reticuloendotheliosis virus and avian leukosis virus subgroup J synergistically increase the accumulation of exosomal miRNAs. *Retrovirology*. (2018) 15:45–56. doi: 10.1186/s12977-018-0427-0

18. Wang GH, Wang ZZ, Zhuang PP, Zhao XM, Cheng ZQ. Exosomes carring gag/env of ALV-J possess negative effect on immunocytes. *Microb Pathogenesis*. (2017) 112:142–7. doi: 10.1016/j.micpath.2017.09.013

19. Wang XM, Zhao YL, Li L, Cheng ZQ, Wang GH. Preparation and application of a monoclonal antibody against chicken TRIM62. *Monoclon Antib Immunodiagn Immunother*. (2018) 37:134–8. doi: 10.1089/mab.2017.0062

20. Kalluri R, Weinberg RA. The basics of epithelial-mesenchymal transition. *J Clin Invest*. (2009) 119:1420–8. doi: 10.1172/JCI39104

21. Ospina Stella A, Turville S. All-round manipulation of the actin cytoskeleton by HIV. *Viruses*. (2018) 10:63–96. doi: 10.3390/v10020063

22. Diaz-Griffero F, Qin XR, Hayashi F, Kigawa T, Finzi A, Sarnak Z, et al. A B-Box 2 surface patch important for TRIM5α self-association, capsid binding avidity, and retrovirus restriction. *J Virol*. (2009) 83:10737–51. doi: 10.1128/JVI.01307-09

23. Li X, Kim J, Song B, Finzi A, Pacheco B, Sodroski J. Virus-specific effects of TRIM5α(rh) RING domain functions on restriction of retroviruses. *J Virol*. (2013) 87:7234–45. doi: 10.1128/JVI.00620-13

24. Chen B, Huo S, Liu W, Wang F, Lu Y, Xu Z, et al. Fish-specific finTRIM FTR36 triggers IFN pathway and mediates inhibition of viral replication. *Fish Shellfish Immunol*. (2019) 84:876–84. doi: 10.1016/j.fsi.2018.10.051

25. Liu BM, Li NL, Wang J, Shi PY, Wang TY, Miller MA, et al. Overlapping and distinct molecular determinants dictating the antiviral activities of TRIM56 against Flaviviruses and Coronavirus. *J Virol*. (2014) 88:13821–35. doi: 10.1128/JVI.02505-14

26. Booth AM, Fang Y, Fallon JK, Yang M Jr, Hildreth JEK, Gould SJ. Exosomes and HIV Gag bud from endosome-like domains of the T cell plasma membrane. *J Cell Biol*. (2006) 172:923–36. doi: 10.1083/jcb.200508014

27. Park IW, He JJ. HIV-1 is budded from CD4+ T lymphocytes independently of exosomes. *Virol J*. (2010) 7:234–39. doi: 10.1186/1743-422X-7-234

28. Stenmark H, Parton RG, Steele-Mortimer O, Lütcke A, Gruenberg J, Zerial M. Inhibition of rab5 GTPase activity stimulates membrane fusion in endocytosis. *EMBO J*. (1994) 13:1287–96. doi: 10.1002/j.1460-2075.1994.tb06381.x

29. Inoue J, Ninomiya M, Umetsu T, Nakamura T, Kogure T, Kakazu E, et al. Small interfering RNA screening for the small GTPase Rab proteins identifies Rab5B as a major regulator of Hepatitis B virus production. *J Virol*. (2019) 93:e00621–19. doi: 10.1128/JVI.00621-19

30. Li L, Zhuang PP, Wang XM, Zhou DF, Xue JW, Cheng ZQ, et al. Effects of miRNA-155 on the cytoskeletal pathways in REV and ALV-J Co-Infection. *Chinese J Cell Biol*. (2018) 40:1706–18. doi: 10.11844/cjcb.2018.10.0223

31. Takada K, Jameson SC. Naive T cell homeostasis: from awareness of space to a sense of place. *Nat Rev Immunol*. (2009) 9:823–32. doi: 10.1038/nri2657

32. Quintas-Cardama A, Post SM, Solis LM, Xiong S, Yang P, Chen N, et al. Loss of the novel tumour suppressor and polarity gene Trim62 (Dear1) synergizes with oncogenic Ras in invasive lung cancer. *J Pathol*. (2014) 234:108–19. doi: 10.1002/path.4385

33. Quintás-Cardama A, Zhang N, Qiu YH, Post S, Creighton CJ, Cortes J, et al. Loss of TRIM62 expression is an independent adverse prognostic factor in acute myeloid leukemia. *Clin Lymphoma Myeloma Leuk*. (2015) 15:115–27.e15. doi: 10.1016/j.clml.2014.07.011

34. Liu TY, Chen J, Shang CL, Shen HW, Huang JM, Liang YC, et al. Tripartite motif containing 62 is a novel prognostic marker and suppresses tumor metastasis via c-Jun/Slug signaling-mediated epithelial-mesenchymal transition in cervical cancer. *J Exp Clin Cancer Res*. (2016) 35:170–90. doi: 10.1186/s13046-016-0445-5

35. Cheng Z, Wei W, Wu Z, Wang J, Ding X, Sheng Y, et al. ARPC2 promotes breast cancer proliferation and metastasis. *Oncol Rep*. (2019) 41:3189–200. doi: 10.3892/or.2019.7113

36. Yoon YJ, Han YM, Choi J, Lee YJ, Yun J, Lee SK, et al. Benproperine, an ARPC2 inhibitor, suppresses cancer cell migration and tumor metastasis. *Biochem Pharmacol*. (2019) 163:46–59. doi: 10.1016/j.bcp.2019.01.017

23

Serological Evidence of Exposure to Peste des Petits Ruminants in Small Ruminants in Rwanda

Anselme Shyaka[1]*, Marie Aurore Ugirabe[1] and Jonas Johansson Wensman[2]*

[1] School of Veterinary Medicine, College of Agriculture, Animal Sciences and Veterinary Medicine, University of Rwanda, Nyagatare, Rwanda, [2] Department of Clinical Sciences, Swedish University of Agricultural Sciences, Uppsala, Sweden

*Correspondence:
Anselme Shyaka
a.shyaka2@ur.ac.rw
Jonas Johansson Wensman
jonas.wensman@slu.se

The status of Peste des Petits Ruminants (PPR) in Rwanda is unknown, despite its prevalence in neighboring countries. A cross-sectional sampling of goats and sheep was carried out in five districts of Rwanda located closer to neighboring countries endemic to PPR. Serum samples were analyzed using a commercial ELISA, to detect antibodies to PPR virus (PPRV). Sixty-eight samples [14.8, 95% Confidence Interval (CI): 11.7–18.4] were seropositive for PPR, of which 17.4% (95% CI: 11.6–24.6; 25/144) were from sheep, whereas 13.6% (95% CI: 10.0–17.9; 43/316) were from goats. Seropositivity ranged from 8.9 to 17.3% (goats) and from 10.5 to 25.8% (sheep) in sampled districts. Seropositivity was slightly higher in males than females in both goats (15.7 vs. 12.4%) and sheep (17.7 vs. 17.1%), and were significantly marked in goats and sheep aged more than 15 months (goats: 17.9, 95% CI: 12.9–24.0; sheep: 22.2, 95% CI: 14.1–32.2) than those between 6 and 15 months (goats: 6.1, 95% CI: 2.5–12.1; sheep: 9.3, 95% CI: 3.1–20.3). Sampling was non-randomized and results are not representative of the true prevalence of PPR antibody in small ruminants. Thus, data does not allow to fully discuss the findings beyond the presence/absence certitude and the comparisons made must be interpreted with caution. The presence of specific antibodies to PPRV may, however, be linked to one or a combination of following scenarios: (1) prevalence and persistence of PPRV in sampled regions which would cause low level of clinical cases and/or mortalities that go unnoticed; (2) introduction of PPRV to herds through movements of livestock from neighboring infected countries, and/or (3) events of disease outbreaks that are underreported by farmers and veterinarians. In addition to strengthen veterinary surveillance mechanisms, further studies using robust sampling methods and integrating livestock and wildlife, should be carried out to fully elucidate PPR epidemiology in Rwanda.

Keywords: small ruminants, Rwanda, PPR, seroprevalence, transboundary diseases

INTRODUCTION

Livestock diseases are recognized global threats to food supply and to livestock industry specifically (1). Peste des Petits Ruminants Virus (PPRV) is a member of the family *Paramyxoviridae*, genus *Morbillivirus*, species *Small ruminant morbillivirus* (2). It primarily affects goats and sheep, but also other domestic animals such as cattle, pigs and camels as well as various wildlife ungulates (3, 4), through contact with infected animals, or indirectly through fecal and/or mucosal secretions (5). The disease caused, Peste des Petits Ruminants (PPR), is highly contagious and is characterized by acute clinical signs in goats and sheep, as well as in wild ruminants (6–8). PPR is associated with a case fatality rate of 15.5% (8) that can reach up to 80–100% in naïve herds (9). PPR is recognized as the most widely distributed infectious disease of domestic small ruminants and wildlife ungulates, and is endemic in most countries of Africa, Middle East and Asia (10). It can negatively impact countries' economy and increase poverty in rural settings where small ruminants are mostly concentrated. In fact, PPR-associated losses are estimated at USD 1.2–1.7 billion annually and a third of this financial burden occurs in Africa (10). In addition, PPR constitutes a growing challenge to biodiversity and wildlife conservation (8, 11).

PPR has affected most countries in East Africa since the last 5 decades and confirmation of the first outbreak in Sudan in 1971–1972 (12), followed by further outbreak reports from Ethiopia in 1989–1990 (13). In Uganda, the major PPR outbreak was reported in 2006–2008, in Karamoja region along with a similar report in neighboring Kenya (14, 15). However, previous reports had suggested presence of PPR through seroprevalence studies carried out in the 1980s in Uganda and Kenya (16), in the 2000s in Uganda (17) and an outbreak reported in Uganda in 2003 (18). In addition, antibodies to PPRV were also detected in Ugandan wildlife in 2004 (19), probably as a consequence of spillover of the virus from livestock. Tanzania had its first confirmation of PPR in 2008 (20), with retrospective serological evidence of earlier circulation (17) and PPR is currently considered endemic, including in Kagera and Kigoma regions close to Rwanda (21). In neighboring Burundi, a first outbreak of PPR occurred in December 2017 to February 2018 (22), but retrospective serological analysis detected antibodies to the virus in samples collected in early 2017. A more recent study highlighted circulation of PPRV in livestock and wildlife living in eastern DRC and western Uganda (19). This brief history shows that PPR has had endemic events in various regions of east Africa surrounding Rwanda, with periodic outbreaks and circulation of the virus in various susceptible animals including detection in wildlife. Phylogenetic analyses of circulating viruses, showed that PPRV lineage II, III, and IV are prevalent in DRC, Uganda, Tanzania, Kenya, and Burundi (22–26).

Rwanda status vis-à-vis PPR is unknown (27). In fact, there has never been any empirical study to establish the prevalence of PPR in the country, despite its occurrence in the neighboring countries (9, 19, 22, 24, 28–31). The presence of this disease in the regional countries, transboundary movements of livestock passing through official and non-official entry/exit points and important wildlife species constitute potential factors for PPRV introduction in the country. In order to strengthen prevention mechanisms against PPR in Rwanda toward eradication of PPR by 2030, it is important to establish systems of surveillance as part of the stage 1 or "Assessment stage" of the Global Strategy for the Control and Eradication of PPR (10). An efficient surveillance stage would give insights on whether the disease is present and passes unnoticed, and provide information for the next steps toward the elimination of PPR. Such surveillance mechanisms

must adopt strategies for the control of PPR in susceptible domestic and wild animals in Rwanda, in order to establish presence, circulation and persistence of the virus. This study investigated the prevalence of specific antibodies to PPRV and aimed at providing baseline data that can be used by concerned regulatory bodies and stakeholders to scale up PPR investigation in Rwanda and set up adequate prevention measures.

MATERIALS AND METHODS

Ethical Approval

Ethical approval for this study was obtained from the College of Agriculture, Animal Sciences and Veterinary Medicine, University of Rwanda (Ethical approval reference: 025/17/DRIPGS). Approved consent forms were distributed and signed prior to the interviews and sampling of animals. Sampling of animals was done following the protocols in conformity with the World Organization for Animal Health (OIE) Terrestrial Animal Health Code 2012 (use of animals in research and education).

Area Description and Study Design

Samples were collected from Bugesera, Kirehe, and Nyagatare districts of the eastern Province in Rwanda, and from Gicumbi and Musanze districts of the Northern Province (**Figure 1**). The five sites sampled are relatively close to borders with Uganda to the north, Tanzania to the east and Burundi to the south.

This cross-sectional study was conducted during a period of 3 months, from January to March 2019. Non-probability convenience samples were collected in farms located in the study area, under guidance of local veterinarians. In addition, a small questionnaire was used to collect information related to animal sampled, herd management and general animal health at the farm and its surrounding. Goats and sheep, apparently healthy, non-vaccinated against PPR and having more than 6 months of age, were recruited into the study. To accurately estimate the age of goats and sheep, the age dentition method was used, according to methods described elsewhere (32, 33). To calculate the sample size, we used a recommended formula for estimating the adequate sample size in prevalence study (34). Thus, assuming a large and homogenous population size with an estimated 50% prevalence (P) that optimizes the sample size, with a confidence level set at 95% and ±5% precision, the formula $n = \frac{z^2 P(1-P)}{d^2}$ recommended 385 samples. Finally, 460 blood samples were drawn from jugular veins of apparently healthy goats and sheep, using Vacutainer needles and sterile plain tubes. Samples were allowed to clot overnight in order to maximize sera collection, which were harvested following a centrifugation at 3,000 rpm for 5 min. The sera were then stored at −20°C until screening was done.

Screening of the Samples

The screening for the presence of PPR was done to detect antibodies to the nucleoprotein of Peste the Petits Ruminants virus, using a commercial competitive ELISA (cELISA) kit (ID screen® PPR competition, IDvet Genetics, Grabels, France) according to the manufacturer's instructions. The sensitivity and

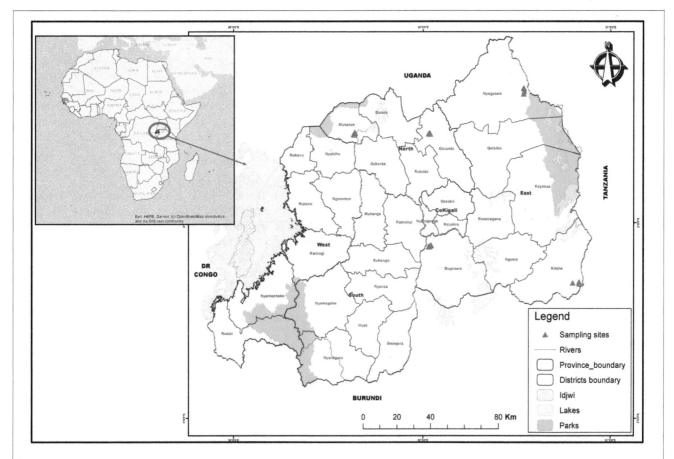

FIGURE 1 | Map of Rwanda districts highlighting sampling sites in East and North areas. The map shows administrative boundaries of districts and provinces. The red triangles highlight sampling sites in Nyagatare, Kirehe and Bugesera districts of the Eastern Province as well as Musanze and Gicumbi districts in the Northern Province.

specificity of this cELISA in sheep and goats, is estimated at 94.5 and 99.4%, respectively, compared to virus neutralization assay (35). The optical densities (ODs) were read using a Thermo Scientific™ Multiskan™ FC Microplate Photometer at a wavelength of 450 nm and the results were expressed as sample positivity percentage (S/N %). Samples were considered positive if the S/N % were ≤50%, negative if ≥60% or doubtful if it was between 50 and 60%. Since the sampled small ruminants had no clinical signs of PPR, doubtful results were finally considered as negative.

Statistical Analyses

The true prevalence in positive animals and herds was estimated by adjusting the apparent prevalence obtained from cELISA results to the sensitivity and specificity of the test, as described by Rogan and Gladen (36). In addition, in order to test for independence between two variables, univariable analysis was done using chi-square test. All the statistical analyses were carried out using R Statistical Software (version 3.6.3; R Foundation for Statistical Computing, Vienna, Austria).

RESULTS

Characteristics of Study Respondents

The descriptions below for study participants and characteristics of farms and small ruminants sampled can be found in **Table 1**.

In total, this study reached 57 households distributed in the 5 districts targeted by this research. Participants were composed of 19 females and 38 males (**Table 1**). The age of respondents ranged between 18 to 87 in females and 16 to 83 in males, with a mean of 44 and 48 years, respectively.

Considering sampled households, 35 of the 57 interviewed (61.4%), reported that small ruminants were managed under a zero-grazing method, in which animals were stall-fed on grasses and food residues. In the remaining herds, 13 and 9 farmers reported to apply open-grazing and semi-zero grazing systems, respectively, in which the small ruminants were allowed to graze freely or go around grazing and get a supplement of food residues once back home. Of the 57 farms targeted, the biggest share (36 out of 57, representing 63.2%) was owning goats, whereas 9 (15.8%) farms had only sheep and 12 (21.1%) had both sheep and goats housed together at farm level. In interviewed farmers, majority (47 of the 57, 82.5%) reported that their animals

TABLE 1 | Characteristics of study respondents and farms sampled (*n* = 45).

Variables		Frequency (%)
District	Nyagatare	6 (10.5)
	Kirehe	18 (31.6)
	Bugesera	7 (12.3)
	Gicumbi	12 (21.1)
	Musanze	14 (24.6)
Gender	Female	19 (33.3)
	Male	38 (67.7)
Age quintiles (years)	<20	5 (8.8)
	21–30	3 (5.3)
	31–40	11 (19.3)
	42–50	17 (29.8)
	>50	21 (36, 8)
Education	No formal education	17 (29.8)
	Primary	28 (49.1)
	Secondary	12 (21.1)
Experience in animal husbandry (years)	<1	1 (1.8)
	1–5	24 (42.1)
	6–10	8 (14.0)
	>10	24 (42.1)
Types of small ruminant owned	Goats only	36 (63.2)
	Sheep only	9 (15.8)
	Goats and Sheep	12 (21.1)
Farming system	Zero-grazing	35 (61.4)
	Semi-zero-grazing	9 (15.8)
	Open grazing	13 (22.8)
Small ruminants disease history	Occurrence of abortions at sampled farms	19 (33.3)
	Occurrence of death at sampled farms	24 (42.1)
Small ruminants disease history in neighboring farms	Report of abortions in neighboring farms	12 (21.1)
	Report of death in neighboring farms	21 (36.8)

were obtained from local livestock markets and others (10/57, making up 17.5%) through various donations. Interestingly, all farmers reported not to observe any quarantine period prior to introduction of new animals in their herds.

Sampled Animals and Occurrence of Small Ruminant Diseases

On a period of 12 months, interviewed farmers reported occurrence of abortions in 19 of their farms, representing 33.3%, whereas 12 farmers (21%) indicated occurrence of abortion incidences in neighboring farms. According to the 19 farmers who experienced abortions, 18 cases occurred in goats whereas 1 case concerned sheep. Also, of the 12 abortion occurrences observed in neighboring farms, all were reportedly observed in goats. Moreover, 24 farms (42.1%) highlighted occurrence of death involving small ruminants at their own farms in the past 12

months, whereas 21 (36.8%) reported events of small ruminant deaths in neighboring farms (**Table 1**).

In total, 316 goats (201 females and 115 males) and 144 sheep (82 females and 62 males) were sampled. Based on age dentition, the goats were classified into three main categories of age: between 6 and 15 months (115 goats), 1.5–3 years (105 goats) and those being more than 3 years (96 goats). Similarly, age estimation in sheep showed that 54 were between 6 and 15 months, 53 were between 1.5 and 3 years, whereas 37 were over 3 years (**Table 2**).

Seroprevalence of PPR

A total of 14.8% (68/460) samples from small ruminants, including 17.4% (25/144) from sheep and 13.6% (43/316) from goats were seropositive for antibodies to PPRV (**Table 3** and **Supplementary Figure 1**). After adjusting to the test specificity and sensitivity, the overall animal-level estimated true prevalence was 15.1% (95% CI: 12.0–18.9), whereas species-level estimated true prevalence was 13.9% (95% CI: 10.3–18.3) and 17.8% (95% CI: 12.2–25.3) in goats and sheep, respectively. Of the 57 farms sampled, 35 had at least one animal seropositive (61.4, 95% CI: 48.4–72.9), giving an estimated farm-level true prevalence of 64.8% (95% CI: 50.9–77.0).

DISCUSSION

Sheep and goats represented 26% of 58,580 metric tons of red meat that was produced in Rwanda in 2017 (37) and this figure is expected to raise to meet growing population. Small ruminants are mainly raised for income generation through sales, but also for meat, wool and manure used in crop fields.

Information generated from this study show that diseases affecting small ruminant and causing deaths and/or abortions are prevalent in the sampled regions. However, due to inadequate veterinary services penetration in rural Rwandan regions, characterized by widespread of less qualified veterinary paraprofessionals (VPP), inadequate veterinary supervision of the VPP (38, 39) and unavailability of supporting laboratory services, diseases that caused abortions were not clearly identified and/or communicated to farmers. PPR is known to cause abortions at all stages of the pregnancy (40). Among possible differential diagnosis, Rift Valley Fever (RVF), another disease that causes abortions in affected animals (41), must be taken into consideration as a possible factor associated to the episodes reported by farmers. In fact, Rwanda has had its first outbreak of RVF declared in 2018 (42) and cases were mainly identified in the eastern region of the country, part of our study area.

This study is the first one to report seroprevalence of PPR in Rwanda. Our laboratory analyses indicated an estimated overall true prevalence of 15.1% (95% CI: 12.0–18.9) and seropositivity of 13.9% (95% CI: 10.3–18.3) and 17.8% (95% CI: 12.2–25.3) in goats and sheep, respectively. These findings of PPRV-specific antibodies circulating in goats and sheep sampled in various areas, constitute evidence of exposure to the disease. Further studies are needed to provide more insights on the epidemiology of PPR in Rwanda. For instance, other investigations should

TABLE 2 | Characteristics of small ruminants sampled.

Characteristics		Goats	Sheep	Total
Sex	Male	115	62	177
	Female	201	82	283
	Total	316	144	460
Age	6–15 months	115	54	169
	1.5–3 years	105	53	158
	>3 years	96	37	133
	Total	316	144	460

TABLE 3 | Seroprevalence of PPR in Small Ruminants according to various disease risk factors.

	Risk factors	Goats				Sheep			
		Total No. of samples	No. of positive samples	Sero-prevalence %	95% CI	Total No. of samples	No. of positive samples	Sero-prevalence %	95% CI
District	Nyagatare	75	13	17.3	(9.6–27.8)	21	4	19.0	(5.4–41.9)
	Bugesera	59	8	13.6	(6.0–25.0)	44	6	13.6	(5.2–27.4)
	Kirehe	70	9	12.9	(6.1–23.0)	29	5	17.2	(5.9–35.8)
	Musanze	56	8	14.3	(6.4–26.2)	31	8	25.8	(11.9–44.6)
	Gicumbi	56	5	8.9	(3.0–19.6)	19	2	10.5	(1.3–33.1)
	Total	316	43	13.6	(10.0–17.9)	144	25	17.4	(11.6–24.6)
Sex	Male	115	18	15.7	(9.5–23.6)	62	11	17.7	(9.2–29.5)
	Female	201	25	12.4	(8.2–17.8)	82	14	17.1	(9.7–27.0)
	Total	316	43	13.6	(10.0–17.9)	144	25	17.4	(11.6–24.6)
Age	6–15 months	115	7	6.1	(2.5–12.2)	54	5	9.3	(3.1–20.3)
	1.5–3 years	105	17	16.2	(9.7–24.7)	53	12	22.6	(12.3–36.2)
	>3 years	96	19	19.8	(12.4–29.2)	37	8	21.6	(9.8–38.2)
	Total	316	43	13.6	(10.0–17.9)	144	25	17.4	(11.6–24.6)
Farming system	Zero grazing	155	18	11.6	(7.0–17.7)	67	14	20.9	(11.9–32.6)
	Semi-zero grazing	37	6	16.2	(6.2–32.0)	20	2	10.0	(1.2–31.7)
	Open grazing	124	19	15.3	(9.5–22.9)	57	9	15.8	(7.5–27.9)
	Total	316	43	13.6	(10.0–17.9)	144	25	17.4	(11.6–24.6)

provide more information on nation-wide prevalence in susceptible domestic and wildlife animals, risk factors associated to PPR prevalence and phylogenetic characterization of circulating viruses in an attempt to determine origin, spread and distribution of various virus lineages and risk factors in Rwanda.

Based on laboratory data from this cross-sectional study, we certainly can confirm the exposure of goats and sheep to PPRV in sampled regions. The comparisons of prevalence with regional findings, should be undertaken carefully. In addition, this study has estimated prevalence of PPR in goats and sheep using non-probability sampling methods. Therefore, it does not allow generalizing the findings at country and small ruminant population level.

PPR is a well-known disease in the region as shown by endemic as well as epidemic events having been reported in Uganda, Tanzania, Burundi and Democratic Republic

of Congo (9, 19, 22, 24, 28, 29, 43). In addition to reports of major outbreak in the region, various retrospective serological analyses, showed positive antibodies to PPRV and confirmed the prevalence of the virus and its circulation before occurrence of all recent outbreaks in above countries (17, 19, 22). Therefore, Rwanda Veterinary Services should strengthen active surveillance mechanisms in order to fully investigate prevalence of the disease and adopt prevention measures before occurrence of large outbreaks in the country.

Future studies on PPR in Rwanda should depict a clearer picture of the epidemiology of the disease in Rwanda. For example, due to limitations inherent to this study, some unanswered questions were for example, the difference in the distribution of PPR across various regions and possible contribution of animal age, sex, and husbandry to the occurrence of PPR.

Our data suggests a correlation between the age of the sampled animals and seroprevalence status within age groups. In fact, small ruminants of more than 15 months were more affected than younger ones. This finding is in conformity with other studies on PPR (28, 44) and can be explained by the facts that older animals have had more exposure time to the virus, especially if this is endemic in the region. In addition, older animals tend to move far from their home in search of greener pastures and water bodies. Some study participants (10 of the 57 interviewed, **Table 1**) reported that their small ruminants were acquired through livestock donating initiatives. Therefore, we cannot rule out the possibility that the livestock were seropositive to PPRV, when gifted to farmers. The presence of antibodies in younger animals is however suggestive of recent virus circulation in Rwanda and this should be investigated further.

Phylogenetic investigations showed that the virus lineages II, III and IV are circulating in the region. Based on limited available sequences, the lineage III seems predominating in western Uganda, eastern DRC and Burundi with sequence similarities in some countries such as DRC and Burundi (19). In addition, the 2017 outbreak of PPR that occurred in various regions in Burundi, followed introduction of Boer goats from potentially infected regions of Uganda and the goats were transported through Tanzania suggesting transboundary movements as possible route of PPRV transmission (22). The regional virus circulation, added to report of PPRV at wildlife-livestock interface in Kabale, Kisoro and eastern DRC; regions close to Rwanda (19), puts an emphasize on the role of movements of livestock across transnational boundaries as well as the role of wildlife animals in the circulation and maintenance of PPRV in the region. Our findings suggest that PPR is prevalent in Rwandan regions close to neighboring countries and areas with recent PPR outbreak events. Rwanda is located in an area characterized by large livestock as well as wildlife populations. In addition, the region is known for important livestock trade between regional countries including Rwanda, and eastern part of DRC (45). The presence of livestock and wildlife and trade movements across countries, could have contributed to the introduction of PPR in north and west parts of Rwanda. Last but not least, Rwanda has experienced large movements of returning citizens from neighboring countries in 1994 and from Tanzania in 2007 as well as Burundian refugees in 2015 (46–48). These movements of people and their livestock could have contributed to the introduction of PPR in various regions of Rwanda. Molecular epidemiology studies and analysis of transboundary livestock movements could shed more insights on PPR epidemiology in Rwanda and the region.

As a preliminary report, this study has several limitations. First, although PPR has never been declared in Rwanda, samples were taken from places relatively close to the borders of the country with countries with known reports of PPR in past years. Due to possible more intense transboundary livestock movements in sampled areas than in other parts of the country, the prevalence found in this study may not necessarily reflect a country-large situation. To minimize this bias, the calculation of needed sample size, assumed a prevalence of 50% which is a condition that maximizes the sample size. Secondly, sampling methods were non-randomized and only a small number of farms was reached. Therefore, without assumption of a homogenous population, the data presented may not be representative of the entire population of small ruminant farmers. Therefore, the current findings do not allow to calculate the true prevalence, analyse the risk factors or to compare prevalence across the study areas. Third, cross-sectional surveys are not suitable for detection of rare, non-endemic diseases such as PPR with an unknown status in Rwanda.

Further studies are needed to collect representative evidence, informative for the eradication and control programs. In this regard, comprehensive studies using probabilistic sampling methods are recommended to investigate PPR at wildlife-livestock interface in Rwandan regions neighboring DRC, Uganda, Tanzania and Burundi. Such studies would help to follow up the occurrence of disease events in small ruminants, and would retrospectively collect evidence of possible endemicity of PPR. This is justified by the possibility of regional circulation of the virus along with livestock transboundary movements as hypothesized by previous studies (19, 22). Rwanda is home to natural parks and forests which may serve as PPRV hotspots at the interface of livestock and wildlife. Therefore, future studies in Rwanda and the region, must take into consideration the livestock and wildlife components, in order to fully understand the epidemiology of PPR.

AUTHOR CONTRIBUTIONS

AS contributed to conceptualization, laboratory analysis, data curation, investigation, methodology, and writing original draft. MU participated in conceptualization, investigation, methodology, and manuscript editing. JW contributed to conceptualization, funding acquisition, supervision, review of the manuscript, and editing conception and design of the study. All authors contributed to the article and approved the submitted version.

ACKNOWLEDGMENTS

We would like to thank Mr. Elysé Ndizeye and Mr. Justin Rucamihigo for their participation in data collection during this study. We would like to thank the Ministry of Agriculture and Animal Resources through the Rwanda Agriculture and Animal Resources Development Board (RAB) for their support in accessing the National Veterinary Laboratory facilities. We are grateful to Dr. Karin Alvåsen from Swedish University of Agricultural Sciences, for valuable discussions.

SUPPLEMENTARY MATERIAL

Supplementary Figure 1 | Percentage Inhibition (PI) distribution based on competitive ELISA results (ID screen® PPR competition, IDvet Genetics, Grabels, France). The distributions are shown by sampled locations (District). Positive samples have below 50% PI and are shown in the graphs with a dark dashed black line.

REFERENCES

1. Boshra H, Truong T, Nfon C, Gerdts V, Tikoo S, Babiuk LA, et al. Capripoxvirus-vectored vaccines against livestock diseases in Africa. *Antiviral Res.* (2013) 98:217-27. doi: 10.1016/j.antiviral.2013.02.016
2. Amarasinghe GK, Ayllón MA, Bào Y, Basler CF, Bavari S, Blasdell KR, et al. Taxonomy of the order Mononegavirales: update 2019. *Arch Virol.* (2019) 164:1967-80. doi: 10.1007/s00705-019-04247-4
3. Munir M. Role of wild small ruminants in the epidemiology of peste des petits ruminants. *Transbound Emerg Dis.* (2014) 61:411-24. doi: 10.1111/tbed.12052
4. Rahman AU, Dhama K, Ali Q, Hussain I, Oneeb M, Chaudhary U, et al. Peste des petits ruminants in large ruminants, camels and unusual hosts. *Vet Q.* (2020) 40:35-42. doi: 10.1080/01652176.2020.1714096
5. Baron MD, Parida S, Oura CAL. Peste des petits ruminants: a suitable candidate for eradication? *Vet Rec.* (2011) 169:16-21. doi: 10.1136/vr.d3947
6. Aziz-ul-Rahman, Wensman JJ, Abubakar M, Shabbir MZ, Rossiter P. Peste des petits ruminants in wild ungulates. *Trop Anim Health Prod.* (2018) 50:1815-9. doi: 10.1007/s11250-018-1623-6
7. Kock R. *Investigation of Peste des Petits Ruminants (PPR) Among Wild Animals and its Potential Impact on the Current PPR Situation in Livestock.* Mission Report 20th January – 1st February 2017. Rome: Crisis Management Centre of the OIE/FAO (2017).
8. Pruvot M, Fine AE, Hollinger C, Strindberg S, Damdinjav B, Buuveibaatar B, et al. Outbreak of peste des petits ruminants virus among critically endangered mongolian saiga and other wild ungulates, Mongolia, 2016-2017. *Emerg Infect Dis.* (2020) 26:51-62. doi: 10.3201/eid2601.181998
9. Torsson E, Kgotlele T, Berg M, Mtui-Malamsha N, Swai ES, Wensman JJ, et al. History and current status of peste des petits ruminants virus in Tanzania. *Infect Ecol Epidemiol.* (2016) 6:32701. doi: 10.3402/iee.v6.32701
10. Food and Agriculture Organization of the United Nations World Organisation for Animal Health. *Global Strategy for the Control and Eradication of PPR.* (2015). Available online at: http://www.oie.int/eng/PPR2015/doc/PPR-Global-Strategy-avecAnnexes_2015-03-28.pdf (accessed January 5, 2021).
11. Aguilar XF, Fine AE, Pruvot M, Njeumi F, Walzer C, Kock R, et al. PPR virus threatens wildlife conservation. *Science.* (2018) 362:165-6. doi: 10.1126/science.aav4096
12. El Hag Ali B, Taylor WP. Isolation of peste des petits ruminants virus from the Sudan. *Res Vet Sci.* (1984) 36:1-4. doi: 10.1016/S0034-5288(18)31991-X
13. Roeder PL, Abraham G, Kenfe G, Barrett T. Peste des petits ruminants in Ethiopian goats. *Trop Anim Health Prod.* (1994) 26:69-73. doi: 10.1007/BF02239901
14. Banyard AC, Parida S, Batten C, Oura C, Kwiatek O, Libeau G. Global distribution of peste des petits ruminants virus and prospects for improved diagnosis and control. *J Gen Virol.* (2010) 91:2885-97. doi: 10.1099/vir.0.025841-0
15. Luka PD, Erume J, Mwiine FN, Ayebazibwe C. Molecular characterization of peste des petits ruminants virus from the Karamoja region of Uganda (2007-2008). *Arch Virol.* (2012) 157:29-35. doi: 10.1007/s00705-011-1135-4
16. Wamwayi HM, Rossiter PB, Kariuki DP, Wafula JS, Barrett T, Anderson J. Peste des petits ruminants antibodies in east Africa. *Vet Rec.* (1995) 136:199-200. doi: 10.1136/vr.136.8.199
17. Karimuribo ED, Loomu PM, Mellau LSB, Swai ES. Retrospective study on sero-epidemiology of peste des petits ruminants before its official confirmation in northern Tanzania in 2008. *Res Opin Anim Vet Sci.* (2011) 1:184-7.
18. AU-IBAR. *Pan African Animal Health Yearbook 2003.* Nairobi, Kenya: Interafrican Bureau for Animal Resources and African Union (2003).
19. Aguilar XF, Mahapatra M, Begovoeva M, Kalema-Zikusoka G, Driciru M, Ayebazibwe C, et al. Peste des petits ruminants at the wildlife-livestock interface in the northern Albertine Rift and Nile Basin, East Africa. *Viruses.* (2020) 12:293. doi: 10.3390/v12030293
20. Kivaria FM, Kwiatek O, Kapaga AM, Swai ES, Libeau G, Moshy W, et al. The incursion, persistence and spread of peste des petits ruminants in Tanzania: epidemiological patterns and predictions. *Onderstepoort J Vet Res.* (2013) 80:593. doi: 10.4102/ojvr.v80i1.593
21. Kgotlele T, Torsson E, Kasanga CJ. Seroprevalence of peste des petits ruminants virus from samples collected in different regions of Tanzania in 2013 and 2015. *J Vet Sci Technol.* (2016) 07:394. doi: 10.4172/2157-7579.1000394
22. Niyokwishimira A, de Baziki J, Dundon WG, Nwankpa N, Njoroge C, Boussini H, et al. Detection and molecular characterization of Peste des Petits Ruminants virus from outbreaks in Burundi, December 2017–January 2018. *Transbound Emerg Dis.* (2019) 66:2067-73. doi: 10.1111/tbed.13255
23. Mahapatra M, Sayalel K, Muniraju M, Eblate E, Fyumagwa R, Shilinde S, et al. Spillover of peste des petits ruminants virus from domestic to wild ruminants in the Serengeti ecosystem, Tanzania. *Emerg Infect Dis.* (2015) 21:2230-4. doi: 10.3201/eid2112.150223
24. Nkamwesiga J, Coffin-Schmitt J, Ochwo S, Mwiine FN, Palopoli A, Ndekezi C, et al. Identification of peste des petits ruminants transmission hotspots in the Karamoja subregion of Uganda for targeting of eradication interventions. *Front Vet Sci.* (2019) 6:221. doi: 10.3389/fvets.2019.00221
25. Misinzo G, Kgotlele T, Muse EA, Van Doorsselaere J, Berg M, Munir M. Peste des petits ruminants virus lineage II and IV from goats in Southern Tanzania During an outbreak in 2011. *Br J Virol.* (2015) 2:1-4.
26. Kgotlele T, Macha ES, Kasanga CJ, Kusiluka LJM, Karimuribo ED, Van Doorsselaere J, et al. Partial genetic characterization of peste des petits ruminants virus from goats in Northern and Eastern Tanzania. *Transbound Emerg Dis.* (2014) 61:56-62. doi: 10.1111/tbed.12229
27. OIE. *Map of PPR Official Status.* OIE - World Organisation for Animal Health (2020). Available online at: https://www.oie.int/animal-health-in-the-world/official-disease-status/peste-des-petits-ruminants/en-ppr-carte/ (accessed August 16, 2020).
28. Torsson E, Berg M, Misinzo G, Herbe I, Kgotlele T, Päärni M, et al. Seroprevalence and risk factors for peste des petits ruminants and selected differential diagnosis in sheep and goats in Tanzania. *Infect Ecol Epidemiol.* (2017) 7:1368336. doi: 10.1080/20008686.2017.1368336
29. Swai ES, Kapaga A, Kivaria F, Tinuga D, Joshua G, Sanka P. Prevalence and distribution of Peste des petits ruminants virus antibodies in various districts of Tanzania. *Vet Res Commun.* (2009) 33:927-36. doi: 10.1007/s11259-009-9311-7
30. OIE. *WAHIS Country report, the Democratic Republic of the Congo.* (2012). Available online at: http://www.oie.int/wahis_2/public/wahid.php/Reviewreport/Review?page_refer=MapFullEventReport%26reportid=11810 (accessed January 6, 2021).
31. Tshilenge GM, Walandila JS, Kikukama DB, Masumu J, Katshay Balowa L, Cattoli G, et al. Peste des petits ruminants viruses of lineages II and III identified in the Democratic Republic of the Congo. *Vet Microbiol.* (2019) 239:108493. doi: 10.1016/j.vetmic.2019.108493
32. Casburn G. *How to Tell the Age of Sheep.* Orange, NSW: NSW Department of Primary Industries (2016)
33. Mitchell T. *How to tell, the age of the domestic animals.* Orange, Australia: NSW Agriculture Agfacts (2003). Available online at: www.agric.nsw.gov.au (accessed August 5, 2020).
34. Wayne WD, Chad LC. *Biostatistics: A Foundation for Analysis in the Health Sciences.* 11th ed. Hoboken, NJ: John Wiley & Sons, Ltd. (2018).
35. Libeau G, Prehaud C, Lancelot R, Colas F, Guerre L, Bishop DHL, et al. Development of a competitive ELISA for detecting antibodies to the peste des petits ruminants virus using a recombinant nucleobrotein. *Res Vet Sci.* (1995) 58:50-5. doi: 10.1016/0034-5288(95)90088-8
36. Rogan WJ, Gladen B. Estimating prevalence from the results of a screening test. *Am J Epidemiol.* (1978) 107:71-6. doi: 10.1093/oxfordjournals.aje.a112510
37. MINAGRI. *Rwanda Livestock Master Plan.* Kigali, Rwanda: MINAGRI (2017). Available online at: http://extwprlegs1.fao.org/docs/pdf/rwa172923.pdf (accessed January 06, 2021).
38. World Organisation for Animal Health. *OIE PVS Evaluation Follow-Up Mission Report, Rwanda.* (2019). Available online at: https://www.oie.int/fileadmin/Home/eng/Support_to_OIE_Members/pdf/20191218_Rwanda_PVS_FU_report_2019_final.pdf (accessed August 8, 2020).
39. Brown C, Havas K, Bowen R, Mariner J, Fentie KT, Kebede E, et al. Animal health in a development context. *Glob Food Sec.* (2020) 25:100369. doi: 10.1016/j.gfs.2020.100369
40. Abubakar M, Ali Q, Khan HA. Prevalence and mortality rate of peste des petitis ruminant (ppr): possible association with abortion in goat. *Trop Anim Health Prod.* (2008) 40:317-321. doi: 10.1007/s11250-007-9105-2

41. Wright D, Kortekaas J, Bowden TA, Warimwe GM. Rift valley fever: biology and epidemiology. *J Gen Virol.* (2019) 100:1187–99. doi: 10.1099/jgv.0.001296

42. OIE. *Rift Valley Fever, Rwanda.* (2018). Available online at: https://www.oie.int/wahis_2/public/wahid.php/Reviewreport/Review?page_refer=MapFullEventReport&reportid=27540 (accessed August 16, 2020).

43. Ruhweza S., Ayebazibwe C, Mwiine F., Muhanguzi D, Olaho W. Seroprevalence of Peste des Petits Ruminants (PPR) virus antibodies in goats and sheep in north-eastern Uganda. *Bull Anim Heal Prod Africa.* (2010) 58:141–6. doi: 10.4314/bahpa.v58i2.62048

44. Mahamat O, Doungous T, Kebkiba B, Oumar HA, Oussiguéré A, Yacoub AH, et al. Seroprevalence, geographical distribution, and risk factors of peste des petits ruminants in the Republic of Chad. *J Adv Vet Anim Res.* (2018) 5:420–5. doi: 10.5455/javar.2018.e293

45. Rweyemamu M, Roeder P, MacKay D, Sumption K, Brownlie J, Leforban Y, et al. Epidemiological patterns of foot-and-mouth disease worldwide. *Transbound Emerg Dis.* (2008) 55:57–72. doi: 10.1111/j.1865-1682.2007.01013.x

46. Nahimana MR, Ngoc CT, Olu O, Nyamusore J, Isiaka A, Ndahindwa V, et al. Knowledge, attitude and practice of hygiene and sanitation in a Burundian refugee camp: implications for control of a Salmonella typhi outbreak. *Pan Afr Med J.* (2017) 28:54. doi: 10.11604/pamj.2017.28.54.12265

47. Kanyamibwa S. Impact of war on conservation: Rwandan environment and wildlife in agony. *Biodivers Conserv.* (1998) 7:1399–406. doi: 10.1023/A:1008880113990

48. Dusabe MC, Wronski T, Gomes-Silva G, Plath M, Albrecht C, Apio A. Biological water quality assessment in the degraded Mutara rangelands, northeastern Rwanda. *Environ Monit Assess.* (2019) 191:139. doi: 10.1007/s10661-019-7226-5

Coinfection and Genetic Characterization of Porcine Astrovirus in Diarrheic Piglets in China from 2015 to 2018

Mingjun Su [1,2†], *Shanshan Qi* [1,2†], *Dan Yang* [1,2], *Donghua Guo* [1,2], *Baishuang Yin* [3] and *Dongbo Sun* [1,2*]

[1] Laboratory for the Prevention and Control of Swine Infectious Diseases, College of Animal Science and Veterinary Medicine, Heilongjiang Bayi Agricultural University, Daqing, China, [2] Heilongjiang Province Cultivating Collaborative Innovation Center for the Beidahuang Modern Agricultural Industry Technology, Daqing, China, [3] College of Animal Science and Technology, Jilin Agricultural Science and Technology University, Jilin, China

*Correspondence:
Dongbo Sun
dongbosun@126.com

[†]These authors have contributed equally to this work

Porcine astrovirus (PAstV) is broadly distributed globally and exists as at least five distinct genotypes. PAstV, which was recently identified as an important pathogen of diarrhea in piglets, is widely distributed in China. However, few studies have investigated the coinfection and genetic characterization of PAstV in diarrheic piglets in China. In this study, 89 PAstV-positive samples were identified in 543 diarrhea samples in China from 2015 to 2018, of which 75.28% (67/89) were coinfected with three to five different porcine pathogens, while none were positive for PAstV only. Among the 543 diarrhea samples, statistical analysis showed that PAstV-induced diarrhea was potentially associated with coinfection of PEV ($p < 0.01$) and GARV ($p < 0.01$). Phylogenetic analysis showed that the 27 identified PAstV strains belong to three different genotypes and that PAstV-2 (81.48%, 22/27) was predominant in diarrheic piglets in China, followed by PAstV-4 (11.11%, 3/27) and PAasV-5 (7.41%, 2/27). Sequence analysis revealed that the 27 RdRp genes identified in this study had nucleotide homologies of 53.8–99.5%. In addition, the RdRp gene of PAstV-4 strain JL/MHK/2018/0115 harbored a unique insert of three nucleotides (GAA) as compared with other known PAstV-4 strains. Furthermore, the genotypes of PAstV varied among different geographical locations, although PAstV-2 was the most widely distributed in China. These data demonstrate that PAstV coinfection with other porcine pathogens was common and there was genetic diversity of PAstV in diarrheic piglets in China.

Keywords: PAstV, coinfection, genetic characterization, diarrhea, piglet

INTRODUCTION

Porcine astrovirus (PAstV), belonging to the family *Astroviridae*, genus *Mamastrovirus*, is a non-enveloped, single-strand, positive-sense RNA virus (1). The PAstV genome consists of three open reading frames (ORFs): ORF1a, ORF1b, and ORF2. ORF1a and ORF1b encode non-structural proteins and the RNA-dependent RNA polymerase (RdRp), and ORF2 encodes the capsid protein (2). PAstV was first identified in diarrheic piglets in 1980 (1). Since then, PAstV has been isolated worldwide, including Europe, Asia, and the Americas (1, 3–6).

Diarrhea of piglets has long been a problem afflicting the global pig industry. Coinfections with more than one porcine pathogen are common and often more clinically severe (7, 8). A previous surveillance study conducted by our group found a high percentage of coinfection among diarrheic piglets (9). PAstV, which has been identified as an important agent of diarrhea (10), and frequently presents as a coinfection with other porcine pathogens (3, 5, 6, 9, 11). However, data regarding coinfections with PAstV in diarrheic piglets in China are limited. Therefore, coinfections with PAstV and other porcine pathogens should be monitored in China.

To date, five genotypes of PAstV (PAstV-1 to PAstV-5) with different prevalences have been identified worldwide. Although all five PAstV genotypes have been reported in Europe, the most common is reportedly PAstV-4 (4), while PAstV-2 and PAstV-4 are the most common throughout Asia (5, 6, 12). However, information available on the genetic characterization of PAstV in China is fairly limited (2, 11). Therefore, it is necessary to investigate the genetic diversity and evolution of PAstV currently in China.

In this study, 89 PAstV-positive diarrhea samples were collected to investigate the prevalence of PAstV coinfection with 12 other porcine pathogens. The obtained RdRp genes were genetically characterized in order to provide insights into the epidemiology of PAstV circulating among diarrheic piglets in China.

MATERIALS AND METHODS

Sample Collection

In our previous study (9), 89 (16.4%) of 543 diarrhea samples collected from 17 provinces or municipalities in China (Anhui, Fujian, Guangdong, Hebei, Heilongjiang, Hubei, Hunan, Jiangxi, Jilin, Liaoning, Shandong, Shaanxi, Shanxi, Sichuan, Shanghai, and the Inner Mongolia Autonomous Region; **Table S1**) from 2015 to 2018 were confirmed as PAstV-positive by reverse-transcription polymerase chain reaction (RT-PCR) and stored at −80°C.

Sequencing and Analysis of the RdRp Gene of PAstV

RNA extraction and cDNA synthesis were performed as previously described by Wang et al. (13). The PAstV RdRp gene was amplified using the nested RT-PCR method described by Chu et al. (14) and then cloned into the vector pMD18-T (TaKaRa Biotechnology Co., Ltd, Dalian, China) in accordance with the manufacturer's protocol. Three positive clones of each amplicon were subjected to Sanger sequencing. Sequence analysis was conducted using the EditSeq tool included with the Lasergene DNASTAR™ 5.06 software package (DNASTAR Inc., Madison, WI, USA). Multiple-sequence alignments were performed using the multiple-sequence alignment tool included with the DNAMAN 6.0 software package (Lynnon BioSoft, Pointe-Claire, QB, Canada).

Phylogenetic Analysis

Sequences of the PAstV RdRp gene retrieved from the GenBank database (https://www.ncbi.nlm.nih.gov/genbank/) were used for sequence alignments and phylogenetic analyses. Multiple-sequence alignments were generated using the ClustalX alignment program included with the MEGA 6.06 software package (15). A phylogenetic tree was constructed from the aligned nucleotide sequences using the p-distance model and 1000 bootstrap replicates and annotated with Interactive Tree Of Life (iTOL) software (http://itol.embl.de/) (16).

Statistical Analysis

The correlation of PAstV infection with other pathogens was assessed with the use of 2 × 2 contingency tables and the chi-square (χ^2) test with confidence limits of 95%. All analyses were performed using IBM SPSS Statistics for Windows, version 22.0 (IBM Corporation, Armonk, NY, USA). Probability (p) values of <0.05 and 0.01 were considered statistically significant and highly significant, respectively. Data regarding the detection of porcine circovirus type 3, porcine group A rotavirus (GARV), mammalian reovirus, porcine bocavirus, porcine deltacoronavirus, porcine enterovirus 9/10 (PEV), porcine kobuvirus (PKV), porcine sapelovirus, porcine torovirus, porcine teschovirus, porcine transmissible gastroenteritis virus (TGEV), and torque teno sus virus 2 in the 543 diarrhea samples (including the 89 PAstV-positive samples) were published in our previous reports (9, 17).

RESULTS AND DISCUSSION

Coinfection of PAstV With Multiple Porcine Pathogens in Diarrheic Piglets

As reported in our previous study, the PAstV-positive rate in diarrheic piglets was 16.39% (89/543), indicating wide distribution in China (9). In the present study, PAstV coinfection with 12 other porcine pathogens in diarrheic piglets was investigated. Of the 89 PAstV-positive diarrhea samples, the rate of PAstV coinfection with 12 other porcine pathogens ranged from 7.87% (7/89) to 85.39% (76/89) (**Figure 1A**). The average number of viruses detected in each sample was 4.12, while 75.28% (67/89) of samples had three to five different viruses, 3.37% (3/89) had seven to eight different viruses, and none were positive for PAstV only (**Figure 1B**). Coinfections of PAstV with other porcine pathogens, such as rotavirus, PEDV, TGEV, porcine circovirus-2 (PCV2), and porcine hemagglutinating encephalomyelitis virus (PHEV), have been reported previously (3, 5, 6, 11). In the present study, the rate of PKV coinfection in PAstV-positive samples was relatively high (85.39%, 76/89), and there was evidence that u shed more PKV than did healthy individuals (18), indicating that PKV may have a potential role in PAstV-induced diarrhea in piglets. PEDV is the major cause of viral diarrheal disease in swine in China (9). Although there was a high prevalence of PEDV in piglets infected with PAstV in our previous study, statistical analysis indicated that PEDV-induced diarrhea was not associated with PAstV coinfection ($p > 0.05$) (9). The pathogenicity of PEV is typically mild in pigs (19), and GARV is among the most common pathogens of diarrhea

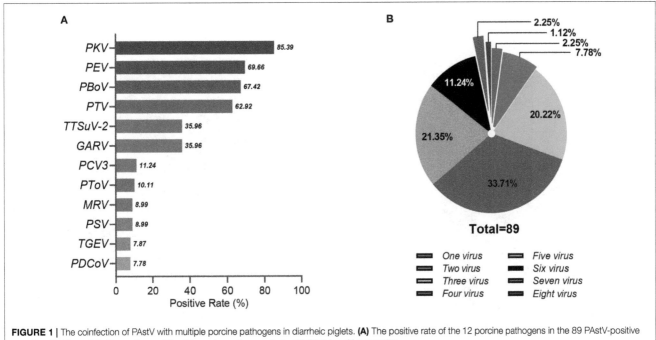

FIGURE 1 | The coinfection of PAstV with multiple porcine pathogens in diarrheic piglets. **(A)** The positive rate of the 12 porcine pathogens in the 89 PAstV-positive samples. **(B)** The coinfection patterns of the 12 porcine pathogens in the 89 PAstV-positive samples.

in piglets (20). In this study, the positivity rates of PEV (69.66%, 62/89) and GARV (35.96%, 32/89) were relatively high in PAstV-positive samples, suggesting a highly significant association of coinfection with PEV ($p < 0.01$) and GARV ($p < 0.01$) in PAstV-positive diarrhea samples of piglets (**Table 1**). However, since evidence of coinfections of PAstV with PEV and GARV causing diarrhea in piglets is somewhat limited, further studies are warranted.

Phylogenetic Analysis of PAstV

In the current study, a total of 27 RdRp genes were successfully sequenced from the 89 PAstV-positive diarrhea samples (**Table S2**). The RdRp gene is widely used to classify the genotype of PAstV (5, 11, 12, 21–23). Here, a phylogenetic tree was constructed based on the RdRp genes of the 27 identified PAstV strains and 115 reference PAstV strains. In the phylogenic tree, 142 PAstV strains were divided into five groups and three distinct genotypes (PAstV-2, PAstV-4, and PAstV-5) (**Figure 2A**). In the phylogenetic analysis, 22 identified PAstV strains and 39 reference strains from nine other countries were placed into the PAstV-2 group and divided into two clusters. With the exception of PAstV strain JX/2015/1224, all other identified PAstV strains and 21 reference PAstV strains formed one cluster in the PAstV-2 group, which shared nucleotide homologies of 84.8–99.5%. PAstV strain JX/2015/1224 and 18 reference PAstV strains shared nucleotide identities of 83.1–90.2% and formed the other cluster in the PAstV-2 group. Two identified PAstV strains, SD/YT/2015/1228b and JX/2015/1221d, which are closely related to a PAstV strain isolated in Croatia, were classified into the PAstV-5 group, which had nucleotide identities of 79.8–94.0%. Three

TABLE 1 | The statistical analysis of correlations of PAstV with other porcine pathogens.

	P-value	Odds ratio (OR)	95% confidence interval (95% CI)
PKV	0.103	1.778	0.908–3.480
PEV	0.000	4.219	2.582–6.896
PBoV	0.193	1.384	0.855–2.240
PTV	0.722	1.115	0.697–1.783
TTSuV-2	0.623	1.149	0.715–1.848
GARV	0.000	2.563	1.563–4.246
PCV3	0.702	1.150	0.556–2.379
PToV	0.393	1.390	0.642–3.009
MRV	0.583	0.747	0.342–1.631
PSV	0.128	1.939	0.835–4.507
TGEV	1.000	0.908	0.393–2.101
PDCoV	0.182	1.852	0.759–4.522

OR, odd ratio; CI, confidence interval.

identified PAstV strains (JL/MHK/2018/0115, SX/XZ/2017/1215, and JX/2015/1221a) and 35 reference strains, which shared nucleotide homologies of 62.1–93.6%, were classified to the PAstV-4 group. Most of the 27 identified PAstV strains were classified to the PAstV-2 group (81.5%, 22/27), indicating that PAstV-2 was predominant in diarrheic piglets in China. Similarly, the high prevalence of PAstV-2 in China was reported by Cai et al. (11) and Qin et al. (22). In contrast, the prevalence of PAstV-4 is reportedly higher than that of PAstV-2 in Thailand, South Korea, and India (5, 6, 12).

Sequence analysis of the 27 RdRp genes identified in this study had nucleotide identities of 53.8–99.5%, indicating

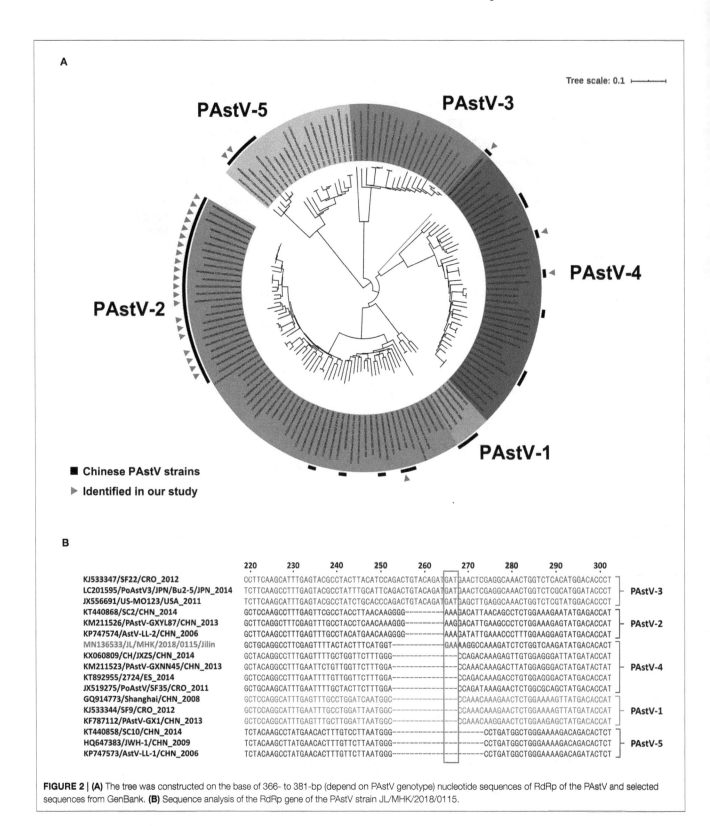

FIGURE 2 | (A) The tree was constructed on the base of 366- to 381-bp (depend on PAstV genotype) nucleotide sequences of RdRp of the PAstV and selected sequences from GenBank. **(B)** Sequence analysis of the RdRp gene of the PAstV strain JL/MHK/2018/0115.

a wide variation at the nucleotide level. PAstV strain JL/MHK/2018/0115 differed genetically from other PAstV-4 strains and formed a unique clade within the PAstV-4 group. Sequence analysis showed that the RdRp gene of strain JL/MHK/2018/0115 had low sequence similarity to the other PAstV-4 strains, with nucleotide identities of 62.1–67.1% and had a unique insert of three nucleotides (GAA) as compared with other PAstV-4 strains (**Figure 2B**). Previous

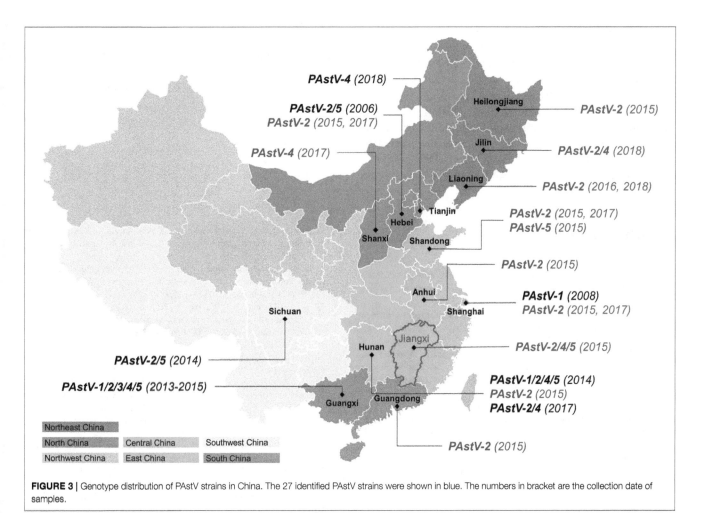

FIGURE 3 | Genotype distribution of PAstV strains in China. The 27 identified PAstV strains were shown in blue. The numbers in bracket are the collection date of samples.

studies have reported a high prevalence of PAstV-4 in other Asian countries, including South Korea (88.46%, 23/26), Thailand (92.00%, 23/25), and India (95.65%, 22/23), as well as European countries (70.4%, 295/419) (4–6, 12). PAstV-4, which was first reported in 2013, is a newly identified genotype in China that has since spread to the provinces of Hunan, Tianjin, Shanxi, Jilin, and Jiangxi (9, 21, 22). In addition, Lv et al. (21) and Zhao et al. (24) reported novel recombinant PAstV-4 strains in China. These data suggest that the Chinese PAstV-4 strains have undergone genetic variations and may have become the predominant strains in diarrheic piglets in China.

Genotype Distribution of PAstV in China

The results of the present study showed that PAstV-2 was circulating in ten different provinces, covering five regions of China (**Figure 3**), suggesting that PAstV-2 is the most widely distributed strain in China, which is supported by recent studies conducted in the provinces of Hebei, Hunan, Sichuan, and Guangxi (11, 21, 22, 25). Previous studies have reported the existence of multiple PAstV genotypes in China. For example,

PAstV-1 was identified in Shanghai as well as the provinces of Hunan and Guangxi (22, 25), while PAstV-3 was identified in Guangxi province only (22), PAstV-4 has been reported in the provinces of Tianjin, Hunan, and Guangxi (22, 24, 25), and PAstV-5 has been detected in the provinces of Hebei, Sichuan, Hunan, and Guangxi (11, 22, 24–26). In the present study, three PAstV-4 strains were identified in the provinces of Jilin, Shanxi, and Jiangxi, and two PAstV-5 strains were identified in Shandong and Jiangxi provinces, respectively. These results suggest the presence of various genotypes of PAstV in different regions of China. Moreover, five PAstV strains identified in Jiangxi province exhibited three distinct genotypes (PAstV-2, PAstV-4, and PAstV-5). Previous studies reported the presence of two or more genotypes of PAstV in the same province of China, such as four different genotypes of PAstV circulating in Hunan province (21, 25), while all five genotypes of PAstV were identified in Guangxi province (22), indicating a remarkable diversity of genotypes of PAstV cocirculating among pig farms in China.

In conclusion, results from the present study provide evidence that coinfection of PAstV with multiple porcine pathogens is common in diarrheic piglets in China, and PAstV-induced diarrhea is potentially associated with PEV and GARV coinfection. Phylogenetic analysis revealed that PAstV-2 was predominant in diarrheic piglets in China and multiple genotypes of PAstV were co-circulating in China from 2015 to 2018. In addition, one PAstV-4 strain was shown to harbor a unique insert within the RdRp gene. These results increase our current understanding of the coinfection and genetic characterization of PAstV in diarrheic piglets in China and provide valuable information for further studies of PAstV.

AUTHOR CONTRIBUTIONS

DS conceived the study. MS, SQ, DY, DG, and BY analyzed the data. MS and SQ wrote the manuscript. All authors contributed to the article and approved the submitted version.

REFERENCES

1. Bridger JC. Detection by electron microscopy of caliciviruses, astroviruses and rotavirus-like particles in the faeces of piglets with diarrhoea. Vet Rec. (1980) 107:532–3.

2. Lan D, Ji W, Shan T, Cui L, Yang Z, Yuan C, et al. Molecular characterization of a porcine astrovirus strain in China. Arch Virol. (2011) 156:1869–75. doi: 10.1007/s00705-011-1050-8

3. Mor SK, Chander Y, Marthaler D, Patnayak DP, Goyal SM. Detection and molecular haracterization of porcine astrovirus strains associated with swine diarrhea. J Vet Diagn Invst. (2012) 24:1064–7. doi: 10.1177/1040638712458781

4. Zhou W, Ullman K, Chowdry V, Reining M, Benyeda Z, Baule C, et al. Molecular investigations on the prevalence and viral load of enteric viruses in pigs from five European countries. Vet Microbiol. (2016) 182:75–81. doi: 10.1016/j.vetmic.2015.10.019

5. Kumthip K, Khamrin P, Saikruang W, Kongkaew A, Vachirachewin R, Ushijima H, et al. Detection and genetic characterization of porcine astroviruses in piglets with and without diarrhea in Thailand. Arch Virol. (2018) 163:1823–9. doi: 10.1007/s00705-018-3806-x

6. Kattoor JJ, Malik YS, Saurabh S, Sircar S, Vinodhkumar OR, Bora DP, et al. First report and genetic characterization of porcine astroviruses of lineage 4 and 2 in diarrheic pigs in India. Transbound Emerg Dis. (2019) 66:47–53. doi: 10.1111/tbed.13058

7. Zhang Q, Hu R, Tang X, Wu C, He Q, Zhao Z, et al. Occurrence and investigation of enteric viral infections in pigs with diarrhea in China. Arch Virol. (2013) 158:1631–6. doi: 10.1007/s00705-013-1659-x

8. Chen Q, Wang L, Zheng Y, Zhang J, Guo B, Yoon KJ, et al. Metagenomic analysis of the RNA fraction of the fecal virome indicates high diversity in pigs infected by porcine endemic diarrhea virus in the United States. Virol J. (2018) 15:95. doi: 10.1186/s12985-018-1001-z

9. Su M, Li C, Qi S, Yang D, Jiang N, Yin B, et al. A molecular epidemiological investigation of PEDV in China: characterization of co-infection and genetic diversity of S1-based genes. Transbound Emerg Dis. (2019) 67:1129–40. doi: 10.1111/tbed.13439

10. Fang Q, Wang C, Liu H, Wu Q, Liang S, Cen M, et al. Pathogenic characteristics of a porcine astrovirus strain isolated in China. Viruses. (2019) 11:1156. doi: 10.3390/v11121156

11. Cai Y, Yin W, Zhou Y, Li B, Ai L, Pan M, et al. Molecular detection of Porcine astrovirus in Sichuan Province, China. Virol J. (2016) 13:6. doi: 10.1186/s12985-015-0462-6

12. Lee MH, Jeoung HY, Park HR, Lim JA, Song JY, An DJ. Phylogenetic analysis of porcine astrovirus in domestic pigs and wild boars in South Korea. Virus Genes. (2013) 46:175–81. doi: 10.1007/s11262-012-0816-8

13. Wang E, Guo D, Li C, Wei S, Wang Z, Liu Q, et al. Molecular characterization of the ORF3 and S1 genes of porcine epidemic diarrhea virus non S-INDEL strains in seven regions of China, 2015. PLoS ONE. (2016) 11:e0160561. doi: 10.1371/journal.pone.0160561

14. Chu DK, Poon LL, Guan Y, Peiris JS. Novel astroviruses in insectivorous bats. J Virol. (2008) 82:9107–14. doi: 10.1128/JVI.00857-08

15. Tamura K, Stecher G, Peterson D, Filipski A, Kumar S. MEGA6: molecular evolutionary genetics analysis version 6.0. Mol Biol Evol. (2013) 30:2725–9. doi: 10.1093/molbev/mst197

16. Letunic I, Bork P. Interactive tree of life (iTOL) v3: an online tool for the display and annotation of phylogenetic and other trees. Nucleic Acids Res. (2016) 44:W242–5. doi: 10.1093/nar/gkw290

17. Qi S, Su M, Guo D, Li C, Wei S, Feng L, et al. Molecular detection and phylogenetic analysis of porcine circovirus type 3 in 21 Provinces of China during 2015-2017. Transbound Emerg Dis. (2019) 66:1004–15. doi: 10.1111/tbed.13125

18. Nantel-Fortier N, Lachapelle V, Letellier A, L'Homme Y, Brassard J. Kobuvirus shedding dynamics in a swine production system and their association with diarrhea. Vet Microbiol. (2019) 235:319–26. doi: 10.1016/j.vetmic.2019.07.023

19. Zell R, Krumbholz A, Henke A, Birch-Hirschfeld E, Stelzner A, Doherty M, et al. Detection of porcine enteroviruses by nRT-PCR: differentiation of CPE groups I-III with specific primer sets. J Virol Methods. (2000) 88:205–18. doi: 10.1016/s0166-0934(00)00189-0

20. Vlasova AN, Amimo JO, Saif LJ. Porcine rotaviruses: epidemiology, immune responses and control strategies. Viruses. (2017) 9:48. doi: 10.3390/v9030048

21. Lv SL, Zhang HH, Li JY, Hu WQ, Song YT, Opriessnig T, et al. High genetic diversity and recombination events of porcine astrovirus strains identified from ill and asymptomatic pigs in 2017, Hunan Province, China. Virus Genes. (2019) 55:673–81. doi: 10.1007/s11262-019-01692-w

22. Qin Y, Fang Q, Li X, Li F, Liu H, Wei Z, et al. Molecular epidemiology and viremia of porcine astrovirus in pigs from Guangxi province of China. BMC Vet Res. (2019) 15:471. doi: 10.1186/s12917-019-2217-x

23. Salamunova S, Jackova A, Mandelik R, Novotny J, Vlasakova M, Vilcek S. Molecular detection of enteric viruses and the genetic characterization of porcine astroviruses and sapoviruses in domestic pigs from Slovakian farms. BMC Vet Res. (2018) 14:313. doi: 10.1186/s12917-018-1640-8

24. Zhao C, Chen C, Li Y, Dong S, Tan K, Tian Y, et al. Genomic characterization of a novel recombinant porcine astrovirus isolated in northeastern China. Arch Virol. (2019) 164:1469–73. doi: 10.1007/s00705-019-04162-8

25. Xiao CT, Luo Z, Lv SL, Opriessnig T, Li RC, Yu XL. Identification and characterization of multiple porcine astrovirus genotypes in Hunan province, China. Arch Virol. (2017) 162:943–52. doi: 10.1007/s00705-016-3185-0

26. Li JS, Li MZ, Zheng LS, Liu N, Li DD, Duan ZJ. Identification and genetic characterization of two porcine astroviruses from domestic piglets in China. Arch Virol. (2015) 160:3079–84. doi: 10.1007/s00705-015-2569-x

Permissions

The contributors of this book come from diverse backgrounds, making this book a truly international effort. This book will bring forth new frontiers with its revolutionizing research information and detailed analysis of the nascent developments around the world.

We would like to thank all the contributing authors for lending their expertise to make the book truly unique. They have played a crucial role in the development of this book. Without their invaluable contributions this book wouldn't have been possible. They have made vital efforts to compile up to date information on the varied aspects of this subject to make this book a valuable addition to the collection of many professionals and students.

This book was conceptualized with the vision of imparting up-to-date information and advanced data in this field. To ensure the same, a matchless editorial board was set up. Every individual on the board went through rigorous rounds of assessment to prove their worth. After which they invested a large part of their time researching and compiling the most relevant data for our readers.

The editorial board has been involved in producing this book since its inception. They have spent rigorous hours researching and exploring the diverse topics which have resulted in the successful publishing of this book. They have passed on their knowledge of decades through this book. To expedite this challenging task, the publisher supported the team at every step. A small team of assistant editors was also appointed to further simplify the editing procedure and attain best results for the readers.

Apart from the editorial board, the designing team has also invested a significant amount of their time in understanding the subject and creating the most relevant covers. They scrutinized every image to scout for the most suitable representation of the subject and create an appropriate cover for the book.

The publishing team has been an ardent support to the editorial, designing and production team. Their endless efforts to recruit the best for this project, has resulted in the accomplishment of this book. They are a veteran in the field of academics and their pool of knowledge is as vast as their experience in printing. Their expertise and guidance has proved useful at every step. Their uncompromising quality standards have made this book an exceptional effort. Their encouragement from time to time has been an inspiration for everyone.

The publisher and the editorial board hope that this book will prove to be a valuable piece of knowledge for researchers, students, practitioners and scholars across the globe.

List of Contributors

Jessica Ruggeri, Cristian Salogni, Stefano Giovannini, Nicoletta Vitale, Maria Beatrice Boniotti and Giovanni Loris Alborali
Istituto Zooprofilattico Sperimentale della Lombardia e dell'Emilia Romagna [Experimental Zooprophylactic Institute of Lombardia and Emilia Romagna], Brescia, Italy

Attilio Corradi
Department of Veterinary Sciences, University of Parma, Parma, Italy

Paolo Pozzi
Department of Veterinary Sciences, University of Torino, Turin, Italy

Paolo Pasquali
Department of Food Safety, Nutrition and Veterinary Public Health, Istituto Superiore di Sanità, Rome, Italy

Li-Xiu Sun, Qin-Li Liang, Xiao-Hui Hu and Xing-Quan Zhu
State Key Laboratory of Veterinary Etiological Biology, Lanzhou Veterinary Research Institute, Chinese Academy of Agricultural Sciences, Lanzhou, China

Zhao Li, Jian-Fa Yang and Feng-Cai Zou
Key Laboratory of Veterinary Public Health of Yunnan Province, College of Veterinary Medicine, Yunnan Agricultural University, Kunming, China

Woo-Hyun Kim and Seongbeom Cho
College of Veterinary Medicine and Research Institute for Veterinary Science, Seoul National University, Seoul, South Korea

Miserach Zeleke, Mussie Girma and Balako Gumi
Aklilu Lemma Institute of Pathobiology, Sefere Selam Campus, Addis Ababa University, Addis Ababa, Ethiopia

Begna Tulu
Aklilu Lemma Institute of Pathobiology, Sefere Selam Campus, Addis Ababa University, Addis Ababa, Ethiopia
Department of Medical Laboratory Sciences, Bahir Dar University, Bahir Dar, Ethiopia

Aboma Zewede
Ethiopian Public Health Institute, Addis Ababa, Ethiopia

Mulugeta Belay, David A. Jolliffe and Adrian R. Martineau
Barts and the London School of Medicine and Dentistry, Queen Mary University of London, London, United Kingdom

Metasebia Tegegn, Fozia Ibrahim, Markos Abebe and Taye Tolera Balcha
Armeur Hansen Research Institute, Addis Ababa, Ethiopia

Henny M. Martineau
Department of Pathology, The Royal Veterinary College, Hatfield, United Kingdom

Gobena Ameni
Aklilu Lemma Institute of Pathobiology, Sefere Selam Campus, Addis Ababa University, Addis Ababa, Ethiopia
Department of Veterinary Medicine, College of Food and Agriculture, United Arab Emirates University, Al Ain, United Arab Emirates

Yalin Wang, Hongxia Wu, Bing Wang, Hansong Qi, Hua-Ji Qiu and Yuan Sun
State Key Laboratory of Veterinary Biotechnology, Harbin Veterinary Research Institute, Chinese Academy of Agricultural Sciences, Harbin, China

Zhao Jin
College of Life Science and Agriculture Forestry, Qiqihar University, Qiqihar, China

Falk Melzer and Heinrich Neubauer
Institute of Bacterial Infections and Zoonoses, Friedrich-Loeffler-Institut, Jena, Germany

Shakeeb Ullah
Faculty of Veterinary and Animal Sciences, Gomal University, Dera Ismail Khan, Pakistan

Qudrat Ullah
Institute of Bacterial Infections and Zoonoses, Friedrich-Loeffler-Institut, Jena, Germany
Faculty of Veterinary and Animal Sciences, Gomal University, Dera Ismail Khan, Pakistan
Department of Theriogenology, Faculty of Veterinary Science, University of Agriculture, Faisalabad, Pakistan

Huma Jamil and Zafar Iqbal Qureshi
Department of Theriogenology, Faculty of Veterinary Science, University of Agriculture, Faisalabad, Pakistan

Stefan Schwarz
Institute of Microbiology and Epizootics, Freie Universität, Berlin, Germany

Tariq Jamil
Institute of Bacterial Infections and Zoonoses, Friedrich-Loeffler-Institut, Jena, Germany
Institute of Microbiology and Epizootics, Freie Universität, Berlin, Germany

Muhammad Saqib
Department of Clinical Medicine and Surgery, Faculty of Veterinary Science, University of Agriculture, Faisalabad, Pakistan

Muhammad Hammad Hussain
Independent Researcher, Bardia, NSW, Australia

Muhammad Aamir Aslam
Institute of Microbiology, Faculty of Veterinary Science, University of Agriculture, Faisalabad, Pakistan

Muhammad Amjad Iqbal
Veterinary Research Institute, Lahore, Pakistan

Usman Tahir
Livestock and Dairy Development, Government of Punjab, Lahore, Pakistan

Bojia E. Duguma, Tewodros Tesfaye, Asmamaw Kassaye and Anteneh Kassa
The Donkey Sanctuary-Ethiopia Office, Addis Ababa, Ethiopia

Stephen J. Blakeway
Director, International Department, The Donkey Sanctuary, Sidmouth, United Kingdom

Young Ji Kim
Infectious Disease Research Center, Korea Research Institute of Bioscience and Biotechnology, Daejeon, South Korea
College of Veterinary Medicine, Chungbuk National University, Chungju, South Korea

Beom Jun Lee
College of Veterinary Medicine, Chungbuk National University, Chungju, South Korea

Sun-Woo Yoon and Dae Gwin Jeong
Infectious Disease Research Center, Korea Research Institute of Bioscience and Biotechnology, Daejeon, South Korea

College of Bioscience, University of Science and Technology, Daejeon, South Korea

Jin Ho Jang
Department of Wildlife Disease, College of Veterinary Science, Jeju National University, Jeju, South Korea
Chungnam Wild Animal Rescue Center, Kongju National University, Yesan, South Korea

Hye Kwon Kim
Department of Microbiology, College of Natural Science, Chungbuk National University, Cheongju, South Korea

Tongwei Ren, Qingrong Mo, Yuxu Wang, Hao Wang, Zuorong Nong, Jinglong Wang, Chenxia Niu, Chang Liu, Ying Chen, Kang Ouyang, Weijian Huang and Zuzhang Wei
Laboratory of Animal Infectious Diseases and Molecular Immunology, College of Animal Science and Technology, Guangxi University, Nanning, China

Kaori Shimizu and Asari Takaiwa
Laboratory of Food and Environmental Hygiene, Cooperative Department of Veterinary Medicine, Gifu University, Gifu, Japan

Shin-nosuke Takeshima
Department of Food and Nutrition, Jumonji University, Saitama, Japan

Ayaka Okada
Laboratory of Food and Environmental Hygiene, Cooperative Department of Veterinary Medicine, Gifu University, Gifu, Japan
Education and Research Center for Food Animal Health, Gifu University (GeFAH), Gifu, Japan

Yasuo Inoshima
Laboratory of Food and Environmental Hygiene, Cooperative Department of Veterinary Medicine, Gifu University, Gifu, Japan
Education and Research Center for Food Animal Health, Gifu University (GeFAH), Gifu, Japan
The United Graduate School of Veterinary Sciences, Gifu University, Gifu, Japan
Joint Graduate School of Veterinary Sciences, Gifu University, Gifu, Japan

Yongzhong Yu, Xuyang Duan, Yuanyuan Liu, Jinzhu Ma, Baifen Song and Yudong Cui
College of Biological Science and Technology, Heilongjiang Bayi Agricultural University, Daqing, China

Zhengxing Lian
College of Animal Science and Technology, China Agricultural University, Beijing, China

Stefano Petrini, Cecilia Righi, Carmen Iscaro, Ilaria Pierini, Cristina Casciari, Claudia Pellegrini, Paola Gobbi, Monica Giammarioli and Gian Mario De Mia
National Reference Laboratory for Infectious Bovine Rhinotracheitis (IBR), Istituto Zooprofilattico Sperimentale Umbria-Marche "Togo Rosati", Perugia, Italy

Patricia König
OIE and National Reference Laboratory for Bovine Herpesvirus Type 1 Infection, Friedrich-Loeffler-Institut, Greifswald, Germany

Zihan Yan, Mingyue Li and Yi Wang
College of Animal Science and Veterinary Medicine, Heilongjiang Bayi Agricultural University, Daqing, China

Dongwei Yuan
College of Animal Science and Veterinary Medicine, Heilongjiang Bayi Agricultural University, Daqing, China
Daqing Center of Inspection and Testing for Agricultural Products Ministry of Agriculture, Daqing, China

Pablo Rodríguez-Hernández and Vicente Rodríguez-Estévez
Department of Animal Production, International Agrifood Campus of Excellence (ceiA3), University of Córdoba, Córdoba, Spain

Lourdes Arce
Department of Analytical Chemistry, Inst Univ Invest Quim Fina and Nanoquim Inst Univ Invest Quim Fina and Nanoquim (IUNAN), International Agrifood Campus of Excellence (ceiA3), University of Córdoba, Córdoba, Spain

Jaime Gómez-Laguna
Department of Anatomy and Comparative Pathology and Toxicology, International Agrifood Campus of Excellence (ceiA3), University of Córdoba, Córdoba, Spain

Claudia Arrieta-Villegas, Enric Vidal and Bernat Pérez de Val
IRTA, Centre de Recerca en Sanitat Animal (CReSA, IRTA-UAB), Campus Universitat Autònoma de Barcelona, Barcelona, Spain

José Antonio Infantes-Lorenzo
Servicio de Inmunología Microbiana, Centro Nacional de Microbiología, Instituto de Investigación Carlos III, Madrid, Spain

Javier Bezos and Lucía de Juan
VISAVET Health Surveillance Center, Universidad Complutense de Madrid, Madrid, Spain
Departamento de Sanidad Animal, Universidad Complutense de Madrid, Madrid, Spain

Miriam Grasa
Agrupació de Defensa Sanitària de Cabrum i Oví Lleter de Catalunya, Barbens, Spain

Irene Mercader
Departament d'Agricultura, Ramaderia, Pesca i Alimentació de la Generalitat de Catalunya, Barcelona, Spain

Mahavir Singh
Lionex Diagnostics and Therapeutics GmbH, Braunschweig, Germany

Mariano Domingo
IRTA, Centre de Recerca en Sanitat Animal (CReSA, IRTA-UAB), Campus Universitat Autònoma de Barcelona, Barcelona, Spain
Departament de Sanitat i Anatomia Animals, Universitat Autònoma de Barcelona (UAB), Barcelona, Spain

Sergio Migliore, Roberto Puleio and Guido Ruggero Loria
Istituto Zooprofilattico Sperimentale Della Sicilia "A. Mirri", Palermo, Italy

Yulong Zhou
College of Animal Science and Veterinary Medicine, Heilongjiang Bayi Agricultural University, Daqing, China

Ye Meng
Department of Heilongjiang Key Laboratory for Animal Disease Control and Pharmaceutical Development, College of Veterinary Medicine, Northeast Agricultural University, Harbin, China

Yachao Ren
Pharmacy Department, Harbin Medical University-Daqing, Daqing, China

Zhiguo Liu and Zhenjun Li
Chinese Center for Disease Control and Prevention, National Institute for Communicable Disease Control and Prevention, Beijing, China

Fanta D. Gutema, Takele B. Tufa, Samson Leta and Zerihun Asefa
College of Veterinary Medicine and Agriculture, Addis Ababa University, Bishoftu, Ethiopia

Getahun E. Agga
U. S. Department of Agriculture, Agricultural Research Service, Food Animal Environmental Systems Research Unit, Bowling Green, KY, United States

Kohei Makita
Department of Veterinary Medicine, School of Veterinary Medicine, Rakukno Gakuen University, Ebetsu, Japan

Rebecca L. Smith
Department of Pathobiology, College of Veterinary Medicine, University of Illinois Urbana-Champaign, Urbana, IL, United States

Monique Mourits
Business Economics Group, Wageningen University, Wageningen, Netherlands

Tariku J. Beyene
Department of Preventive Veterinary Medicine, Ohio State University, Columbus, OH, United States

Beksissa Urge
Ethiopian Institute of Agricultural Research, Addis Ababa, Ethiopia

Emeli Torsson and Mikael Berg
Department of Biomedical Sciences & Veterinary Public Health, Swedish University of Agricultural Sciences, Uppsala, Sweden

Tebogo Kgotlele and Gerald Misinzo
Department of Veterinary Microbiology and Parasitology, Sokoine University of Agriculture, Morogoro, Tanzania

Oskar Karlsson Lindsjö
Department of Animal Breeding and Genetics, Swedish University of Agricultural Sciences, Uppsala, Sweden

Nathalie Meijerink, Daphne A. van Haarlem and Christine A. Jansen
Division Infectious Diseases and Immunology, Department Biomolecular Health Sciences, Faculty of Veterinary Medicine, Utrecht University, Utrecht, Netherlands

Francisca C. Velkers and J. Arjan Stegeman
Division Farm Animal Health, Department Population Health Sciences, Faculty of Veterinary Medicine, Utrecht University, Utrecht, Netherlands

Jannigje G. Kers
Division Farm Animal Health, Department Population Health Sciences, Faculty of Veterinary Medicine, Utrecht University, Utrecht, Netherlands
Laboratory of Microbiology, Wageningen University & Research, Wageningen, Netherlands

Hauke Smidt
Laboratory of Microbiology, Wageningen University & Research, Wageningen, Netherlands

David M. Lamot
Cargill Animal Nutrition and Health Innovation Center, Velddriel, Netherlands

Jean E. de Oliveira
Cargill R&D Center, Vilvoorde, Belgium

Victor P. M. G. Rutten
Division Infectious Diseases and Immunology, Department Biomolecular Health Sciences, Faculty of Veterinary Medicine, Utrecht University, Utrecht, Netherlands
Department of Veterinary Tropical Diseases, Faculty of Veterinary Science, University of Pretoria, Pretoria, South Africa

Yumiko Shimizu, Yoko Hayama, Yoshinori Murato, Kotaro Sawai, Emi Yamaguchi and Takehisa Yamamoto
Viral Disease and Epidemiology Research Division, National Institute of Animal Health, National Agriculture and Food Research Organization, Tsukuba, Japan

Ling Li, Jie Yang, Ziqiang Cheng and Guihua Wang
College of Veterinary Medicine, Shandong Agricultural University, Tai'an, China

Dongyan Niu
Veterinary Medicine, University of Calgary, Calgary, AB, Canada

Jianmin Bi
China Animal Husbandry Industry Co., Ltd., Beijing, China

Lingjuan Zhang
Penglai City Animal Epidemic Prevention and Control Center, Penglai, China

Anselme Shyaka and Marie Aurore Ugirabe
School of Veterinary Medicine, College of Agriculture, Animal Sciences and Veterinary Medicine, University of Rwanda, Nyagatare, Rwanda

Jonas Johansson Wensman
Department of Clinical Sciences, Swedish University of Agricultural Sciences, Uppsala, Sweden

Mingjun Su, Shanshan Qi, Dan Yang, Donghua Guo and Dongbo Sun
Laboratory for the Prevention and Control of Swine Infectious Diseases, College of Animal Science and Veterinary Medicine, Heilongjiang Bayi Agricultural University, Daqing, China
Heilongjiang Province Cultivating Collaborative Innovation Center for the Beidahuang Modern Agricultural Industry Technology, Daqing, China

Baishuang Yin
College of Animal Science and Technology, Jilin Agricultural Science and Technology University, Jilin, China

Index

Printed in the USA
CPSIA information can be obtained
at www.ICGtesting.com
JSHW051625061123
51533JS00005B/103

9 781641 168427